The Art and Science of Midwifery

The Art and Science of Midwifery

Louise Silverton

Head of Maternal and Child Health,
Nightingale and Guy's College of Health,
London, UK

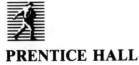

PRENTICE HALL
New York   London   Toronto   Tokyo   Sydney   Singapore

First published 1993 by
Prentice Hall International (UK) Ltd
Campus 400, Maylands Avenue
Hemel Hempstead
Hertfordshire, HP2 7EZ
A division of
Simon & Schuster International Group

Typeset in 10/12pt Times
Mathematical Composition Setters Ltd, Salisbury, Wiltshire.

Printed in Great Britain by
Redwood Books, Trowbridge, Wiltshire

Library of Congress Cataloging-in-Publication Data

Silverton, Louise, 1956-
    The art and science of midwifery/Louise Silverton.
        p.   cm.
    Includes bibliographical references and index.
    ISBN 0-13-046707-3 : $35.99
    1. Obstetrics. 2. Midwives. I. Title.
    RG542.S537 1992
    618.2--dc20   92-9561
                                                                CIP

British Library Cataloguing in Publication Data

A catalogue record for this book is available
from the British Library

ISBN 0-13-046707-3 (pbk)

2 3 4 5   97   96   95   94

Contents

Preface   xv

1 The midwife   1

History of midwifery   1
Definition of the role of the midwife   10
Midwifery practice in the United Kingdom   12
Supervision of midwifery   16
Midwifery in other countries   17
References   20

2 The midwife in the community   25

Place of work   25
The primary health care team   26
Equipment   27
Place of birth   30
The role of the midwife in the community   34
Notification and registration of birth   37
References   38

3   Indicators of health in relation to maternity care   40

Collection of data   40
What is health?   41
Statistics and maternity care   42
References   48

4   Planning a healthy pregnancy   51

Preconception care   51
References   55

5   Conception and early development   57

The female genital tract   57
The uterus during pregnancy   65
The menstrual cycle   68
Fertilisation   71
Diagnosis of pregnancy   78
References   80

6   Adaptation to pregnancy   82

Physiological adaptation   82
Cerebrovascular system   88
Muscoloskeletal system   89
Cardiovascular system   90
The skin   90
Diet   90
Psychological and social adjustment   93
References   97

7   Antenatal care   102

History   102
Aims of antenatal care   104
Types of care available   105
Who provides antenatal care?   107
The booking visit/interview   109
Definitions   113
Subsequent care   116
Progress of the pregnancy   120
References   121

8   Fetal growth and well-being   125

Techniques for detecting problems   125
Abdominal examination   126
Terminology   127
Examination techniques   130
Fetal activity   136
Cardiotocography   136
Hormone assays   138
Ultrasound   138
References   139

9   Parent education   142

Parent education classes   142
Parent education curriculum   145
Exercise in pregnancy   146
Birth plans   147
References   148

10   Early teenage pregnancy   150

Numbers of early teenage pregnancies   150
Obstetric aspects   151
Finance   153
Housing   154
Education   154
Social aspects   156
References   157

11   Bleeding in early pregnancy   159

Causes of bleeding   160
Abortion   163
Effects of early fetal loss on parents   167
Therapeutic abortion   168
References   170

12   Hypertensive disorders in pregnancy   174

Blood pressure   174
Hypertensive disease in pregnancy   176
Effects of hypertension   179
Labour and delivery   182
Postnatal eclampsia   183
References   183

13 Medical disorders and childbirth   187

The role of the midwife   187
Diabetes mellitus   188
Cardiac disease   192
Chronic renal disease   195
Epilepsy   197
Cystic fibrosis   198
References   199

14 Antepartum haemorrhage   203

Maternal and fetal blood loss   203
Abruptio placentae   204
Placenta praevia   208
References   212

15 Anaemia in pregnancy   215

Physiological changes in blood composition   215
Causes of anaemia in pregnancy   216
Iron deficiency anaemia   216
Folic acid deficiency   218
Haemoglobinopathies   219
Thalassaemias   219
Sickle cell disease   220
References   221

16 Multiple pregnancy   224

Incidence   224
Causes of multiple pregnancy   225
Diagnosis of multiple pregnancy   226
Pregnancy complications   227
Antenatal care   228
Labour   229
Postpartum care   231
Psychological problems   231
References   232

17 Infectious disease in pregnancy   235

Normal vaginal secretions   235
Bacterial discharges   236
Fungal infections   238
Parasitic infections   239
Viral infections   240
Hepatitis   241

Human immunodeficiency virus (HIV)   242
Cervical cytology   245
References   247

18 Risk in pregnancy   251

The older mother   251
The grande multipara   252
Risk assessment in pregnancy   253
Employment and pregnancy   254
Antenatal care of rhesus-negative women   254
Abnormalities of liquor   255
Hyperemesis gravidarum   257
References   258

19 Physiology of labour   261

Definition of labour   261
Progress of labour   262
Mechanism of labour   264
Onset of labour   271
The first stage of labour   273
The mechanism of normal labour   276
The third stage of labour   280
References   282

20 The first and second stages of labour   286

Onset of labour   286
Planning care in labour   289
Progress in labour   290
Maternal well-being   299
Maternal care in labour   300
Fetal well-being   308
Conduct of the second stage   309
Conduct of delivery   311
Resuscitation of the newborn   314
References   318

21 Management of the third and fourth stages
of labour   324

History   324
Clinical trials of treatments   325
Physiological management   326
Active management   327
The fourth stage of labour   333

Record keeping   335
Initial examination of the neonate   337
References   339

22 Active management of labour   342

Acceleration of labour   342
Disordered uterine action   345
Induction of labour   348
Maternal distress in labour   353
Fetal distress and monitoring   354
Assessing fetal well-being   355
References   357

23 Preterm labour and delivery   363

Causes   363
Diagnosis of preterm labour   365
Management of preterm labour   365
Preterm delivery   368
References   370

24 Malpositions and malpresentations   373

Malpresentation   373
Abnormal pelves   374
Pelvic assessment   378
Occipito-posterior position   380
Breech position   383
Management of breech presentation   385
Brow presentation   391
Shoulder presentation   392
Compound presentation   393
References   393

25 Instrumental and operative delivery   396

Instrumental delivery   396
Caesarean section   399
Trial of labour/trial of scar   404
References   404

26 Postpartum haemorrhage and complications
of the third stage of labour   407

Postpartum haemorrhage   407
Bleeding from the placental site   408
Causes of atonic uterus   409

Treatment   411
Secondary postpartum haemorrhage   414
References   415

27 Shock and obstetric emergencies   417

Emergencies   417
Shock   418
Disseminated intravascular coagulation (DIC)   421
Obstetric emergencies   423
Hazards of general anaesthesia   427
Fetal emergencies   428
References   430

28 Postnatal care   433

The puerperium   433
Reception on the postnatal ward   435
Physiological changes in the puerperium   436
Psychological changes in the puerperium   439
Midwifery care of the postnatal woman   440
References   446

29 Complications of the puerperium   449

Psychological disturbances in the puerperium   449
Adaptation to motherhood   450
Postnatal depression   451
Puerperal psychosis   453
Infection in the puerperium   454
Urinary tract disturbances in the puerperium   457
Thromboembolic disorders   458
References   460

30 Family planning   463

History of contraception   463
Choice of contraceptive method   466
Provision of family planning services   468
Contraceptive methods   469
Sterilisation   476
References   476

31 Loss and grief in midwifery practice   480

Grief   480
Maternity and loss   482
Termination of pregnancy   484

Stillbirth   484
Maternal death   487
Sudden infant death syndrome   488
References   490

32 Adaptation of the newborn to extra-uterine life   493

Initiation of respiration   493
Fetal circulation and changes at birth   495
Thermoregulation   497
Neonatal cold injury   499
The urge to care   499
Birth injuries   499
Neonatal reflexes   500
References   501

33 Care of the normal newborn baby   504

Daily examination of the newborn baby   504
The umbilical cord   507
Sore buttocks   507
Weight   508
The fetal skull   508
The scalp   515
Screening tests   516
Sleep   516
Crying   517
Baby care   517
References   518

34 Infant feeding   520

Advantages of breast feeding   520
Constituents of breast milk   521
Who are the breast feeding mothers?   523
Factors influencing choice of feeding method   524
Anatomy of the breasts and changes in pregnancy   526
Physiology of breast feeding   528
Management of breast feeding   530
Problems while feeding   534
Contra-indications to breast feeding   537
Stopping feeding   537
Artificial feeding   538
Weaning   541
References   542

35   Jaundice   547

Physiology   547
Causes of jaundice   549
Haemolytic disease of the newborn   551
Physiological jaundice   554
Management of jaundice   554
Management of rhesus disease   556
Management of exchange transfusion   557
Reference   558

36   The low birthweight baby   561

Classification of low birthweight   561
The preterm baby   563
The small-for-gestational-age baby   568
Sequelae of low birthweight   570
Involving the parents   570
References   571

37   The newborn requiring extra care   575

The infant of the diabetic mother   575
The neurologically disturbed baby   577
The infant of the drug-dependent mother   580
Infection of the newborn   582
Transplacental infections   583
References   588

38   The malformed baby   591

Causes of abnormalities   591
Prevention of congenital abnormalities   595
Detection of abnormalities   595
Types of congenital abnormality   597
Abnormalities of the alimentary tract   599
Congenital dislocation of the hip   600
Talipes   601
Congenital heart disease   601
Chromosomal abnormalities   602
Inborn errors of metabolism   603
Cystic fibrosis   605
Hypothyroidism   605
Effect of malformation upon parents   606
References   606

39   Child abuse   610

Background   610
Types of abuse   611
References   617

Index   619

Preface

This book was originally planned primarily for qualified midwives, particularly those undertaking the Advanced Diploma in Midwifery. However, advances in midwifery education during the last 5 years have been such that it will now be relevant to student midwives, especially those undertaking courses at diploma level.

Throughout the book I discuss the research base for practice and question assumptions which can easily be perpetuated if non-research-based texts are consulted. In many areas there is a considerable body of research-based knowledge which needs to be evaluated. Regrettably, in other areas the task of compiling objective evidence remains. This was most obvious when I wrote Chapter 24 on malpositions and malpresentations where I found major omissions from the knowledge base.

Whilst the role of the midwife remains central to this book, many issues relating to the practice of obstetrics have also been included. It is important for midwives to be aware of the rationale for the actions of the obstetrician. This in no way diminishes the importance of supporting the woman and her partner through the process of care (whatever form that may take). This book cannot provide the answer to every question; it is intended to stimulate debate, further knowledge and improve professional practice. Hopefully it is a text that will mature and grow with the years.

Finally I would like to thank all those who have assisted me with the writing of this book, not all of whom can be mentioned here. In particular my thanks are due to my long-suffering editor Cathy Peck who never thought she would see the book completed, to Ann Thomson who provided expert advice and encouragement, to Patricia Al-Salihi and Shelia Morgan who typed the early drafts before I became computer-literate, to my students who constantly questioned midwifery practice, and lastly to my mother and husband who kept me going when I was ready to give up. In addition this book is dedicated to the memory of my late father and of the late Molly B Staples who fired my interest in midwifery and in the achievement of the best possible care for mothers and babies.

Louise Silverton

19.2.92

1   The midwife

This chapter examines the history and development of midwifery. The legislation which regularised British midwifery practice will be discussed, together with present day statutory controls in the United Kingdom. This leads on to a discussion of the role of the British midwife in relation to the World Health Organization definition of a midwife. Whilst this chapter will concentrate on midwifery in the United Kingdom, there will be consideration of midwifery in The Netherlands, New Zealand and the United States, together with a description of the role of the traditional birth attendant in more traditional societies.

History of midwifery

Midwives have evolved through the ages to serve the society to which they belonged (Arney 1982). In prehistory women may have given birth alone or have been assisted by their partner (Chamberlain 1981). As man became less nomadic and settled more in groups, the mother could be attended in labour by a kinswoman (Gelis 1991). Through experience and exchange of knowledge such women would develop skills which could be used for the good of the community. Whilst their knowledge base could be extended, illiteracy and isolation meant that information was not easily disseminated (Chamberlain 1981).

The first record of training for midwives comes from ancient Greece. There appeared to be two types of midwives, those with lesser skills who dealt with normal births and a superior group permitted and able to give care to abnormal ones (Towler and Bramall 1986). Midwives enjoyed a high position in the society. Roman writings by Soranus (150 AD) indicate that midwifery was well established, with literate practitioners who could utilise his work on obstetrics and gynaecology.

Records of the role and work of midwives exist in the papyri and tomb paintings of ancient Egypt and in the Old Testament (Chamberlain 1981). The latter records how the Hebrew midwives (Shiprah and Puah) found favour in the eyes of the Lord by failing to carry out the instructions of the Pharaoh to kill male children as they were delivered. The explanation they gave for their lack of obedience was that the Hebrew women, being more active and vigorous than their Egyptian counterparts, had given birth before the midwives arrived (Exodus 1: 15-20). By this time women healers and midwives had lost much of their status and independence. Female domination of the healing arts predominantly through priestesses intervening with female goddesses had been superseded by male 'scientific' medicine and male gods. This was continued in Greek, Roman and Hebrew societies where male domination of the healing arts became the norm, although most caring was still undertaken by women under male direction (Chamberlain 1981). With the decline of the Roman Empire most knowledge was lost as Europe entered the Dark Ages (Donnison 1988). The developing Christian church regarded the involvement of women in healing as a malevolent force, being viewed as paganism and later as sorcery. This was possibly because health was seen as being divinely ordained and women healers were not under the control of the local priest (Chamberlain 1981). Throughout the ages poor people have continued to consult female healers to obtain herbs and potions to relieve suffering as their only affordable form of health care (Chamberlain, 1981).

In medieval Britain, midwives were traditional birth attendants (TBAs) who passed what little knowledge and skills they possessed from mother to daughter (Biller 1986). In the Middle Ages, some of these traditional midwives who had healing skills were denounced as witches and subsequently burnt at the stake (Ehrenreich and English 1973). Explanations for the association of witchcraft with midwifery centre around the midwife's access to material (such as the placenta) which could be used for ceremonies of black magic (Ehrenreich and English 1973) and because they were not amenable to male control, especially that of the priest (Chamberlain 1981). Midwives were also viewed as a threat to men who were seeking to establish themselves as the sole holders of the healing arts (Ehrenreich and English 1973). To the church, with its teachings about sin surrounding female sexuality, midwives represented a threat by their interference with fertility (Oakley 1976).

From the fourteenth century records exist in England of pensions which were paid to royal midwives in recognition of service given. Such midwives were held in high esteem and were well rewarded by their employers (Dewhurst 1983). In the sixteenth century licensing of British midwives began; this had existed in France for the previous 150 years (Biller 1986). This licensing could be performed by secular authorities but was more commonly under the authority of the church (Donnison 1988). The clergy needed to be assured of the moral character of the midwife, that she would not procure or condone abortions, that she would baptise any sickly babies and that she would report the name of the father of any illegitimate baby (Donnison 1988). There was little assessment of the midwife's skills or knowledge which in a time of widespread illiteracy were often scant.

It was the seventeenth century which saw the rise of the 'man-midwife', a medical practitioner who specialised in childbirth (Arney 1982). Such moves were not without resistance since normal birth was still seen as an entirely female preserve (Donnison 1988). William Harvey, best known for his description of the circulation of the blood, wrote the first British book on midwifery, which was originally published in Latin in 1651 (Donnison 1988). The seventeenth century saw the spread to England of the French scientific approach to childbirth, with the body being viewed as a 'machine' whose constituent parts contributed to the action of the whole (Arney 1982). This view allowed for intervention in the processes of birth in order to keep the 'machine' in working order, giving legitimacy to the then current British interventionist practices. Conversely, in France this same theory was used to limit interventions especially those which could interfere with the workings of the machine, resulting in the natural processes being left alone (Arney 1982). The British 'medical' model with its mechanistic philosophy did not take account of the individual's environmental and social circumstances in the way adopted by empirical healers, such as traditional midwives, who learnt through trial and error (Chamberlain, 1981)

Percival Willoughby a 'man-midwife' advocated the teaching of female midwives and assisted his own daughter in her practice (Donnison 1988). This was usually achieved by subterfuge with him giving his aid out of sight under a blanket unseen by the mother and other birth companions (Donnison 1988). During the latter half of the eighteenth century many changes occurred in both the organisation of society and in the position of the midwife (Arney 1982). The beginning of industrialisation saw a migration of people from the country to the towns with an accompanying rise in the birthrate (Donnison 1988). The developing and socially ambitious middle classes followed the wealthier groups in society in employing men-midwives to attend their wives in labour (Arney 1982). Although the men charged more for their services (this was part of their attraction since their engagement indicated the possession of wealth), it was the use of obstetric forceps and an increased knowledge base which helped to maintain their position (Arney 1982). The advent of male birth attendants (and their increasing acceptance in an area previously considered a female preserve) was accompanied by a change in birthing position from the stool to the bed, allowing better visibility and the easier use of forceps (Gelis 1991). An increasing number of men were competing for the custom of the well-to-do in order to ensure their continuing custom for medical care (Arney 1982). The licensing system for midwives was breaking down and this, combined with their poor levels of literacy and education, did little for their social standing (Donnison 1988). Many midwives were trying to do their best for the poor who often could not afford to pay for their services (Donnison 1988).

At the same time as these social changes, there was an explosion in medical knowledge, especially in the areas of anatomy and physiology. William Smellie, a Scottish doctor, did much to advance the role of the obstetrician. Unable, due to the resistance of local midwives, to gain much practice in the conduct of normal births he moved to London and then to Paris in order to gain experience (Donnison 1988). He established a training centre for men-midwives which also provided a service to the poor in return for using their deliveries as teaching experience (Arney 1982). Smellie had a rather condescending attitude to midwives and was critical of their practice, resulting in some feelings of hostility from the midwives (Towler and Bramall 1986). Eventually Smellie recognised the importance of training for midwives and established classes for them. These were quite separate from those for men, as Smellie thought that they had very different roles (Towler and Bramall 1986).

The eighteenth century also saw the rise of some English midwives who were well learned and able to pass on their knowledge through the books that they wrote (Donnison 1988). Unfortunately few of the women they were trying to teach were able to read and so most remained in ignorance (Donnison 1988). Amongst the major figures was Mrs Sarah Stone who in 1737 published the *Complete Practice of Midwifery*. She emphasised the importance of a thorough knowledge of relevant anatomy and recommended attendance at dissections (Chamberlain 1981). In order to counter the rise of the man-midwife she suggested that midwives should show their abilities in abnormal cases, or the public would send for a man in the first place (Donnison 1988).

Another key figure was Elizabeth Nihell who had studied at the Hôtel-Dieu in Paris. She wrote a *Treatise on the Art of Midwifery* in 1760 in which she ridiculed the teachings of William Smellie, especially his use of models and dolls as teaching aids (Donnison 1988). She unfortunately harmed her case against the use of obstetric forceps by stating that they were never necessary (Towler and Bramall 1986).

The late eighteenth and early nineteenth centuries saw the establishment of lying-in hospitals usually supported by charities (Abel-Smith 1964). The first such hospital in England was founded in 1739 by Sir Richard Manningham, in 1809 becoming Queen Charlotte's Hospital (Lewis 1989). The first lying-in hospital was established in the United States in 1799 in New York (Speert 1980). Some of these hospitals had as their express purpose the training of doctors and midwives. However this was often too expensive for the midwives to afford, especially in relation to the fees they received, which were a fraction of those given to doctors (Abel-Smith 1964; Donnison 1988). Many midwives continued to have a poor reputation which was not aided by their portrayal in literature, notably as Sairey Gamp in Dicken's *Martin Chuzzlewit*, although she was a monthly nurse rather than a midwife (Donnison 1988). The first provision for formal training for midwives was in Scotland, with examinations and licensing being established in Edinburgh from 1726 and in Glasgow from 1740 (Marshall 1983).

The start of the nineteenth century saw battles for the regulation of medical practice and in the fight for power and position doctors sought (as happened in the United States) to establish childbirth as their special preserve (Arney 1982; Donnison 1988). Although they wished to control childbirth themselves, many doctors recognised the need for female help during labour and the puerperium (Donnison 1988). To this end a 3 month training period was established in 1824 for monthly nurses who would give care during labour, assist the doctor at the delivery and support the mother during the puerperium, often undertaking domestic duties as well (Towler and Bramall 1986). During the century there were many attempts by interest groups (including the apothecaries) to gain control over midwives, without significant success (Donnison 1988).

Puerperal fever was common despite the discovery of its cause and prevention by Semmelweis in Vienna (Semmelweis 1881), haunting many lying-in hospitals. Outbreaks led to closure of some lying-in hospitals and disruption to the training of any midwives working there (Chamberlain 1981).

As opportunities grew for the education of girls from wealthier families some of them turned their attention to charitable work which included nursing and midwifery (Abel-Smith 1960; Donnison 1988). Impetus was given to more formal training which required literacy. In the United States women could gain admittance to private medical schools, thus denying their talents to the advancement of nursing and midwifery (Arney 1982).

Attempts were made by the London Obstetrical Society in 1870 through Parliament to enforce training and registration of midwives (Donnison 1988). Other bodies such as the British Medical Association lobbied the Government to introduce controls of practice because midwives were seen as a threat to their livelihood (Arney 1982). In early 1880 an educated group of midwives joined together to form The Matron's Aid Society later renamed the Midwives' Institute (and later to become the College of Midwives) (Cowell and Wainwright 1981). The aim of the Institute was to obtain legislation which would regulate the education and practice of midwives. They also arranged lectures, ran a library and in 1888 first published *Nursing Notes* which was later to become the *Midwives' Chronicle* (Cowell and Wainwright 1981). The lectures and journal were both introduced by Miss (later Dame) Rosalind Paget, a recently qualified member of the Institute (Rivers 1981). The fight for registration took until 1902, following the unsuccessful introduction of 8 bills in the previous 11 years (Donnison 1988). Some of these failed due to opposition from the medical profession who felt that if the bill became law they would be deprived of part of their income from obstetrics. In addition, the British Medical Association wanted the restriction of midwifery practice with the regulations being under their own control (Donnison 1988). In the end, the 1902 Midwives' Act put midwifery under the control of the Privy Council (Donnison 1988). The Act was not designed to protect the profession of the practitioners but to protect the general public from untrained and unregulated midwives (Donnison 1988).

The 1902 Midwives' Act which applied in England and Wales legislated for the establishment of the Central Midwives' Board (CMB) and for the local supervision of midwifery practice. Membership of the first CMB consisted of:

1. Four doctors (one nominated by each of the Worshipful Company of Apothecaries, the Midwives' Institute and the Royal Colleges of Physicians and of Surgeons).

2. Two people (one of whom had to be a woman) nominated by the President of the Privy Council.
3. One representative each from the Royal British Nurses' Association, Queen Victoria's Jubilee Institute for Nurses and the Association of County Councils (Donnison 1988).

Although there was no provision within the Act for there to be any midwives on the CMB, there were three midwives on the first board, two representing each of the two nursing organisations and another as a Privy Council nominee (Towler and Bramall 1986). The CMB was empowered to:

1. Arrange for the certification of midwives and to maintain a roll of those certified. Certification could be achieved either by undertaking CMB approved training and passing their exam or, before 1 April 1905, by those midwives in possession of recognised midwifery certificates (such as those awarded by the London Obstetrical Society) who could apply for certification together with midwives of good character who had been in practice for a minimum of a year. Following this date, entry to the midwives' roll was only by training and examination, with the title of midwife being the preserve of those on the roll.
2. Arrange for midwifery training and for the holding of qualifying examinations. From 1903 the period of training was three months and in 1905 the first schools of midwifery were approved in Manchester and Sheffield (Towler and Bramall 1986).
3. Frame rules relating to the workings of the CMB, admission to the roll, regulating and supervising practice, and suspension from practice. The first rules were published in 1903.
4. Determine protocol and conduct hearings in cases of misconduct and if proven to remove the midwife's name from the roll. It was not until the 1919 Act that midwives could be suspended from the roll for lesser misdemeanours or whilst awaiting a hearing.
5. Appoint local supervising authorities who would assess midwives' practice and ensure that the rules were being observed. The inspectors of midwives appointed included medical officers, sanitary inspectors and health visitors. Their jurisdiction was originally only over domiciliary midwives, a situation which was not regularised to include hospital practice until 1942 (Bent 1982).

Other legislation and reports which have affected midwifery in the twentieth century include:

1910: Uncertified midwives were no longer permitted to practise habitually or for gain except under direct supervision of a medical practitioner. This loophole was not finally closed until 1936 when these women were prohibited from practising as monthly nurses even under supervision (Robinson 1990).
1911: The introduction of the National Insurance Act gave the working man access to medical care for himself and to maternity benefits for his wife.

Despite this if a midwife had to call a doctor she would often have to undertake to meet his costs herself before he would agree to visit (Chamberlain 1981).

1915: Notification of birth was made a statutory duty. This was usually undertaken by the midwife, although it was not until 1919 that she was reimbursed for the cost of postage (Towler and Bramall 1986).

1916: Midwifery training was lengthened to 6 months with a remission of 2 months to those with a nursing qualification. Antenatal care was included in the syllabus for the first time.

1919: The Midwives' Act placed upon local authorities the responsibility of paying a doctor's fees and then seeking to reclaim them from the family (Donnison 1988). Prior to this doctors had often refused to attend when summoned unless their fees were guaranteed. This could result in the midwife having to pay him despite the fact that his fees were in excess of those received by the midwife or for the summons to be delayed too long (Towler and Bramall 1986). Midwives under this Act could be suspended from practice for disobeying the rules.

The establishment of the Ministry of Health gave an impetus to local authorities who wished to provide antenatal services on the rates, although this provision was not compulsory. This was resisted to some extent by general practitioners who feared that they were losing custom to local authority clinical medical officers (Oakley 1984). Most midwives were still in independent practice in the community, doing home confinements and carrying out varying amounts of antenatal care. Midwives were reluctant to refer their clients to the local clinics for fear that a hospital confinement would be advised and the midwife's fees lost (Oakley 1984).

1923: The report into the training of midwives recommended that training be lengthened to 6 months for qualified nurses and 1 year for non-nurses (Campbell 1923).

1924: Enquiry into maternal mortality headed by Dame Janet Campbell. This was established to discover why maternal mortality remained high despite 20 years having passed since the regulation of midwifery. It was noted that mortality rates were higher amongst better-off women who were attended in labour by doctors who may themselves have been inadequately trained (Loudon 1986). Untrained midwives were still able to practise under medical supervision and were doing so until declared illegal under the 1936 Midwives' Act. The enquiry highlighted the poor working conditions and fees received by many midwives (Campbell 1924). Due to the poverty of many of their clients, midwives could not demand high fees and were therefore finding problems surviving financially (Towler and Bramall 1986).

In 1924 the Midwives' Institute began instruction for midwives who wished to teach and in 1926 the first specific course for midwife teachers was provided (Cowell and Wainwright 1981).

1926: The third Midwives' Act allowed for the roll of midwives to be split into two parts, those who were practising and those who were not (Towler and Bramall 1986).

1936: The Midwives' Act recognised the difficulties of midwives in independent practice in relation to uncertainty of income. Because of this midwives were often reluctant to refer mothers to local authority antenatal clinics for fear of losing their fee (Donnison 1988). There were also difficulties attracting newly qualified midwives (especially those who were also nurses) to practise as a result of the precarious financial situation (Towler and Bramall 1986). There were a number of rural areas with few if any midwives available, other than those who were unqualified. As a way of reducing the still high rate of maternal mortality it was decided to establish a salaried midwifery service under the control of the local authority. Midwives were given the opportunity of joining this scheme or of remaining in private practice. They could also surrender their certificates and retire, being given some severance pay (Donnison 1988).

The 1936 Act also reviewed the education of midwives, it made provision for the CMB to establish the Midwife Teacher's Diploma and for the provision of a five-yearly refresher course in addition to establishing regulations regarding return to practise after a period away from midwifery (Towler and Bramall 1986). The role and qualifications of the supervisor of midwives were established to prevent unsuitable individuals being appointed to the post.

1938: Midwifery training was split into two parts. The first part consisted of the theory of normal and abnormal midwifery and neonatal paediatrics whilst the practical experience was hospital based. Part two was partly or wholly based in the community. Each part would take 6 months for qualified nurses and 1 year for non-nurses. It was hoped that the split in training would reduce the numbers of nurse who qualified as midwives whilst never practising (Towler and Bramall 1986).

1941: The Midwives' Institute became the College of Midwives and in 1947 it received a Royal Charter (Cowell and Wainwright 1981).

1948: National Health Service (NHS) established. This entitled every woman to free maternity care; now that doctors did not need to be paid directly, women were more likely to use them for care (Robinson 1990). In addition the midwife was less likely to be the first professional consulted when the woman knew she was pregnant (Bent 1982). Despite the fact that only a third of general practitioners (GPs) had been involved in maternity care at the end of the Second World War, they negotiated that all GPs would be able to undertake maternity care in the NHS regardless of qualifications and experience despite the opposition of the Royal College of Obstetricians and Gynaecologists (Robinson 1990).

1952: The membership of the CMB was increased from 14 (as established in 1929) to 16 as follows

1. Six members appointed by the Ministry of Health.
2. Four members appointed by the Royal College of Midwives.
3. One member appointed by each of the Royal Colleges of Obstetricians and Gynaecologists, Surgeons and Physicians, by the County Councils

Association, the Society of Medical Officers of Health and the Association of Municipal Corporations (Towler and Bramall 1986).

1959: The Cranbrook Committee (Ministry of Health 1959) recommended that 70% of births should take place in hospital.

1970: The Peel Report (Department of Health and Social Security 1970) recommended that 100% of births should take place in hospital. The limited evidence used by the committee to formulate their recommendations was flawed by including unplanned together with planned home births in the statistics (Tew 1990; see Chapter 2 of this book).

1974: The reorganisation of the NHS brought together the three elements of maternity care under one authority. Domiciliary midwifery (controlled by the local authority), hospital maternity services (controlled by local hospital boards) and general practitioner services (controlled by the local executive council) would all be under the control of newly established health authorities. This was supposed to permit continuity of care and assist in interprofessional communications and relationships, although in practice all that happened is duplication of care (Oakley and Houd 1990). The 1960s and 1970s saw the rise of technological obstetrics, resulting in a move away from home birth and a loss of autonomy for the midwife (Arney 1982).

1975: The Sex Discrimination Act and a 1976 ruling from the European Community removed the bar on men becoming midwives (Towler and Bramall 1986). Two pilot training schemes were started in 1977.

1983: Midwifery education programmes were lengthened to 18 months for nurses and three years for non-nurses.

1983: The Central Midwives' Board was replaced by four national boards for nurses, midwives and health visitors and the United Kingdom Central Council (UKCC), each body to have a midwifery committee. Problems have occurred due to the wording of the 1979 Nurses, Midwives and Health Visitors Act, which states that the National Boards shall consult their Midwifery Committees but does not compel them to follow the wishes of the midwives, who can be outvoted on the Boards. The UKCC cannot overule the wishes of its Midwifery Committee on issues related to midwifery. For the first time Midwives' Rules and Code of Practice have been released on an all United Kingdom basis preventing inconsistencies between countries.

Oakley (1989) has advanced a theory for the disparity between medical and midwifery philosophies of child bearing based on their different conceptual domains.

Midwives...Obstetricians   Emotion...Reason
Women...Men   Intuition...Intellect
Health...Disease   Nature...Culture
Normality...Abnormality   Feminine...Masculine
Art...Science   Community...Institution

Social...Medical	Family...Work
Subjective...Objective	Private...Public
Experience...Knowledge	Care...Control
Observation...Intervention	"Soft"..."Hard"
Practice...Theory	(Oakley 1989, p. 215)

The essential difference between doctors and midwives is apparent in the passivity of a midwife caring for a labouring woman. The midwife will watch, wait, observe for problems and support the woman as required. The doctor however often feels impelled to justify his presence by doing something, most commonly by intervening in the labour (Arney 1982). Kirkham (1986) sums up this situation when she states that:

> Perhaps the difference between being the ring-master and being the safety net is really the difference between midwives and doctors. (Kirkham 1986, p. 36)

Modern medicine is based upon intervention, viewing illness as relating solely to the body and not to environmental or social factors. The doctor seeks to cure or manipulate the individual rather than to prevent illness or to encourage natural healing (Chamberlain 1981).

Definition of the role of the midwife

The definition jointly agreed by the World Health Organization, the International Confederation of Midwives and the International Federation of Gynaecologists (FIGO) is:

> A midwife is a person who, having been regularly admitted to a midwifery educational programme, duly recognised in the country in which it is located, has successfully completed the prescribed course of studies in midwifery and has acquired the requisite qualifications to be registered and/or legally licensed to practise midwifery.
>
> She must be able to give the necessary supervision, care and advice to women during pregnancy, labour and the postpartum period, to conduct deliveries on her own responsibility and to care for the newborn and the infant. This care includes preventative measures, procurement of medical assistance and the execution of emergency measures in the absence of medical help. She has an important task in health counselling and education, not only for the patients, but also within the family and the community. The work should involve antenatal education and preparation for parenthood and extends to certain areas of gynaecology, family planning and child care. She may practice in hospitals, clinics, health units, domiciliary conditions or in any other service. (United Kingdom Central Council 1989, pp 1–2.)

Unfortunately although this definition is accepted within the United Kingdom, the actual role of the midwife may be very different. The increasing medical involvement in the processes of childbirth has eroded the role and independence of the midwife (Robinson 1989a), a process which began in the nineteenth century with the medical profession attempting to limit midwifery practice (Arney 1982). The change in practice from that of midwife to 'obstetric nurse' has been accompanied by a loss in confidence in the midwife's skills and intuition (Robinson 1989b). This is a possible explanation for the unwillingness of midwives who have not been practising their role to the full to engage in initiatives in care which are aimed at restoring the midwife's autonomy (Donley 1990). The decline in the independence of the midwife can be seen in their historical development from private practice to salaried employee (Towler and Bramall 1986). It has also been argued that the 'nursing' culture with its hierarchies, uniforms and subservience to medical staff has been a contributory factor (Flint 1984, 1987). This is one of the reasons advanced for favouring preregistration midwifery programmes over those for qualified nurses (Downe 1986, 1987). The decline in the number of home births, the availability of free medical advice following the establishment of the NHS (Bent 1982) and the public belief that the medical profession can control all natural processes for the common good have aided the decline (Wagner 1987). Most damaging to the position of the midwife has been the change in the definition of normality in childbirth. Whereas previously a pregnancy and birth were regarded as normal until proved otherwise, medical management states that normality can only be defined in retrospect (Kirkham 1986). Midwives thus lost their place as practitioners of the normal and also as the individual who identified deviation from normality before calling in assistance (Donnison 1988).

Even within medicine in the last 30 years there has been a considerable change in the way that the processes of childbirth have been viewed. Most notably this has included the change from a natural and physiological process to one of potential pathology which can only be classified as normal in retrospect (Schwarz 1990). This change in philosophy has provided justification for the interventionist policies (most notably in labour) of the 1960s and early 1970s including ultrasound scanning, artificial rupture of the membranes, induction of labour and intrapartum fetal monitoring (Schwarz 1990). The usefulness of the application of these techniques and technologies to the care of normal mothers and babies has not been demonstrated, making their continued use of doubtful value given their potentially adverse effects on morbidity (World Health Organization 1985; Chalmers *et al.* 1989). Such technologies and activities require careful protocols for their application, resulting in a loss of decision-making for midwives who still care for the large majority of women during birth (Robinson 1989b).

Increasing medical involvement in the supervision of childbearing women most notably by general practitioners who see themselves, rather than midwives, as the practitioners of the normal has further marginalised midwives (Robinson 1989a). As Robinson (1989a) demonstrated in her survey into the role of the midwife, most doctors were happy with their role in the care of childbearing women; although they realised that junior medical staff were not always the most appropriate to conduct antenatal examinations, this was important as a part of their training. The use of obstetric units to train medical staff can result in a further diminution of midwives' responsibilities as doctors in training wish to be in control of the pregnancy and labour (Kitzinger *et al.* 1990). In a scheme where the middle grade of obstetrician (registrar) was absent from a sample of maternity units. The results were better relationships between midwives and consultants and an increase in midwives' autonomy (Kitzinger *et al.* 1990). The reports of the Maternity Services Advisory Committee (1982, 1984, 1985) recommend that the skills of midwives should be used to the full, that duplication of care should be reduced and that the obstetrician should devote his efforts to the care of women thought to be at high risk of complications. Robinson (1990) showed considerable underuse of midwifery skills and duplication of effort. The latest National Audit Office Report (1990) into the maternity services is most critical of this waste of resources and talent. Mothers now often expect to be cared for by doctors even during labour, and they may regard midwives in hospital as nurses, a situation perpetuated by the use of named grades similar to those in the nursing hierarchy and the wearing of 'nursing' uniforms including belts and caps (Flint 1984; Kirkham 1986).

Areas where midwifery skills were not being properly utilised in Robinson's survey (1990) carried out in 1979 (the results from which have been substantiated in later studies (Askham and Barbour 1987; Garcia and Garforth 1990)) included the antenatal care of normal women, support and supervision of labour of normal women and postpartum care including the transfer of normal mothers home from hospital. Some initiatives in midwifery care have been developed and will be discussed below.

Midwifery practice in the United Kingdom

This section considers developments in the patterns of midwifery care which seek to re-establish the role of the midwife, in addition to some thoughts about the future in relation to changes in the provision of health care in the United Kingdom. The outcome of some of these schemes has been evaluated (both in the United Kingdom and abroad) and they have been shown to be at least as good as those for similar women receiving medical care with the advantage of being cheaper and more acceptable to the mothers (Humphrey 1985; Thompson 1986; van Alten *et al.* 1989; Flint 1991; Tew and Damstra-Wijmenga 1991). Indeed Chng *et al.* (1980) have shown that midwives may be more accurate than doctors in detecting deviations from the normal. Some of the midwifery initiatives have centred on areas of care which are of little interest to the medical profession such as care of the bereaved (Collins, 1986), support for mothers of low birthweight infants (Hughes, 1986) and schemes to aid poorer women (Davies and Evans 1991).

Midwives' clinics

In many areas of the United Kingdom midwives are giving total antenatal care to normal women, often alongside an obstetric clinic (Stuart and Judge 1984). These are small changes though, which do not affect the underlying problems of the position of the midwife. They do however provide an educational opportunity for students (Thomson 1991), a more psychologically supportive service for the mother (DeVries 1989) and a potential reduction in the number of care givers (Flint 1991), although these last two points were not supported in Thomson's (1991) study. Murphy (1990) has described an as yet unevaluated scheme where a midwives' antenatal clinic has been established in a 'drop-in' centre used by other health professionals and sited in an inner city area. Women can attend by appointment or they can simply drop-in during the hours that the midwives are based there. This provision is aimed at women who might not normally attend for care, often those with poor social circumstances such as homelessness. The use of the time the women are there is maximised by having the clinic at the same time as a health vistor-run well baby clinic. This has also increased liaison between the two professional groups (Murphy 1990).

Midwifery beds

A number of schemes to re-establish the role of the midwife in the total care of normal women have been developed. In one scheme low technology labour rooms have been established on postnatal wards to permit the mothers to have the same care givers during labour and the early postpartum period (Drayton personal communication). Only those women assessed as being at high risk of complications are cared for in the labour ward. In another design for midwifery care, women experiencing a normal pregnancy are selected antenatally receiving antenatal intrapartum and postnatal care (shared with the GPs) from hospital and community midwives (Prout and Pearson 1989; Waterhouse 1989).

Protocols have been established to permit midwives to undertake the augmentation of labour and to request the siting of an epidural from the anaesthetists (Waterhouse 1989). This scheme originated with the closure of four GP units (three isolated and one integrated) which had previously provided care for women experiencing a normal pregnancy, labour and puerperium (Prout and Pearson 1989). The resultant increase in workload on the obstetric staff was the ideal opportunity for such a change. Whilst 40% of women in the district receive either obstetric and midwifery care (if they are classed as being at high risk of complications) or GP and midwifery care (if at low risk), 60% of mothers (approximately 4000/year) are cared for antenatally by the midwife in conjunction with the GP and by the midwife solely during labour and the postnatal period (Prout and Pearson 1989; Waterhouse 1989). The results of this pattern of care are currently under evaluation. The involvement of the GP in antenatal care needs to be questioned especially regarding duplication of care when midwives are qualified and able to care specifically for this group of women.

The Know Your Midwife Scheme

In the early 1980s an innovative project to assess the effect of midwifery care on normal mothers was established (Flint 1991). Women classified as being at low risk of complications were selected early in pregnancy and randomly allocated to receive midwifery or standard medical care. The women in the midwifery group were cared for by a group of 4 midwives throughout the remainder of their antenatal care (with the exception of a medical examination at 36 weeks gestation), during labour and the puerperium in hospital and at home. In all 460 women were cared for by the midwives over a 2 year period. The mothers cared for by midwives were statistically less likely to be admitted to hospital in the antenatal period, to use analgesia in labour, to have less chance of intervention and to have a greater chance of a normal birth. They were also much more likely to receive care during labour from a midwife known to them. The outcome for perinatal mortality showed that the midwifery group experienced more deaths (8 compared to 4) although these were all due to recognised causes which could not be affected by the care received (Flint 1991). Flint's (1991) original scheme has been used as a basis for others where hospital and community staff remain separate although members of the same team (Frohlich and Edwards 1989) or where the project is totally community based as in the Rhondda Valley in South Wales. Both these schemes are currently being evaluated.

Independent midwifery

Dissatisfaction with the segmented and medically dominated hospital midwifery practice has led a small number of midwives to establish themselves in private practice (Weig 1984; Isherwood 1989). Few midwives working in the United Kingdom have the opportunity to care for the same woman throughout her pregnancy, labour and puerperium (Robinson 1989a). Private midwifery practice is difficult within the British health care system which, although it encourages private medicine, has no provision (through insurance schemes) for payment for normal midwifery care. The independent practice of midwifery is totally legal within the UK so long as the UKCC's Midwives' Rules (1986) are adhered to (Isherwood 1989). Such midwives often have a precarious financial situation although they achieve considerable satisfaction through the total midwifery care they are able to give. The mothers approach the midwives personally through 'word of mouth' knowledge although limited advertising of their services is allowed under the UKCC's 'Code of Professional Conduct' (United Kingdom Central Council 1984, 1985). Care is usually given in the woman's own home and involves antenatal supervision, preparation for labour, care during labour and birth and postpartum care up until 28 days (Isherwood 1989). The independent midwife must notify the local supervisor of midwives that she is undertaking the care of a woman in that district and she must fulfil her legal duties with respect to notification of birth. Currently most independent midwives are practising in the South East of England; some of them work with a partner (Kargar 1987). Independent midwifery provides one possible model for the practice of midwifery following the forthcoming changes within the National Health Service (Meyer 1990).

Midwifery education is changing

There are seven centres in England offering preregistration midwifery education (to non-nurses) with others being developed throughout the United Kingdom. In 1989 the first preregistration midwifery degree commenced in Oxford, a further two courses are being developed. These changes (together with those occurring in post-registration midwifery education) are needed to reflect the altered expectations placed upon midwives by society. If midwifery is to prosper it must foster articulate, intelligent and perceptive midwives who can represent midwifery to other professional groups, government agencies and to the general public. Their practice must be based upon sound research, giving the midwife the ability to argue the rationale for her management from a strong theoretical base. Midwives must be responsive to the needs of mothers and families. No longer are most women happy just to end childbirth unscathed with a live baby. There is a need amongst all women to be involved in the decisions surrounding birth (Kirkham 1986). To this end the information gained during antenatal examinations (for example) should be shared with the woman. This applies to women from all social groups. One cannot assume that simply because a woman does not ask direct questions that she simply does not want to know (Kirkham 1986).

Midwifery after the changes within the NHS

These changes move away from central control towards local management of hospitals. Health authorities who no longer run the service are placed in the position of purchasers of care which is provided by a number of services including 'opted-out' NHS hospitals and the private sector. In some situations GPs may be in the position of negotiating the provision of maternity services for the women in their care. This may not be to the benefit of the women or of midwifery if the practice simply chooses to refer all their pregnant women to the local consultant unit. It must be asked what knowledge is possessed by the GP (who often has been prepared through high-technology hospital obstetrics) of the available alternative forms of care and of the women to whom they are appropriate? However the GPs may be persuaded that a midwifery service could offer better value for money in providing the care of normal women. The hospital providing the service may offer a two-tier operation with a differential rate for the care of normal women and those classed as being at high risk. Midwives could provide the former service along the lines of the model suggested by Waterhouse (1989). Some areas may even establish that the midwife is the first professional seen by the pregnant woman and that it is with her that the woman can discuss the options available to her and the pattern of care which is appropriate and which she would prefer along the lines suggested by the Royal College of Midwives (1987). One could foresee a future where the pattern of midwifery practice within the United Kingdom is markedly different from now. In the worst-case scenario, midwives remaining in hospital employment with clinical directorate management system led by doctors could be working as obstetric nurses under strict medical control.

In another vision, midwives who have demonstrated that they can provide high quality care at lower costs than doctors (Flint 1991), could establish themselves into teams within health organisations or as independent cooperatives to provide care at competitive rates. Such a scheme based on Flint's (1991) work on the 'Know Your Midwife' scheme could negotiate access to hospital facilities where necessary, might engage medical staff to provide the necessary obstetric cover and could offer a service tailored to the needs of each woman and her family. Intermediate patterns of care could see midwives acting as independent contractors selling their services to the opted-out hospitals in a smiliar way to that currently utilised by the hospital consultants. All these schemes would require midwives to work across the full range of their skills and not, as present, to be in one particular sphere (such as postpartum care) (Robinson 1989a).

Supervision of midwifery

The 1902 Midwives' Act made provision for the supervision of midwifery practice by medical and non-medical supervisors appointed by the local supervising authority (usually the local council). There were no specific qualifications established for the non-medical supervisor, leading to the appointment of unsuitable individuals who could antagonise the midwives (Towler and Bramall 1986). This was amended in the 1936 Act which stated that the supervisor should have adequate experience of midwifery. It was also stated that there should be a distinction between the supervisor and the senior manager of midwives employed by an authority (Welsh National Board 1987). In 1983 the UKCC stated that the supervisor must have had at least 3 years' experience as a midwife (with not less than one year being in the previous two) and that they must have undertaken an induction course as supervisor or that they undertake a course within 1 year of their appointment (United Kingdom Central Council 1991).

The supervisor of midwives was originally established to assess the standard of midwifery care in the area (as a safeguard to the public), to ensure that the midwives' rules were being adhered to and to act as the 'counsellor and friend of the midwives' (Towler and Bramall 1986). In addition to this role of supporter and help to the midwife her functions today are as follows:

1. To notify the UKCC annually of the details of all midwives practising in the district.
2. To ensure that all midwives in the district have attended an approved statutory refresher course within the last 5 years.
3. To ascertain the facts surrounding allegations of malpractice, misconduct or negligence and to submit a report to the local supervising authority (health authority or board).

4. To suspend a midwife from practice where she is at risk of spreading infection.

5. She may suspend a midwife from practice pending investigation of misconduct by a National Board or by the Professional Conduct or Health Committees of the UKCC.

6. She must arrange training for a midwife needing to acquire new skills.

7. Ensure that there are local policies to support a midwife caring for a woman having a home birth.

8. She must ensure that appropriate detailed contemporary records are kept. Where a midwife leaves the area or is unable to care for her own records these should be kept by the supervisor.

9. She must examine at least annually the equipment, register of cases and drugs and the case notes of any independent midwives working in the area.

10. She must ensure that the regulations governing the supply, administration and storage of controlled drugs by midwives in her district are complied with.

11. She must investigate the circumstances involving a midwife related to any occurrence of perinatal or maternal death in the area (Welsh National Board 1987).

Midwifery in other countries

The Netherlands

Eighty per cent of midwives working in The Netherlands today are not nurses, but undertake a three year education programme in midwifery (Smulders and Limburg 1988).

Midwives play a major role in the provision of Dutch maternity care (van Teijlingen 1989). Over one-third of babies are born at home under the care of the midwife, a third are born under a scheme similar to the Domino style of care in the United Kingdom and the rest, those mothers classified as being at a high risk of complications are delivered in hospital (van Teijlingen 1989). The Dutch system of health insurance for maternity services only provides reimbursement to the parents of the cost of hospital care if the mother is not at low risk (van Teijlingen 1989) thus providing no choice for this group of women (Oakley and Houd 1990). Midwives caring for mothers at home are supported in their work by the maternity aide who assists in the care during labour and in the postnatal care of mothers and their families (Kloosterman 1984) whilst providing necessary social support which is not available in the United Kingdom (Oakley and Houd 1990).

Recent examination of the Dutch perinatal mortality statistics according to place of birth and care giver has demonstrated that midwives acheive better outcomes for all births after 32 weeks of gestation for all levels of risk assessment than either general practitioners or obstetricians (Tew and Damstra-Wijmenga 1991). The low-technology care given by midwives in the home and to a lesser extent in hospital results in significantly lower perinatal mortality than the interventionist medical care. Babies born at home under the care of the midwife have a mortality rate 12 times less than that for babies born in hospital under medical supervision. Only for a baby born at less than 32 weeks gestation does hospital-based medical care achieve a similar result to that obtained by midwifery care (Tew and Damstra-Wijmenga 1991). The authors conclude by stating that there appears to be little support for the stated advantages of high technology as opposed to the less interventionist care given by midwives and that this study supports others (Campbell and Macfarlane 1987; Tew 1990) which question the supposed greater safety of hospital birth (Tew and Damstra-Wijmenga 1991).

The United States

Midwifery in the United States was almost destroyed by the opposition of the medical profession (Arney 1982). New immigrants into the United States brought their midwives with them but as the population became more prosperous they sought out the services of doctors whose engagement indicated that the family were getting on in the world (Ehrenreich and English 1973). Lay midwives continued to care for poor, rural communities most notably in the southern states and in New Mexico (Gaskin 1988). Midwifery was declared illegal in many states (Arney 1982) following the lobbying of doctors who saw lucrative opportunities in obstetric care (Ehrenreich and English 1973). All the outlawing of lay midwifery achieved in many cases was to deny poor women any assistance and support during childbirth. Such women were unable to pay the fees demanded by doctors even in less affluent areas (Ehrenreich and English 1973). Some nurses were trained as midwives and employed in public hospitals in New York in the 1920s but their widespread use was opposed by doctors (Gaskin 1988).

Mary Breckinridge who had seen midwives working in Europe trained in the United Kingdom before returning to Kentucky to establish the Frontier Nursing (sic) Service (FNS) to serve an impoverished rural community (Breckinridge 1981). Initially midwives were attracted from the United Kingdom but with the outbreak of the Second World War they returned home and a local school to train nurses as midwives was established. The work of the midwives in reducing a very high perinatal mortality rate to well below the national average for the United States whilst acknowledged by the Metropolitan Life Insurance Company (Raisler 1985) did not receive much publicity and did little to advance the cause of American midwifery (Gaskin 1988). A modern example of the effectiveness of midwifery care in Southern California in the 1960s (Levy et al. 1971) was not allowed to continue due to opposition from doctors within the state. When medical care (rather than midwifery care) was reinstated, there was a significant rise in the rates of preterm birth and neonatal mortality (Levy et al. 1971). More recent evidence of the effectiveness of midwifery care has been provided by statistics from the North Central Bronx Hospital in New York. This serves a disadvantaged, ethnically diverse, inner city population. All mothers of whatever degree of risk are cared for by midwives, with an obstetrician to manage obstetric problems which arise. Despite serving a deprived population, the midwifery service achieves better maternal and infant outcomes (mortality and morbidity rates, levels of intervention and operative delivery) than do most private hospitals in the United States (Haire 1990).

The American College of Nurse Midwives was established in 1955 with the aim of making the practice of nurse-midwifery legal (Gaskin 1988). Nurse-midwifery is seen very much as a branch of nursing with most of the midwives practising in institutional settings (DeVries 1989). Nurse-midwives care for medically indigent women in public hospitals, in nurse-midwifery practices in birth centres and Health Maintenance Organizations with a small number being in private practice (Silverton 1988). Midwives (of all types) deliver less than 5% of American babies (Kitzinger 1988). Nurse-midwifery is legal in 49 states (Gaskin 1988).

Licensed (or non-nurse) midwives have undertaken a course of training which is often combined with an apprenticeship to an experienced midwife. These schools had their origins in the Women's Movement of the 1960s aided by the extremely interventionist attitudes of American obstetricians which included the use of 'twilight sleep' to anaesthetise the woman and routine forceps delivery (Gaskin 1988). The early midwives were often self-taught, gaining their knowledge from experience, textbooks or sympathetic physicians (Gaskin 1988). The licensed midwife takes a holistic approach to the woman and her family and she is less likely to follow the medical model of care adopted by many nurse-midwives (Silverton 1988). Licensed midwifery is legal in fewer states than nurse-midwifery. Licensed midwives may practice in institutions such as birth centres and also in private practice (Myers-Ciecko 1988).

Lay midwives, although illegal in many areas of the United States, continue to provide a service for their own social groups, such as amongst the Native Americans in New Mexico. They learn their skills through an apprenticeship system being taught by experienced lay midwives. In some states these midwives have been outlawed resulting, in the case of Alabama, in a large group of poor women having no access to any care or support during labour and delivery (Gaskin 1988). Midwifery care during pregnancy and birth remains a minority experience in the United States. Most mothers are under the supervision of obstetricians whilst receiving care in labour and the postpartum period from maternity nurses, their babies being looked after by paediatric nurses (DeVries, 1989).

New Zealand

Midwifery has not existed in New Zealand for the last 20 years. Midwives have not been permitted to take responsibility for care during normal pregnancy and birth but have worked under medical direction as obstetric nurses; indeed midwifery training ceased in 1979 (Donley 1990). Fifty years of free access to medical care during childbirth had resulted in the loss of the midwives' role in large institutions, although midwives continued to practice in small maternity units. However centralisation of services had led to the closure of these units further jeopardising the future of midwifery (Donley 1990). Intense lobbying by the newly formed New

Zealand College of Midwives in partnership with women concerned at the level of control exerted by the medical profession resulted in an amendment to the law. This permitted midwives to once again have equal status with doctors regarding responsibility for care during childbirth (Guilliland 1990). This change allows women to choose midwifery care should they so wish and it frees midwives from medical control. As in The Netherlands, midwives can be reimbursed by the state for care they give (Guilliland 1990). In addition to the new educational programmes which are being established for nurses and non-nurses who wish to become midwives (Guilliland 1990), the skills of the midwife lost during the years of medical control will need to be rediscovered and relearned (Donley 1990). Alternative models of midwifery care including those which are community based are being explored, these will need to be evaluated.

The developments in New Zealand brought about by a failure of the medical profession to produce satisfactory outcomes, the increasing cost of medical care and intense consumer pressure will provide an ideal opportunity to evaluate the outcomes of midwifery care with its low-technology and non-interventionist approach.

Traditional Birth Attendants (TBAs)

The TBA is the most common person present at a birth in poor countries. They are a part of the community they serve often with skills being handed-on orally. The World Health Organization has suggested that countries undertake training programmes for their TBAs which encourage helpful practices (such as an upright posture for birth), discouraging those which have been shown to be dangerous, such as the application of dung to the recently cut umbilical cord (Royston and Armstrong 1989). The TBA can also be instructed in how to recognise abnormalities early, so the women can be transported perhaps a considerable distance in order to obtain the required help. An example of such a screening test is a wooden pole with an attached piece of wood which can be used to detect women of abnormally small stature (Bryar, personal communication). The WHO has been encouraging the use of a birthing kit which includes a piece of soap for hand washing, a sharp instrument (or a stone) for cutting the umbilical cord, a woven rush or leaf mat which can provide a clean area for the birth and some matches (to light a fire, sterilise equipment and as a light source). The kits must be simple, easy to use and replacements should be readily available locally at minimal cost.

References

Abel-Smith B (1960) *A History of the Nursing Profession* Heinemann: London
Abel-Smith B (1964) *The Hospitals 1800–1948* Heinemann: London

van Alten D, Eskes M, and Treffers P E (1989) 'Midwifery in The Netherlands, The Wormerveer Study; selection, mode of delivery, perinantal mortality and infant morbidity' *British Journal of Obstetrics and Gynaecology* 96 (6): 656–62

Arney W R (1982) *Power and the Profession of Obstetrics* University of Chicago Press: Chicago

Askham J and Barbour R S (1987) 'The role and responsibilities of the midwife in Scotland' *Health Bulletin* 45 (3): 153–9

Bent E A (1982) 'The growth and development of midwifery' in P Allan and M Jolley (eds) *Nursing, Midwifery and Health Visiting Since 1900* Faber and Faber: London

Biller P (1986) 'Childbirth in the Middle Ages.' *History Today* 36(8): 42–9

Breckinridge M (1981) *Wide Frontiers: A story of the Frontier Nursing Service* University Press of Kentucky: Kentucky

Campbell J (1923) *Reports on Public Health and Medical Subjects No 21: The training of midwives* HMSO: London

Campbell J (1924) *Maternal Mortality* Reports on Public Health and Medical Subjects 25 HMSO: London

Campbell R and Macfarlane A (1987) *Where to be Born* National Perinatal Epidemiology Unit: Oxford

Chalmers I, Enkin M and Kierse M J N C (eds) (1989) *Effective Care in Pregnancy and Childbirth* Oxford Medical: Oxford

Chamberlain M (1981) *Old Wives' Tales: Their history, remedies and spells* Virago: London

Chng P, Hall M and MacGillivray I (1980) 'An audit of antenatal care: the value of the first antenatal visit' *British Medical Journal* 281: 1184–6

Collins M (1986) 'Health care for families following still-birth and first week deaths' *Midwives Chronicle* 99: (Suppl) xiii–xv

Cowell B and Wainwright D (1981) *Through the Blue Door* Royal College of Midwives: London

Davies J and Evans F (1991) 'Newcastle inner city midwifery support project' in S Robinson and A M Thomson (eds) *Midwives, Research and Childbirth Vol 2* 104–39 Chapman and Hall: London

Department of Health and Social Security (1970) *Report of the Sub-Committee on Domiciliary and Maternity Bed Needs* HMSO: London

DeVries R G (1989) 'Caregivers in pregnancy and childbirth' in I Chalmers, M Enkin and M J N C Kierse (eds) *Effective Care in Pregnancy and Childbirth* 143–61 Oxford Medical: Oxford

Dewhurst J (1983) 'Royal midwives of former times' *Midwife, Health Visitor and Community Nurse* 19(10): 386–92

Donley J (1990) 'Midwives' dilemma' *Proceedings of the International Confederation of Midwives 22nd International Congress* 59–61 Midwives' Division of the Japanese Nurses' Association/Japanese Midwives' Association: Tokyo

Donnison J (1988) *Midwives and Medical Men (2nd edn)* Historical Publications: London

Downe S (1986) 'Dispelling the myths on direct entry training' *Nursing Times* 82 (Sept 10): 63–4

Downe S (1987) 'Can midwives deliver?' *Midwives Chronicle* May: 141–4

Ehrenreich B and English D (1973) *Witches, Midwives and Nurses—A history of women healers* The Feminist Press, City University of New York: New York

Flint C (1984) 'Symbols of servility' *Nursing Times* 80 (Oct 10): 50–1

Flint C (1987) 'Conflicting allegiances' *Nursing Times* 83: 24

Flint C (1991) 'The know your midwife scheme' in S Robinson and A M Thomson (eds) *Midwives, Research and Childbirth Vol 2* 72–103 Chapman and Hall: London

Frohlich J and Edwards S (1989) 'Team midwifery for everyone–Building on the 'Know your midwife' scheme' *Midwives Chronicle* 102: 66–70

Garcia J and Garforth S (1990) 'Parents and new-born babies on the labour ward' in G Garcia, R Kilpatrick and M Richards (eds) *The Politics of Maternity Care* 163–82 Clarendon Paperbacks: Oxford

Gaskin I M (1988) 'Midwifery reinvented' in S Kitzinger (ed) *The Midwife Challenge* 61–86 Pandora: London

Gelis J (1991) *History of Childbirth: Fertility, pregnancy and birth in early modern Europe* Polity Press: Cambridge

Guilliland K (1990) 'Women and midwives: A partnership in progress' *Proceedings of the International Confederation of Midwives 22nd International Congress* 121–3 Midwives' Division of the Japanese Nurses' Association/Japanese Midwives' Association: Tokyo

Haire D (1990) 'Reducing intervention improves high risk care' Proceedings of the International Confederation of Midwives 22nd International Congress 163 Midwives' Division of the Japanese Nurses' Association/Japanese Midwives' Association: Tokyo

Hughes P (1986) 'Neonatal community liaison visiting' *Midwives Chronicle* 99: (Suppl) xi–xii

Humphrey C (1985) 'The community midwife in maternity care' *Midwife, Health Visitor and Community Nurse* 21(10): 349–55

Isherwood K (1989) 'Independent midwifery in the UK' *Midwife, Health Visitor and Community Nurse* 25(7): 307–9

Kargar I (1987) 'Independent midwives: threat or stimulus?' *Nursing Times* 83(45): 69

Kirkham M (1986) 'A feminist perspective in midwifery' in C Webb (ed) *Feminist Practice in Women's Health Care* 35–49 Wiley: Chichester

Kitzinger J, Green J and Coupland V (1990) 'Labour relations: Midwives and doctors on the labour ward' in G Garcia, R Kilpatrick and M Richards (eds) *The Politics of Maternity Care* 149–62 Clarendon Paperbacks: Oxford

Kitzinger S (1988) *The Midwife Challenge* Pandora: London

Kloosterman G J (1984) 'The Dutch experience of domiciliary confinements' in L Zander and G Chamberlain (eds) *Pregnancy Care for the 1980's* 116–25 Macmillan: London

Levy B, Wilkinson R and Marine W (1971) 'Reducing neonatal mortality rate with nurse-midwives' *American Journal of Obstetrics and Gynecology* 109: 50–8

Lewis T (1989) 'Happy birthday Queen Charlotte's' *Midwife, Health Visitor and Community Nurse* 25(7): 277–8

Loudon I (1986) 'Obstetric care, social class and maternal mortality' *British Medical Journal* 293: 606–8

Marshall R (1983) 'Birth of a profession' *Nursing Mirror* Nov 30 (Suppl): i–vii

Maternity Services Advisory Committee (1982) *Maternity Care in Action Part I: Antenatal Care* HMSO: London

Maternity Services Advisory Committee (1984) *Maternity Care in Action Part II: Care During Childbirth* HMSO: London

Maternity Services Advisory Committee (1985) *Maternity Care in Action Part III: Care of the Mother and Baby* HMSO: London

Meyer J (1990) 'Options for midwives after the NHS review' *Midwife, Health Visitor and Community Nurse* 26(1): 37–8

Ministry of Health (1959) *Report of the Maternity Services Committee* HMSO: London

Murphy L (1990) 'Midwives' drop-in centre' *Midwife Health Visitor and Community Nurse* 26(1): 18–20

Myers-Ciecko J A (1988) 'Direct-entry midwifery in the USA' in S Kitzinger (ed) *The Midwife Challenge* 87–98 Pandora: London

National Audit Office (1990) *Maternity Services* HMSO: London

Oakley A (1976) 'Wisewoman and medicine man: Changes in the management of childbirth' in J Mitchell and A Oakley (eds) *The Rights and Wrongs of Women* Penguin: Harmondsworth

Oakley A (1984) *The Captured Womb* Basil Blackwell: Oxford

Oakley A (1989) 'Who cares for women? Science versus love in midwifery today' *Midwives Chronicle* 102: 214–21

Oakley A and Houd S (1990) *Helpers in Childbirth: Midwifery Today* Hemisphere Publishing Corporation: New York

Prout S and Pearson L (1989) 'Practising midwifery' *Nursing Times* 85(48): 41–3

Raisler J (1985) 'Improving pregnancy outcome with nurse-midwifery care.' *Journal of Nurse Midwifery* 30: 189–91

Rivers J (1981) *Dame Rosalind Paget DBE, ARRC* Royal College of Midwives: London

Robinson S (1989a) 'Caring for childbearing women: the interrelationship between midwifery and medical responsibilities' in S Robinson and A M Thomson (eds) *Midwives, Research and Childbirth Vol I* 8–41 Chapman and Hall: London

Robinson S (1989b) 'The role of the midwife: opportunities and constraints' in I Chalmers, M Enkin and M J N C Kierse (eds) *Effective Care in Pregnancy and Childbirth* 162–80 Oxford Medical: Oxford

Robinson S (1990) 'Maintaining the independence of the midwifery profession: a continuing struggle' in G Garcia, R Kilpatrick and M Richards (eds) *The Politics of Maternity Care* 61–91 Clarendon Paperbacks: Oxford

Royal College of Midwives (1987) *Towards a Healthy Nation – a policy for the maternity services* RCM: London

Royston E and Armstrong S (1989) *Preventing Maternal Deaths* WHO: Geneva

Schwarz E W (1990) 'The engineering of childbirth: A new obstetric programme as reflected in British obstetric textbooks 1960–80' in G Garcia, R Kilpatrick and M Richards (eds) *The Politics of Maternity Care* 47–60 Clarendon Paperbacks: Oxford

Semmelweis I P (1881) 'Childbed fever: classics in infectious diseases' *Reviews of Infectious Diseases* 3(4): 53–5

Silverton L I (1988) *Midwifery Education in the USA* School of Social Studies, University College of Swansea

Smulders B and Limburg A (1988) 'Obstetrics and midwifery in the Netherlands' in S Kitzinger (ed) *The Midwife Challenge* 235–50 Pandora: London

Speert H (1980) *Obstetrics and Gynecology in America: A History* American College of Obstetrics and Gynecology: Chicago

Stuart B and Judge E (1984) 'The return of the midwife?' *Midwives Chronicle* 97: 8–9

Tew M (1990) *Safer Childbirth? A critical history of maternity care* Chapman and Hall: London

Tew M and Damstra-Wijmenga S M I (1991) 'Safest birth attendants: recent Dutch evidence' *Midwifery* 7(2):55

Thompson J B (1986) 'Safety and effectiveness of nurse-midwifery care: Research review' in H P Rooks and J E Haas (eds) *Nurse-Midwifery in America* American College of Nurse-Midwives Foundation: Washington

Thomson A M (1991) 'Providing care at a midwives'antenatal clinic' in S Robinson and A M Thomson (eds) *Midwives, Research and Childbirth Vol II* 140–175 Chapman and Hall: London

Towler J and Bramall J (1986) *Midwives in History and Society* Croom Helm: London

United Kingdom Central Council (1984) *Code of Professional Conduct for the Nurse, Midwife and Health Visitor* UKCC: London

United Kingdom Central Council (1985) *Advertising by Registered Nurses, Midwives and Health Visitors* UKCC: London

United Kingdom Central Council (1989) *A Midwife's Code of Practice (2nd edn)* UKCC: London

United Kingdom Central Council (1991) *Handbook of Midwives Rules* UKCC: London

van Teijlingen E R (1989) 'Going Dutch?' *Midwife, Health Visitor and Community Nurse* 25(4): 146–7

Wagner M (1987) 'Home birth today – an international perspective' *Paper given at the first International Home Birth Conference* Wembley, London 24.10.87

Waterhouse I L (1989) 'Oh to be a midwife: the Reading model' *Midwife, Health Visitor and Community Nurse* 25(9): 395–6

Weig M (1984) 'An independent streak' *Nursing Times* 80 (Jan 25): 16–18

Welsh National Board for Nursing, Midwifery and Health Visiting (1987) *All Wales Guidelines for Supervision of Midwives* WNB: Cardiff

World Health Organization (1985) *Having a Baby in Europe* WHO: Copenhagen

2 The midwife in the community

This chapter will consider the role and working patterns of the midwife in the community in the United Kingdom, including her position in the primary health care team (independent practice and midwifery in the United States and The Netherlands having been considered in Chapter 1). There will then be a discussion of the work of the midwife antenatally, intrapartum and postnatally. This will be related to the choice of antenatal care and place of birth. The subject of home birth will be covered, including the statutory duties of the midwife. Although the work of the community midwife should not be separated from that of the midwife in hospital, there is value in examining the differences in the organisation of non-institutional midwifery care.

Place of work

The midwife in the community may work alone or as part of a larger group of midwives. In many cases she and a partner will cover each other's days off (Cronk and Flint 1989); this can help reduce fragmentation of care (Humphrey 1985). The midwife may be a member of the primary health care team if one is established in her area (Marsh 1985a). In some rural settings the midwife may undertake double or triple duties as a district nurse and/or a health visitor (Smith 1989). Such positions are being phased-out in all but the most isolated areas, as the different priorities of each role can result in the needs of some client groups not being met. It can be difficult for such a professional to maintain her level of skill in areas as diverse as home birth, terminal care and developmental screening. Midwifery practice in poorer countries can also involve the adoption of many different roles including that of public health educator.

Community midwives may work from home, from a health authority clinic, community centres and bases, a health centre, a general practitioner's surgery or from a hospital. In some areas midwives rotate on a regular basis between hospital and community. This has advantages since the midwife remains in touch with the normal family-centred aspects of midwifery. The disadvantages are that families may not experience continuity of care and the community midwife will not be well known in her working area. The 'Know Your Midwife' scheme (Flint 1991) overcomes some of the difficulties by demonstrating the worth of a small team of midwives caring for a specific group of women in hospital and the community.

In urban areas the midwife may be attached to specific general practitioner practices or to practices in a health centre, whereas in more sparsely populated parts of the country she is often responsible for a defined geographical area. This is to prevent unnecessary travelling, loss of time and expense. It is not unusual for midwives in such areas to drive over 100 miles a day when women at the periphery of their 'patch' need care.

Whatever the allocation of case load it is vital that the midwife develop a good working relationship with the doctors to whose 'patients' (*sic*) she is giving care, with the hospital midwives and with other members of the primary health care team (Cronk and Flint 1989). This can prevent duplication of effort, misunderstandings and animosity developing. The GP sees him/herself as responsible for the care of his/her patient and for the continuing care of the whole family (Klein and Zander 1989). Recently qualified GPs will have little experience of normal midwifery and even less of out of hospital births (McKendrick 1985). His/her recent experience of obstetrics is often 6 months as a junior doctor seeing almost entirely abnormal cases (Klein and Zander 1989). It is little wonder that following medical school teaching about the risks of childbirth he/she is reluctant to undertake more than 'shared antenatal care'.

The primary health care team

Primary health care refers to the preventative actions, screening, emergency care and minor treatments undertaken in the community for a well population. Acute illness is not primarily the responsibility of the primary health care team; after initial treatment if the situation has not resolved, the individual is referred to hospital. Following resolution, the person returns to the community. If the condition becomes chronic, tertiary care is given in the community or alternatively, in long-stay non-acute institutions.

Table 2.1 Classification of health care

Care	Primary	Secondary	Tertiary
Setting	Community	Hospital	Community/long-stay institutions
Health status	Health	Acute illness	Chronic illness

The primary health care team provides screening for referral care, emergency treatment, care in the health centre and at home, health education and medicosocial care. They also play a role in determining health needs and the processes necessary to maintain and improve the health of the community. The make-up of the team will depend on the needs in its catchment area. If on a new housing estate with young couples, there will be an increased demand for midwives and health visitors. On the other hand, if the area has many elderly people, more district nurses and a chiropodist may be needed (Marsh and Kaim Caudle 1976). In some deprived and inner city areas a social worker could be of help together with interpreters (as are advised by the Asian Mother and Baby Campaign) (Wilcox 1988).

The team always includes clerical staff and medical professionals (possibly with a trainee), district nurse(s), health visitor(s) and a midwife. The midwife may be a member of more than one team. In addition there may be a practice nurse, a social worker and an administrator (Marsh 1985a). The team should meet on a regular basis to discuss progress and strategy. For some team members meetings may be daily (Marsh 1985a). There may be separate meetings for team members involved in maternity care. These should include the health visitor who may already know the family and who will observe the development of the baby after birth. The practice nurse (employed by the GP) has little role in maternity care unless she is qualified (and practising) in midwifery or family planning (Wilcox 1988). Marsh (1985a) comments that the team should not be hierarchical but must work on a democratic basis. Leadership should change to the member most suitable to coordinate the management of the current problem. The doctor should not automatically assume that he or she is the team leader. Most team members are independent professionals who could view such leadership with resentment. It is better if all team members are aware of their specific roles in maternity care. This prevents both duplication of provision and underuse of skills. The women know from whom they will be receiving care at any particular stage in their pregnancy, labour and puerperium. Antenatal midwives' clinics can make the best use of the midwives' skills and free the doctor to care for his/her more needy patients (Marsh 1985b). It could be argued that the obstetric experience of the GP does not provide him/her with the skills to care for a woman experiencing a normal pregnancy.

Equipment

Since the midwife is mobile and she may be working at some distance from her base it is vital that she has with her everything necessary to cope, including in emergency situations (Cronk and Flint 1989). She keeps in contact with her base by regular telephone calls, a bleeper or by a two-way radio. If a mother's telephone is used, payment must be made. Since the midwife is an invited guest in the house she should not abuse this privilege (Cronk and Flint 1989). Equipment which should be carried includes:

For antenatal care

Fetal stethoscope
Tape measure
Portable sphygmomanometer and stethoscope
Urine test strips
Sterile containers for midstream specimen of urine
Syringes, needles and blood tubes
Appropriate forms and records; maternity certificates

For intrapartum care usually only the delivery pack is carried plus equipment marked '*'. If the midwife has a mother booked for home birth all the equipment is carried.

* Delivery pack
* Sterile gloves
* Two clinical thermometers
* Plastic apron
  Nail brush
* Urinary catheter(s)
* Cord clamps
* Disposable mucus extractor
  Entonox cylinder
* Disposable needles and syringes
* Tape measure
* Sterile cotton wool
  Baby resucitation equipment including neonatal naloxone (narcan) and oxygen
* Obstetric antiseptic cream
  Lotions for antisepsis
* Labour records and birth notification forms
* Sterile scissors
  Suture pack
  Drugs: Pethidine (obtained on a supply order)
* Syntometine, Ergometrine, vitamin K, Lignocaine

Postpartum care
as above plus:

Baby scales
Equipment for neonatal screening tests

Sterile cotton wool and normal saline
Bacteriology swabs
Suture removal equipment
Cord clamp removers
Alcohol wipes (if used locally for
cord care)
Postnatal record charts and paediatric
records (Adapted from Flint 1986 and
Cronk and Flint 1989).

The midwife is responsible for the maintenance of her equipment, maternity records and for the standard of her professional practice as laid down in Midwives' Rules 43(1):

A practising midwife shall give to her supervisor of midwives, the relevant Board and the local supervising authority, every reasonable facility to inspect her methods of practice, her records, her equipment and such part of her residence as may be used for professional purposes. (United Kingdom Central Council 1986, p. 17)

The Code of Practice (United Kingdom Central Council 1989) goes on to state that the equipment carried must meet the appropriate standard as laid down by her local supervising authority.

Record keeping

The midwife wherever she is working is bound by the Midwives' Rules (United Kingdom Central Council 1986) to maintain detailed contemporaneous records. These include:

Visits made – antenatal and postnatal.
Care given – antenatal and postnatal.
Intrapartum care – labour and delivery records.
Medicines and drugs administered including controlled drugs and prescription-only medicines.

The purpose of record keeping is to protect the midwife in the case of queries about the care given. These records should be periodically audited by the supervisor of midwives with special reference to the ordering, storage, usage and disposal of controlled drugs and prescription-only medicines (United Kingdom Central Council 1989). All records must be kept for at least 25 years from the time they were made. The records must not be destroyed. If the midwife leaves her employment, retires or in the case of an independent midwife leaves the area these records should be handed over to the local superivising authority and the transfer recorded as appropriate (United Kingdom Central Council 1989). Such records include formal records and the midwife's diary or other informal notes as used in specific areas. Attempts are being made to standardise these records.

Place of birth

Approximately 98% of British babies are born in hospital (Tew 1990). This figure includes those babies born in GP units in isolation or attached to consultant units (Tew 1990). Depending on facilities in her area the pregnant woman has the following choices regarding place of birth:

1. Birth in a consultant unit.
2. Birth in a GP unit.
3. Domino delivery.
4. Home birth.

In (2)–(4) listed above, antenatal care is given by the GP and/or midwife with referral to an obstetrician as and when required (Klein and Zander 1989). For a woman having a consultant unit delivery, antenatal care is usually shared between the hospital and the GP. Community midwifery involvement is variable. Although the woman has a theoretical choice of place of confinement, this is not always true in practice. She may be referred to hospital by her GP without being consulted about the matter or she may be offered a choice but be unsure what her alternatives are (Beech and Claxton 1983). GP units and Domino births are not available in all areas. (Domino refers to DOMiciliary IN and Out.) Care in early labour occurs at home and it is given by the community midwife. When labour is progressing the mother is transferred to hospital. The baby is born under the care of the midwife, who then transfers the mother home between 2 and 24 hours after birth (Cronk and Flint 1989)). The mother may be ignorant of her right to have a home birth, especially if her doctor is reluctant to undertake domiciliary care (Beech and Claxton 1983).

In addition to the mother's wishes, her suitability for the chosen place of birth must be considered. Previous obstetric difficulties, maternal and fetal well-being in this pregnancy and pre-existing medical conditions are all important factors which can increase the risks of home birth (Chamberlain *et al*. 1978). For the mother considered too high a risk for home birth, a Domino delivery can be a helpful compromise. It should be remembered that the mother must be fully consulted and that she should be in full agreement with her provision of care (Beech and Claxton, 1983). Where births occur unplanned at home because of the lack of take-up of antenatal care, concealed pregnancy or precipitate birth, perinatal mortality rates have been shown to average 196/1000 as opposed to 4.1/1000 for those booked for home delivery and 12.8/1000 in GP units (Campbell *et al*. 1984). Both Tew (1984, 1985 and 1990) and Campbell and Macfarlane (1987) have determined that low-risk women have better perinatal outcomes when birth occurs at home or in GP or small obstetric units than when cared for in large consultant units. This is contrary to advice given in numerous government reports (Ministry of Health 1970; House of Commons Social Services Committee 1980) which assumed that centralisation of maternity care increases safety. Kloosterman (1982) regards as most important the disruption in normal physiological processes which occurs when a woman is transferred from a known, safe environment (home) to one which is strange, threatening and over which she has no control (hospital). Being attended in labour by a familiar professional and supported by a close friend or relative can alleviate but not remove the effects of these disturbances (Keirse *et al.* 1989). Mothers giving birth attended by a known midwife under the 'Know Your Midwife' scheme were more likely to rate their experience as positive and statistically less likely to require an episiotomy, acceleration of labour and epidural or systemic analgesia (Flint 1991).

Guidelines for selection for home birth

Although it is every woman's right to have her baby at home, there are some women considered to be at too high a risk. They should be encouraged to consider an alternative such as a Domino delivery or birth in an attached or integrated GP unit (Tew 1990). These risk factors include:

1. Significant pre-existing medical disorders including diabetes, essential hypertension, cardiac disease, thyrotoxicosis and renal disease (Department of Health 1989). To these should be added known drug abuse (Shearer 1986).
2. Abnormalities in past obstetric history such as postpartum haemorrhage, retained placenta, operative delivery, or a history of uterine surgery (including cone biopsy or myomectomy) and difficult forceps delivery (Shearer 1986).
3. Maternal indications. Most obstetricians would not recommend a primiparous woman to have a home birth although Stirratt (1983) would consider them if they were between the ages of 18 and 30 years. The rationale for excluding older first-time mothers who are physically fit and well-supported financially is not stated. It is not ideal to care for women who have had more than 4 babies or who are aged over 35 years at home because they have an increased risk of complications and a higher maternal mortality rate (Department of Health 1989). Also it is advisable to exclude women under 5'1" in height who are more likely to experience cephalopelvic disproportion (Shearer 1986).
4. Complications in this pregnancy. Whilst the woman may be suitable for a home birth at the start of pregnancy, certain conditions may develop which put mother and fetus at risk. These include rhesus issoimmunisation, antepartum haemorrhage, preterm labour, multiple pregnancy, malpresentation, cephalopelvic disproportion, hypertensive disease of pregnancy and a gestation in excess of 42 weeks.

How to obtain a home birth

The mother wanting a home birth should inform her GP on her first visit to him/her (Beech and Claxton 1983; Flint 1986). She may experience a hostile reaction or find herself referred to the consultant unit anyway. Where her GP is unhelpful the woman can obtain midwifery care by writing to her local supervisor of midwives (via the health authority) requesting that a midwife should call to begin making arrangements (Beech and Claxton 1983). If her GP is unwilling or unable to provide obstetric care the mother should not sign the Maternity Services Payment Form but should write to the local family health service authority requesting to be given the name of a GP who will give such care (Beech and Claxton 1983). She can transfer her registration for the period of her pregnancy and puerperium. If no doctor is available and willing to give care, an approach should be made to the consultant unit for them to provide cover via the obstetric flying squad. It is not necessary for the mother to have any medical care or for a doctor to be in attendance at delivery (Beech and Claxton 1983). However, the GP will often agree to undertake a full medical examination of the mother to exclude abnormalities and to assess suitability for inhalational analgesia (Flint 1986). The midwife is capable of giving all antenatal, intrapartum and postpartum care. The mother's efforts to obtain medical cover should be recorded by the midwife and relayed to her supervisor. Where emergency medical assistance is required the midwife can call the GP with whom the mother is registered; if he/she is unavailable she can call any GP on the obstetric list (who is then obliged to attend) or summon the hospital flying squad. The Midwives' Code of Practice (United Kingdom Central Council 1989) gives the following advice regarding home birth:

4 HOME CONFINEMENTS

4.1 A midwife attending a mother having a home confinement should ascertain whether or not a registered medical practitioner is available for referral, to attend or be on call if required. The registered medical practitioner should preferably be from the obstetric list in those parts of the United Kingdom where such a list is held. In situations where the support of a registered medical practitioner is not available the midwife records appropriate arrangements to provide advice and support when necessary.

4.2 In a situation where the midwife considers that home confinement is inappropriate and the mother refuses to take the advice of the midwife to receive care in a maternity unit the midwife must continue to give care and consult with her supervisor of midwives, making an appropriate record.

4.3 In some instances a midwife may require medical assistance for a mother booked for a home confinement but the mother or her partner may refuse to have the registered medical practitioner in attendance. If this situation arises the midwife must continue the care of the mother and consult as soon as possible with her supervisor of midwives, making an appropriate record.

4.4 It is the duty of the supervisor of midwives to ensure that agreed local policies are easily available to all practising midwives within their supervisory jurisdiction. The local policy should provide support for the midwife in the above or other difficult situations associated with home confinements, and enable the best possible arrangements to be made for the care of the mother and her baby. (United Kingdom Central Council 1989, 10–11). (Reproduced by permission of the United Kingdom Central Council)

Advantages and disadvantages of home birth

Advantages
- The mother is in control in her own environment (Kitzinger 1978).
- She is free to have as many labour companions present as she wishes (Kitzinger 1978).
- Her children can be present.
- She can have full mobility during labour (Kitzinger 1978).
- Availability of a light diet.
- Less need for pain relief (O'Brien 1978).
- No strangers present at the delivery.
- Safer for low-risk mothers and babies (Campbell and Macfarlane 1987; Tew 1990).

Disadvantages
- Lack of availability of emergency obstetric team in cases of harmorrhage, neonatal asphyxia and cord prolapse.
- Midwives may not be familiar with birth at home (Cronk and Flint 1989).

Preparations for a home birth

There are certain home conditions which are required for a home birth although, since the mother is already living there, one could argue that the very minimum required is a waterproof roof. However the ideal conditions include the provision of adequate heating (especially in the winter), hot and cold running water and somewhere the mother can bathe or shower (Cronk and Flint 1989). The midwife should discuss with the mother arrangements for the care of other children and who will do the housework in the early puerperium. The place of birth, ideally adjacent to the bathroom and toilet, should be decided. Good lighting should be available with some form of back-up in case the electricity should fail (Cronk and Flint 1989). If a bed is to be used it should be firm and permit access from either side.

Whilst the midwife will bring most of the equipment required the mother should supply the following items:

In the area for delivery the midwife will require a large flat surface (protected by cloths or newspapers) on which to arrange her equipment:

Three towels (one for mother, one for midwife, one for baby)
A washing up bowl
Bin liners and dustbin bags for waste
Flannels
Soap on a saucer
A bucket or bedpan if the toilet is not near
Antiseptics
A new inexpensive nail brush
A jam jar for antiseptic solution
Old towels or incopads for the mother to sit on
Old sheets for the bed
A plastic cover for the bed/delivery area (preferably heavy polythene)
A nightdress or shirt to wear during labour
Sanitary towels and belt or old underpants
Cotton wool
A hot water bottle and old sheet (to wrap the baby after delivery)
Clothes for the baby
A large saucepan (to boil instruments if not already sterilised)
Baby clothes
A torch and spare batteries (for emergency lighting) (Flint 1986; Cronk and Flint 1989).

The role of the midwife in the community

Antenatal care

The midwife in the community can give antenatal care in the GP's surgery, GP unit or in the woman's own home (Cronk and Flint 1989). She will also undertake follow-up care of defaulters from hospital antenatal clinics. Marsh (1985a) recommends that whenever the GP and midwife are giving antenatal care their responsibilities should be carefully set out to prevent duplication of care. It is necessary to determine whether there will be separate midwives' clinics or if care is given jointly. In some areas the community midwife undertakes the initial antenatal interview in the woman's own home. This allows the midwife to get to know the mother in her own home and to find out how the woman feels about her pregnancy. For the woman it saves time travelling to and waiting in clinics whilst she has her first contact with the maternity services on her own territory (Cronk and Flint 1989). A later home visit allows the midwife to assess arrangements for home birth (including when and how to contact the midwife) if most care is being given in the GP's surgery or for early postnatal transfer from hospital. The visit can also be used to help the woman and her partner complete the birth plan or to discuss welfare benefits.

Intrapartum care

- Home birth. The woman summons the midwife when she thinks labour has begun. The midwife can often assess whether labour is established by the woman's manner on the telephone and how she copes with contractions. On arrival in the woman's home the midwife sits with the woman to assess her contractions before performing a full examination to determine progress in labour (Cronk and Flint 1989). If it is unclear whether labour has begun or if the mother is in the latent stage of labour the midwife may leave the mother to continue with her other duties. The woman must not be left alone. The midwife will arrange to return to reassess the woman usually in 1–2 hours time. Arrangements must be made to allow the mother to contact the midwife quickly where necessary (Cronk and Flint 1989). The midwife should complete a full record of her visit and the care given.

  If the woman is in labour the midwife can commence the labour progress records. The woman is free to adopt any position in which she feels most comfortable. In early labour she might find that keeping busy around the house, playing with children, or watching television helps the time to pass. She is free to have a bath or shower whenever she feels the need. Observations and record-keeping occur as for any first stage of labour and care includes physical and emotional support. If not already discussed the conduct of the birth should be agreed upon including the management of the third stage, clamping of the umbilical cord and the immediate care of the baby.

  The birth occurs according to the wishes of the parents. If the GP wishes to be present and the parents agree to his/her presence he/she should be summoned as the second stage approaches having been previously informed that the woman is in labour. Following the birth the baby is weighed and examined and the mother is washed and made comfortable. (If she wishes she can be assisted to have a bath or a shower.) The mother and baby can get to know each other and the baby can be put to the breast whilst the midwife checks and weighs the placenta. The room is tidied and any soiled linen and disposables taken care of. Syringes, needles and sharps should be carefully removed. The records should then be completed including the Notification of Birth form. The placenta should be disposed of by burying, burning or returning it to the hospital for incineration. Since it is the property of the mother, her agreement should be received as to the method of disposal.

The midwife remains with the mother for an hour or two after delivery. During that time careful observations are made on the condition of mother and baby. When she leaves the family must know how to contact her in an emergency and when she will be returning. The midwife returns 4–6 hours later to carry out the first postnatal examination. If the mother has not already passed urine she is helped to the toilet. If the mother feels well enough she can have a bath or shower. The baby should be observed with special attention being given to his/her temperature and breathing. Assistance can be given with breast feeding.

If an emergency occurs at any time during a home birth the midwife should remain with the woman whilst sending a reliable person to summon assistance. In most circumstances the obstetric flying squad should be summoned. Precise instructions as to the location of the house should be given while the house is made noticeable for example, by switching on lights. It may be helpful to station someone outside to direct the ambulance. The midwife must record why, how and when she summoned assistance and what actions she took whilst awaiting its arrival.

- Domino delivery. Care is similar to that for a home birth. Once the mother is in established labour she is transferred to hospital. The community midwife accompanies the woman to hospital and continues the care of the woman there. Depending on the woman's wishes and her condition she and the baby are transferred home between 2–24 hours after birth.
- GP Units. Some GP units are staffed by their own midwives. Others are staffed in rotation by community midwives who give intrapartum and postnatal care.

Postnatal care

Where a mother is transferred home from hospital less than 48 hours after birth or where she has had a home birth the midwife will visit twice daily for the first 3 days and usually daily until 10 days, as necessary. Later visits can be arranged up until 28 days.

The mother is questioned as to her well-being before she is given a full postnatal examination. This allows the midwife to assess how the mother is feeling, her adaptation to motherhood and her worries about the baby. The mother is usually examined first because she is less likely to relax if the baby has been disturbed and is crying. The baby is then examined with particular attention being paid to his temperature. If upset by him being disturbed, the mother may wish to feed the baby to help him to settle. This gives the midwife an opportunity to observe her feeding technique and to offer help if required. The midwife can provide teaching on infant feeding and bathing as appropriate. She may arrange to be present to give help with feeds, especially for the mother breast feeding for the first time. Between 6 and 10 days after birth, blood is taken from the baby to screen for inborn errors of metabolism such as phenylketonuria. Parental permission is needed before this test is performed.

Rest after delivery is important. It is part of the midwife's role to ensure that the mother is being relieved of the normal burdens of childcare and housework. The midwife is there as a support for the mother, someone who can answer her questions and offer advice (see Chapter 28). Towards the end of her visiting period she should offer advice on family planning. The health visitor will visit on or after the eleventh day to begin her surveillance of infant well-being and development. Depending on local arrangements, where the midwife visits up until 28 days the health visitor may delay her initial visit.

Throughout the postnatal period the midwife must complete records on the mother and baby. This should include any advice or treatment given and whether the GP has been informed about or summoned to deal with any abnormalities. This prevents conflicting advice should a different midwife call on another occasion. Before leaving the midwife should arrange an approximate time for the next visit so the family are not inconvenienced.

Notification and registration of birth

Statutory notification of birth was introduced in the United Kingdom in 1915 as a method of alerting the developing health and welfare services that a birth had occurred. Prior to this time although there was provision for the birth to be notified, many stillbirths and neonatal deaths were not recorded. It is the duty of the father, or any person in attendance at the delivery or who is present within 6 hours of the birth to notify the appropriate medical officer in the area in which the delivery occurred. This must be carried out in writing within 36 hours of birth. Notification includes live births of whatever gestation and stillbirths after the twenty-fourth completed week of pregnancy. In practice the notification is usually completed by the midwife present at the delivery.

The notification includes information about the mother such as age, parity, marital status, address and her GP. Information about the baby includes gestational age, birthweight and the presence of any visible congenital abnormalities. Copies of the notification are sent by the medical officer to the local Registrar of Births, Marriages and Deaths, to the Office of Population Censuses and Survey and to the health visiting services so that they can arrange to call after the tenth day.

Registration of a birth in the United Kingdom must take place within 42 days of the birth (21 days in Scotland). Registration of a birth has been mandatory in England and Wales since 1837 (Delamothe 1987). The registration normally takes place in the office serving the district where the delivery occurred. It is usually performed by one of the parents. If the mother is not married to the father of the child but they wish the father's name to be recorded on the certificate, they should register the birth together or a written declaration of paternity must be submitted. The parents are presented with a free short birth certificate which gives details of the baby's name and the date and place of birth. The full certificate can be obtained on payment of the set fee. This contains more detail such as the names and address of the parents and the father's occupation.

Should the parents fail to register the birth they may be liable to a small fine. Other people who are responsible for the child can also register the birth.

A stillbirth is normally registered by one of the parents who takes the certificate of stillbirth to the local registrar. The registrar will then issue a certificate of burial which can be taken to an undertaker or to the hospital depending on who the parents have chosen to arrange the funeral.

References

Beech B A and Claxton R (1983) *Health Rights Handbook for Maternity Care* Community Rights Project: London

Campbell R, Macdonald Davies I, Macfarlane A and Beral V (1984) 'Home births in England and Wales, 1979: perinatal mortality according to intended place of delivery' *British Medical Journal* 289: 721–4.

Campbell R and Macfarlane A (1987) *Where to be Born* National Perinatal Epidemiology Unit : Oxford.

Chamberlain G, Philipp E, Howlett B and Masters K (1978) *British Births 1970 Vol 2 Obstetric Care* Heinemann: London

Cronk M and Flint C (1989) *Community Midwifery* Heinemann: Oxford.

Delamothe T (1987) 'The OPCS: many (more) happy returns?' *British Medical Journal* 295: 1–2

Department of Health (1989) *Report on Confidential Enquiries into Maternal Deaths in England and Wales* 1982–4 HMSO: London

Flint C (1986) *Sensitive Midwifery* Heinemann: Oxford.

Flint C (1991) 'The know your midwife scheme' in S Robinson and A M Thomson (eds) *Midwives, Research and Childbirth Vol 2* 72–103 Chapman and Hall: London

House of Commons Social Services Committee (1980) *Perinatal and Neonatal Mortality: Second Report from the Social Services Committee 1979–80* HMSO: London

Humphrey C (1985) 'The community midwife in maternity care' *Midwife, Health Visitor and Community Nurse* 21(10): 349–55

Keirse M J N C, Enkin M and Lumley J (1989) 'Social and professional support during childbirth' in I Chalmers, M Enkin and M J N C Keirse (eds) *Effective Care in Pregnancy and Childbirth* 805–14 Oxford Medical: Oxford

Kitzinger S (1978) 'Women's experiences of birth at home' in S Kitzinger and J A Davis (eds) *Birth at Home* 135–56 Oxford University Press: Oxford

Klein M and Zander L (1989) 'The role of the family practitioner in maternity care' in I Chalmers, M Enkin and Keirse M J N C (eds) *Effective Care in Pregnancy and Childbirth* 181–91 Oxford Medical: Oxford

Kloosterman G J (1982) 'The universal aspects of childbirth: human birth as a socio-psychosomatic paradigm' *Journal of Psychosomatic Obstetrics and Gynaecology* 1: 35–41

Marsh G N (1985a) 'The primary health care team in obstetrics' in G N Marsh (ed) *Modern Obstetrics in General Practice* Ch 12 172–84. Oxford Medical : Oxford

Marsh G N (1985b) '"New style" obstetric care.' in G N Marsh (ed) *Modern Obstetrics in General Practice* Ch 12 172–84 Oxford Medical: Oxford.

Marsh G N and Kaim Caudle P (1976) *Team Care in General Practice* Croom Helm: London

McKendrick M (1985) 'The training and continuing education of the general practitioner in maternity care' in G N Marsh (ed) *Modern Obstetrics in General Practice* 407–12 Oxford Medical: Oxford.

Ministry of Health (1970) *Domiciliary Midwifery and Maternity Bed Needs: the Report of the Standing Maternity and Midwifery Advisory Committee* HMSO: London

O'Brien M (1978) 'Home and hospital: a comparison of the experiences of mothers having home and hospital confinements' *Journal of the Royal College of General Practitioners* 28: 460–66

Shearer M (1986) 'Delivering babies in the mother's home' *Midwife, Health Visitor and Community Nurse* 22(11): 398–403.

Smith S (1989) 'Taking the high road...' *Nursing Times* Community Outlook 85(Jan): 10–12

Stirratt G M (1983) 'The general practitioner's role in obstetrics' *Update* 1:1, 26–37

Tew M (1984) 'Understanding intranatal care through mortality statistics' in L Zander and G Chamberlain (eds) *Pregnancy Care for the 1980's* Ch 12 105–14 Macmillan: London

Tew M (1985) 'Safety in intranatal care – the statistics' in G N Marsh (ed) *Modern Obstetrics in General Practice* 413–33 Oxford Medical: Oxford

Tew M (1990) *Safer Childbirth? A critical history of maternity care* Chapman and Hall: London

United Kingdom Central Council (1986) *Handbook of Midwives Rules* UKCC: London

United Kingdom Central Council (1989) *A Midwives Code of Practice (2nd edn)* UKCC: London

Wilcox S (1988) 'Response from the inner city' *Midwives Chronicle* Jan: 16–19

3 Indicators of health in relation to maternity care

This chapter will review how statistics can be used as indicators of health with particular reference to the outcome of pregnancy. The World Health Organization's definitions of health will be criticised together with other definitions. Health indicators and inequalities of provision and outcome will be considered. The statistics referred to will be those with special reference to midwifery including birth rate, stillbirth, perinatal, neonatal, infant and maternal death rates. Initiatives aimed at reducing mortality rates will be mentioned. Finally the mechanisms of notification and registration of birth will be considered.

Collection of data

In this century data have been collected in order to assess the health of the nation and to determine priorities for the allocation of resources (Delamothe 1987). The national organisation which performs this function in the United Kingdom is the Office of Population Censuses and Surveys (OPCS) (Delamothe 1987). This body receives notifications and information from district registrars, district medical officers and chief administrative medical officers relating to births, deaths, congenital abnormalities, abortions, infectious diseases and hospital discharges. The OPCS is also responsible for conducting the 10-yearly census and for compiling the annually produced report, Social Trends which assesses the socio-economic well-being of the nation. After analysis, age, sex and class-specific rates for the occurrence of particular diseases can be produced (Delamothe 1987).

Death is an event commonly utilised by statisticians because unlike illness or state of health it is easily defined (Cartwright 1983). Death rates are a very insensitive measure of the health of a community (Martini *et al.* 1977). Problems can occur due to inaccuracies in recording or determining the cause of death, especially where the precipitating event is different from the underlying illness (Whitehead 1987). For example, neonatal death rates from intraventricular haemorrhage give little guide to the number of infants who survive this condition and their degree of handicap if any. Death rates in the United Kingdom are usually used together with the Hospital Activity Analysis to assess disease prevalence (Coulter 1987); however it must be remembered that it is only those with serious illness who are referred to hospital and such data take no account of common complaints or of chronic illnesses whose sufferers may never receive specialist advice (Coulter 1987).

Morbidity is extremely difficult to assess because it relies upon agreed deficits in activities or uniformity of symptoms which themselves are culturally based (Seedhouse 1986). It must also be remembered that statistics themselves are not value-free. The type of information sought (or even more importantly what is ignored), and the categories into which it is organised, reflect the underlying ideology of the organisation commissioning the analysis or of the individual statistician (Chalmers 1985).

Most statistical indices demonstrate social class and geographical differences in their occurrence rates (Whitehead 1987). For example, in 1988 the infant death rate (deaths before the age of 1 year/1000 live births) was 10.2 in West Midlands Regional Health Authority but only 6.9 in the East Anglian Region (Office of Population Censuses and Surveys 1989). In 1986, the same indicator amongst legitimate births was 7.2 for babies whose father was in social class I but 11.2 in class V (Office of Population Censuses and Surveys 1988a). These social class gradients with the lowest occurrence in social class I persist throughout the whole range of health indices from stillbirth rates to premature death rates and overall life expectancy (Townsend and Davidson 1982; Whitehead 1987). In addition, access to primary health care such as screening services, health centres and dentists tends to be worst in the inner city areas just where the need for them is the greatest (Townsend and Davidson 1982). The richer groups in society make much greater use of preventive health services such as cervical screening and vaccination programmes (Smith and Jacobson 1988).

What is health?

The role of the World Health Organization

In 1978 in Alma Ata a conference organised by the World Health Organization on primary health care made a declaration of the necessity for the governments and peoples of the world to work towards the achievement of Health For All by the Year 2000. The first part of this declaration was the reaffirmation that

> 'health which is a state of complete physical, mental and social wellbeing, and not merely the absence of disease or infirmity, is a fundamental human right and that the attainment of the highest possible level of health is a most important world-wide social goal whose realisation requires the action of many other social and economic sectors in addition to the health sector.' (World Health Organization 1978)

This definition has been criticised as being too idealistic, standardised and unobtainable (Ewles and Simnett 1985; Seedhouse 1986). The definition assumes that any individual with an infirmity or social problem cannot be considered to be healthy because health is an absolute standard (Seedhouse 1986). Other definitions of health have similarly been far from problem-free. Parsons (1951) defined health in terms of whether the individual was able to fulfil his or her role in society. This though depends very much on what that role may be and does not take any account of why the individual cannot function as expected. In addition this definition reinforces the *status quo* and does not provide much incentive for improvement (Seedhouse 1986). The medical view is that health is a commodity, something which can be bought and provided (Seedhouse 1986). This tends to minimise any effects which can be brought about by the individual, since a return to health can come about without any effort (Sacks 1982). Illich (1977) is critical of the medical model which interferes with an individual's ability to adapt in times of stress. The improvements in health which have occurred over the last century are seen as a result of social measures such as the provision of clean water rather than as a result of science; the major infectious diseases were on the decline well before the introduction of immunisation programmes (Illich 1977).

To take account of the diversity of health problems, the provision of health care and of economic development, regional targets have been set by WHO to encourage all areas to participate (World Health Organization 1986). In Europe the targets include that by the year 2000:

1. There should be no indigenous measles, polio, neonatal tetanus, congenital rubella, diphtheria, congenital syphilis or indigenous malaria in the region.
2. Life expectancy at birth in the region should be at least 75 years.
3. Infant mortality in the region should be less than 20/1000 live births.
4. Maternal mortality in the region should be less than 15/100 000 live births (World Health Organization 1986).

Statistics and maternity care

Birthrate

This is the number of births occurring in each calendar year divided by the total population in the area (usually estimated in the middle of the year). It is usually expressed per 1000 of the population. In 1988 the birthrate in England and Wales was 13.8/1000 (Office of Population Census and Surveys 1989). Birthrate is a useful statistic because it can show whether the population is increasing or falling when compared with death rates. Kenya has the highest birthrate in the world at 53/1000; it will double its population in 17 years if the rate of growth continues. The average number of births for each Kenyan mother is more than 8 (Loraine 1985).

Using birthrate it is difficult to differentiate between countries of similar birthrate where one has a small population of women of reproductive age who are having large families and another with a larger group who have few children (Fathalla *et al.* 1990). Fertility rates which are calculated by dividing the number of births by the female population of childbearing age, usually 15–44 years, provide a more useful picture.

Stillbirth rate

A stillbirth as defined by the 1953 Births and Deaths Registration Act is

> 'A baby who has issued forth from its mother after the 28th week of pregnancy and has not at any time after being completely expelled from its mother breathed or shown any sign of life...' (United Kingdom Central Council 1989).

This definition is to be altered in view of the change to 24 weeks in 1992.

The stillbirth rate is calculated by dividing the number of stillbirths by the total number of births both live and still. It is usually expressed per 1000 total births. In 1988 in England and Wales the rate was 4.9/1000 births (Office of Population Censuses and Surveys 1989). The causes of stillbirth are similar to those of death in the first week of life (Wigglesworth 1980) and will be discussed with perinatal death below.

Perinatal death rate

This is a very sensitive indicator of the standard of provision of obstetric and early neonatal care and of the socio-economic well-being of the community (Townsend and Davidson 1982). The perinatal death rate is calculated by combining the numbers of registered stillbirths and of those babies who die in the first week of life; the total is then divided by the number of births both live and still in each year (Bradford Hill 1977). The rate is expressed per 1000 total births. In 1988 in England and Wales the rate was 8.7/1000 births (Office of Population Censuses Surveys 1989).The main causes of perinatal death are:

1. Low birthweight. This is the major cause in the United Kingdom; it includes early delivery both spontaneous and induced, multiple birth and intrauterine growth retardation (Chamberlain 1981; Mutch 1986).

2. Congenital abnormality. Major anomalies can result in either stillbirth or early neonatal death (Wigglesworth 1980). Much effort has been expended in trying to reduce the number of abnormal babies who are born by antenatal screening and the availability of therapeutic abortion (see Chapter 38). This has had some effect in cutting the numbers born but it has not always reduced the incidence. Genetic counselling for couples at risk and modern techniques of detecting gene probes may prove more effecʌive in the future (Donnai 1986). The incidence of neural tube defects has reduced to a much greater extent than can be accounted for by the screening programme; it is thought that improvements in diet and social conditions may be responsible (Eurocat Working Group 1987).

3. Asphyxia and anoxia. This can occur during pregnancy, for example, antepartum haemorrhage can cause premature separation of the placenta: in labour, uteroplacental insufficiency is worsened by contractions which further reduce the blood supply or in the neonatal period as in cases of respiratory disease of the newborn (Chamberlain 1981).

In some cases it is impossible to attribute death to one of the above causes, although a combination of the following factors are known to increase the risk of perinatal death. They include:

1. Maternal age, the extremes of reproductive age increase the risks of perinatal death (Craig 1985).
2. Parity, the first pregnancy and delivery is to some extent a trial of the mother's reproductive ability. Hazards in the first pregnancy include pregnancy-induced hypertension and cephalopelvic disproportion (Chamberlain 1981). For both mother and baby the second delivery is the safest with the risks to both increasing thereafter (Caporto et al. 1987; Department of Health 1989b).
3. Socio-economic class. As previously stated, the perinatal mortality rate is at its lowest in social class I and its highest in class V (Office of Population Censuses and Surveys 1988a). The rate is even greater for women in the unclassified group without a stable partner (Whitehead 1987).
4. Smoking is associated with a lowering of average birthweight, an increased incidence of preterm delivery and a higher rate of perinatal death (Sexton 1986).

Perinatal mortality rates are used as one of the measures for an international comparison of the health of nations (Knox et al. 1986). National differences in the collection of data or in the classifications used can confuse simple comparison (Mugford 1983). Amongst the developed nations, Britain has a high perinatal mortality rate (Whitehead 1987), but as Chamberlain (1981) argues, this could be partly accounted for by our non-homogeneous population as regards both socio-economic status and ethnic origin. The proportion of low birthweight babies and the high incidence of lethal congenital abnormalities place a large obstacle in the way of the United Kingdom in its efforts to improve its international placing in the league of perinatal mortality rates (Macfarlane 1988). The countries with the lowest rates are in Scandanavia with their high standard of living and integrated systems of health and social welfare (Macfarlane 1988).

Efforts and initiatives aimed at reducing the perinatal mortality rate have attempted to improve obstetric and neonatal care rather than affecting the economic, social and educational level of the community (Chamberlain 1981). Much of the recent improvement in the perinatal mortality rate has been due to major technological advances in neonatal care and a reduction in congenital abnormalities (Alberman 1984; Yu 1987). There is no evidence that the move towards 100% hospital confinements has contributed significantly (if at all) to the improvement (Campbell and Macfarlane 1987).

UK government enquiries such as the Short Reports (the Social Services Committee on Perinatal and Neonatal Mortality, House of Commons Social Services Committee 1980, 1984), have done much to stimulate awareness but without a research base to their recommendations or adequate funding of their initiatives little action can result. The major recommendations in respect of improving perinatal outcome are as follows:

1. There should be continued moves towards centralising deliveries in large obstetric units.
2. Continuous fetal heart rate monitoring in labour should be an increasing part of labour ward management.
3. Every delivery suite should have a minimum of 24 hour obstetric, anaesthetic and paediatric cover immediate access to a suitable operating theatre proper on site facilities for the care of sick babies.
4. There should be an immediate increase in the provision of neonatal intensive care cots.
5. Every region should have one or two referral units equipped to provide intensive care facilities for mother, fetus and neonate (House of Commons Social Services Committee 1980)

In addition to United Kingdom initiatives, regional and local enquiries such as the Welsh Perinatal Mortality Initiative can be instrumental in highlighting deficiences and detailing local plans of action. It is necessary if such exercises are to be seen to be credible that the recommendations result from accurate information obtained by detailed research.

Neonatal mortality

This is the number of deaths occurring in the first 4 weeks of life per 1000 live births per year. It is usually divided into early neonatal deaths (those occurring in the first week of life whose causes are similar to those of stillbirth) and late neonatal deaths (in the second, third and fourth weeks of life). The latter include some babies who survive low birthweight, anoxia or congenital anomaly only to succumb after the first week (Knox *et al.* 1986). Other causes include infection and sequelae of prematurity such as necrotising enterocolitis and intraventricular haemorrhage. In 1988 in England and Wales the neonatal mortality rate was 4.9/1000 live births (Office of Population Censuses and Surveys 1989).

Infant mortality

This is the number of infants who die in the first year of life per 1000 live births per year. It includes all neonatal deaths with the remainder being termed postneonatal deaths. The rate for England and Wales in 1988 was 9.0/1000 live births (Office of Population Censuses and Surveys 1989). The causes of postneonatal death include infections (such as respiratory tract and gastroenteritis), non-accidental injury, accidents and sudden infant death syndrome (Sunderland *et al.* 1986). For many of these causes poor parental socio-economic circumstances are a predisposing factor (Macfarlane 1988).

There was much controversy surrounding the announcement of the 1986 infant mortality rate which had risen from 9.4/1000 live births in 1985 to 9.6 (Office of Population Censuses and Surveys 1987). This rise was eventually attributed not to deficiencies in the Health Service provision but rather to public health problems (Macfarlane 1988). These were thought to be related to unemployment, poor housing conditions and low pay for some of those with work (Macfarlane 1988). The Social Services Committee report on perinatal, neonatal and infant mortality has suggested that an inquiry process be established to review stillbirths and infant deaths highlighting areas of substandard practice. The government has supported these recommendations (Department of Health 1989a).

Maternal mortality

The World Health Organization (WHO) (1977) defines maternal death as:

> '..the death of a woman while pregnant or within 42 days of termination of pregnancy, irrespective of the duration and site of the pregnancy, from any cause related to or aggravated by the pregnancy or its management but not from accidental or incidental causes.' (World Health Organization 1977)

The rate is expressed per 100 000 births. In the United Kingdom, deaths within 1 year of childbirth or abortion are counted for statistical purposes with those occurring after 42 days being considered as 'late deaths' (Chamberlain 1985).

In the United Kingdom there exists a procedure for confidential enquiries into the causes of maternal deaths. This has been in place since the early 1930s prompted by Dame Janet Campbell's report into maternal mortality published in 1924 making it one of the earliest established forms of medical audit. Reports have been produced for England and Wales and for the next period from 1985 they include Scotland and

Northern Ireland. The system of confidential enquiry is voluntary, relying upon a confidential report from the local district or Chief Administrative Medical Officer (Chamberlain 1985). The information is collected by the regional obstetric assessor. Only one copy is kept of all documents and statements; this is destroyed once the final report has been prepared (Chamberlain 1985). Any details which could identify the mother or hospital concerned are removed. No copies of the report or any documents relating to it are included in the case notes. None of the information given can be passed on to a court of law or any other authority. The Committee of the confidential enquiry examine each case to determine whether or not the death was preventable. They look for omissions and commissions on the part of obstetricians, anaesthetists, general practitioners, midwives, administrative services and by the mother and her immediate family. Where elements of substandard care exist recommendations are made to suggest good practice (Chamberlain 1985). In such cases it does not necessarily follow that if the care had been up to standard the death would not have occurred (Chamberlain 1985).

In the Report on Confidential Enquiries, deaths are divided into three categories:

1. Direct obstetric deaths which result from complications of pregnancy, labour and the puerperium or from treatments or omissions.
2. Indirect obstetric deaths are due to a pre-existing disease or to one which first occurred in pregnancy but which was not due to direct obstetric causes but which was made worse by pregnancy (e.g. cardiac disease)
3. Fortuitous deaths are those due to other causes which happen to occur during pregnancy, e.g. road traffic accidents or suicide.

The enquiry is mainly concerned with direct deaths. The major causes are shown in Table 3.1.

Table 3.1 Major causes of maternal death in England and Wales 1976–1984 and in the United Kingdom 1985–1987

	ENGLAND AND WALES			UK
Triennium	1976–8	1979–81	1982–4	1985–7
Hypertensive diseases of pregnancy	29	36	25	25
Pulmonary embolism	43	23	25	24
Abortion	14	14	11	6
Haemorrhage	24	14	9	10
Anaesthesia	27	22	18	5
Ectopic pregnancy	21	20	10	11
Amniotic fluid embolism	11	18	14	9
Sepsis excluding abortion	15	8	2	6
Ruptured uterus	14	4	3	5
Other direct	19	19	21	20
Total	217	178	138	121

Internationally the situation regading maternal deaths is somewhat bleak. Instead of death rates of 8.6/100 000 births (Department of Health 1989b) as occurs in the United Kingdom, in less developed countries they can be between 100 and 300/100 000 (Rosenfield and Main 1985; Royston and Armstrong 1989). WHO estimate that 500 000 women die every year from the complications of pregnancy childbirth and abortion in developing countries (Royston and Armstrong 1989). In addition, for every woman who dies in childbirth, many more are handicapped or suffer severe illness as a result (Kwast 1991). The Safe Motherhood Initiative was launched by WHO with the aim of improving this catastrophic situation through the spacing of pregnancies, education of mothers and the training of all levels of health personnel from midwives to traditional birth attendants (Kwast and Bentley 1991). Major causes of death are haemorrhage, illegal abortion, pregnancy-induced hypertension, sepsis and obstructed labour (Rosenfield and Maine 1985). The situation is exacerbated by poor communication systems, a lack of suitably trained personnel and concentration of health care expenditure on western-style provision in urban centres (Royston and Armstrong 1989).

References

Alberman E (1984) 'Perinatal mortality rates' in G Chamberlain (ed) *Contemporary Obstetrics* 259–66 Butterworth: London

Bradford Hill A (1977) *A Short Textbook of Medical Statistics* Hodder and Stoughton: London

Campbell J (1924) *Maternal Mortality* Reports on Public Health and Medical Subjects 25 HMSO: London

Campbell R and Macfarlane A (1987) *Where to be Born: the debate and the evidence* National Perinatal Epidemiology Unit: Oxford

Caporto A, Battarino O, Donatiello A and Giannatempo A (1987) 'The grand multipara: always an actual problem' *Surgery, Gynecology and Obstetrics* 165(10): 99–100

Cartwright A (1983) *Health Surveys in Practice and in Potential* King's Fund: London

Chalmers I (1985) 'Short, Black, Baird, Himsworth, and social class differences in fetal and neonatal mortality rates' *British Medical Journal* 291: 231–3

Chamberlain G V P (1981) 'The epidemiology of perinatal loss' in J Studd (ed) *Progress in Obstetrics and Gynaecology Vol I* Ch 1: 3–17 Churchill Livingstone: Edinburgh

Chamberlain G V P (1985) 'Confidential enquiry into maternal deaths' in J Studd (ed) *Progress in Obstetrics and Gynaecology Vol V* Ch 12: 179–94 Churchill Livingstone: Edinburgh

Coulter A (1987) 'Measuring morbidity' *British Medical Journal* 294: 263–4

Craig G M (1985) 'The increased risk of childbirth with increasing maternal age' *Maternal and Child Health* 3: 88–94

Delamothe T (1987) 'The OPCS: many (more) happy returns' *British Medical Journal* 295: 1–2

Department of Health (1989a) *Perinatal, Neonatal and Infant Mortality: Government reply to the first report of the Social Services Committee session 1988–89* HMSO: London

Department of Health (1989b) *Report on Confidential Enquiries into Maternal Deaths in England and Wales 1982–4* HMSO: London

Department of Health (1991) *Report on Confidential Enquiries into Maternal Deaths in the United Kingdom 1985–7* HMSO: London

Donnai D (1986) 'Genetic aspects' in G Chamberlain and J Lumley (ed) *Prepregnancy Care: A Manual for Practice* 11–29 Wiley: London

Dubos R (1959) *The Mirage of Health* Harper and Row: New York

Eurocat Working Group (1987) 'Prevalence of neural tube defects in 16 regions of Europe, 1980–1983' *International Journal of Epidemiology* 16(2): 264–51

Ewles L and Simnett I (1985) *Promoting Health: A practical guide to health education* Wiley: Chichester

Fathalla M F, Rosenfield A, Indriso C, Sen D K and Ratnam S S (1990) *Reproductive Health: Global Issues* Parthenon: Carnforth

House of Commons Social Services Committee (1980) *Second Report: perinatal and neonatal mortality* HMSO: London

House of Commons Social Services Committee (1984) *Third Report: perinatal and neonatal mortality: follow-up session 1983–4* HMSO: London

Illich I (1977) *Limits to Medicine* Penguin: Harmondsworth

Knox E G, Lancashire R and Armstrong E H (1986) 'Perinatal mortality standards: construction and use of a health care performance indicator' *Journal of Epidemiology and Community Health* 40: 193-204

Kwast B E (1991) 'Maternal mortality: the magnitude and the causes' *Midwifery* 7(1): 4–7

Kwast B E and Bentley J (1991) 'Introducing confident midwives: midwifery education-action for safe motherhood' *Midwifery* 7(1): 8–19

Loraine J A (1985) 'Overpopulation' *Midwife Health Visitor and Community Nurse* 21(12): 438–42

Macfarlane A (1988) 'The downs and ups of infant mortality' *British Medical Journal* 296: 230–1

Martini C J M, Allan G J B, Davison J and Backett E M (1977) 'Health indices sensitive to medical care intervention' *International Journal of Health Services* 7: 293–309

Mugford M (1983) 'International comparisons of definitions of vital events' *World Health Statistics Quarterly* 36: 201–12

Mutch L M M (1986) 'Epidemiology, perinatal mortality and morbidity' in N R C Roberton (ed) *Textbook of Neonatology* 3–19 Churchill Livingstone: Edinburgh

Office of Population Consenses and Surveys (1987) *Infant and Perinatal Mortality 1986 (DH3 87/4)* OPCS: London

Office of Population Censuses and Surveys (1988) *Infant and Perinatal Mortality 1987* (Series DH3) OPCS: London

Office of Population Censuses and Surveys (1989) *Infant and Perinatal Mortality 1988: DHAs* OPCS: London

Parsons T (1951) *The Social System* Glencoe: Illinois

Rosenfield A and Maine D (1985) 'Maternal mortality–a neglected tragedy; Where is the M in MCH?' *Lancet* ii: 83–5

Royston E and Armstrong S (1989) *Preventing Maternal Deaths* WHO: Geneva

Sacks O (1982) *Awakenings* Pan Books: London

Seedhouse D (1986) *Health: The foundations of achievement* Wiley: Chichester

Sexton M (1986) 'Smoking' in G Chamberlain and J Lumley (eds) *Prepregnancy Care: A manual for practice* 141–64 Wiley: Chichester

Smith A and Jacobson B (1988) *The Nation's Health: A strategy for the 1990's* King's Fund: London

Sunderland R, Gardner A and Gordon R R (1986) 'Why did postperinatal mortality fall in the 1970s' *Journal of Epidemiology and Community Health* 40: 228–31

Townsend P and Davidson N (1982) *Inequalities in Health: The Black Report* Penguin: Harmondsworth

United Kingdom Central Council (1989) *A Midwives's Code of Practice (2nd edn)* UKCC: London

Whitehead M (1987) *The Health Divide: Inequalities in Health in the 1980's* The Health Education Council: London

Wigglesworth J (1980) 'Monitoring perinatal mortality: a pathophysiological approach' *Lancet* i: 684–6

World Health Organization (1977) *International Classification of Diseases. Manual of the Internatiomal Statistical Classification of Diseases, Injuries and Causes of Death* (9th revision) WHO: Geneva

World Health Organization (1978) *Alma-Ata 1978: Primary Health Care:report of an international conference* WHO: Geneva

World Health Organization: Regional Office for Europe (1986) *Targets for Health for All: Implications for Nursing/Midwifery* WHO: Geneva

Yu V Y H (1987) 'Survival and neurodevelopment outcome of preterm infants' in V Y H Yu and E C Wood (eds) *Prematurity* 223–45 Churchill Livingstone: Edinburgh

4   Planning a healthy pregnancy

Preconception care

Recent interest has developed in ensuring that parents are in the best possible state of health at the time of conception. Lumley and Astbury (1989) argue that this change in focus has occurred because care during pregnancy has failed to have an effect on the rate of preterm deliveries or the occurrence of congenital abnormalities. It should also be pointed out that one of the main risk factors for perinatal mortality is low socio-economic status (Townsend and Davidson 1982; Whitehead 1987). Preconception advice has always existed; the newlyweds of ancient Carthage were prohibited from taking alcohol for fear that any children would be malformed (Haggard and Jellinek 1942); women with medical disorders or poor obstetric histories and couples with a risk of congenital abnormality have received specialist advice aimed at calculating the risks for a future pregnancy (Steel and Johnstone 1986).

A randomised trial to evaluate the effects of preconception information, support, advice and screening is currently in progress in Australia (Lumley and Astbury 1989). Although preconception care is now being made available to the general public, its effectiveness for a fit, well-nourished population with no underlying medical disorders has yet to be determined (Chamberlain 1986). As with any prophylactic measure in health care (such as cervical screening), those who are first to take advantage are more often those highly educated and well-motivated people who already care for their health and have good outcomes (Smith and Jacobson 1988). It was thought that preconception care may provide a route through which the more deprived members of society could improve their perinatal mortality and morbidity rates; unfortunately the gap between the 'haves' and the 'have-nots' has remained constant and in some indices may even have widened (Smith and Jacobson 1988).

The advice given as preconception care is wholly applicable to life in general (Chamberlain 1986). For such a programme to be effective, it requires great motivation from the couple, especially since it should be started before pregnancy is attempted and conception may need to be delayed. The concept of preconception care implies that pregnancies are planned or at the very least diagnosed early. Cartwright (1988) reported that over a quarter of the mothers in her survey described their pregnancy as unintended, whilst for many couples, by the time they are aware of the pregnancy organogenesis is well advanced and any damage may already have occurred (Lumley and Astbury 1989).

The rationale for preconception care is to seek to reduce those factors which have been implicated in the causation of prematurity, low birthweight and congenital abnormality (Wynn 1985). Because there is a significant multifactorial element in these conditions it may not be possible to remove every factor. By lessening the effect of those which are amenable to change it is hoped that the scales will be tipped in favour of normality rather than abnormality.

Pickard (1984) has produced a countdown to a healthy pregnancy which is elaborated upon as follows:

10. Give yourselves time. For both partners it is a good idea not to rush into a pregnancy but to consider their general fitness and well-being. It is known that short intervals between births which do not allow the woman's body to recover sufficiently and build up nutrient stores are associated with an increased risk of prematurity and intrauterine growth retardation (United States, National Center for Health Statistics 1980; Wynn and Wynn 1981).

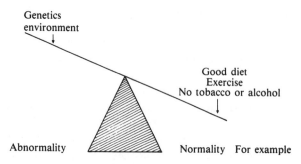

Figure 4.1 The balance between normality and abnormality as a result of influences on the pregnancy.

This however may only be of importance where the woman's overall nutritional status is poor.

9. Eat good food. Pickard (1984) advises a balanced diet based on fresh ingredients which are varied to provide the essentials for body maintenance and growth. Such a diet would be rich in fibre, minerals and vitamins and low in fat with the majority of energy coming from complex carbohydrates (bread and potatoes, for example). There is no evidence that general dietary advice has resulted in a reduction in the occurrence of malformation or low birthweight (Rush 1986). In addition, Chamberlain (1986) questions whether such advice is specific to pregnancy stating that it is related to general health. It has been suggested however that a deficiency in the B group of vitamins could be associated with an increase in cases of neural tube defects amongst susceptible people (Smithells *et al.* 1983). Information from times of famine has shown a reduction in conception rates and increased proportions of spontaneous abortions and stillbirths for babies conceived during the food shortage (Stein *et al.* 1975). Rush (1986) questions how far such observations are generalisable to a healthy population.

8. Check your weight. Being underweight is associated with amenorrhoea, subfertility and intrauterine growth retardation. Overweight women have an increased incidence of pregnancy complications such as diabetes and hypertension (Pickard 1984). To check one's weight a guide called the Quetlet or Q index is used; this is a body weight to height ratio:

$$Q \text{ index} = \frac{\text{Weight in kilogrammes}}{\text{Height in metres squared}}$$

Q indices

Under 20 – This is underweight; it is associated with amenorrhoea, infertility and can be a long-term health hazard

20–25 – The ideal range for pregnancy and long-term health

25–29.9 – Moderate obesity. Slight risk to health but it may lead to severe obesity.

Over 30 – Severe obesity; there is an increasing risk of menstrual problems and pregnancy complications. A health hazard (Pickard 1984).

7. Protect your baby from infections. It is known that the presence of some active infections such as rubella may harm the baby (Gregg 1941). Effects range from particular structural anomalies to spontaneous abortion (Hibbard 1988). There are particular infections such as rubella against which immunisation can be offered; the woman should have her immunity checked and if necessary be immunised before attempting a pregnancy (Horstmann 1982). A 3 month interval between immunisation and conception is vital if abnormalities are not to arise (Horstmann 1982). Other infectious diseases which either affect the pregnancy or the fetus/newborn infant are hepatitis, HIV and herpes simplex.

6. Check contraception. In order for the body to return to normal after a period of oral contraception it is recommended that 3 months should elapse before a pregnancy is attempted (Pickard 1984). The couple should be advised to use an alternative family planning method for the 3 months. Pregnancies which have occurred whilst the woman is taking oral contraception (due to stomach upsets which affect absorption or to missed pills) have shown an increase in fetal anomaly which could be due to exogenous hormones in early pregnancy (Elliot 1983). No other studies have substantiated this finding.

5. See your doctor about drugs. Some prescribed drugs and others available over the counter are known to cause teratogenesis (fetal abnormality). For women on long-term therapy such as for epilepsy or hypertension it may be necessary for them to alter their medication to a type known to be safe for use in pregnancy (de Swiet 1986). Doctors and dentists ask their clients to inform them if the woman thinks she may be pregnant or is planning a pregnancy; this allows suitable treatment to be given. Drugs which can be bought over the counter such as simple analgesics or anti-inflammatory agents should not be used before discussion with the pharmacist (Pickard 1984). Homeopathic remedies are quite safe.

4. Stop smoking. Smoking is associated with increased rates of spontaneous abortion, antepartum haemorrhage and prematurity (Sexton 1986). It is thought that these effects are due to alterations in the maternal immune system which make the mother less able to retain her fetus (Altschuler et al. 1975). In the male, smoking lowers both the sperm count and the proportion of sperm which are motile (DeMarini 1983). The birthweight of babies born to mothers who smoke is on average 200 g lighter than that of babies whose mothers are non-smokers (Lumley and Astbury 1989; see Chapter 7 of this book).

3. Cut down on alcohol intake. Whilst it is known that drinking during pregnancy can be associated with a reduction in birthweight and with fetal alcohol syndrome, it is difficult to show that specific quantities of alcohol produce certain effects (Jones et al. 1974). Some women drink heavily throughout pregnancy and deliver a normal baby whereas an occasional drinker may have a badly affected child especially where a session of binge drinking coincides with a crucial period of development (Jones et al. 1974). Advice ranges from cutting down on alcohol intake to stopping all drinking. Until more research is available the latter appears to be the more sensible step (Pickard 1984).

2. Have enough exercise and rest. It is better to begin pregnancy fit and full of energy than to expect to become fit during it. Many women find pregnancy itself rather tiring, especially in the later stages. Physical fitness is a great help in labour especially if the woman wishes to be mobile.

1. Check any dangers at work. Although hazardous occupations such as mining or construction are rarely undertaken by women some of the most innocuous can be a danger in pregnancy. It has been shown that theatre nurses and anaesthetists have an increased spontaneous abortion rate especially if no

'scavenger' system is employed to retrieve waste gases (Cohen *et al.* 1974). Another risk occupation occurs amongst women who work with dry-cleaning fluids (Holmberg 1979). If possible it is helpful if such women could change their jobs but this may be unrealistic in this time of high unemployment and dependency on the woman as wage earner. Physical exertion whether outside or inside the home has been associated with an increased risk of small-for-gestational-age births (Launer *et al.* 1990). This physical work can include manual labour, standing for long periods (which increased the frequency of preterm births) and caring for three or more children at home (Launer *et al.* 1990).

Much discussion has occurred as to the best time and place to give preconception advice. By the time the midwife sees the woman it is too late, as the pregnancy is established. It is possible however to give preconception advice for the next pregnancy whilst giving post-natal care. Advice could be offered through family planning clinics or GP's surgeries but the best opportunity would be to include it as part of the 'healthy living' programme given in schools. This might also be an opportunity to introduce the midwife to talk about her role in normal childbirth and to encourage early diagnosis of pregnancy. Until more research is carried out as to the effectiveness of preconception care, it is doubtful if the service will become widespread and available to those who most require it.

References

Altschuler G, Russell P and Ermocilla R (1975) 'The placental pathology of small for gestational age infants' *American Journal of Obstetrics and Gynecology* 121: 351–9

Cartwright A (1988) 'Unintended pregnancies that lead to babies' *Social Science and Medicine* 27(3): 249–54

Chamberlain G (1986) 'Pregnancy care' in G Chamberlain and J Lumley (eds) *Prepregnancy Care: A Manual for Practice* Ch1 1–10 Wiley: Chichester

Cohen E N, Brown B W, Bruce D L, Cascorbi H F, Corbett T H, Jones T W and Whitcher C E (1974) 'Occupational disease among operating room personnel: a national study' *Anesthesiology* 41: 321–40

DeMarini D M (1983) 'Genotoxicity of tobacco smoke and tobacco condensate' *Mutation Research* 114: 59–89

de Swiet M (1986) 'Pre-existing medical diseases' in G Chamberlain and J Lumley (eds) *Prepregnancy Care: A Manual for Practice* Ch 5 69–112 Wiley: Chichester

Elliot E (1983) 'Post coital use of the pill' *Foresight the Next Generation: Avoiding damage before birth* Foresight: London Ch14 77

Gregg N M (1941) 'Congenital cataract following German measles in the mother' *Transactions of the Ophthalmological Society of Australia* 3: 35

Haggard H W and Jellinek E M (1942) *Alcohol Explored* Doubleday, Doran and Company: New York

Hibbard B M (1988) *Principles of Obstetrics* Butterworths: London

Holmberg F C (1979) 'Central nervous system defects in children born to mothers exposed to organic solvents during pregnancy' *Lancet* ii: 177–9

Horstmann D M (1982) 'Viral infections' in G N Burrow and T F Ferris (eds) *Medical Complications During Pregnancy (2nd edn)* Ch 4 Saunders: Philadelphia

Jones K L, Smith D W and Streissguth A P (1974) 'Outcome in offspring of chronic alcoholic women' *Lancet* I: 1076–8

Launer L J, Villar J, Kestler E and De Onis M (1990) 'The effect of maternal work on fetal growth and duration of pregnancy' *British Journal of Obstetrics and Gynaecology* 97: 62–70

Lumley J and Astbury J (1989) 'Advice for pregnancy' in I Chalmers, M Enkin and M J N C Keirse (eds) *Effective Care in Pregnancy and Childbirth* Ch 16 237–54 Oxford Medical: Oxford

Pickard B (1984) *Eating Well for a Healthy Pregnancy* Sheldon Press: London

Rush D (1986) 'Nutrition in the preparation for pregnancy' in G Chamberlain and J Lumley (eds) *Prepregnancy Care: A Manual for Practice* Ch 6 113–40 Wiley: Chichester

Sexton M (1986) 'Smoking' in G Chamberlain and J Lumley (eds) *Prepregnancy Care: A Manual for Practice* Ch 7 141–64 Wiley: Chichester

Smith A and Jacobson B (1988) *The Nation's Health* King's Fund: London

Smithells R W, Nevin N C, Seller M J, Shepherd S, Harris R, Read A P, Fielding D W, Walker S, Schorah C J and Wild J (1983) 'Further experience of vitamin supplementation for prevention of neural tube defect recurrences' *Lancet* i: 1027–31

Steel J M and Johnstone F D (1986) 'Prepregnancy management of the diabetic' in G Chamberlain and J Lumley (eds) *Prepregnancy Care: A Manual for Practice* Ch 8 165–82 Wiley: Chichester

Stein Z, Susser M, Saenger G and Marolla F (1975) *Famine and Human Development* Oxford University Press: Oxford

Townsend P and Davidson N (1982) *Inequalities in Health: The Black report* Penguin: Harmondsworth

United States, National Center for Health Statistics (1980) *Factors Associated with Low Birthweight*: USA 1976 Series 11 No. 37

Whitehead M (1987) *The Health Divide: Inequalities in Health in the 1980's* The Health Education Council: London

Wynn A (1985) 'Pre-pregnancy health and counselling' in J Studd (ed) *Progress in Obstetrics and Gynaecology Vol 5* Ch 5 78–88 Churchill Livingstone: Edinburgh

Wynn M and Wynn A (1981) *The Prevention of Handicap of Early Pregnancy Origin* Foundation for Education and Research in Childbearing: London

5   Conception and early development

The female genital tract

External genitalia

External genitalia are known as the vulva (see Figure 5.1) which consists of the following structures:

1. The mons veneris − a mound of fatty tissue lying over the symphysis pubis and in the adult covered with pubic hair.
2. The labia majora, two large folds of skin, the outer surface after puberty is covered with hair, whereas the inner surface is smooth containing sweat and sebaceous glands. Anteriorly the labia majora meet at the mons veneris; posteriorly they merge with the perineal body.
3. The smaller labia minora are smooth with some sweat and sebaceous glands. Anteriorly the labia minora meet as two separate folds of skin − one fold surrounds the clitoris and is called the prepuce, the lower fold passes under the clitoris and is called the frenulum. Posteriorly the labia minora meet to produce the thin area of skin known as the fourchette. The area contained within the labia minora is called the vestibule.

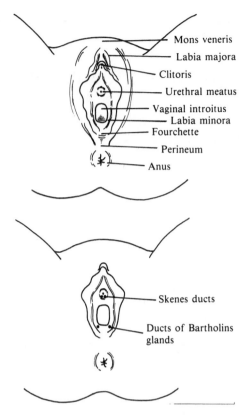

Figure 5.1 External female genitalia.

4. The clitoris is a small sensitive structure made of erectile tissue. The clitoris, which is the female counterpart of the penis, becomes enlarged and engorged when the female is sexually stimulated. In certain North and Central African countries (such as Sudan) the clitoris is excised along with the labia minora during the rite of female circumcision causing much scarring. The extent of the excision is dependent on local custom; as the operation is often performed by an untrained village women there is considerable morbidity (Cutner 1985). The procedure which is performed as a traditional rite of passage is said to preserve the girl's virginity until marriage (Cutner 1985). Bilateral or an anterior and a posterior episiotomy may be needed to permit delivery.

5. Within the vestibule the following structures are as follows:

   (a) the urethral meatus;
   (b) the openings of Skene's tubules on either side of the urethral meatus;
   (c) the introitus or opening to the vagina. In a virgin this is partially covered by a thin membrane known as the hymen. Remnants of the hymen may be seen as skin tags called carunculae myrtiformes;

(d) the opening of Bartholin's glands. These are racemose glands lying on either side of the vagina which secrete mucus to keep the external genitalia lubricated.

Blood supply to the external genitalia is from branches of the femoral arteries – the external and internal pudendal arteries. Venous drainage is via the corresponding veins. Nerve supply is provided by the pudendal and ilioinguinal nerves.

The pelvic floor

It is important for both the midwife and the mother to have a knowledge of the structure and functions of the pelvic floor. For the midwife this is necessary to assist her in the conduct of labour and delivery, for the repair of perineal trauma and in the teaching of postnatal exercises. For the mother such knowledge assists her in understanding the mechanisms of labour.

The pelvic floor fills the outlet of the pelvis with a muscular layer providing support for the pelvic and abdominal organs (Smout et al. 1969). The pelvic floor is not as the name suggests flat, it is a sloping 'gutter' shape, being higher at the front than at the back. The plane of the pelvic floor is related to the angle of inclination of the pelvis. In the woman, the pelvic floor is pierced by three structures, the urethra, the vagina and the rectum (Smout et al. 1969). From above moving downwards, the pelvic floor comprises six layers of tissue:

1. The pelvic peritoneum which covers the uterus and fallopian tubes. Anteriorly to the uterus it forms the uterovesical pouch which covers the upper surface of the vagina. Posteriorly it falls behind the posterior vaginal fornix to form the pouch of Douglas (Smout et al. 1969).
2. The next is a layer of pelvic fascia which is connective tissue thickened to form the uterine supporting ligaments (Smout et al. 1969).
3. The deep muscle layer consists of three pairs of muscles, all of which are inserted around the coccyx. They are known collectively as the levator ani muscles (see Figure 5.2). Individually the muscles are:

   (a) the iliococcygeus passing posteriorly from a point on the ilium to the coccyx;
   (b) the ischiococcygeus runs from each ischial spine downwards and inwards to the coccyx and the lower border of the sacrum;
   (c) the pubococcygeus runs from the pubic bone posteriorly surrounding the urethra, vagina and rectum before attaching to the coccyx.

The levator ani form a strong muscular sling which provides the main strength of the pelvic floor (Smout et al. 1969).

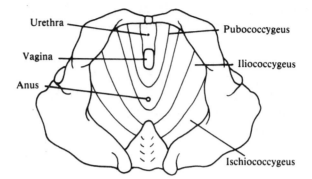

Figure 5.2 The levator ani seen from below.

4. The superficial muscles serve to further strengthen vulnerable areas of the pelvic floor. Unlike the deep muscles they do not form a complete layer. They consist of three pairs of muscles and two sphincters (see Figure 5.3):

(a) The transverse perineal muscles pass from each ischial tuberosity meeting in the centre of the perineal body.

(b) The bulbocavernosus start in the centre of the perineum passing anteriorly on either side of the vagina and urethra (thus encircling the orifices) before being inserted into pubic bones.

(c) The ischiocavernosus muscles run from the ischial tuberosities to the pubic bones.

(d) The external anal sphincter is a ring of muscle which is attached posteriorly to the coccyx and anteriorly to the perineal body.

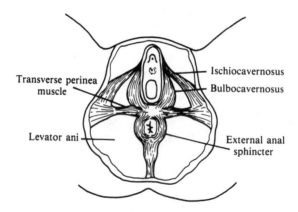

Figure 5.3 Superficial pelvic floor muscles seen from below.

(e) The membranous sphincter of the urethra is formed by two bands of muscle passing from one pubic bone to the other whilst encircling the urethra (Smout *et al.* 1969).

5. The two final layers of the pelvic floor consist of fat and skin (Smout *et al.* 1969).

The perineal body is a pyrimidical-shaped mass of fibrous and muscular tissues lying between the anal canal and the lower portion of the vagina (see Figure 5.4). It is a key area of the pelvic floor which, if damaged, can seriously undermine pelvic integrity. The perineal body consists of an outer layer of skin with the bulbo-cavernosus and transverse perineal superficial muscles and the deep pubo-coccygeus muscle. It is of great importance in childbirth and in defaecation. Overstretching can weaken the pelvic floor causing possible incontinence and prolapse of pelvic organs (Smout *et al.* 1969).

In the performance of an episiotomy it is the perineal body which is incised. In the United Kingdom it is usual to perform a mediolateral episiotomy whereas in the United States a midline is more common (Sleep *et al.* 1989) (see Figure 5.5 and Chapter 21). A mediolateral incision has the advantage of it being unlikely should

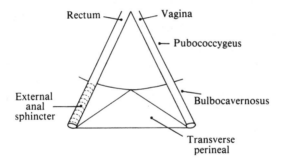

Figure 5.4 Cross-section demonstrating muscles forming the perineal body.

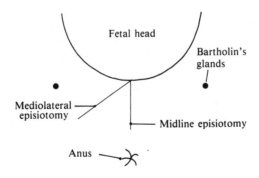

Figure 5.5 Direction of episiotomy incisions in the perineum.

an extension occur to the episiotomy, of it affecting the rectum, although this type of incision is more complex to repair. A midline incision if extended has a high risk of causing a third-degree tear but it is easier to repair and is said to cause less discomfort (Cunningham *et al.* 1989) although there is limited research which demonstrates this.

The pelvic floor plays a vital role in supporting the pelvic and abdominal organs. Its flexibility allows compensation to be made for changes in intra-abdominal pressure which occur, for example, when sneezing or lifting heavy loads. During pregnancy, under the influence of the hormones oestrogen and relaxin, the pelvic floor softens and relaxes. This permits the stretching required to facilitate passage of the fetus to occur. Gordon and Logue (1985) have shown that the strength of the pelvic floor is determined more by a woman's level of fitness and the amount of exercise she takes than by the presence or absence of a history of trauma associated with childbirth (see Chapter 21 for the care of the pelvic floor during labour).

Internal genitalis

The uterus

The uterus is a thick-walled muscular organ lying within the pelvic cavity (see Figure 5.6). The non-pregnant uterus is anteverted and anteflexed (see Figure 5.7) with the uterine body lying above the bladder. The non-pregnant uterus is a pear-shaped organ weighing about 60 g (50–70 gms in primigravidae and over 80 g in multigravidae (Langlois 1970)), and measuring 7.5 cm long (6–8 cm in primigravidae and 9–10 cm in multigravidae (Cunningham *et al.* 1989)), 5 cm wide and 2.5 cm thick. There are six main areas of the uterus (see Figure 5.8):

1. The cornua – the area where the fallopian tubes are inserted into the uterus.

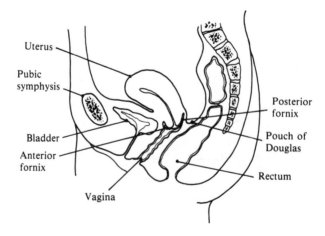

Figure 5.6 Sagittal section through the female pelvis.

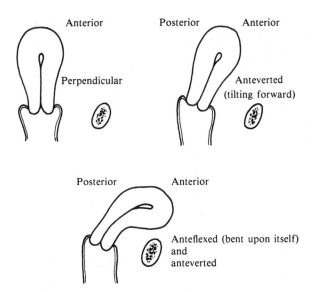

Figure 5.7 Inclination of the uterus.

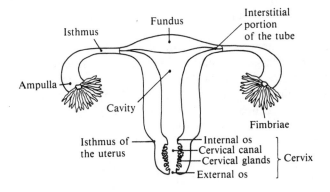

Figure 5.8 The uterus and fallopian tubes.

2. The fundus – the top of the uterus between the two cornua.
3. The corpus – the main body of the uterus including all the area above the cervix.
4. The cavity – the hollow in the centre of the uterus.
5. The cervix – the lower third of the uterus.
6. The isthmus – a narrow strip of tissue lying between the corpus and the cervix.

The uterus consists of three areas of tissue: an inner lining or endometrium, a layer of muscle cells or myometrium and an outer layer called the perimetrium.

The endometrium lines the uterine cavity and varies in thickness and structure according to the stage in the menstrual cycle. Cells are of columnar epithelium with a basal layer which is not shed during menstruation.

The myometrium comprises three sets of muscle fibres: an inner circular layer present throughout the uterus but especially around the cornua, isthmus and cervix (this is the weakest of the muscle layers permitting cervical dilatation); a middle layer of oblique fibres arranged in a figure-of-eight configuration in the body of the uterus (see Figure 5.9) (these are the major muscle fibres involved in contraction and retraction during labour and for the control of bleeding after expulsion of the placenta); and an outer layer of longitudinal fibres extending from the fundus to the cervix, the function of which is to assist in shortening of the cervix.

The perimetrium is the name given to the peritoneum which covers the posterior and the upper two-thirds of the anterior surface of the uterus, where the peritoneum covers the fundus. It is draped over the fallopian tubes in a double fold known as the broad ligament.

Blood supply to the uterus is via the ovarian and uterine arteries. The vessels are twisted so that as the pregnant uterus grows, they can expand to meet the increasing demand for blood. Venous drainage is via the ovarian veins which drain on the left side of the body into the renal vein and into the inferior vena cava on the right. Nerve supply is from the Lee Frankenhauser plexus (also known as paracervical) which lies just behind the cervix.

The uterus has various supports which maintain its position. These include:

- The round ligament extending from each cornua to the tissues of the labia minora. This helps to maintain anteversion and anteflexion.
- The transverse cervical or cardinal ligament which extends from the cervix at the level of the internal or to the side walls of the pelvis.
- The pubo-cervical ligament runs from the cervix at the level of the os to the posterior aspect of the pubic bones.

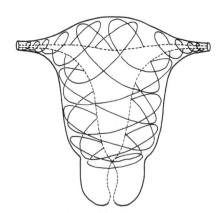

Figure 5.9 Diagrammatic representation of oblique muscle fibres in the body of the uterus.

● The uterosacral ligaments extend from the cervix at the level of the internal os to the sacrum.

The uterus during pregnancy

The uterus grows to accommodate the growing fetus, becoming globular in shape; by 12 weeks it is no longer a pelvic organ (Cunningham *et al*. 1989). At term the uterus weighs about 1100 g (Cunningham *et al*. 1989) and measures 30 × 25 × 20 cms on average. In pregancy the uterus is dextrorotated (twisted to the right) rather than anteverted and anteflexed.

The isthmus, which measures 7 mm prior to pregnancy, grows to about 22 mms at term and together with the cervix will form the lower segment from 28 weeks gestation. The endometrium is known as the decidua during pregnancy when it becomes thicker (5–10 mm) and more vascular (Cunningham *et al*. 1989). Muscle fibres in the myometrium increase in length (up tenfold) and in width (up to 3 times) in addition to new fibres which are formed. At term the corpus of the uterus is at least 1.5 cms thick (Cunningham *et al*. 1989).

The cervix

This forms the lower third of the uterus projecting into the vagina at right angles. It is barrel-shaped being approximately 2.5 cm long. Through the cervix runs the cervical canal with the internal os at the opening into the uterus and the external os opening into the vagina. Like the corpus of the uterus, the cervix consists of three main types of tissue. The endometrium which, unlike that lining the corpus, is not shed during menstruation, contains some ciliated epithelium and numerous racemose glands. This lining is arranged in a series of folds called the arbor vitae (tree of life). The myometrium has two layers of muscle cells which make up 10% of the tissue (Buckingham *et al*. 1965), an inner circular and an outer longitudinal layer of fibres. Peritoneum covers the cervix except where it is in contact with the base of the bladder.

During pregnancy, increased blood flow to the cervix (in early pregnancy) and changes in the collagen content (in the final trimester) make the cervix softer. The cervical glands secrete a mucus plug known as the operculum which helps prevent the spread of infection into the genital tract. During the period of prelabour the operculum may be shed as a mucus plug as the cervix begins to dilate.

The vagina

The vagina is the female organ of sexual intercourse; it also forms the birth canal through which the fetus passes during birth. It runs upwards and backwards from the vulva to the cervix in the same plane as the pelvic brim. As the walls of the vagina are arranged in folds which are usually in apposition, it is sometimes referred to as a potential tube. In order to accommodate the fetus at delivery the vagina is capable of great distension. The anterior wall of the vagina is 8 cm long on average, the posterior wall 10 cm. Where the cervix projects into the vagina there are four fornices of which the posterior is the largest.

The walls of the vagina are arranged in folds known as rugae. There are four layers to the vaginal wall:

- A lining of stratified squamous epithelium. At the junction with the cervix this changes to columnar cells − the squamo-columnar junction from which cell samples are taken for a cervical smear.
- A vascular layer of elastic connective tissue.
- A muscle layer consisting of inner circular fibres and outer longitudinal ones.
- An outer layer of connective tissue which is part of the pelvic fascia. This contains blood vessels, lymphatics and nerves.

The vagina does not contain any glands; it is kept moist by cervical mucus and a transudate of fluid from the vaginal wall. Doderlein's bacilli which normally live in the vagina act upon glycogen stored in the stratified squamous epithelium (Larsen and Galask 1980). The lactic acid which is produced helps to keep the vagina acid (pH 4.5) and free from infection. During pregnancy due to changes in the effects of oestrogen, there is less glycogen stored, the vagina is less acid and therefore more liable to colonisation by pathogens (Emens 1983).

Blood supply to the vagina is from the vaginal, uterine, haemorrhoidal, inferior vesical and pudendal arteries which are all branches of the internal iliac arteries. Venous drainage is via the corresponding veins and the nerve supply is from the Lee Frankenhauser plexus.

The fallopian tubes

The fallopian tubes (see Figure 5.10) extend on each side of the uterus from the cornua, run towards the side walls of the pelvis, turning downwards and backwards in a curve at their extremities. The fallopian tubes are contained within the folds of the broad ligament. The lumen of each tube connects the peritoneal cavity to the uterine cavity. The tubes are approximately 10 cm long (range 8–14 cm; Cunningham *et al.* 1989) with a diameter of about 3 mm. The tubes are divided into 4 parts (see Figure 5.6).

1. Interstitial (1 cm long) lying within the wall of the uterus.
2. Isthmus (2.5 cm long) the narrowest portion with a diameter of 2–3 mm (Cunningham *et al.* 1989).
3. Ampulla (5 cm long) the widest part (diameter 5–8 mm; Cunningham *et al.* 1989) where fertilisation occurs.

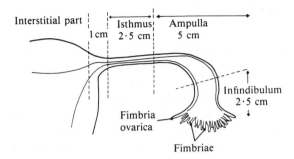

Figure 5.10 Gross structure of the fallopain tube showing areas and dimensions.

4. Infindibulum (2.5 cm) the fimbriated end whose finger-like processes surround the opening of the tube. One of these fimbriae called fimbria ovarica, is longer than the others and is thought to guide the ovum from the ovary into the tube.

The tubes are lined with ciliated epithelium which together with peristaltic action moves the ovum into the ampulla (Thibault 1972). To retain the fertilised ovum within the fallopian tube, permitting maturation and early development, there is antiperistaltic action in the isthmus. As the oestrogen level falls and that of progesterone rises this action is lessened and the embryo passes into the uterine cavity (Croxatto *et al*. 1978). Beneath this lining there is connective tissue, a two-layer muscle coat and the peritoneal covering. Folds of the broad ligament form the infundibulo-pelvic ligament which runs from the infundibulum of the tube to the side wall of the pelvis.

The ovaries

The ovaries lie in a small depression in the posterior wall of the broad ligament; they are attached to the uterus by the ovarian ligament. Suspended above each ovary is the fimbriated end of the fallopian tube. The ovaries themselves are pearly-grey in colour and almond-shaped with a wrinkled surface. They are about 3 cm long, 2 cm wide and 1 cm thick. The ovaries consists of an outer cortex and an inner medulla the whole being contained within a fibrous coat – the tunica albuginea, and a layer of modified peritoneum known as germinal epithelium. The cortex contains primordial follicles each containing a primitive ovum from which follicles develop to expel mature ova into the tubes. The scars of previous follicles can be seen on the surface as the remains of the corpus luteum and corpus albicans. The medulla contains blood vessels, nerves and lymphatics and ovarian hormones (oestrogen and progesterone) which pass into these blood vessels (ovarian vein) before entering the general circulation.

The menstrual cycle

The menstrual cycle lasts on average 28 days. With great variations, cycles can be as short as 21 days or as long as 4 months. Gunn *et al.* (1937) analysing the menstrual cycles of 479 normal British women found that most had a difference of 8 or 9 days between the lengths of their shortest and longest cycles. In 30% of women this difference was more than 13 days and in none of the study group was this variation less than 2 days (Gunn *et al.* 1937). Longer cycles are more common in women at the beginning and the end of their reproductive lives (Arey 1939). During the cycle an ovum matures and the uterus prepares to receive it should fertilisation occur. These two areas will be considered separately.

The menstrual cycle is under the control of the higher centres of the brain (the cerebrum). As these areas are also concerned with emotions, psychological upset can alter menstrual regularity. The cerebrum influences the hypothalamus to produce releasing factors (FSHRH and LHRH) necessary for the production of follicle stimulating hormone (FSH) and luteinising hormone (LH) from the anterior pituitary gland (see Figure 5.11). The anterior pituitary is also sensitive to feedback mechanisms governed by hormone levels produced by other endocrine glands.

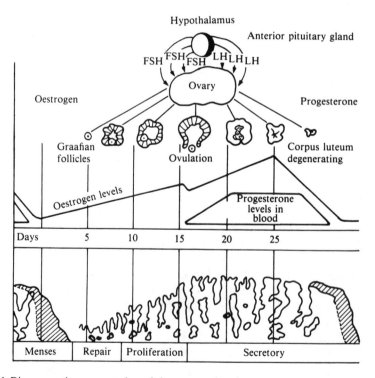

Figure 5.11 Diagrammatic representation of the menstrual cycle.

The hormones produced by the anterior pituitary gland have the following functions:

- Follicle stimulating hormone (FSH). From puberty this hormone stimulates primordial follicles (created during the embryonic life of the woman) in the ovarian cortex to develop and the ova within them to mature. When a number of follicles are so stimulated one will develop faster than the others, which will then atrophy. As growth of the follicle continues there is a great increase in protein-rich follicular fluid causing the follicle to bulge out on the surface of the ovary. This follicle is referred to as a Graafian follicle.
- Luteinising hormone (LH) is necessary for the final stage of follicular growth and maturation. Approximately 48 hours before ovulation there is a surge in LH production. The Graafian follicle swells rapidly whilst the granulosa and theca cells are altered into lutein cells which produce progesterone and reduce their secretion of oestrogen. The surge of LH is vital for ovulation. The wall of the follicle becomes weakened due to the effects of proteolytic enzymes and the pressure from follicular fluid. Rupture occurs with the ovum (surrounded by the corona radiata) and follicular fluid being expelled into the peritoneal cavity. Following ovulation the remaining granulosa and theca cells complete the process of luteinisation to produce the corpus luteum which will secrete oestrogen and progesterone (see Figure 5.12).

If conception occurs the corpus luteum continues to function (under the influence of human chorionic gonadotrophin (hCG) producing large amounts of progesterone and oestrogen until the placenta is mature enough (at about 12 weeks) to carry out this function (Cunningham *et al.* 1989). Should fertilisation not occur, one week after ovulation the corpus luteum degenerates to form the small white scar known as the corpus albicans (Cunningham *et al.* 1989).

Ovarian hormones are required to prepare the uterus to receive the fertilised ovum.

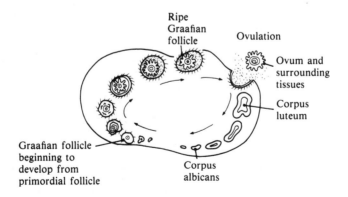

Figure 5.12 Diagrammatic representation of the development of a Graafian follicle within the ovarian cortex.

- Oestrogens. During the proliferative phase of the menstrual cycle oestrogens cause rapid proliferation of cells in the endometrium until it is about 2 – 3 mm thick. Further growth occurs in the third part of the cycle. Oestrogens also control the release of FSH by a negative feedback mechanism. When oestrogen levels are low FSH is released and the developing follicle produces oestrogen which at a certain level inhibits FSH production.
- Progesterone is produced mainly in the second half of the menstrual cycle – the secretory phase. Under its influence the endometrium becomes more vascular.

The menstrual cycle has three phases; the days given are for an 'average' 28 day cycle. Ovulation usually occurs 14 days before the onset of menstruation but it can occur between 12 and 16 days prior to the menses. Allen *et al.* (1930) isolated mature unfertilised ova from the genital tracts of women 12, 15 and 16 days after the start of the menstrual cycle. The first day of bleeding is regarded as the start of the cycle.

The menstrual phase lasts 4–6 days and occurs due to degeneration of the corpus luteum following a fall in oestrogen and progesterone production. The endometrium disintegrates and is shed leaving the basal layer from which the next cycle's endometrium will form.

In the proliferative phase, with low levels of circulating oestrogen, the hypothalamus is stimulated to produce FSHRH resulting in release of FSH, stimulating the developing Graafian follicle to produce oestrogen which causes growth of the endometrium. Ovulation occurs at the end of this phase on about day 14 of the cycle (12–16 days before menstruation (Allen *et al.* 1930)). The ovum is capable of fertilisation for 12 – 24 hours. Sperm can remain within the uterus and fallopian tubes and they are capable of fertilisation for up to 72 hours.

In the secretory phase the corpus luteum produces oestrogen and progesterone causing the endometrium to thicken further, becoming more vascular as it does so. This produces an environment into which the fertilised ovum can implant and obtain nourishment. If fertilisation does not occur hormone levels fall and menstruation begins.

Structure of a Graafian follicle

The functions of the Graafian follicle (see Figure 5.13) are to bring the ova to maturity and to produce oestrogen and progesterone (Cunningham *et al.* 1989). A primordial follicle within the cortex of the ovary develops into a Graffian follicle which consists of:

- The ovum. A large cell in the centre of the follicle about 0.133 mm in diameter (Allen *et al.* 1930). The large nucleus contains 46 chromosomes but prior to ovulation this is reduced to 23 by reduction division, resulting in the formation of the first polar body (Cunningham *et al.* 1989).

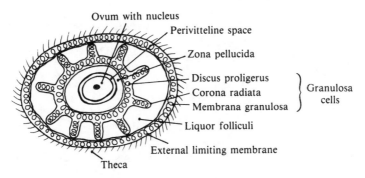

Figure 5.13 Structure of a Graafian follicle.

- The ovum is surrounded by the perivitteline space into which the extra chromosomes are passed.
- The zona pellucida contains nutritive substances which sustain the ovum after ovulation and fertilisation.
- Surrounding the zona pellucida are the granulosa cells which are in three layers. The discus proligerus and corona radiata surround the ovum after ovulation. The membrana granulosa lines the follicle and contains the follicular fluid which is rich in protein.
- The theca cells are formed from the stroma of the cortex which is compressed to form a capsule consisting of a vascular and a fibrous layer (Cunningham *et al.* 1989).

The Graafian follicle grows to a diameter of 10–12 mm before rupture at ovulation (Cunningham *et al.* 1989).

Fertilisation

Fertilisation (see Figure 5.14) occurs in the ampulla of the fallopian tube (Eddy and Pauerstein 1980). The ovum is capable of fertilisation for 12–24 hours after ovulation, whereas sperm can survive for up to 72 hours. Before the sperm can fertilise the ovum they must have been within the genital tract for about 7 hours for capacitation to occur. This is a conditioning process involving the removal of the protective covering over the acrosome (on the head of the sperm) allowing for the escape of digestive enzymes if the sperm should encounter the ovum. These enzymes digest a path through the corona radiata and the zona pellucida, allowing the head of the sperm to become attached obliquely to the ovum. Fusion of the cell membranes occurs so that the two cells are now one. The contents of the sperm move into the substance of the ovum to await maturation of the female nucleus. A reduction division reducing the female chromosome number from 46 to 23 occurs, the spare chromosomes known as the second polar body then migrating into the perivitaline space (Longman 1990) (see Figure 5.6).

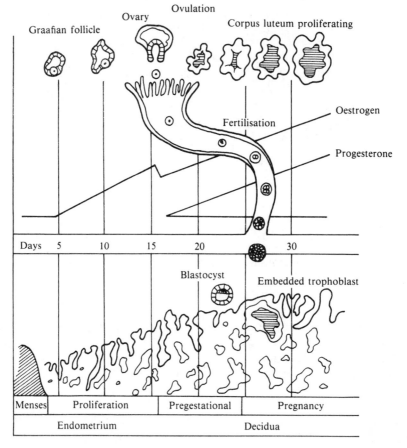

Figure 5.14 Diagrammatic representation of the menstrual cycle during which fertilisation occurs.

Once the sperm has attached itself to the ovum there are alterations in the ovum's metabolism. Changes occur in the ovum's cell membrane rendering it impervious to other sperm. Oxygen consumption and protein synthesis increase as the dormant ovum becomes activated initiating production of the second polar body. Once this has occurred the two sets of 23 chromosomes (one set from each parent), line up in the centre of the cell. The fertilised ovum now has its full complement of 46 chromosomes (Jeffcoate 1975). This process has taken approximately l0 hours from the first contact of the sperm with the ovum.

Early embryonic development

The fertilised ovum, which is referred to as a zygote, splits to form two cells; further divisions occur to form a cluster of cells known as the morula (latin for mulberry) (Moore 1973; see Figure 5.15). Up until this time (day four) the zygote has not been able to grow in size as the cells are contained within the zona pellucida, each cell division producing ever smaller cells (Moore 1973). The cell membrane starts to disappear as the morula enters the uterine cavity and at this stage fluid enters the morula producing two areas of cells, an outer cell mass or trophoblast and a centrally placed group, the inner cell mass (Hertig *et al.* 1954). This structure is now known as a blastocyst (Moore 1973).

Development of the placenta

The blastocyst remains free in the uterine cavity for about 2 days until the zona pellucida has disappeared and the cells are ready for implantation (Hertig and Rock 1944). It is thought that many potential pregnancies are lost at this stage. Around 6 days after fertilisation the blastocyst attaches itself to the endometrium. Enzymes in the primitive trophoblast erode the endometrium and at this time the woman may experience a small amount of blood loss vaginally. This spotting is known as implantation bleeding and is caused by enzymes dissolving the walls of vessels and glands in the endometrium. A process called decidual reaction prevents implantation of the blastocyst through the basal cells of the endometrium. The trophoblast cells proliferate rapidly and are differentiated into two layers (see Figure 5.16):

1. An outer syncitiotrophoblast made of cells with no distinct cell membranes. These cells form finger-like projections (villi) which penetrate the endometrium and increase the surface area available for exchange of nutrients.
2. An inner cytotrophoblast which is a single layer of cuboidal cells surrounding the blastocyst (Moore 1973).

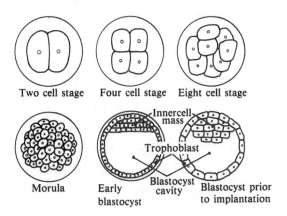

Figure 5.15 Early stages of development.

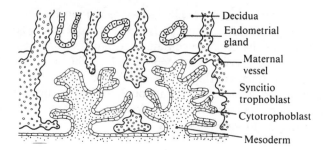

Decidua
Endometrial gland
Maternal vessel
Syncitio trophoblast
Cytotrophoblast
Mesoderm

Figure 5.16 Diagrammatic representation showing cell types which make up chorionic villi.

At this stage the lining of the uterus is referred to as the decidua, that surrounding the implanted blastocyst is referred to as the decidua capsularis and the small area of decidua beneath the blastocyst (where it first implanted) is known as the decidua basalis (Hamilton *et al.* 1945). Breakdown of vessels and glands in the decidua results in the blastocyst being surrounded with a rich nutritive medium from which nourishment can pass through the permeable trophoblast (Boyd and Hamilton 1970). As the blastocyst grows, the blood supply to the decidua capsularis is cut resulting in atrophy of the villi in that area. This part of the blastocyst is smooth and is known as the chorion laeve (Cunningham *et al.* 1989).

The villi in the decidua basalis continue to proliferate and spread producing the chorion frondosum which is the forerunner of the mature placenta. Up until the fourteenth week of gestation, trophoblast cells grow out from the placenta into the adjoining decidua and myometrium replacing the endothelium, invading and destroying the musculoelastic tissue and producing fibrinoid changes in the vessel wall (Fox 1991). From the sixteenth week onwards trophoblast cells migrate down into the intramyometrial segments of the spiral arteries (maternal blood vessels within the myometrium) producing similar changes to those described above. The end result of both these changes is that the thick-walled muscular spiral arteries become 'flaccid sac-like uteroplacental vessels' which are capable of expansion to accommodate the necessary increased blood flow (Fox 1991). It is known that amongst women who develop pregnancy-induced hypertension or give birth to a growth retarded fetus these changes in the arterial walls of maternal vessels are partial (in the case of the decidual part of the vessel) or absent (in the myometrial portion) (Khong *et al.* 1986).

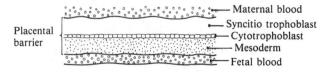

Placental barrier

Maternal blood
Syncitio trophoblast
Cytotrophoblast
Mesoderm
Fetal blood

Figure 5.17 Schematic representation of the placental barrier.

In the mature placenta there are three layers of cells lying between maternal and fetal circulation (two types of trophoblast cells and the mesoderm) (Wislocki and Dempsey 1955). They form the placental 'barrier' across which all gases and nutrients must pass. This barrier prevents large molecules and bacteria from passing from mother to fetus (Cunningham *et al*. 1989, see Figure 5.17).

Functions of the placenta

The placenta is the lifeline of the fetus and has to provide for all fetal needs. The functions are as follows:

1. Respiration. Oxygen passes from the mother's circulation to the fetus by a simple process of diffusion down a concentration gradient (Page 1957). Fetal uptake is assisted by the higher affinity of fetal haemoglobin for oxygen and high fetal haemoglobin levels (Pearson 1976). Carbon dioxide diffuses quickly across the placenta aided by changes in maternal respiratory control which result in a lowering of her blood carbon dioxide levels (Morriss and Boyd 1988).
2. Nutrition. Glucose is the major source of fetal energy and is assisted in its transfer across the placenta (Morriss and Boyd 1988). Amino acids are freely transferred across the placenta in addition to being synthesised in the trophoblast (Lemons 1979). The fetus has higher serum-amino acid levels than the mother. Free fatty acids pass easily from mother to fetus (Szabo *et al*. 1969), other lipids are synthesised from carbohydrates by the fetus. Vitamins and minerals are actively transported; there is some suggestion that the placenta may act as a store until they are required.
3. Excretion. All waste products are excreted via the placenta and then through the mother's own excretory systems (Page 1957); the major products are urea and bilirubin.
4. Secretion. The placenta produces large quantities of hormones necessary to maintain the pregnancy and ensure fetal growth. The main hormones are human chorionic gonadotrophin (hCG), progesterone and the oestrogens (Cunningham *et al*. 1989). Assays of these have been used as an assessment of fetal well-being.
5. Protection. The placenta prevents drugs and other substances of high molecular weight or bacteria crossing the placenta. Viruses pass easily across the placenta. The liquor protects the fetus from bumps as well as providing an environment of stable pressure allowing free fetal movements.

Cell differentiation

Simultaneously with implantation cell differentiation begins to occur (Figure 5.18). A layer of cells known as the germinal disc appears on the surface of the inner cell

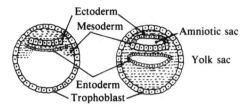

Figure 5.18 The beginning of cell differentiation.

mass (Hamilton *et al.* 1945). There are three layers of cells, the ectoderm, mesoderm and entoderm which will be formed into various parts of body systems (Figure 5.18). The mesoderm grows outwards until it eventually lines the whole cavity of the blastocyst (Moore 1973). The combination of mesoderm and trophoblast cells is known as the chorion; this will line the inside of the uterus and cover the fetal surface of the placenta. Cavities appear in the cell layers formed of the ectoderm and entoderm which are destined to become the amniotic and yolk sacs, respectively (Moore 1973). The two small spheres with their surrounding mesoderm move to the centre of the blastocyst cavity being connected to the edge of the blastocyst by the mesodermal stalk. The two opposing layers of entoderm and ectoderm together with the mesoderm between are known as the embryonic area and will form the embryo (Moore 1973, see Figure 5.19).

The amniotic sac expands to fill the whole of blastocyst. In doing so it enfolds the yolk sac, part of which is incorporated in the embryo whilst the remainder forms a vestigial tube attached to the mesodermal stalk (Moore 1973; see Figure 5.20). Blood vessels develop rapidly within the mesoderm; these vessels grow from the chononic villi through the connecting stalk (mesodermal stalk plus some yolk sac) towards the embryo to form the umbilical arteries and vein. Within the embryo further cell differentiation occurs, cells derived from the three primary layers develop as follows:

Ectoderm: Skin and appendages. The central nervous system including the adrenal medulla. Glands such as the pituitary and salivary.

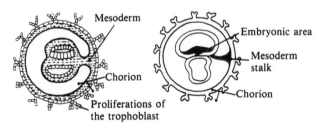

Figure 5.19 Further cell differentiation.

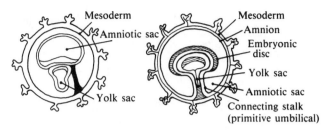

Figure 5.20 Formation of the embryonic disc.

Mesoderm: Bone, muscle, cartilage, connective tissue and serous linings. The cardiovascular system, the kidneys and most of the genital tract.

Entoderm: Gastrointestinal tract, the liver, gall bladder, biliary tree and pancreas. The respiratory tract. Germ cells of the gonads (Hamilton *et al.* 1945).

The process of embryonic development and cell differentiation occur first at the cephalic end of the embryo. By 4 weeks after conception (sixth week of gestation), the head of the embryo can be distinguished; by 6 weeks the heart is formed and beating, and primitive limb buds are visible (Moore 1973). By 10 weeks after conception (12 weeks of gestation) all the organ systems of the fetus are formed and all that is required is for them to increase in size and to mature (Moore 1973; see Figure 5.21).

All body systems develop in similar ways, either from a sheet of tissue which folds to create a shallow tube or groove or from groups of cells which cluster together to form pockets or rods (Hamilton and Mossman 1972; Longman 1990). The neural tube develops on the eighteenth day after conception from a thickened area of ectoderm cells (Moore 1973; Figure 5.22a). This neural plate folds inwards to form a neural groove with folds on either side (Figure 5.22b). By day 20 these neural folds

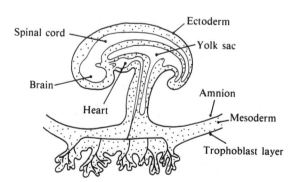

Figure 5.21 The embryo 7 weeks after conception.

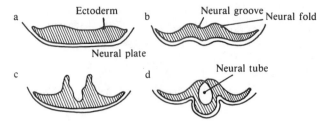

Figure 5.22 Development of the neural tube.

begin to move together (Figure 5.22c) and on the twenty-sixth day they fuse converting the neural plate into a neural tube (Figure 5.22d). Further development of the lateral walls of the tube occurs with the laying down of nerve cells destined to become grey and white matter (Hamilton *et al.* 1945).

Diagnosis of pregnancy

The signs and symptoms of pregnancy are many and varied; they have been utilised with differing degrees of accuracy to diagnose pregnancy. For the purpose of this chapter the traditional approach of defining the sign or symptom as a presumptive, probable or positive diagnosis of pregnancy has been adopted.

Presumptive evidence

Presumptive evidence is usually based upon the woman's subjective reports of signs and symptoms (Cunningham *et al.* 1989). The main sign in this category is amenorrhoea. If fertilisation has occurred, the corpus luteum continues to produce oestrogen and progesterone inhibiting both menstruation and ovulation. If the hormone levels are not sufficiently high some women experience a small amount of bleeding around the time of the expected menstrual period (Speert and Guttmacher 1954). Pregnancy is not the only cause of amenorrhoea which can also be due to anorexia, emotional upset (especially if the woman is worried she may be pregnant), hormone imbalances, severe anaemia and the menopause (Cunningham *et al.* 1989).

Morning sickness may occur from 6 weeks after the last menstrual period. It is thought to be caused by one or more of the following (although there is no conclusive research evidence as to these effects): high levels of oestrogen, rapidly increasing amounts of human chorionic gonadotrophin (hCG) or altered carbohydrate metabolism. Whilst it is most common upon rising, the nausea can occur at any time of the day. Other causes of nausea and vomiting include gastric upset and hiatus hernia. Frequency of micturition from polyuria is thought to be due to a disruption in the centre controlling osmolality, another presumption sign of pregnancy. Due to the incidence of urinary tract infections amongst women of reproductive age, it is not a very reliable sign.

Breast changes due to increases in levels of oestrogen and progesterone are often noticed. These include tingling, tenderness, venous engorgement and later on in pregnancy, pigmentation and the development of Montgomery's Tubercles. Many women experience similar early breast changes in the days before their menstrual period commences. These changes are most noticeable in primiparous women (Chamberlain 1989).

Probable evidence

This group includes those signs which would be discovered by the midwife upon examination of the woman; they are almost all related to the increase in pelvic blood supply and the growth of the uterus. Uterine enlargement can be felt abdominally after 12 weeks when the uterus is no longer within the pelvic cavity. Prior to that internal examination will reveal an increase in uterine size (Cunningham et al. 1989).

The most commonly used sign to diagnose a pregnancy is the immunological pregnancy test. This detects hCG levels in urine by using the specific monoclonal antibody to beta hCG. This test is swift, accurate and specific (Jovanovic et al. 1987). The tests which are commercially produced are designed to be used with an early morning specimen of urine (Bandi et al. 1987). Mixing the urine in the provided test-tube causes particles in the mixture to aggregate and if left to stand produce a noticeable ring or colour change. These tests are sensitive and can be performed shortly after the day of the expected period. On investigation of the accuracy of these tests when conducted by women at home, Doshi (1986) found that whilst 83% of the positive results were correct this was true of only 56% of those shown to be negative. Results obtained via home testing are subject to operator error and should be treated with caution especially if negative. As levels of hCG rise in cases of hydatidiform mole and other gonadotrophins increase during the menopause and with certain malignant diseases, this test is not a positive sign of pregnancy (Cunningham et al. 1989).

Positive evidence

If one of these signs is present then a pregnancy exists. There is no other cause for these manifestations other than pregnancy (Cunningham et al. 1989). Such signs include hearing the fetal heart or seeing it on ultrasound, seeing the fetus on ultrasound or the observer feeling fetal parts or fetal movements. The fetal heart can be auscultated from as early as 17 weeks (Jimenez et al. 1979) and it can be detected using echocardiography from as early as 48 days after the first day of the last menstrual period (Robinson 1972). Real-time sonography can demonstrate both fetal movement and the fetal heart from as early as the second month of pregnancy. As regards fetal movements O'Dowd and O'Dowd (1985) discovered a large variation in the gestations at which mothers perceive fetal movements, the range was 15–22 weeks for primiparous women and 14–22 weeks for multiparous women.

References

Allen E, Pratt J P, Newell Q U and Bland L J (1930) 'Human tubal ova: Related early corpora lutea and uterine tubes' *Contributions to Embryology* 22: 45

Arey L B (1939) 'The degree of normal menstrual irregularity: An analysis of 20,000 calendar records from 1,500 individuals' *American Journal of Obstetrics and Gynecology* 37: 2

Bandi Z L, Schoen I and DeLara M (1987) 'Enzyme-linked immunosorbent urine pregnancy tests: Clinical specificity studies' *American Journal of Clinical Pathology* 87: 236

Boyd J D and Hamilton W J (1970) *The Human Placenta* Heffer: Cambridge

Buckingham A C, Buethe R A and Danforth D N (1965) 'Collagen-muscle ratio in clinically normal and clinically incompetent cervices' *American Journal Obstetrics and Gynecology* 91: 232

Chamberlain G (1989) 'Prepregnancy care' in A Turnbull and G Chamberlain (eds) *Obstetrics* Ch 13 207–17 Churchill Livingstone: Edinburgh

Croxatto H B, Ortiz M E, Diaz S, Hess R, Balmaceda J and Croxatto H-D (1978) 'Studies on the duration of egg transport by the human oviduct' *American Journal of Obstetrics and Gynecology* 132: 629–34

Cunningham F G, MacDonald P C and Gant N F (1989) *William's Obstetrics* (18th edn) Prentice Hall: London

Cutner L P (1985) 'Female genital mutilation' *Obstetrical and Gynecological Survey* 40(7): 437–43

Doshi M L (1986) 'Accuracy of consumer performed in-home tests for early pregnancy detection' *American Journal of Public Health* 76: 512

Eddy C A and Pauerstein C J (1980) 'Anatomy and physiology of the fallopian tube' *Clinics in Obstetrics and Gynecology* 23: 1177

Emens M J (1983) 'The diagnosis and treat ment of vaginitis and vaginal discharge' in J Studd (ed) *Progress in Obstetrics and Gynaecology Vol 3* Ch 17 213–30 Churchill Livingstone: Edinburgh

Fox H (1991) 'A contemporary view of the human placenta' *Midwifery* 7: 31–9

Gordon H and Logue M (1985) 'Perineal function after childbirth' *Lancet* ii 123–5

Gunn D L, Jenkin P M and Gunn A L (1937) 'Menstrual periodicity: Statistical observations on a large sample of normal cases' *Journal of Obstetrics and Gynaecology of the British Empire* 44: 839

Hamilton W J, Boyd J D and Mossman H W (1945) *Human Embryology* W Heffer and Sons: Cambridge

Hamilton W J and Mossman H W (1972) *Clinical Embryology* Macmillan: London

Hertig A T and Rock J (1944) 'On the development of the human ovum with special reference to the trophoblast of the previllous stage' *American Journal of Obstetrics and Gynecology* 47: 149

Hertig A T, Rock J, Adams E C and Mulligan W J (1954) 'On the preimplantation stages of the human ovum' *Contributions to Embryology* 35: 199

Khong T Y, de Wolf F and Robertson W B (1986) 'Inadequate maternal vascular response to placentation in pregnancies complicated by preeclampsia and by small for gestational age infants' *British Journal of Obstetrics and Gynaecology* 93: 1049–59

Jeffcoate T N A (1975) *Principles of Gynaecology* (4th edn) Butterworth: London

Jimenez J M, Tyson J E, Santos-Ramos R and Duenhoelter J H (1979) 'Comparison of obstetric and pediatric evaluation of gestational age' *Pediatric Research* 13: 498

Jovanovic L, Singh M, Saxena B B, and Mills J L (1987) 'Verification of early pregnancy tests in a multicentre trial' *Proceedings of the Society for Experimental Biological Medicine* 184: 201

Langlois F L (1970) 'The size of the normal uterus' *Journal of Reproductive Medicine* 4: 220

Larsen B and Galask R P (1980) 'Vaginal microbial flora: Practical and theoretical relevance' *Obstetrics and Gynecology* 55: 100

Lemons J A (1979) 'Fetal placental nitrogen metabolism' *Seminars in Perinatology* 3: 177

Longman, J C (1990) *Medical Embryology* (6th edn) Williams and Wilkens: Baltimore

Moore K L (1973) *The Developing Human: Clinically Orientated Embryology* Saunders: Philadelphia

Morriss F H and Boyd R D H (1988) 'Placental transport' in E Knobil and J Neill (eds) *The Physiology of Reproduction* 2053 Raven Press: New York

Page E W (1957) 'Transfer of materials across the placenta' *American Journal of Obstetrics and Gynecology* 74: 705–14

Pearson J F (1976) 'Maternal and fetal acid-balance' in R Beard and P W Nathaniels (eds) *Fetal Physiology and Medicine* Ch 25 Saunders: London

O'Dowd, M J and O'Dowd T M (1985) 'Quickening – a re-evaluation' *British Journal of Obstetrics and Gynaecology* 192: 1037–9

Robinson H P (1972) 'Detection of fetal heart movement in first trimester of pregnancy using pulsed ultrasound' *British Medical Journal* 4: 66

Sleep J, Roberts J and Chalmers I (1989) 'Care during the second stage of labour' in I Chalmers, M Enkin and M J N C Keirse (eds) *Effective Care in Pregnancy and Childbirth* Ch 66 1129–44 Oxford Medical: Oxford

Smithells R W, Nevin N C, Seller M J, Shepherd S, Harris R, Read A P, Fielding D W, Walker S, Schorah C J and Wild J (1983) 'Further experience of vitamin supplementation for prevention of neural tube defect recurrences' *Lancet* i: 1027–31

Smout C F V, Jacoby F and Lille E W (1969) *Gynaecological and Obstetrical Anatomy (4th edn)* H K Lewis: London

Speert H and Guttmacher A F (1954) 'Frequency and significance of bleeding in early pregnancy' *Journal of the American Medical Association* 155: 172

Szabo A J, Grimaldi R C D and Jung W F (1969) 'Palmitate transport across perfused human placenta' *Metabolism* 18: 406

Thibault C (1972) 'Physiology and physiopathology of the fallopian tube' *International Journal of Fertility* 17: 1–13

Wislocki G B and Dempsey E W (1948) 'The chemical histology of human placenta and decidua with reference to mucoproteins, glycogen lipids and acid phosphatase' *American Journal of Anatomy* 123: 133

Wislocki G B and Dempsey E W (1955) 'Electron microscopy of the human placenta' *Anatomical Record* 123: 133

Bibliography

Grabowski, C T (1983) *Human Reproduction and Development* Saunders College Publishing

Moore, K L (1977) *Before we are Born – Basic Embryology and Birth Defects* W B Saunders

6   Adaptation to pregnancy

For the pregnancy to have a successful outcome, changes have to occur in the mother's physiology. These alterations are not always specifically aimed at their target organ(s); other, more general effects, can occur. These are known as the 'minor disorders' of pregnancy. The medical profession pays little attention to these nuisances, but to the women concerned they can be very disruptive. Much of the midwife's time during the antenatal period is spent advising the pregnant woman how she may lessen the effects of any minor disorders. These will be discussed following coverage of the effects of pregnancy on maternal physiology.

Physiological adaptation

Body water

As pregnancy progresses, the total amount of water in the body increases by as much as 6 l (Hytten 1980a). Some of the increase is as a result of increasing levels of oestrogen which encourages water retention (Hytten 1980a). A similar phenomenon can be seen (but to a lesser extent) during the last few days of the menstrual cycle. Manifestations of the increase in body water include swelling of the gums and alterations in the cornea (Milldoot 1977). Oedema is a common occurrence during pregnancy, being present in 40% of normal healthy women (Thomson *et al.* 1967).

Blood

Part of the increase in body water is accounted for by an approximately 50% rise in plasma volume; for primigravid women the prepregnant plasma volume of 2600 ml is increased by on average 1250 ml and in subsequent pregnancies by 1500 ml (Hytten and Leitch 1971). The increase starts very early in pregnancy, reaching its fastest rate of growth by 12–16 weeks gestation, a maximum level being achieved by 32–34 weeks (Letsky 1980). There is no relation between a woman's prepregnancy blood volume and the percentage by which it increases during pregnancy (Hytten and Paintin 1963). The actual rise in volume varies between individuals, a smaller amount being associated with poor fetal outcome (Pirani *et al.* 1973). Primigravid women have smaller increases in blood volume than multipara; even greater increases occur in multiple pregnancies (Rovinsky and Jaffin 1965; Gibson 1973). The growth in plasma volume is required to supply the new circulation which is established within the placental bed (Cunningham *et al.* 1989) and to allow for raised renal blood flow to remove fetal waste products.

Letsky (1980) reviewing research on changes in red cell volumes reports average increases in red cell volume of 240 ml (18%) where no iron supplementation was given and 400 ml (30%) where the woman received iron. Red cell production during pregnancy becomes more rapid, but there is no alteration in the lifespan of the cells (Pritchard and Adams 1960). As the rise in the number of cells is less than the increase in plasma volume, haemodilution occurs, lowering the haemoglobin levels (Letsky 1984). To correspond with the peak in plasma volume at 34 weeks, haemoglobin concentration reaches its lowest level at this time.

Clotting factors, especially VII, VIII, X and plasma fibrinogen increase during pregnancy (Letsky 1980). By term, plasma fibrinogen has risen from a prepregnant level of 2.5–4.0 g/1 to as much as 6 g/l (Letsky 1980). Given the rise in plasma volume, total plasma fibrinogen can reach double prepregnant levels by term (Letsky 1985). Although the platelet count is occasionally reduced during pregnancy, blood clots more easily. Letsky (1985) comments that this reduction in platelet numbers may be due to a small amount of persistent coagulation in the uteroplacental circulation. She sees this as being physiological. Increased coagulability of the blood is helpful to control bleeding from the placental site after delivery (Letsky 1985; see Chapter 21 for more details).

Cardiac output

The rise in cardiac output occurs early in pregnancy, reaching a maximum by about 14 weeks gestation (Walters *et al.* 1966). The increase is from a prepregnant level of 4.5 l/min up to 6 l/min (Walters *et al.* 1966). Larger rises can be found in women who have multiple pregnancies (Rovinsky and Jaffin 1966). During labour, further increases occur; these are especially marked in the second stage when they can amount to a further 2 l/min (Bleker *et al.* 1975). This increase is achieved by both increasing the heart rate (by approximately 15 beats/min) and the stroke volume (de Swiet 1980). Most women can cope with these changes but care should be taken where there is pre-existing cardiac disease (Hankins *et al.* 1983). Towards the end of pregnancy, women should avoid lying supine as the weight of the uterus and its contents can compress the inferior vena cava, producing hypotension (Howard *et al.* 1953).

The increased blood flow is directed towards the uterus, placenta, kidneys, lungs and skin (de Swiet 1980). Renal flow can have reached twice prepregnant levels by 16 weeks gestation, increasing by as much as 400 ml/min (Dunlop 1981). Skin blood flow rises (especially to the hands and feet) and can be between twice and five times the prepregnant level, helping to disperse heat produced by the fetus (Spetz 1964). This accounts for the fact that some pregnant women rarely feel the cold (de Swiet 1980).

Blood pressure

Diastolic and to a lesser extent systolic blood pressure fall during pregnancy (MacGillivray *et al.* 1969). This is partly due to a reduction in peripheral resistance caused by the effects of progesterone on smooth muscle (Bader *et al.* 1955). The mean fall of diastolic blood pressure recorded with the woman sitting was 15 mmHg (MacGillivray *et al.* 1969), whereas Holmes (1960), showed that when the woman was supine 70% had a fall of at least 10% in their diastolic blood pressure and in 8% of women it falls by 30–50%. The fall has occurred by 12–16 weeks gestation, pressure then gradually rises to reach prepregnant levels by term (MacGillivray *et al.* 1969). Systolic pressure falls little, but diastolic can drop by as much as 15 mmHg (MacGillivray *et al.* 1969). Blood pressure is discussed at greater length in Chapter 12.

The renal tract

Pregnancy produces alterations in renal anatomy and physiology. The kidneys enlarge by approximately 1 cm in length, their average combined weight increasing from 250 g in non-pregnant women to 307 g during pregnancy (Sheehan and Lynch 1973). In 90% of pregnant women, the renal pelvis, calyces and ureters are dilated (Bailey and Rolleston 1971). This is due to the effect of progesterone and to partial obstruction of the ureters at the pelvic brim by the gravid uterus (Bellina *et al.* 1970). Reflux of urine from the bladder can occur due to the relaxed vesicoureteric sphincter or due to alteration of the relative position of entry of the ureters into the repositioned bladder (Mattingly and Borkowf 1978). These changes can predispose to urinary tract infections, especially in those women with asymptomatic bacteruria (a bacterial count of more than 10 organisms/ml of urine in the absence of symptoms) (Kass 1956). It can take the urinary tract as long as 3 months post-partum to return to its prepregnant state. Investigations of any abnormality should be delayed until after this time (Davison 1980).

In addition to the increase in renal blood flow, the glomerular filtration rate rises by 30–50% over prepregnant values (of approximately 120 ml/min) (Davison 1974). Excretion rates of uric acid increase from a prepregnancy clearance of 6–12 ml/min to 12–20 ml/min (Dunlop and Davison 1977). Creatinine clearance is similarly improved, blood levels fall from a prepregnant level of 73–65 μmol/l in the first trimester, 51 μmol/l in the second and 47 μmol/l in the third (Kuhlback and Widholm 1966). For this reason, non-pregnant parameters should not be used in assessing renal function during pregnancy. The kidneys become less efficient at re-absorbing glucose, resulting in an increased frequency of glycosuria amongst normoglycaemic women (Davison and Hytten 1975). There is also a loss of amino acids and vitamins via the kidneys (Davison 1975).

Renal function during pregnancy is influenced by posture. Where the pregnant woman lies on her side there is an increase in the flow of urine, a possible contributory cause of frequent nocturia (Chesley and Sloan 1964) which can normally occur up to four times nightly (McFadyen et al. 1973). Other contri-butory factors include polydypsia during the day and the transfer of fluid from oedematous tissues to the general circulation when the woman is recumbant (McFadyen 1989).

The alimentary tract

Between 50 and 100% of pregnant women experience gums which feel 'spongy' and bleed more easily (Manson 1971). Gingivitis is more common, as the gums are more reactive to any dental plaque present. Pre-existing gum disease is worsened (Johnson 1985). Although ptyalism (excess production of saliva) has been reported (often associated with pregnancy nausea) Hytten (1980b) states that there is no evidence to support its occurrence, one possible explanation being that the saliva is not swallowed, due to nausea (Hytten 1990b). The acidity of gastric secretions is reduced mid-trimester, but rises again before the end of pregnancy (Murray et al. 1957). Gastric tone and motility are reduced, resulting in an increase in gastric emptying time (Davison et al. 1970). Glucose absorption appears slower than with the non-pregnant woman; this is possibly due to the high osmolality of glucose solutions used in testing (Davison and Hytten 1975). Stomach capacity is reduced in later pregnancy by the growing fetus and uterus which press upon it. Reduced competence of the cardiac sphincter of the stomach predisposes to reflux of stomach contents and heartburn (Hey et al. 1977). Passage of food through the small intestine is slowed (Parry et al. 1970). In the large intestine there is an increase in water absorption, which can predispose to constipation. It has been postulated that the cause is the increased levels of angiotension and aldosterone in pregnancy (Parry et al. 1970).

Respiration

During pregnancy oxygen consumption increases by approximately 45 ml/min (Alaily and Carrol 1978), a rise over the prepregnant level of 18% (de Swiet 1984). Ventilation increases by up to 40% (de Swiet 1984); to achieve this rise the tidal volume (the volume of air exchanged during normal respiration) increases from 500 to 700 ml (Cugell et al. 1953). During pregnancy the residual volume (the volume of air remaining in the lungs on expiration) is progressively reduced (Cugell et al. 1953). There is little change in the respiratory rate (Pernoll et al. 1975).

Anatomical changes occur early in pregnancy, with the diaphragm rising by up to 4 cm, long before any increase in abdominal size which could mechanically raise the diaphragm (Mobius 1961). The subcostal angle increases as pregnancy progresses, widening from 68° in early pregnancy to 103° at term (Thomson and Cohen 1938). Women are aware of this change in mid-pregnancy when their clothes may feel tight on the diaphragm.

Weight gain

Weight gain varies considerably between individuals and cultures depending on standards of nutrition (Hytten 1990c). In the developing world some women start pregnancy thin, gaining little weight, due to physical labour and scarce food supplies. Most authorities cite a gain of 2–3 kg in the first 20 weeks, (even allowing for a loss during the period of morning sickness), and a further 0.5 kg/week up until term, giving a total increase of 12–13 kg. Thomson and Billewicz (1957) demonstrated that women gain 0.36 kg/week from 16 to 18 weeks, this increases to 0.45 kg/week up until 26–28 weeks, reducing to a weight gain of 0.36–0.41 kg/week until term. The same authors recorded the average weight gain amongst 2868 normotensive primigravidae as 11.4 kg from 13 weeks gestation (Thomson and Billewicz 1957), whilst Humphreys (1954) measured an average of 11.7 kg from 12 weeks in a group of 1000 normal women.

The overall gain is more important than individual recordings which can suffer distortion, due to events such as holidays. Hytten (1990a) states that because of the inaccuracies surrounding accurate weighing (relating to the weighing machines themselves and differences in the woman's clothing between visits) there is little point in using this parameter to measure fetal growth, especially since its value is dependent on prepregnancy weight and any oedema present (see Table 6.1). A larger woman who gains little weight may be living off reserves whilst the baby is growing normally.

Minor disorders of pregnancy

These include a number of conditions regarded as minor by doctors which can cause so much irritation and discomfort for the mother-to-be that they blight the whole

Table 6.1 Distribution of weight gain

Fetus	3.4 kg
Placenta	0.6 kg
Amniotic fluid	0.8 kg
Increase in uterus	0.9 kg
Increase in breasts	0.4 kg
Increase in blood volume	1.3 kg
Extracellular fluid	1.7 kg
Fat	3.4 kg
Total	12.5 kg

Adapted from Hytten (1980a) p. 221.

pregnancy. Much of the midwife's time is spent in explanation of these disorders and in trying to reduce their effects. Most are caused by one or more of the following:

1. Increased levels of oestrogen: this causes the body to retain salt and water (Cain *et al.* 1971); it may induce nausea.
2. Increased levels of progesterone: this relaxes smooth muscle especially in the uterus, alimentary tract and skeletal system (Marshall *et al.* 1966).
3. Mechanical effects of the growing uterus which displaces other organs and causes pressure.

The gastrointestinal tract

Morning sickness

This is experienced by over half of pregnant women usually between 7 and 14 weeks gestation (Klebanoff and Mills 1986). Symptoms of nausea and vomiting are more common in the mornings, but can occur all day (Cunningham *et al.* 1989). Many women find that the smell of food makes them feel sick (Cunningham *et al.* 1989). Three possible explanations have been put forward: firstly, that the nausea is a reaction to the rapid rise in oestrogen levels up until the twelfth week; or secondly, it is due to the high levels of human chorionic gonadotrophin which reach a maximum at 12 weeks; or lastly that it is caused by an alteration in carbohydrate metabolism causing hypoglycaemia. It has been said that morning sickness is a sign of a well-functioning placenta since spontaneous abortion occurs more commonly where there is no nausea (Masson and Gordon 1985).

As the condition is usually self-limiting, treatment is symptomatic. Hibbard (1988) states that fewer than 1–2 women/1000 will require admission to hospital as a result of excess vomiting. Small frequent meals are helpful to maintain blood glucose levels. Starches are fairly well tolerated and are absorbed better than sugars, so biscuits are preferable to chocolate (Hibbard 1988). Some women find a snack before bedtime with tea and toast on rising to be of help. Adequate fluid intake should be ensured to avoid dehydration (Hibbard 1988). If cooking or food smells induce nausea these should be avoided if possible – this may not be easy if there are other children or if the woman is employed in the food industry. If the condition is excessive or has not resolved itself by 14–15 weeks, a medical opinion should be sought. Dundee *et al.* (1988) demonstrate the relief of the symptoms of morning sickness in a randomised trial of acupressure (the control group applied pressure to a 'non-active' dummy area away from the meridien).

Oesophageal reflux (heartburn)

This is a common and intractable problem caused by repeated regurgitation of acid stomach contents into the oesophagus (Hytten 1980b). The cardiac sphincter of the stomach is relaxed, permitting reflux of gastric contents (Feeney 1982). Heartburn is experienced more severely in heavier women (Brock-Utne *et al.* 1981). Posture is a precipitating factor; recumbancy results in many women experiencing disturbed sleep (Hart 1978). Foods which delay gastric emptying should be avoided, including fatty and spicy foods. Extra pillows can help, or even putting a pillow under the head of the mattress to avoid the woman lying flat at night (Hibbard 1988). Some sufferers find a degree of relief by moving the main meal of the day to lunchtime; others eat small frequent snacks to avoid distending the stomach after a large meal. Milk can be soothing and antacids can be given. Care should be taken with the latter, as frequent use can disrupt digestion and induce flatulence (Enkin and Chalmers 1982). Heartburn disappears totally after delivery.

Constipation

This can be troublesome, especially in the final trimester. The risk of developing constipation depends on prepregnant bowel action, amount of physical exercise, dietary and fluid intakes (Greenhalf and Leonard 1973). Some iron tablets can induce constipation. The management involves discussing diet and activity. If this fails to produce an improvement, fibre supplements or vegetable laxatives may be prescribed. Lubricants such as liquid paraffin are contraindicated due to their effects on the absorption of fat soluble vitamins A and D (Hibbard 1988). Laxatives should only be used for a short time, as their use can interfere with normal bowel action (Enkin and Chalmers 1982). Constipation can precipitate or worsen haemorrhoids.

Cerebrovascular system

Varicosities

These are caused by venous dilatation and reduced peripheral resistance due to the action of progesterone. It is thought that women who experience varicosities have a congenital predisposition to them (Cunningham *et al.* 1989). The valves in the veins become less competent and pooling of blood can occur, especially in the lower limbs. This can be exacerbated by the increase in uterine size, which together with the large blood flow from the uterus and placenta impedes venous return from the lower limbs. During pregnancy blood flow from the lower limbs is retarded except when the woman is lying laterally (Wright *et al.* 1950).

1. Varicose veins of the legs are experienced to some degree by 10% of pregnant women. The veins subside after delivery but worsen with each pregnancy. Long periods of standing or sitting should be avoided if possible (Cunningham *et al.* 1989). Walking or ankle and calf exercises help venous return and may ease the dull aching. Any constriction of the calves such as is caused by tight boots should be avoided, as there is a risk of deep venous thrombosis from increased coagulability of the blood (Hibbard 1988). Sitting with the legs elevated gives relief, together with the wearing of support tights (Cunningham *et al.* 1989). If the condition is severe these can be obtained on prescription. Tights should be put on before rising to avoid trapping pooled blood.

2. Vulval varicosities can be seen as large tortuous blood vessels running down the labia majora in the vulva sometimes crossing the perineum. They increase in severity with each pregnancy. Vulval varicosities can be painful and distressing – a perineal pad may give support and comfort (Cunningham *et al.* 1989). Care should be taken at delivery, since rupture of a varicosity can give rise to massive haemorrhage.

3. Haemorrhoids. These are varicose veins of the anal margin and are exacerbated by constipation (Hibbard 1988). Soothing creams may give relief, but a high fibre diet with plenty of fluids is the best prevention and this can also ease the problems of a relaxed large bowel, caused by the action of progesterone on smooth muscle. If the woman is taking iron pills it should be ascertained that these are not the cause of the constipation. Haemorrhoids worsen in the second stage of labour and can be particularly troublesome in the puerperium.

Muscoloskeletal system

Backache

Incorrect posture which produces strain on muscles is often the cause of backache especially in multiparous women who have lax abdominal muscles, allowing the weight of the uterus to fall forward as it enlarges. A compensatory lordosis develops which together with an increased angle of inclination of the pelvic brim help to maintain balance but produce strain in the small of the back (Hibbard 1988). Women report that the wearing of high heels or carrying heavy loads, both of which can alter posture, may cause more pain.

Occasionally in the later months of pregnancy painful sacroiliac joints or a tender symphysis pubis can be experienced. The hormone relaxin softens the symphysis pubis and relaxes the sacroiliac joints to increase pelvic flexibility prior to labour (Hibbard 1988; Sherwood 1988). There is no specific treatment other than the reassurance to be gained from an explanation. Posture may be improved with guidance or with help from an obstetric physiotherapist.

Cardiovascular system

Cramp

Leg cramps, especially at night, are experienced by 50% of pregnant women and are troublesome in 10% (Hibbard 1988) giving rise to considerable distress (Salvatore 1961). The cause is far from clear although low serum calcium in later pregnancy has been blamed without supporting evidence (Niswander 1982). Trials of calcium supplements have given inconclusive results, especially since many trials have not been adequately controlled (Enkin and Chalmers 1982). Massage and stretching of the affected limb has been found to be helpful (Shervington 1974).

The skin

Striae gravidarum

The stretch marks (striae) appear as purplish-red streaks on abdomen, breasts, buttocks and thighs (Wong and Ellis 1984). They are similar to those seen in non-pregnant people after weight loss. Although excess uterine enlargement (for example in cases of multiple pregnancy or polyhydraminos) can precipitate them, Poivedin (1959) demonstrated that striae can develop without significant stretching of the skin.

Braverman (1988) suggests that the cause of striae is related more to the mother's particular skin type than to the amount and rate of uterine enlargement, although the two factors may combine. None of the proprietary creams have been shown to be effective. After pregnancy striae will fade to silver.

Diet

The content of the diet is governed by social, cultural and religious influences, in addition to personal preference and money. Advice about diet can conflict with a person's self-image and if so is often resisted (Rodwell-Williams 1985). McKnight and Merrett (1987) in their study of the eating habits of pregnant women in Belfast showed that those with an unbalanced or inadequate diet were the least likely to follow dietary advice. The role for health educators is to educate the woman as to how she can easily and gradually alter her present diet to approach the 'ideal'. Dietary changes recommended for everyone in the UK by the National Advisory Committee on Nutrition Education (NACNE) (1983) include eating less fat (especially of the saturated variety), sugar and salt to help prevent heart disease, obesity and hypertension, respectively. More fibre (at least 30 g/day) should be included to aid digestion. To this end, change can be brought about by grilling foods rather than frying, reducing salt and sugar used in cooking gradually so that the change is not noticed, and substituting wholemeal cereals for refined ones (Walker and Cannon 1984). The type of diet advised must take into account the woman's income level, social environment and willingness to implement change (Rodwell-Williams 1985). Wholemeal bread is often more expensive than white and may not be readily available in all areas (Walker and Cannon 1984). Where a young girl is living at home, suggesting a diet at variance with that of her parents may create conflict (Rodwell-Williams 1985).

Diet in pregnancy

Protein

Metabolism during pregnancy is mainly anabolic, that is, concerned with the building of tissues (Worthington-Roberts and Vermeesch 1985). Protein is required for growth of the baby, development of the placenta, increase in maternal tissues such as uterus and breasts, expansion of maternal blood volume and for amniotic fluid (Rodwell-Williams 1985). The Food and Nutrition Board of the National Research Council (NRC) of the United States in 1980 recommended that the average 5' 4" woman should, when pregnant, increase her daily protein intake from 44 g/day to 74 g/day. This figure differs very significantly from that calculated by Hytten (1990c) which is 8.5 g/day to provide growth in fetal tissues of 6 g/day. This amount of extra protein is easily obtained if the woman eats the extra 350 kcal needed to meet daily energy requirements (Hytten 1990c).

Supplementation

Grieve *et al.* (1979) studied the effects of high-protein low-carbohydrate diets on pregnancy outcome. Possibly due to protein being used as a source of calories rather than for tissue growth, there was an average reduction in birthweight of 400 g – a figure only surpassed amongst the babies born during the siege of Leningrad during World War II. A system of protein and/or calorie supplementation has been used for women considered to be at risk of a low birthweight baby (Campbell Brown 1983). The women were selected because they were in the lowest 25% for weight gain between 20 and 30 weeks gestation. Supplements received included 299 kcal/day of carbohydrate and 15.9 g/day of protein. Whilst maternal weight gain and fetal size were larger than in a matched control group, the results were not statistically significant (Campbell Brown 1983).

Calories

The increased energy requirement of pregnancy has been calculated as 80 000 kcal, although this does not take account of energy savings from reduction in the level of physical activity (Hytten 1980a). The woman will gain weight (as stored fat) in the early months which can be metabolised when required in later pregnancy under the influence of human placental lactogen (Hytten 1980a, 1983). Whilst the NRC (1980) recommend an extra 300 kcal/day, Durnin *et al.* (1985) found increases in intake amongst pregnant women of as low as 50 kcal/day in the first 34 weeks rising to 150 kcal/day by delivery. Illingworth *et al.* (1987) demonstrated that women become significantly more energy efficient during pregnancy therefore reducing the need for extra calories. Restriction of fluid and calories over a short period of time may provoke labour, as shown by Kaplan *et al.* (1983) who report a rise in the delivery rates amongst orthodox Jewish women in the day following the 24 hour fast of Yom Kippur. Women considering fasting for any reason should be warned of the possible risks. Most religions which advocate fasting as a part of their observances make provision for the exemption of pregnant and nursing mothers. Many women however prefer to join their family in the fasting and not to delay as is permitted, for example for Moslem women during Ramadan.

Vitamins and minerals

The NRC (1980) recommend that vitamin A intake should increase from 800 RE to 1000 RE /day and vitamin C from 60 mg to 80 mg/day; both vitamins are vital for general tissue growth. Vitamin D is vital for growth of bones and the laying down of teeth (Worthington-Roberts and Vermeesch 1985) and intake during pregnancy should increase from 5 to 10 μg/day (National Research Council 1980). Care should be taken with women from the Indian subcontinent as their diet, especially when vegetarian, may be deficient in vitamin D (Abraham 1983). In addition because of their style of dress and the Northern European climate they may form little vitamin D from sunlight.

There has been much interest in vitamin deficiency and the incidence of neural tube defects. Both Smithells *et al.* (1981) (using a multivitamin compound) and Laurence *et al.* (1981) (using folate) have demonstrated a reduction in the incidence of these defects (when compared with matched control groups) where women at risk received supplements although there are flaws in the methodologies used. For example Laurence *et al.* (1981) in their trial did not control for the fact that neural tube defects were still most common amongst women with poor diets, despite dietary advice being given. This bias, together with the fact that they demonstrated a barely significant reduction in neural tube defects, highlights flaws in their methodology. Questions have also been raised regarding Smithells *et al.* (1981) study because 45% of their control group came from Northern Ireland (an area with a high incidence of neural tube defects), compared with only 20% of the group who chose to take the extra vitamins.

Calcium is necessary for bones and teeth. Problems may occur where the prepregnant diet is deficient in this mineral or where pregnancies are closely spaced and insufficient time is allowed to replenish stores (Worthington-Roberts and Vermeesch 1985). The daily intake in pregnancy should increase from 800 to 1200 mg (National Research Council 1980). Hytten and Leitch (1971) have estimated the iron costs of pregnancy as 750 mg, taking into account amenorrhoea. The majority of iron is used for the increase in maternal blood volume and for growth of the fetus including its iron stores (Letsky 1980).

When the woman is vegetarian, she needs to take great care to ensure an adequate supply of all nutrients, especially protein and vitamins. It is often the case, however, that such women are more nutritionally aware than the general population (Rodwell-Williams 1985). Care must therefore be taken not to be patronising. Some Asian women adhere to the ancient custom of hot and cold foods. Each state of the body is classified as hot or cold. Therefore, in order to ameliorate the condition, food from the opposite category will be eaten (Anderson 1987). Pregnancy is a 'hot' state and lactation 'cold', and as a result, many women will avoid first-class proteins in pregnancy but will eat them during the puerperium. The midwife must find out what the woman's preferences are before giving any suggestions.

Whilst many hospitals in the United Kingdom employ a dietician to see all pregnant women, dietary advice during pregnancy and the puerperium is a major part of the role of the midwife (in some places the dieticians teach the midwives). Good habits established during this time, if perpetuated, will result in a better diet for the whole family and the best foundation for the health of future generations (Smith and Jacobson 1988). Advice should always be tailored for the individual and provide a diet as varied as possible. The recommended diet may however take up a disproportionate amount of household income. For example in 1984 the Maternity Alliance calculated that the cost of a diet recommended by many hospitals was (in February 1984) 9% of average earnings, 16% of income for families eligible for family income supplement, 32% of the amount payable to a couple living on supplementary benefit and 49% of the allowance for a single householder. A similar situation was found in the 1988 update of this study. They state that the Government recommended diet in pregnancy is just too expensive for many women (Maternity Alliance 1984).

Finally, some women experience cravings during pregnancy for non-food items such as coal or clay; this is known as pica (Bronstein and Dollar 1974). Far more mothers develop a taste for spicy foods not present prior to pregnancy. An aversion to previously preferred foods is also common, and this may include tea and coffee (Worthington-Roberts and Vermeesch 1985).

Psychological and social adjustment

Society adopts a less hypocritical attitude than previously towards women and pregnancy; it is still expected of those who are married (or in a stable relationship) but less so where the woman is single and unsupported (Greer 1984). Western society has however come a long way since the nineteenth century when the unmarried woman and her child were sometimes left to fend for themselves, being cast out of their community (Lomax 1985), although this still occurs in the United Kingdom amongst some groups.

Western culture regards childhood as a separate state with its own rights and conditions (Davis and Strong 1976). Having children is seen (especially by men) as fulfilling the woman's natural role (Oakley 1980; Adams and Laurikietis 1980) and as important for marriage (Peel and Carr 1975). Motherhood is often idealised; the Freudian view is that women who do not enjoy pregnancy or complain about minor disorders are rejecting their role as mother (Oakley 1980). To avoid extreme pressure being placed upon them by family and friends, the couple who choose to remain childless may use spurious subfertility as an acceptable explanation of their state (MacIntyre 1976; Reading 1983). Childlessness is still only condoned in some groups of society if it is involuntary (Newill 1974).

Since women in the Western world are having fewer children, pregnancy is becoming a relatively rarer event (William and Jellife 1972). Indeed the first baby a woman holds may well be her own (Kitzinger 1984). Couples who desire a large family can be made to feel guilty for contributing to world overpopulation. A failure of contraception may be blamed (Kitzinger 1978).

Commenting upon the concept of adapting to pregnancy, Oakley (1980) asks "'adaptation' or 'adjustment' to what?" (p. 60). She questions the value of earlier work on this topic which seeks to demonstrate that motherhood is a part of femininity, arguing that it is not natural that all women should like and enjoy being mothers with all the constraints that this puts on 'normal life'. Breen (1975) from her study of the birth of the first child developed two contrasting views of pregnancy. The first states that it is an obstacle to be overcome, that a great strain is put upon the woman and that it is pathological rather than physiological (a standpoint taken by many obstetricians). The second explanation is that birth allows a woman to become fully developed. Reviewing previous psychological analyses of childbirth Breen (1975) comments that as these studies made no distinction between cultural influences and physiological changes, their findings are of limited use.

The idealising of motherhood (sometimes by men) has led to some particularly feminine women experiencing difficulties in striving to be 'the perfect mother' (Breen 1975). Those women who are often seen as rejecting traditional femininity in favour of 'Women's Lib' rarely aspire to perfection and adjust well to motherhood; they sometimes become advocates of natural childbirth and prolonged breast feeding (Breen 1975). Kitzinger (1984) has noted that where a woman is unprepared for the changes in her role, she may attempt to delay the time at which the pregnancy becomes obvious by selecting clothes which hide her vanishing waistline. Women may also delay publically acknowledging the pregnancy whilst they are waiting for the results of antenatal screening tests such as amniocentesis (Kitzinger 1984).

Educated and professional women may regard childbearing as a break in their 'real lives' of employment (Lopata 1971). Most diagnoses of pregnancy are accompanied by feelings of ambivalence, however much the child is desired (Price

1988). Childbirth (especially the first time) ranks high in the list of life events which can produce stress and give rise to depression (Brown and Harris 1978). Pregnancy results in changes in the woman's lifestyle, independence, financial status and position within society. The woman may have little control over events in her pregnancy, a situation reinforced by the power exercised by obstetricians (Oakley 1980).

A first pregnancy produces the greatest change. If the woman has been in employment she has to decide whether to continue after the birth. Can the couple afford to lose one income and, if so, which; how will she keep in contact with friends and colleagues? Will they still have anything in common? Komarovsky (1953) likens the situation to male retirement with all its anxieties and loss of status. After the birth the woman may feel lonely and isolated, deprived of social contacts and independence (Kitzinger 1978). A non-working mother can be regarded as a 'non-person' by a society which views paid employment as being of much higher status than childcare (Oakley 1980). Miller (1977) argues that only by raising the status of the producing and rearing of children will women be able to distance themselves from the male definitions of her position in society.

Pregnancy is increasingly being regarded as something abnormal (Arney 1982), something to be suffered. Women find their state of health being enquired after, implying that they should be looking and feeling unwell (Kitzinger 1978). This is despite the fact that many feel full of energy (at least in the middle part of pregnancy) and bursting with health (Kitzinger 1984). Discomfort can occur as the fetus grows larger, leaving the woman feeling ungainly (Rubin 1984). She may worry that her partner will no longer find her attractive (Kitzinger 1984). Additional concerns include apprehension as to how she will cope with labour and whether she will make a good mother (Price 1988). It is not often that such disquiet is openly expressed, but the midwife should be aware that the woman may be in need of explanation, support and reassurance (Reading 1983; Kitzinger 1984).

Where a woman has already had children she may fear a repetition of a previous unpleasant experience, for example during labour (Raphael-Leff 1991). The couple may be unable to afford another child or their accommodation may already be overcrowded and unable to fit in another person. If they are living in public sector rented accommodation a new baby may mean that the family qualifies for a move to better housing. The majority of pregnant women are concerned about the well-being of their baby, whether it will be all right and that it should not come to any harm through the mother's actions (Raphael-Leff 1991). Some women even dream that their baby is born dead, which can produce great anxiety (Kitzinger 1984).

Many women enjoy being pregnant, they feel well and relish the whole experience, being untroubled by worries or minor disorders. It is seen by some as fulfilling their role in life; they expect no problems and therefore find none (Oakley 1980). Others have the contrary view, (although rarely for the whole pregnancy), especially if troubled by minor disorders and other worries such as accommodation or money (Oakley 1980). They suffer in comparison with their happier sisters. The whole process of attending a big antenatal clinic can be frightening, as it may be the first time the woman has been in a hospital (Kitzinger 1984). Local or GP antenatal clinics may be seen by some women as more welcoming. The hospital clinic is full of efficient-looking people who rush around, talk in jargon and seem to write in hieroglyphics (Kitzinger 1978). Lack of awareness of welfare benefits and employment rights (including time off for clinic attendance) can add to physical, psychological and emotional stresses (Daniels 1980; Rodwell and Smart 1982). The situation is worsened where the woman has a poor knowledge of English or feels like an object on a conveyor belt (Kitzinger 1984).

Some so-called 'minor' disorders of pregnancy are culturally linked, especially in the case of morning sickness. Certain societies regard it as normal but only for the first pregnancy whereas others see it as signifying rejection of the child. In our Western society, nausea is considered to be a positive sign implying pregnancy (Mead 1962). In poorer societies where there is little access to health care, pregnancy is only considered to begin when quickening (fetal movement) is felt (Mead 1962). Klaus and Kennell (1976) regard the mother's perception of fetal movements as an important milestone in the development of maternal feelings. Another aspect in beginning the process of the formation of the maternal–infant bond is 'seeing' the baby during an ultrasound scan (Reading *et al.* 1982). This has also been shown to increase compliance with antenatal advice.

The role of the father in our society is changeable (Bedford and Johnson 1988). Many are delighted, whilst unsure of what is to come. Others are unaware of the pregnancy, or do not want to know. (Kitzinger 1984). It may bring the couple closer together, the pregnancy being seen by the man as evidence of his masculinity. In other circumstances the man may dislike the physical and psychological changes occurring in his partner (Rubin 1984). He may later resent having to share her time and affection with an unrewarding third party (Kitzinger 1984).

Siblings vary in their reaction to the forthcoming child. Where the baby will be a half-brother or sister, the older child may use its presence as a subconscious way of relieving conflicts with parent or step-parent. Some younger children expect a playmate of their own size and age, others do not relish the future of having to share bedroom, toys or parental time and affection.

No firm statements can be made regarding social and psychological adaptation to pregnancy. The midwife must not assume that the woman is pleased to be pregnant – she should make herself available so that the woman can voice her fears and discuss her problems with someone who will not pass judgement or give unsolicited advice.

References

Abraham R (1983) 'Ethnic and religious aspects of diet' in D M Campbell and M D G Gillmer (eds) *Nutrition in Pregnancy* Royal College of Obstetrics and Gynaecologists: London 23–9

Adams C and Laurikietis R (1980) *The Gender Trap II. Sex and Marriage* Virago: London

Alaily A B and Carrol K B (1978) 'Pulmonary ventilation in pregnancy' *British Journal of Obstetrics and Gynaecology* 85: 518–24

Anderson E N (1987) 'Why is humoral medicine so popular?' *Social Science and Medicine* 25(4): 331–7

Arney W R (1982) *Power and the Profession of Obstetrics* University of Chicago Press: Chicago

Bader R A, Bader M E, Rose D J and Braunwald E (1955) 'Haemodynamics at rest and during exercise in normal pregnancy as studied by cardiac catheterisation' *Journal of Clinical Investigation* 34: 1524

Bailey R R and Rolleston G L (1971) 'Kidney length and ureteric dilation in the puerperium' *Journal of Obstetrics and Gynaecology of the British Commonwealth* 78: 55

Bedford V A and Johnson N (1988) 'The role of father' *Midwifery* 4(4): 190–5

Bellina J A, Bougherty C M and Mickal A (1970) 'Pyelo-ureteral dilatation and pregnancy' *American Journal of Obstetrics and Gynecology* 108: 356

Bleker O P, Kloosterman G J, Mieras D J, Oosting J and Salle H J A (1975) 'Intervillous space during uterine contractions in human subjects: an ultrasound study' *American Journal Of Obstetrics and Gynecology* 123: 697

Braverman I M (1988) 'The skin in pregnancy' in G N Burrow and T F Ferris (eds) *Medical Complications During Pregnancy (3rd edn)* Ch 22 526–39 W B Saunders: Philadelphia

Breen D (1975) *The Birth of a First Child* Tavistock: London

Brock-Utne J G, Dow T G B and Dimopoulos G E (1981) 'Gastric and lower oesophageal sphincter pressures in early pregnancy' *British Journal of Anaesthesia* 53: 381–4

Bronstein E S and Dollar J (1974) 'Pica in pregnancy' *Journal of the Medical Association of Georgia* 63: 332

Brown G W and Harris T (1978) *Social Origins of Depression: A Study of Psychiatric Disorder in Women* Free Press: New York

Cain M D, Walters W A W and Catt K J (1971) 'Effects of oral contraceptive therapy on the renin-angiotensin system' *Journal of Clinical Endocrinology and Metabolism* 33: 671

Campbell Brown M (1983) 'Protein energy supplements in primigravid women at risk of low birthweight' in D M Campbell and M D G Gillmer (eds) *Nutrition in Pregnancy* Royal College of Obstetricians and Gynaecologists: London 85–98

Chesley L C and Sloan D M (1964) 'Changes in renal function in late pregnancy' *American Journal of Obstetrics and Gynecology* 89: 754

Cugell D W, Frank N R, Gaesnsler E A and Badger T L (1953) 'Pulmonary function in pregnancy. 1 Serial observations in normal women' *American Review of Tuberculosis* 67: 568–97

Cunningham F G, MacDonald P C and Gant N F (1989) *William's Obstetrics* (18th edn) Prentice Hall: London

Daniels W W (1980) *Maternity Rights and the Experience of Women* Policy Studies Institute: London

Davis A G and Strong P M (1976) 'Aren't children wonderful?' in M Stacey (ed) *The Sociology of the NHS* Sociological Review Monograph No 22: University of Keele

Davison J M (1974) 'Changes in renal function and other aspects of homeostasis in early pregnancy' *Journal of Obstetrics and Gynaecology of the British Commonwealth* 81: 1003

Davison J M (1975) 'Renal nutrient excretion with emphasis on glucose' *Clinics in Obstetrics and Gynaecology* 2: 365

Davison J M (1980) 'The urinary system' in F E Hytten and G Chamberlain (eds) *Clinical Physiology in Obstetrics* Blackwell Scientific: London Ch 11 289–327

Davison J S, Davison M C and Hay D M (1970) 'Gastric emptying time in late pregnancy and labour' *Journal of Obstetrics and Gynaecology of the British Commonwealth* 77: 37

Davison J M and Hytten F E (1975) 'The effect of pregnancy on renal handling of glucose' *Journal of Obstetrics and Gynaecology of the British Commonwealth* 82: 374

de Swiet M (1980) 'The cardiovascular system' in F E Hytten and G Chamberlain (eds) *Clinical Physiology in Obstetrics* 3–42 Blackwell Scientific: London

de Swiet M (1984) 'Diseases of the respiratory system' in M de Swiet (ed) *Medical Disorders in Obstetric Practice* Ch 1 1–34 Blackwell Scientific: Oxford

Dundee J W, Sourial F B R, Ghaly R G and Bell P F (1988) 'P6 acupressure reduces morning sickness' *Journal of the Royal Society of Medicine* 81(8): 456–7

Dunlop W and Davison J M (1977) 'The effect of normal pregnancy upon renal handling of uric acid' *British Journal of Obstetrics and Gynaecology* 84: 13

Dunlop W (1981) 'Serial changes in renal haemodynamics during normal human pregnancy' *British Journal of Obstetrics and Gynaecology* 88: 1

Durnin J V G A, McKillop F M, Grant S and Fitzgerald G (1985) 'Is nutritional status endangered by virtually no extra intake during pregnancy?' *Lancet* ii: 823–5

Enkin M and Chalmers I (1982) 'Symptomatic treatment in pregnancy: Antiemetics, antacids, laxatives and calcium supplements' in M Enkin and I Chalmers (eds) *Effectiveness and Satisfaction in Ante Natal Care* Spastics International: London 122–31

Feeney J G (1982) 'Heartburn in pregnancy' *British Medical Journal* 1: 1138–9

Gibson H M (1973) 'Plasma volume and glomerular filtration rate in pregnancy and their relation to differences in fetal growth' *Journal of Obstetrics and Gynaecology of the British Commonwealth* 80: 1067

Greer G (1984) *Sex and Destiny; The Politics of Human Fertility* Secker and Warburg: London

Greenhalf J O and Leonard H S (1973) 'Laxatives in the treatment of constipation in pregnant breast feeding mothers' *Practitioner* 210: 259–63

Grieve J F K, Campbell Brown M and Johnstone F D (1979) 'Dieting in pregnancy' in M W Sutherland and J M Stowers J M (eds) *Carbohydrate Metabolism in Pregnancy* Springer Verlag: Berlin 518–33

Hankins G D V, Wendel G D, Whalley P J and Quirk J G (1983) 'Cardiovascular monitoring in high risk pregnancy' *Perinatology and Neonatology* 7: 29

Hart D M (1978) 'Heartburn in pregnancy' *Journal of International Medical Research* 6 (Suppl 1): 1–5

Hey V M F, Cowley D J, Ganguli P C, Skinner L D, Ostick D G and Sharp D S (1977) 'Gastro-oesophageal reflux in late pregnancy' *Anaesthesia* 32: 372

Hibbard B M (1988) *Principles of Obstetrics* Butterworth: London

Holmes F (1960) 'Incidence of supine hypotensive syndrome in late pregnancy' *Journal of Obstetrics and Gynaecology of the British Empire* 67: 254–8

Howard B K, Goodson J H and Mengert W F (1953) 'Supine hypotensive syndrome in late pregnancy' *Obstetrics and Gynecology* 1: 371

Humphreys R C (1954) 'An analysis of the maternal and foetal weight factors in normal pregnancy' *Journal of Obstetrics and Gynaecology of the British Empire* 61: 764

Hytten F E (1980a) 'Weight gain in pregnancy' in F E Hytten and G Chamberlain (eds) *Clinical Physiology in Obstetrics* 193–233 Blackwell Scientific: London

Hytten F E (1980b) 'Nutrition' in F E Hytten and G Chamberlain (eds) *Clinical Physiology in Obstetrics* 163–92 Blackwell Scientific: London.

Hytten F E (1983) 'Nutritional physiology during pregnancy' in D M Campbell and M D G Gillmer (eds) *Nutrition in Pregnancy* 4–8 Royal College of Obstetricians and Gynaecologists: London

Hytten F E (1990a) 'Is it important or even useful to measure weight gain in pregnancy?' *Midwifery* 6(1): 28–32

Hytten F E (1990b) 'The alimentary system in pregnancy' *Midwifery* 6(4): 201–4

Hytten F E (1990c) 'Nutritional requirements in pregnancy. What happens if they are not met?' *Midwifery* 6(3): 140–5

Hytten F E and Leitch I (1971) *The Physiology of Human Pregnancy (2nd edn)* Blackwell Scientific: London 429

Hytten F E and Paintin D B (1963) 'Increase in plasma volume during normal pregnancy' *Journal of Obstetrics and Gynaecology of the British Commonwealth* 70: 402

Illingworth P J, Jung R T, Howie P W and Isles T E (1987) 'Reduction in postprandial energy expenditure during pregnancy' *British Medical Journal* 294: 1573–6

Johnson A (1985) 'Dental care during pregnancy' *Nursing Times* 81(51) (Dec 11): 28–35

Kaplan M, Eidelman A I and Aboulafia Y (1983) 'Fasting and the precipitation of labour: the Yom Kippur effect' *Journal of the American Medical Association* 250: 1317

Kass E H (1956) 'Asymptomatic infections of the urinary tract' *Transactions of the Association of American Physicians* 60: 56–63

Kitzinger S (1978) *Women as Mothers* Martin Robertson: Oxford

Kitzinger S (1984) *The Experience of Childbirth* (5th edn) Penguin Books: Harmondsworth

Klaus M H and Kennell J H (1976) *Maternal Infant Bonding* Mosby: St Louis

Klebanoff M A and Mills J L (1986) 'Is vomiting during pregnancy teratogenic?' *British Medical Journal* 292: 724–6

Komarovsky M (1953) *Women in the Modern World* Little, Brown: Boston

Kuhlback B and Widholm O (1966) 'Plasma creatinine in normal pregnancy' *Scandinavian Journal of Clinical and Laboratory Investigation* 18: 654

Laurence K M, James N, Miller M H, Tennant G B and Campbell H (1981) 'Double-blind randomised controlled trial of folate treatment before conception to prevent recurrence of neural tube defects' *British Medical Journal* 282: 1509–11

Letsky E (1980) 'The haematological system' in F E Hytten and G Chamberlain (eds) *Clinical Physiology in Obstetrics* 43–78 Blackwell Scientific: London

Letsky E (1984) 'Blood volume, haematinics, anaemia' in M de Swiet (ed) *Medical Disorders in Obstetric Practice* Ch 2 35–69 Blackwell Scientific: Oxford

Letsky E (1985) *Coagulation Problems During Pregnancy* Churchill Livingstone: Edinburgh

Lomax E (1985) 'Outcasts from society: The tribulations of the 19th century unmarried mother and her newborn baby' *Maternal and Child Health* 10(5) 138–42

Lopata H Z (1971) *Occupation: Housewife* OUP: New York

MacGillivray I, Rose G A and Rowe B (1969) 'Blood pressure survey in pregnancy' *Clinical Science* 37: 395–407

MacIntyre S (1976) 'Who wants babies? The social construction of "instincts"' in A Q Barker and Allen (eds) *Sexual Divisions and Society* Tavistock: London

Manson J D (1971) *Periodontics* Henry Kimpton: London

Mantle M J, Greenwood R M and Currey H L F (1977) 'Backache in pregnancy' *Rheumatology and Rehabilitation* 16: 95–101

Marshall S, Lyon R P and Minkler D (1966) 'Ureteral dilatation following use of oral contraceptives' *Journal of the American Medical Association* 198: 206

Masson G and Gordon A (1985) 'Morning sickness' *British Journal of Obstetrics and Gynaecology* 92(3) 221–225

Maternity Alliance (1984) *Poverty in Pregnancy* Maternity Alliance: London

Mattingly R F and Borkowf H I (1978) 'Clinical implications of ureteral reflux in pregnancy' *Clinical Obstetrics and Gynecology* 21: 863

McFadyen I R, Eykyn S J and Gardner N H N (1973) 'Bacteruria in pregnancy' *Journal of Obstetrics and Gynaecology of the British Commonwealth* 80: 385–405

McFadyen I R (1989) 'Maternal changes in normal pregnancy' in A Turnbull and G Chamberlain G (eds) *Obstetrics* Ch 10 151–71 Churchill Livingstone: Edinburgh

McKnight A and Merrett D (1987) 'Nutrition in pregnancy – a health education problem' *The Practitioner* 231: 530–8

Mead M (1962) *Male and Female* Penguin Books: Harmondsworth

Milldoot M (1977) 'The influence of pregnancy on the sensitivity of the cornea' *British Journal of Opthalmology* 61: 646

Miller J B (1977) *Towards a New Psychology of Women* Beacon Press: Boston

Mobius W V (1961) 'Abrung und Schwangershaft' *Munchener medizinische Wokenshrift* 103: 1389

Murray F A, Erskine J P and Fielding J (1957) 'Gastric secretion in pregnancy' *Journal of Obstetrics and Gynaecology of the British Empire* 64: 373

National Advisory Committee on Nutrition Education (NACNE) (1983) *A Discussion Paper on Proposals for Nutrition Guidelines for Health Education in Britain* Health Education Council: London

National Research Council (NRC) (1980) *Recommended Dietary Allowances* (edn 9) National Academy of Sciences: Washington DC US Government Printing Office

Newill R (1974) *The Infertile Marriage* Penguin Books: Harmondsworth

Niswander K R (1982) 'Prenatal care' in R C Benson (ed) *Current Obstetric and Gynecologic Diagnosis and Treatment* 616–29 Large: California

Oakley A (1980) *Women Confined* Martin Robertson: Oxford

Parry E, Sheilds R and Turnbull A C (1970) 'The effect of pregnancy on colonic absorption of sodium, potassium and water' *Journal of Obstetrics and Gynaecology of the British Commonwealth* 77: 616

Peel J and Carr G (1975) *Contraception and Family Design* Churchill Livingstone: Edinburgh

Pernoll M L, Metcalfe J, Kovach P A, Wachter R and Dunham M J (1975) 'Ventilation during rest in pregnancy and postpartum' *Respiration Physiology* 25: 295

Pirani B B K, Campbell D M and MacGillivray I (1973) 'Plasma volume in normal first pregnancy' *Journal of Obstetrics and Gynaecology of the British Commonwealth* 80: 884

Poivedin L O S (1959) 'Striae gravidarum. Their relation to adrenal cortical hyperfunction' *Lancet* ii: 436

Price J (1988) *Motherhood: What it Does to Your Mind* Pandora: London

Pritchard J A and Adams R H (1960) 'Erythrocyte production and destruction during pregnancy' *American Journal of Obstetrics and Gynecology* 79: 750

Raphael-Leff J (1991) *Psychological Processes of Childbearing* Chapman and Hall: London

Reading A (1983) *Psychological Aspects of Pregnancy* Longman: London

Reading A E, Campbell S, Cox D N and Sledmere C M (1982) 'Health beliefs and health care behaviours in pregnancy' *Psychological Medicine* 12: 379–83

Rodwell S and Smart E (1982) *Pregnant at Work: The experiences of women* Open University Press: Milton Keynes

Rodwell-Williams S (1985) 'Nutritional guidance in prenatal care' in B S Worthington-Roberts, J Vermeesch and S Rodwell-Williams (eds) *Nutrition in Pregnancy and Lactation (3rd edn)* Ch 4 132–68 Mosby: St Louis

Rovinsky J J and Jaffin H (1965) 'Cardiovascular hemodynamics in pregnancy. I Blood and plasma volumes in multiple pregnancy *American Journal of Obstetrics and Gynecology* 93: 1

Rovinsky J J and Jaffin H (1966) 'Cardiovascular hemodynamics in pregnancy. II Cardiac output and left ventricular work in multiple pregnancy' *American Journal of Obstetrics and Gynecology* 95: 781

Rubin R (1984) *Maternal Identity and the Maternal Experience* Springer: New York

Salvatore C A (1961) 'Leg cramp syndrome in pregnancy' *Obstetrics and Gynecology* 17: 634–9

Sheehan H L and Lynch J B (1973) *Pathology of Toxaemia of Pregnancy* 47 Churchill Livingstone: Edinburgh

Shervington P C (1974) 'Common pregnancy disorders and infections' in D F Hawkins (ed) *Obstetric Therapeutics* 231–73 Balliere Tindall: London

Sherwood O D (1988) 'Relaxin' in E Knobil and J Neil (eds) *The Physiology of Reproduction* 585 Raven Press: New York

Smith A and Jacobson B (1988) *The Nation's Health* King's Fund: London

Smithells R W, Sheppard S, Schorah C J, Sellar M J, Nevin N C, Harris R, Read A P and Fielding D W (1981) 'Apparent prevention of neural tube defects by periconceptual vitamin supplementation' *Archives of Diseases in Childhood* 56: 911–18

Spetz S (1964) 'Peripheral circulation during pregnancy' *Acta Obstetrica et Gynaecologica Scandanavica* 43: 309

Thomson K J and Cohen M E (1938) 'Studies on the circulation in pregnancy II. Vital capacity observations in normal pregnant women' *Surgery, Gynecology and Obstetrics* 66: 591

Thomson A M and Billewicz W Z (1957) 'Clinical significance of weight trends during pregnancy' *British Medical Journal* i: 243

Thomson A M, Hytten F E and Billewicz W Z (1967) 'The epidemiology of oedema during pregnancy' *Journal of Obstetrics and Gynaecology of the British Commonwealth* 74: 1

Walker C and Cannon G (1984) *The Food Scandal* Century: London

Walters W A W, MacGregor W G and Hills M (1966) 'Cardiac output at rest during pregnancy and the puerperium' *Clinical Science* 30: 1

William C and Jellife O B (1972) *Mother and Child Health: Delivering the services* Oxford University Press: Oxford

Wong R C and Ellis C N (1984) 'Physiologic skin changes in pregnancy' *Journal of the American Academy of Dermatology* 10: 929

Worthington-Roberts B S and Vermeersch J (1985) 'Physiological basis of nutritional needs' in B S Worthington-Roberts, J Vermeesch and S Rodwell-Williams (eds) *Nutrition in Pregnancy and Lactation (3rd edn)* Ch 3 61–131 Mosby: St Louis

Wright H P, Osborn S B and Edmonds D G (1950) 'Changes in rate of flow of venous blood in the leg during pregnancy, measured with radioactive sodium' *Surgery, Gynecology and Obstetrics* 90: 481

7   Antenatal care

History

Formal provision of antenatal care is a relatively recent innovation (Oakley 1984). In line with world-wide developments, the first regular clinics were established in the United Kingdom during the time of the First World War but it was only during the Second World War that over 50% of pregnant women received any antenatal care. Prior to this time there were many customs and beliefs applied to pregnancy (for example, regarding diet) and some women had access to medical care (Oakley 1984). Because the study of diagnosis and treatment during pregnancy was not mandatory in the medical syllabus until 1923 (Oakley 1984) and due to the small knowledge base at that time, such care and advice which was given did not have a scientific basis.

At the turn of the century in the United Kingdom the first time the midwife met the pregnant woman was often when called out to attend her in labour (Donnison 1988). The 1911 National Insurance act which provided health insurance for working men also included a 30 shilling maternity benefit for their wife, the first time that the labouring classes had any provision to pay for maternity care (Oakley 1984). The first UK hospital facility designated for antenatal women was in 1901 when Ballantyne secured the endowment of a bed in Edinburgh for the prevention of antenatal pathology and fetal malformations (Oakley 1984). The first regular antenatal clinic in the United Kingdom was also started in Edinburgh in 1915 by Haig Ferguson as part of a national and international movement.

Concern had been expressed about the poor physical condition of recruits for the Boer War and this led in part to the establishment of infant welfare provision (Davies 1915) and the setting up of schools for mothers. In 1914 the Board of Education stated that the health of the adult depends on the health of the child, which in turn depends upon the health of the mother and infant. It was, however, the huge loss of life during the First World War which gave a spur to antenatal care as a method of reducing infant and maternal mortality by improving both the quality and quantity of the population. The 1918 Maternal and Child Welfare Act made provision for local authorities to establish an antenatal care service, although this was not compulsory (Oakley 1982). Midwives who were self-employed were sometimes reluctant to advise women to attend these municipal clinics for fear that the woman would be selected for hospital confinement and the midwife lose her fee (Donnison 1988). The 1936 Midwives' Act allowed for the establishment of a salaried midwifery service which ensured the midwife's remuneration for giving complete care to the mother (Donnison 1977).

In the early days of antenatal surveillance, the care given was very rudimentary, consisting mainly of advice with possible urinalysis and abdominal examination (Campbell 1923). In 1930 the Departmental Committee (of the Ministry of Health) on Maternal Mortality and Morbidity recommended the addition of measurement of the mother's blood pressure and external assessment of the pelvis.

It was quickly recognised that whilst the provision of antenatal care was an apparently simple remedy to the problems of mortality, it would not be truly effective without the political will to alter the make-up of society through reducing social deprivation, poverty, disease and ignorance which were the major causes of perinatal and maternal death (Lancet 1934).

In 1930 the Ministry of Health laid down guidelines for the minimum number of antenatal examinations during pregnancy; these were not based on research but upon a survey of some of the existing provision for antenatal care (Oakley 1984). They have remained, almost unchanged, to this day. Diagnosis of pregnancy was still not easy and the first antenatal visit to a municipal clinic was expected to take place at about 16 weeks of gestation, with further examinations usually in the mother's home at 24 and 28 weeks, every two weeks until 36 weeks and weekly thereafter. The report however suggested that only the first examination and those at 32 and 36 weeks would be carried out by a doctor, the remainder being the province of the midwife. These guidelines were written following evidence from the British Medical Association who were keen to protect the livelihood of their members and resisted the establishment of the midwife as an independent practitioner (Oakley 1984).

The uptake of antenatal care increased slowly until, during the Second World War, there was a general improvement in rates of attendance, since it was necessary to have a certificate confirming pregnancy to obtain the extra rations available for expectant mothers. Pregnant and nursing mothers were a high priority for evacuation to a place of safety. Dietary supplementation and control of prices did much to improve the health of the general population, reducing the extent of social inequality, none more so than for the pregnant woman and her child (Titmuss 1950; Winter 1979). The wartime care and surveillance given to mothers resulted in a fall in perinatal and maternal mortality rates (Ferguson and Fitzgerald 1954).

With the formation of the National Health Service in 1948 the provision of antenatal care was shared between the hospital service, the local authorities (who supplied domiciliary midwives) and the executive councils (who controlled the GPs); these services were partly united when the municipal responsibility for providing community care was removed with the 1974 reorganisation of the NHS. As the number of hospital confinements increased, the involvement of GPs and community midwives reduced. In 1970 the report of the Standing Maternity and Midwifery Advisory Committee (the Peel Report) recommended the integration of the GP and hospital midwifery services and a move towards 100% hospital confinements. These recommendations were not based upon scientific evidence as to the safety of hospital births, but on a misunderstanding of the high mortality which resulted when women who had received no antenatal care gave birth unattended at home (Tew 1990). There are some moves to reverse these trends but, given the increasing numbers of interventions and tests carried out during the antenatal period, it remains to be seen whether technology will move to the health centre, or, if there will be a return to the full use of the clinical skills of the midwife and GP.

Aims of antenatal care

The Maternity Services Advisory Committee (1982) (Maternity Care in Action I) stated that:

> The aim of antenatal care must be to ensure as far as possible the health and wellbeing of the woman and her unborn child. (Para 1.3)

This would include making sure that the woman is in the best possible state of general health in addition to monitoring maternal and fetal well-being for the first sign of any complications. The report recognises the great opportunity for health education provided by pregnancy (Maternity Services Advisory Committee 1982). Care geared to maximising the mother's emotional well-being combined with relevant theoretical input can best prepare the parents (especially the mother) for labour and the responsibilities of childrearing. Hall (1984) divides antenatal care into routine care given to asymptomatic women, education and 'reassurance' for pregnant women and out- or in- 'patient' care for those women with specific problems. Routine care is aimed at the prediction of problems on the basis of history and physical examination, whilst using prophylactic measures to prevent problems and treating any which occur (Hall 1984). Hall (1984) questions whether the premises underpinning the planning and provision of antenatal care are valid. She states that these are:

1. That antenatal care does good rather than harm.

2. That since it does good, the more care the woman receives and the earlier this care begins the better.
3. This care is given best and most efficiently by highly trained and skilled professionals (Hall 1984).

These assumptions are, she states, far from totally proven. Although risk in many cases can be predicted and recognised it cannot be eliminated. Too much time is spent with skilled professionals giving care to low-risk women. The expectations of the professions, the public and the government regarding the possible achievements of antenatal care may be unrealistic (Hall 1984).

Types of care available

Both *The Vision* (Association of Radical Midwives (ARM) 1986) and *Towards a Healthy Nation* (Royal College of Midwives (RCM) 1987) recommend that the first point of contact for the pregnant woman with the primary health care team and the maternity services should be the midwife. With flexibly timed local services, the pregnant woman would call to see the midwife who could, if necessary, arrange tests to confirm the pregnancy and then discuss the options available for antenatal care, delivery and the puerperium. Unfortunately this ideal does not yet exist and for many women their first point of contact is via their own GP who sees them during normal surgery hours. Choice as to the place of antenatal care and of confinement are not often given and the woman is usually referred to the local hospital without an awareness of alternative forms of care. Whilst not all of the following options are available in every area, it is rare for there to be no flexibility at all; the provision of antenatal care is related to the place and type of delivery and whether the setting is rural or urban.

1. Antenatal care at home, usually by the midwife who calls by appointment. Advice of the GP can be sought where necessary. This type of care is usually given for the woman planning a home confinement or a DOMINO delivery (Beech 1987).
2. Joint care by the GP and the midwife, who see the woman in the surgery or health centre. For this to be most effective the midwife must be treated as an equal, carrying out antenatal examinations on her own responsibility (Robinson 1989a). This type of care is often received by women delivering in GP units or cottage hospitals, some women having home confinements and those who have opted for a DOMINO delivery; (to recap: DOMINO – DOMiciliary IN and OUT; the antenatal care is as above, but once the woman thinks that she is in labour she contacts the midwife who visits the house and assesses the situation. When labour is established the midwife accompanies the woman to the place of confinement, usually a GP or a consultant unit, delivers her and looks after her and the neonate until transfer home 6–48 hours later (Beech 1987)). Such care is said by mothers to combine the best parts of a home

confinement – early labour at home, known care giver – with the safety of medical back-up if required.)

3. Shared care. The pregnant woman attends the hospital antenatal clinic and then receives care from her GP/midwife until returning to the hospital at a stated date. For this pattern of care to be successful, it is necessary that all care givers and the mother are aware of what is being done, why it is being done and the results of care. The woman should preferably carry her own antenatal records to avoid duplications or omissions in care (Draper *et al.* 1986) and to ensure that she has her records with her when she is admitted in labour (Zander *et al.* 1978). Shared care is the most frequent pattern of antenatal care provision in the United Kingdom (Keirse *et al.* 1989).

4. Total care in a consultant or regional referral unit. Only women supposedly thought to be at high obstetric risk usually receive such care (Maternity Services Advisory Committee 1982), but they may include some who find visiting the hospital more convenient. High-risk women would include the insulin-dependent diabetic who ideally should see the obstetrician and the physician on every visit (Murphy *et al.* 1984).

5. There are some alternative schemes of care which are not yet widely available but are being introduced experimentally into some areas:

   (a) The Sighthill Scheme (Boddy *et al.* 1980) was designed to provide care for a socially deprived area on the outskirts of Edinburgh. There is a health centre where GPs and midwives give most of the antenatal care supported by a consultant obstetrician who visits every 3 weeks and to whom women with problems can be referred. Such a scheme of care has the benefits of continuity, reduced travelling and waiting times and lowered frequencies of non-attendance and late booking (McKee 1984). A record card giving presence of risk factors is recorded after each visit, giving a clearly visible pattern of the onset of complications.

   (b) The Know Your Midwife Scheme (Flint 1990). In this scheme women of low obstetric risk were selected to receive a package of antenatal, intrapartum and postnatal care from a team of midwives. The mothers were seen by an obstetrician at booking and again at 36 weeks gestation. Women receiving this type of care had more continuity (met fewer care givers), reduced clinic waiting times, fewer interventions in labour including epidural anaesthesia and increased satisfaction with the care they received.

   (c) The Newcastle Community Midwifery Care Project (Davies and Evans 1990). Midwives were based in a poor area of Newcastle to give support to pregnant women and new mothers in their own homes. The project showed how mothers with many socio-economic and obstetric risk factors could be targeted and given extra support. The women were satisfied with the 'enhanced' midwifery care they received, there were improved rates of attendance at parent education classes (which were specifically designed for the client group) and there was a reduction in the rate of low-birthweight babies born to women who had previously given birth to a small baby (Davies and Evans 1990).

Who provides antenatal care?

The midwife

A midwife is qualified to take responsibility for the antenatal care of women experiencing a normal pregnancy, to detect any deviations from the normal and to refer the woman to other professionals for medical care. Robinson (1989b) conducted a survey involving a quarter of all the health districts in England and Wales. Questionnaires were given to all midwives, health visitors, GPs and obstetric staff in these districts. In all, 4248 midwives replied to the request, 19% of the total in practice at the time. Robinson (1989b) discovered that midwives were being underused in antenatal care; they were acting as chaperones, testing urine or having their examinations repeated by medical staff who were often less experienced. Most midwives felt that their role had been eroded by increasing involvement of medical staff in the care of normal women. This underuse of midwifery skills is a waste of both money and resources (Robinson 1989a). The midwife is ideally placed to provide individualised care, to view the mother as part of a family and a social group and to answer fully all questions whilst giving health education or parent education information (Flint 1986). In order to dispel a woman's fears or anxieties it is helpful if she has trust in a midwife she knows. The midwife has time to talk to the mother, especially since midwifery is founded upon normality rather than pathology. In some hospitals, midwives' clinics are being established, which run alongside obstetric clinics, with the midwife having her own case load, arranging return appointments and referring problems directly to the consultant if necessary (Flint 1990).

The general practitioner

Although the pregnant woman can go directly to a midwife, it is usually the GP who is the woman's first contact with the maternity services. He/she acts as a gatekeeper controlling access to maternity care and other NHS services with the exception of clinics for the treatment of sexually transmitted diseases. At this stage he/she should discuss with the woman the options available to her for antenatal care and place of delivery. The GP has a very important role as he/she will already know the woman and her family and has the responsibility of looking after the new family member (Klein and Zander 1989). GPs can work well with midwives where the latter have some autonomy and the doctor gives credit for their observations and decisions. Recently qualified GPs may have a limited knowledge of normal midwifery, having spent 6 months as a GP trainee working in a pathology-orientated hospital obstetric unit (McKendrick 1985). The role of the GP/family doctor in providing care in pregnancy has declined considerably since the 1950s (Klein and Zander 1989).

It could be argued that since the midwife is the practitioner of the normal, there is no role for the GP in the antenatal care of normal women, and should complications arise, these should be referred by the midwife directly to the obstetrician.

The obstetrician

The obstetrician is experienced in the management of abnormal childbirth. It has never been shown that care from an obstetrician can improve outcomes for normal healthy women (Keirse 1989); indeed there may be a morbidity associated with some of the tests and interventions which are becoming commonplace in obstetric care (Williams and Studd 1980). The Maternity Services Advisory Committee (1982) stated:

> 'The obstetrician is a scarce resource; the skills of the consultant team should be devoted primarily to the care of those women in greatest need of specialist advice.' (Para 1.5)

Ideally the obstetrician is capable, in conjunction with the midwife and GP, of deciding the risk category for the pregnant woman and of planning the woman's care accordingly. It must be remembered that some women may only be at a high risk of complications for part of their pregnancy, for example, until the chance of spontaneous abortion has passed, and can then be recategorised. The whole concept of risk assessment in relation to pregnancy is fraught with difficulty and no one scheme has been demonstrated to be of proven value (Alexander and Keirse 1989). The community midwife should be free to refer women in her care direct to the obstetrician for specialist advice whilst informing the GP of her actions.

The health visitor

The health visitor has the responsibility of caring for the under fives, monitoring their progress and well-being and in conjunction with the midwife of providing teaching on topics related to child-care and general health. She may already know the family and can continue the supervision of the care of the baby and other children under five.

Advice on diet

In many centres the pregnant woman is seen by the dietician on her first hospital visit; in others this role may be taken by the midwife. This is useful, as general dietary advice can be given in addition to suggesting ways to reduce the effects of minor disorders of pregnancy such as heartburn. Such an approach means that the woman does not feel she is being singled out for special treatment; normal dietary habits can be ascertained and advice can be personalised to take account of religious requirements and personal preferences. Some mothers may need specialist advice but it is vital to determine the woman's dietary history before giving any advice (Methven 1989). Davies and Evans (1990) demonstrated the teaching of simple cooking techniques to women in their project was vital to supplement dietary advice.

The obstetric physiotherapist

The obstetric physiotherapist is qualified to teach exercises in the antenatal and postnatal period. However, the effectiveness of these is questionable. In the puerperium, pelvic floor exercises have not been shown to reduce the occurrence of urinary incontinence (Sleep and Grant 1987). The effectiveness of the pelvic floor musculature is related more to the individual's state of general fitness and the exercise they take than to any effects of childbirth (Gordon and Logue 1985).

The booking visit/interview

During the Second World War, due to poor home conditions and social disruption, there was an increase in childbirth occurring in institutions (Oakley 1984). The rate of births in institutions increased from 40% in 1937 to 58% in 1946 (Chamberlain et al. 1975). With the start of the National Health Service in 1948, there was an increasing demand for hospital deliveries (Oakley 1984). This came from most areas of society; the working class mothers wished to deliver away from poor home conditions whereas middle class women wanted access to medical supervision (Lewis 1990). Hospital facilities were limited, so that those women with an uncomplicated pregnancy who wanted a hospital confinement had to present early for antenatal care in order to reserve or 'book' a bed. The first visit to the antenatal clinic became known as the booking visit.

Depending on the type of care chosen there may or may not be a booking visit. For the majority of women having hospital or shared care they will receive an appointment to attend the antenatal clinic between 10 and 14 weeks gestation. As Flint (1986) comments, these letters give very little information; for the well woman who has never attended hospital before, an antenatal clinic can come as something of a shock. Waiting time, especially for the first visit, can be long, facilities such as a tea bar or a creche are not universally available, hospital gowns are revealing and depersonalising and the woman may no longer feel like an individual (McIntyre 1981). Graham and McKee (1979) reported that only 31% of first and second time mothers in their study actually enjoyed attending the antenatal clinic. Improvements are being made by using an appointment system to cut waiting time (Tranter 1989). In some areas community midwives conduct the booking interview in the woman's own home (Scott et al. 1987). This however does not permit continuity of care, nor does it allow the midwife to give total care. An appointment system for home visits has helped to reduce embarrassment for the woman who for the time being does not wish her pregnancy to be widely known. Flint (1986) suggests informing the woman in the letter accompanying her appointment about the exact whereabouts of the clinic, how long the visit will take and what will happen. An appointment preferably at a time away from the general antenatal clinic may be one solution.

The booking interview is invariably carried out by the midwife, sometimes in a cramped area with little privacy. Methven (1989) discovered that midwives were not taking advantage of the opportunity to talk to the woman and plan individualised care (such as her reaction to the pregnancy or her eating habits) but they were simply undertaking a task of form filling. The midwives were simply asking about medical details without deviating from the questions or their order on the person's record sheet. The questioning was almost entirely closed, that is, requiring a simple answer (often yes or no) and not permitting the woman to elaborate on her answers. Methven (1989) comments that the majority of interviews followed a style practised by the interviewer, taught to students and perpetuated through the system. She suggests changes in the orientation and tone of the interview to improve the quality of midwifery information obtained and the woman's level of satisfaction. It is vital that such an interview takes place in a private area without barriers (such as desks) and in a relaxed fashion (Methven 1989). Ideally it should occur in the woman's own home where she is at ease and feels free to ask questions, although there is a risk of interruption from other family members. Using personal details, such as reaction to pregnancy, an individualised care plan can be established. Methven (1989) recommends using Orem's (1980) categories for health in planning care – sufficient intake of air, water and food; elimination of waste; balance between activity and rest, solitude and social interaction; prevention of hazards to life; and the promotion of individual well-being and personal development. These allow the midwife to discover the woman's normal behaviour (e.g. alcohol intake), her social interaction and how the pregnancy will affect her.

When considering what questions to ask, it is necessary to understand the importance of each piece of information. In many cases such knowledge is needed to determine the risk category into which the woman falls and thus decide her programme for antenatal care. Fawdry and Mutch (1986) analysed booking record sheets from all the teaching hospitals in the UK and discovered a wide variation in information required. They produced a basic minimum of questions to be asked (with some amendments). Following these is an indication of the type of information which Methven (1989) recommends should be included as part of the planning of individualised care.

Hospital name, Consultant

Expectant mother: Full name.
                     Date of birth, age   Telephone numbers
                     Address, telephone and   assist if urgent
                     postcode   contact is
                     Change of address, unit   required

	number	
	Marital status (or whether supported financially and emotionally), religion, occupation, ethnic origin, country of birth	Ethnic origin may indicate whether specific tests such as for sickle cell disease are required
Next of kin:	Name, telephone number, relationship	
Husband/partner:	One parent family, occupation	Gives an indication of social circumstances
GP:	Name, address, telephone number	
Past medical history:	Heart disease, rheumatic fever, TB, diabetes epilepsy. Previous surgery: gynaecological, cervical cytology, infertility. Accidents (e.g. fractured pelvis), allergies, blood transfusions	These may give rise to problems during the current pregnancy
Contraception:	Most recent. When ceased.	(Was the last menstrual period a withdrawl bleed?)
Past obstetric history: (for each pregnancy)	Date, place, gestational age, mode of delivery, sex, birthweight	To these could be added the following: antenatal complications. Labour spontaneous or induced. Reason for mode of delivery. Analgesia. Labour complications: First, second, third stage. Name of child. Mode of feeding. Current health of the child(ren).
Family history:	Hypertension, diabetes, congenital abnormalities, twins	These may occur in pregnancy or in later life.

| Present pregnancy: | Last menstrual period: sure/unsure. Menstrual cycle estimated date of delivery. Bleeding since pregnant. Date of quickening. Drugs and medications taken. Smoking and alcohol intake. Intention regarding infant feeding. | Important to assess the accuracy of the expected date of delivery. |

(Adapted from Fawdry and Mutch, 1986)

The following information may be requested to organise a programme of individualised care (Methven 1989).

1. *The number of children at home*   In these days when divorce and remarriage are common, a primiparous woman may already be caring for children whereas a multiparous may have none at home. This, together with whether the pregnancy was planned, gives an indication as to how the woman will cope after the birth; whether she will require help at home or whether a nursery place will need to be found for an older child to reduce the strain.

2. *Type and size of housing*   The housing may already be overcrowded or of a poor standard and housing worries cause stress which is detrimental to health (McCarthy *et al*. 1985; Paterson and Roderick 1990). The new baby may make the family a priority for rehousing or if homeless improve their changes of finding accommodation depending on local circumstances and the length of the waiting list.

3. *Occupation*   Is the woman the breadwinner for the family? With high unemployment and the frequency of part-time work many families rely on the woman's earnings. If in part-time work she may not have been employed for long enough to be entitled to maternity leave; does she intend to return to work and if so, when? What arrangements are being made to look after the new baby – creche, childminder, family, baby's father? Is the occupation hazardous to the pregnancy (McCloy 1989)? The woman may be anxious about this but unable to stop work as the money is vital. Legislation permitting maternity leave for women in paid employment varies between countries. In the European Community, Denmark allows 28 weeks of leave (18 weeks at 90% of salary and 5 months at 50%), the United Kingdom 40 weeks (if employed full time for more than 2 years, 90% of salary for 6 weeks and a further 13 weeks at a flat rate) and France 16 weeks (on 90% of earnings) (Labour Research Department 1987).

4. *Dietary habits*   To assess a person's diet it is helpful to ask what they ate the previous day; people's definitions of a good or adequate diet vary greatly. At

this time information about smoking and drinking alcohol can be obtained, for the latter ask about the previous week. After this advice regarding diet, alcohol and smoking can be given paying attention to the person's lifestyle, social circumstances and motivation. Maternal smoking (Butler and Alberman 1969), alcohol intake (Council Report 1983) and use of non-prescribed drugs (Fraser 1983) are all known to reduce optimal outcome.

5. *Information required about present pregnancy*   When asking if the woman has any queries, the midwife can discover how the woman feels about this pregnancy, whether she is troubled by so-called 'minor' disorders and also any worries from previous confinements. This subject should be approached in an open fashion allowing the woman to ask questions freely and talk about whatever is on her mind.

The above are guidelines for taking a woman's history; as women are individuals they may wish to give different information and it is here that the midwife must use her judgement and discretion. Previous pregnancies about which the partner is unaware, for example, should be handled carefully. Since most women have a maternity services cooperation card and some carry their own notes, it is advisable to define a way of denoting such circumstances.

Definitions

Parity – the number of times a woman has given birth after 28 weeks gestation or any live births occurring before that time.
Gravidity – the number of times a woman has been pregnant.
Primiparous – giving birth for the first time.
Primigravida – pregnant for the first time.

For example:-

Joan Smith	Gravida 0	Para 0	Never been pregnant.
Mary Brown	Gravida 2	Para 0 also Para 0 + 1	Pregnant this time (previous spontaneous abortion or termination of pregnancy).
Susan Jones	Gravida 2	Para 1 also Para 1 + 0	Given birth once. Pregnant now.
Ann Evans	Gravida 4	Para 2 or Para 2 + 1	Two previous births, one spontaneous abortion or termination of pregnancy, pregnant now

Following the booking interview there is the booking examination, the thought of which makes many women quite anxious. If the booking history is carried out in the woman's home, there will be a delay before this occurs and the midwife can help by explaining what will be done and why. The aims of this examination, carried out by the obstetrician or GP are to assess the woman's general state of health, to confirm the pregnancy and its gestation, to provide baseline recordings for later in pregnancy and to detect any complications. In the United States women receiving midwifery care will have these examinations performed by the nurse-midwife. To avoid fragmentation of care it is helpful if all the parts of this examination take place in the same room. It is not necessary for the woman to be undressed although, if this occurs, it is important that the hospital gowns provided maintain modesty, especially if the woman has to move outside the examination room.

General state of health

Weight	Some women will have lost weight due to morning sickness.
Height and/or shoe size	Gives an indication as to the adequacy or otherwise of the pelvis. In the Cardiff Birth Survey (Andrews *et al*. 1985), small maternal height was associated with higher incidences of perinatal mortality, low birthweight and abnormal delivery.
Urinalysis and MSSU	To detect underlying medical conditions (diabetes, renal disease) and the presence of an asymptomatic infection (a bacterial count above 10 000/ml) which may predispose to later more serious infection such as pyelonephritis with its risks of preterm delivery or kidney diseases in later life (Kass 1962).
Blood pressure	Baseline for later recordings.
Full general medical examination	Examination of the heart, lungs, breasts, abdomen (enlarged liver or spleen). Observation for operation scars. Neurological integrity.

Obstetric examination

Abdominal examination	The uterus should be palpable abdominally from 12 weeks gestation.
External genitalia	For signs of oedema or redness (possible infection), herpes lesions, genital warts or scarring (episiotomy or circumcision).
Cervix	A speculum is passed to visualise the cervix and a cervical smear is taken, unless the woman has had one in the last year, when a note is made to take the smear at the postnatal clinic.
Pelvic examination	For the following reasons: 1. To confirm pregnancy and that the gestation accords with period of amenorrhoea. 2. Whether the uterus is anteverted and anteflexed or whether it is retroverted.

3. To detect uterine abnormality, e.g. double uterus or fibroids.
4. Any other deviation from normal, e.g. ovarian cysts, ectopic pregnancy.

Although a general impression of the size of the pelvis can be obtained, it is unusual to perform pelvimetry at this stage, since the woman is often tense. If pelvimetry is required, it is better performed in late pregnancy when the pelvic joints and ligaments have relaxed.

Blood tests
The midwife should explain to the woman the rationale for these tests, how the results can be obtained and state that they are performed as routine on all women.

Haemoglobin	Baseline for later recordings. Some areas assess serum ferritin as a guide to iron stores. Whilst the woman may have a satisfactory haemoglobin, there may be insufficient iron stores to cope with the demands of pregnancy, with resultant anaemia (Fenton *et al.* 1977).
ABO and rhesus	All blood is grouped, the rhesus factor determined and a Coomb's test performed for rhesus antibodies. This is in case blood is required in an emergency. Rhesus-negative women require special treatment (see Chapter 35) as do those with antibodies.
Rubella immunity	Rubella can cause severe fetal malformation if caught during pregnancy (Hanshaw *et al.* 1985). Antibody titres measure resistance; if not immune, vaccine is given in the postnatal period, the woman should ensure she does not become pregnant for a further three months (Horstmann 1982).
Sexually transmitted diseases	The gonococcal fixation test and the treponema pallidum haemaglutination test are performed to check for gonorrhoea or syphilis. Gonorrhoea can give rise to neonatal infection, whilst syphilis can cause congenital abnormalities. Women are also being offered testing for the presence of antibodies to human immunodeficiency virus (HIV).
Abnormal haemoglobins	Women in susceptible ethnic groups are screened for sickle cell trait and thallassaemia (see Chapter 15 for more details). People of African descent should be screened for the presence of sickle cell disease/trait (Tuck and White 1981) and those of Mediterranean or Far Eastern origin for the thallassaemias (Perkins 1971).
Fetal Screening	At 16 weeks gestation, if the mother so wishes, blood can be taken for serum alphafeto protein (AFP) levels. If raised, there is a risk of open neural tube defects, diagnosis is confirmed by ultrasound scan and/or amniocentesis. Chorion villus sampling is permitting even earlier testing in pregnancy (see Chapter 8 for more details).

This completes the booking examination. In some centres an ultrasound scan is routine at this stage, in others it is only advocated if the gestation or viability of the pregnancy is in doubt (Campbell and Pearce 1985). The rationale for the difference in policies is far from clear. It is important to inform the woman of the outcome of these examinations especially if the findings are normal; anxiety may result from the woman being unaware of the rationale for or findings of various examinations. The midwife should inform the woman about available parent education groups, including an early class, which describe the process of pregnancy and explain minor disorders. The woman should receive her certificate of expected confinement which will entitle her to free prescriptions and dental care whilst she is pregnant and for one year after the birth.

Subsequent care

The assumption that antenatal care is good and that more antenatal care is better has been challenged by Hall *et al.* (1980). By careful selection of women at risk, the 'normal' woman can have fewer visits and examinations, and each will have a specific purpose (Hall 1984). For this to be successful there must be an informal process by which women who are worried can contact the midwife and seek advice. As many community midwives have certain fixed arrangements during the week, such as clinics, all that would be needed is that they should be free to see women who drop in at a certain specified time.

In 1930 the Ministry of Health established a recommended pattern for antenatal care. The woman would be seen first at 16 weeks, with subsequent visits at 24 and 28 weeks, fortnightly examinations until 36 weeks and weekly thereafter. This pattern although based on no scientifc evidence, is still followed in the United Kingdom with women averaging 12 or 13 visits for antenatal care (Blondel *et al.* 1985). Blondel *et al.* (1985) studied variations in the pattern of antenatal care throughout Europe and found that the number of examinations ranges from 5 in Luxembourg to 14 in Finland with little proven benefit for any pattern and unclear rationales behind their planning.

Before discussing some of the visit patterns for the provision of antenatal care, it is necessary to define risk. There is agreement that women with pre-existing medical disorders or poor obstetric history require intensive antenatal care and surveillance; what is more contentious is the application of such principles to women who are at potentially low risk. It must be remembered that at any time during pregnancy or labour the risk category can change from high to low.

The following are risk categories used by midwives to decide which women are suitable for midwifery care. They are somewhat more stringent than those which would be employed by a GP to decide which women he/she should refer to obstetric care. Callis (1983) (in an unevaluated project) used the following three risk categories to decide the care that women would receive. Low-risk women would see the midwife except at the 28–32 week and 37–38 week visits and post-term when care would be from an obstetrician (who had made the initial risk selection). Women in high- and intermediate-risk categories usually saw the midwife on alternate visits to the clinic (which does not provide continuity of care) or saw both the midwife and the obstetrician.

The following could be used to classify risk:

- *High Risk*

- Factors known to be associated with poor outcomes

| Maternal disease, e.g. hypertension, diabetes | | These have a significant bearing on the outcome of pregnancy |

| Multiple pregnancy | (Aumann and Baird 1986) | |
| Abnormal presentation Small stature | (Andrews et al. 1985) | |

| Chronic Anaemia Threatened abortion Previous perinatal Death Previous abnormality of pregnancy/delivery/ puerperium | (Shapiro et al. 1968). | Problems which have occurred in a previous pregnancy may recur |

- *Intermediate risk*

Woman who has factors associated with obstetric problems

- Factors which may in susceptible individuals or in the presence of more than one of them adversely affect outcome

e.g. age

Social class

Heavy smoker
Primigravida

● *Low Risk*

● These groups
have been shown
by Butler and
Alberman (1969)
and by Andrews
et al. (1985)
to have the best
chance of a good
outcome

{
Age 18–30
Social class I, II or III

No maternal disease

No significant family history (of disease)

Average weight

Non-smoker
Happily married
One or two previous normal
pregnancies and deliveries (Callis 1983)
}

Flint (1990) used similar but simpler criteria to select women for the 'Know Your Midwife' scheme study:

Over five feet tall.
No serious medical conditions.
No previous uterine surgery.
No more than two miscarriages or terminations of pregnancy.
No previous intrauterine growth retardation.
No previous stillborn babies or neonatal deaths.
No previous preterm labours.
No rhesus antibodies.

For low-risk women Marsh (1985) a GP has suggested the following pattern of care for nulliparous and multiparous women; visits are shared between midwife and GP, who discuss their findings at the end of each clinic. Marsh (1985) argues that such schemes remove the necessity for low-risk women to travel to hospital for antenatal care (see Table 7.1); however an extension of this argument would question why the woman are not receiving all their care from a midwife, since they were categorised as normal.

Once the schedule of visits has been decided upon, it is important to consider what observations will be made.

Maternal well-being

At every visit the midwife should make enquiries as to the presence of any of the following; the efficacy of any previous advice should be evaluated before giving any further advice and explanation and instituting the correct treatment or referral.

Table 7.1 New style antenatal programme for low-risk women

Gestation (Weeks)	Examiner	Nulliparous	Primiparous	Reason
8	Midwife and GP			Booking
8–12	Midwife and GP			Booking
12	Midwife			Results of booking tests
16	Hospital			Scan. Alphafeto protein test
22	Midwife			Weight gain. Blood pressure, presence of twins, parentcraft, involving lay groups-NCT
26	Midwife			As 22 weeks
30	Midwife and GP			Fetal size. Blood pressure, weight, blood tests, detect IUGR
34	Midwife and GP			Presentation. Pelvic assessment, blood pressure, urinalysis
36	Midwife and GP			BP Urinalysis.
	Family planning nurse			Presentation, discussion of birth plan and contraception
38	Midwife and GP			Clinical assessment as 36 weeks. Engagement of fetal head
40	Midwife and GP			As 38 weeks
41	Midwife and GP			Confirm normality. As 38 weeks
42	Midwife and GP			As 41 weeks. Double check dates
Total number of examinations by GP:				
Traditional scheme		15	15	
New scheme		8	6	

- Nausea, vomiting or heartburn
- Abdominal pain or backache
- Constipation or diarrhoea
- Frequency of micturition or dysuria
- Any vaginal bleeding
- Fetal movements
- General state of health and well-being, e.g. appetite, sleeping.

If women forget what they wish to ask, it is useful to suggest that they write their queries down to jog their memory when the time comes. In addition to the above indicators of maternal well-being the following are usually assessed:

1. Blood pressure. Blood pressure falls up until 16–18 weeks and then rises to reach prepregnancy levels by term. In the antenatal period the following are significant and require reporting to the GP or obstetrician:

   A rise of 15 mmHg in diastolic pressure, 30 mmHg in the systolic or a B.P. above 140/90. (MacGillivray *et al.* 1969) (See Chapter 12 of this book for more details.)

   Many women experience labile hypertension exacerbated by waiting times, worry and crowded clinics; if remeasured after the woman has rested, a significant number of cases will have returned to normal (Hibbard 1988).

2. Urinalysis. Normal urine is straw coloured, clear, odourless and without protein, glucose or ketones being present. Where the woman has severe morning sickness the urine may be dark and concentrated, containing ketones.

   The presence of protein can be due to contamination, infection, renal disease or pre-eclampsia. This last is unusual before 26–28 weeks gestation and in the absence of other symptoms. A midstream specimen of urine should be obtained to eliminate contamination and look for infection. If the woman brings the specimen with her, ask at what time of day it was passed and whether the container was thoroughly cleaned beforehand.

   Glucose may be present due to the lowered renal threshold for glucose in pregnancy (or because the woman has just had a large meal) (Jowett and Nicol 1986), to contamination from the container or to diabetes or prediabetes (see Chapter 13). The presence of more than a trace of glucose on two or more occasions should be reported to the medical staff. A random blood sugar estimation may be performed or a glucose tolerance test ordered.

3. Blood tests. Haemoglobin is assessed at booking, 28–30 weeks and 34–36 weeks, to check for anaemia. Iron tablets are rarely given routinely (Hibbard 1988). Rhesus-negative women usually have checks made for the presence of antibodies at the same time as haemoglobin estimations. Many centres now offer serum alphafeto protein levels. This is assessed at 16 weeks gestation to detect open neural tube defects. If raised, the test is repeated, followed by an ultrasound scan and/or amniocentesis if performed, to finalise the result. If the result is still positive the couple should be counselled as to the implications and the choices involved in management including the option to terminate the pregnancy.

Progress of the pregnancy

1. Weight gain. The pregnant woman should gain approximately 12 kg throughout the pregnancy, 2 kg in the first 20 weeks and 0.5 kg/week

thereafter (see Chapter 6). This is a rough guide though; many women lose weight in early pregnancy. Some centres no longer weigh women routinely during antenatal care (Hytten 1990).

2. Oedema. Oedema in dependent areas is a common sign which is not pathological, the midwife must observe for oedema in non-dependent areas such as the face and abdomen. The hands and feet are common areas for oedema, especially as the day progresses, although physiological oedema resolves overnight following a period with the lower limbs raised.

3. Abdominal examination. There are three parts to this inspection, palpation and auscultation; these are described in detail in the following chapter.

Assessment of individual need

Ample time and opportunity must be made available for the woman to ask questions and receive answers at a level suitable for her individual case. Women who do not wish to attend parent education classes can receive some of the information in an informal manner from the midwife during antenatal visits. Although antenatal care as currently provided may not be ideal nor achieve all of the aims, there are certain factors which may provide an improvement:

- Proximity of the place of care to the woman's home or place of work (Williams *et al.* 1989)
- Facilities for amusing small children (Maternity Services Advisory Committee 1982).
- Clinic times related to available public transport
- Strict appointment systems, no block bookings (Williams *et al.* 1989).
- Refreshment facilities (Maternity Services Advisory Committee 1982)
- Health education/parentcraft information displays (Maternity Services Advisory Committee 1982)
- Using waiting time for parentcraft discussions.
- Continuity of care – arranging for the woman to see the same person(s) at each visit (Williams *et al.* 1989)
- Performing investigations and examinations for a specific purpose (World Health Organization 1985)
- Improving privacy in clinics – curtained cubicles are not soundproof (Williams *et al.* 1989)
- Professionals attending the clinics on time or sending a deputy (Maternity Services Advisory Committee 1982)

References

Alexander S and Keirse M J N C (1989) 'Formal risk scoring during pregnancy' in I Chalmers, M Enkin and M J N C Keirse (eds) *Effective Care in Pregnancy and Childbirth* Ch 22 345–65 Oxford Medical: Oxford

Andrews J, Davies K, Chalmers I and Campbell H (1985) 'The Cardiff Birth Survey: development, perinatal mortality, birthweight and length of gestation' in P S Harper and E Sunderland (eds) *Genetic and Population Studies in Wales* University of Wales Press: Cardiff

Association of Radical Midwives (1986) *The Vision* ARM: Ormskirk Lancashire

Aumann G M E and Baird M M (1986) 'Screening for the high risk pregnancy' in R A Knuppel and J E Drukker (eds) *High Risk Pregnancy* Saunders: Philadelphia

Beech B L (1987) *Who's Having Your Baby?* Camden Press: London

Blondel B, Pusch D and Schmidt E (1985) 'Some characteristcs of antenatal care in 13 European countries' *British Journal Of Obstetrics and Gynaecology* 92: 565–8

Board of Education (1914) *Annual Report for 1913* HMSO: London

Boddy K, Parboosingh I J T and Shepherd W T (1980) *A Schematic Approach to Prenatal Care* University of Edinburgh: Edinburgh

Butler N R and Alberman E D (1969) *Perinatal Problems* E and S Livingstone: Edinburgh

Callis P (1983) 'Midwives'clinics' *Midwives' Chronicle* Nov(Suppl): 2–4

Campbell J M (1923) *The Training of Midwives. Ministry of Health Reports on Public Health and Medical Subjects No. 21* HMSO: London

Campbell S and Pearce J M F (1985) 'Ultrasound in obstetrics and gynaecology' in R R MacDonald (ed) *Scientific Basis of Obstetrics and Gynaecology* Ch 10 Churchill Livingstone: Edinburgh

Chamberlain R, Chamberlain G, Howlett B and Claireaux A (1975) *British Births 1970, Vol 1* Heinemann: London

Council Report (1983) 'Fetal effects of maternal alcohol abuse' *Journal of the American Medical Association* 249: 2517–21

Davies M L (1915) *Maternity: Letters From Working Women* G Bell and Sons, Reprinted 1978, Virago: London

Davies J and Evans F (1990) 'The Newcastle Community Midwifery Care project' in S Robinson and A M Thomson (eds) *Midwives, Research and Childbirth Vol 2* 104–39 Chapman and Hall: London

Departmental Committee on Maternal Mortality and Morbidity (1930) *Interim Report* HMSO: London

Donnison J (1977) *Midwives and Medical Men* Heinemann: London

Donnison J (1988) *Midwives and Medical Men: the history of the struggle for the control of childbirth* Historical Publications: London

Draper J, Field S, Thomas H and Hare M J (1986) 'Should women carry their antenatal records?' *British Medical Journal* 292: 603

Fawdry R D S and Mutch L M M (1986) 'Antenatal history taking: what are we asking?' *MIDIRS* Information pack No. 3

Fenton V, Cavill K and Fisher J H (1977) 'Iron stores in pregnancy' *British Journal of Haematology* 37: 145–9

Ferguson S M and Fitzgerald H (1954) *Studies on the Social Services* HMSO: London

Flint C (1986) *Sensitive Midwifery* Heinemann: London

Flint C (1990) 'Know your midwife scheme' in S Robinson and A M Thomson (eds) *Midwives, Research and Childbirth Vol 2* Chapman and Hall: London

Fraser A C (1983) 'The pregnant drug addict' *Maternal and Child Health* 8(11): 461–3

Gordon H and Logue M (1985) 'Perineal muscle function after childbirth' *Lancet* ii: 123–5

Graham H and McKee L (1979) *The First Months of Motherhood* University of York: York

Hall M H (1984) 'Are our accepted practices based on valid assumptions?' in L Zander and G Chamberlain (eds) *Pregnancy Care for the 1980's* 3–8 Macmillan: London

Hall M H, Chng P K and MacGillivray I (1980) 'Is routine antenatal care worthwhile?' *Lancet* i: 78–80

Hanshaw J B, Dudgeon J A and Marshall W C (1985) *Viral Diseases of the Fetus and the Newborn (2nd edn)* Saunders: Philadelphia

Hibbard B M (1988) *Principles of Obstetrics* Butterworth: London

Horstmann D M (1982) 'Viral infections' in G N Burrow and T F Ferris (eds) *Medical Complications During Pregnancy (2nd edn)* Ch 14 Saunders: Philadelphia

Hytten F (1990) 'Is it important or even useful to measure weight gain in pregancy?' *Midwifery* 6(1): 28–32

Jowett N I and Nicol S G (1986) 'Gestational diabetes – Are the right women being screened?' *Midwifery* 2(2): 98–100

Kass E H (1962) 'Pyelonephritis and bacteruria' *Annals of Internal Medicine* 56: 46

Keirse M J N C (1989) 'Interaction between primary and secondary care during pregnancy and childbirth' in I Chalmers, M Enkin and M J N C Keirse (eds) *Effective Care in Pregnancy and Childbirth* Ch 13 197–201 Oxford Medical: Oxford

Klein M and Zander L (1989) 'The role of the family practitioner in maternity care' in I Chalmers, M Enkin and M J N C Keirse (eds) *Effective Care in Pregnancy and Childbirth* Ch 11 181–191 Oxford Medical: Oxford

Labour Research Department (1987) *Time Off for Childcare* Labour Research Department: London

Lancet, Notes and Comments (1934) 'Antenatal care on trial' *Lancet* ii: 1204.

Lewis J (1990) 'Mothers and maternity policies in the twentieth century' in J Garcia, R Kilpatrick and M Richards (eds) *The Politics of Maternity Care* Ch 1 1–14 Clarendon Paperbacks: Oxford

Marsh G M (1985) 'A new programme of antenatal care in general practice' *British Medical Journal* 291: 646–8

Maternity Services Advisory Committee (1982) *Maternity Care in Action. Part 1 – Antenatal Care* HMSO: London

MacGillivray I, Rose G A and Rowe B (1969) 'Blood pressure survey in pregnancy' *Clinical Science* 37: 385–407

MacIntyre S (1981) *Expectations and Experiences of First Pregnancy* University of Aberdeen Institute of Medical Sociology Occasional paper No 5

McCarthy P, Byrne D, Harrison S and Keithley J (1985) 'Respiratory conditions: effects of housing and other factors' *Journal of Epidemiological Community Health* 39: 15–19

McCloy E C (1989) 'Work, environment and the fetus *Midwifery* 5: 53–62

McKee I H (1984) 'Community antenatal care: the Sighthill community antenatal scheme' in L Zander and G Chamberlain (eds) *Pregnancy Care for the 1980's* Ch 5 32–40 Macmillan: London

McKendrick M (1985) 'The training and continuing education of the general practitioner in maternity care' in G N Marsh (ed) *Modern Obstetrics in General Practice* Ch 30 407–12 Oxford Medical: Oxford

Methven R (1989) 'Recording an obstetric history or relating to a pregnant woman? A study of the antenatal booking interview' in S Robinson and A M Thomson (eds) *Midwives, Research and Childbirth Vol 1* Ch 3 42–71 Chapman and Hall: London

Ministry of Health (1930) *Memorandum on Antenatal Clinics; Their Conduct and Scope* HMSO: London

Murphy J, Peters J, Morris P, Hayes T M and Pearson J F (1984) 'Conservative management of pregnancy in diabetic women' *British Medical Journal* 288: 1203–5

Perkins R P (1971) 'Inherited disorders of hemoglobin synthesis and pregnancy' *American Journal of Obstetrics and Gynecology* 111: 120–59

Oakley A (1982) 'The origins and development of antenatal care' in M Enkin and I Chalmers *Effectiveness and Satisfaction in Antenatal Care* 1–21 Spastics International: London

Oakley A (1984) *The Captured Womb. A History of the Medical Care of Pregnant Women* Blackwell: Oxford

Orem D (1980) *Nursing: Concepts of Practice* McGraw Hill: New York

Paterson C M and Roderick P (1990) 'Obstetric outcome in homeless women' *British Medical Journal* 301: 263–6

Robinson S (1989a) 'The role of the midwife: opportunities and restraints' in I Chalmers, M Enkin and M J N C Keirse (eds) *Effective Care in Pregnancy and Childbirth* Ch 10 162–80 Oxford Medical: Oxford

Robinson S (1989b) 'Caring for childbearing women: the interrelationship between midwifery and medical responsibilities' in S Robinson and A M Thomson (eds) *Midwives, Research and Childbirth Vol 1* Ch 2 8–41 Chapman and Hall: London

Royal College of Midwives (1987) *Towards a Healthy Nation* RCM: London

Scott R M, Tustain J, Campbell S, Millis P, Ordili R, Stephens Y and Hammond J (1987) 'Waiting time in the antenatal booking history' *Midwives Chronicle* Sept: 286–7

Shapiro S, Schlesinger E R and Nesbitt R E L (1968) *Infant, Perinatal, Maternal and Childhood Mortality in the United States* Harvard University Press: Cambridge, Massachusetts

Sleep J and Grant A (1987) 'Pelvic floor exercise in postnatal care' *Midwifery* 3: 158–64

Standing Maternity and Midwifery Advisory Committee (1970) *Domiciliary Midwifery and Maternity Bed Needs* (Peel Report) HMSO: London

Tew M (1990) *Safer Childbirth? A critical history of maternity care* Chapman and Hall: London

Titmuss R M (1950) *Problems of Social Policy* Longman: London

Tranter S (1989) 'Reducing the wait' *Nursing Times* 85(51): 39–41

Tuck S M and White J M (1981) 'Sickle cell disease' in J Studd (ed) *Progress in Obstetrics and Gynaecology Vol 1* Ch 6 Churchill Livingstone: Edinburgh

Williams R and Studd J (1980) 'Induction of labour' *Maternal and Child Health* 5(1): 16–21

Williams S, Dickson D, Forbes J, McIlwaine G and Rosenberg K (1989) 'An evaluation of community antenatal care' *Midwifery* 5(2): 63–8

Winter J M (1979) 'Infant mortality, maternal mortality and public health in Britain in the 1980's' *The Journal of European Economic History* 8(2): 439–62

World Health Organization (1985) *Having a Baby in Europe* WHO: Copenhagen

Zander L I, Watson M, Taylor R W and Morrell D C (1978) 'Integration of general practitioner and specialist care' *Journal of the Royal College of General Practitioners* 28: 455

8   Fetal growth and well-being

Techniques for detecting problems

One of the main aims of antenatal care is to assess the well-being of the fetus. Whilst this is difficult to measure directly, the techniques attempt to determine the rate of fetal growth (abdominal examination and ultrasound), level of fetal activity (kick charts), response to stimuli (cardiotocography) or the functioning of the placenta (new placental proteins and hormones) (Pearson 1981). A combination of methods is often advised to increase accuracy, especially since all the procedures have their particular disadvantages. The biophysical profile combines assessment of fetal activity (movements and breathing) with recording of the fetal heart and estimation of amniotic fluid volume (Baskett 1989). With the exception of ultrasound and hormone assays, the procedures are part of the midwife's provision of antenatal care.

The main emphasis of the techniques is on detection of the growth-retarded fetus (one whose weight is in the lowest 10% for babies in that community and of that gestational age (Kitchen 1968) and therefore on an assessment of placental functioning. Detection of the growth-retarded fetus is difficult; the diagnosis can only be confirmed after delivery. Where the fetus is also preterm, the diagnosis can be confused by innaccuracies such as an uncertain period of gestation (Beischer *et al.* 1984). In addition, the centiles for detecting the lowest 10% of babies vary between communities and different ethnic and social groups (McFadyen 1985). Hall *et al.* (1980) pointed out that many of the tests used to diagnose intrauterine growth retardation (IUGR), rather than detecting the actual condition, predict that there is an increased risk of it being present. In the United Kingdom 6–7% of neonates weigh less than 2.5 kg and a third of these babies will have suffered from IUGR (that is, they are small for gestational age); the remainder of low birthweight babies are preterm. Babies whose birthweight is below 2.5 kg account for two thirds of deaths in the first week of life (Wallis and Harvey 1986). Growth retardation is the third most common cause of perinatal death after prematurity and major malformations (Beischer *et al.* 1984).

Many of the tests of fetal well-being are not diagnostic but indicate that the fetus is or may be at risk of compromise. Hall *et al.* (1980) showed that a significant number of women were falsely thought to have IUGR, whilst a proportion of actual cases were missed completely. In their study, only 44% of cases of IUGR were detected antenatally and there were 2.5 false-positive cases for every true one. One of the best predictors for growth retardation is the woman's history; a previously affected baby, medical disorders, smoking and poor socioeconomic status are all factors in the incidence of IUGR (Beischer *et al.* 1984). Where these risk factors occur together with complications of pregnancy such as hypertensive disease, the chances of IUGR occurring are increased. In our multiethnic society it is important to remember the influence of race on birthweight, with the infants of Asian mothers tending to be smaller than those of European or Afro-Caribbean origins (McFadyen 1985).

Abdominal examination

Abdominal examination is one of the oldest methods of assessing fetal growth although it is of limited value and accuracy (Altman and Hytten 1989). It forms a major part of the midwife's examination of the pregnant woman, although as Robinson (1989) demonstrated, it is often repeated by the medical staff with little if any account being taken of the midwife's findings. In addition to any information obtained (which should be shared with the mother), it provides reassurance through touch and demonstrates concern for the welfare of mother and baby. Traditionally, the abdominal examination has three main components:

1. Inspection
2. Palpation: Uterine size.
   Fundal palpation ⎫   To determine the number of
   Lateral palpation ⎬   fetuses present, their size,
   Pelvic palpation ⎭   presentation and position.

3. Auscultation (to which a fourth should be added: Recording of the findings and their explanation to the woman and her partner).

Terminology

Lie: This refers to the way in which the fetus is lying in the mother's uterus with respect to the maternal spine. The lie can be longitudinal, oblique or transverse (see Figure 8.1), by term 99% of babies have a longitudinal lie (Scheer and Nubar 1976). Scheer and Nubar (1976) have shown that after 32 weeks gestation when the volume of liquor reduces, the fetal lie becomes more dependent on the shape of the uterus. Since this is usually pyridiform, the fetus most often adopts a longitudinal lie with the bulky breech in the wider fundus.

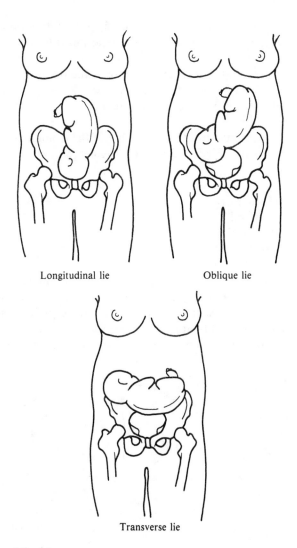

Longitudinal lie   Oblique lie

Transverse lie

Figure 8.1 The lie of the fetus.

Attitude: This term is used to describe the relationship of the fetal head and limbs to the trunk. The vast majority of fetuses have a flexed attitude but some are deflexed or extended, giving rise in labour to a possible malposition or malpresentation (see Figure 8.2). It is possible to determine attitude on abdominal palpation if the woman is slim.

Presentation: Refers to that part of the fetus lying in the lower pole of the uterus. By 34 weeks gestation the vast majority of fetuses have a cephalic (head first) presentation (White 1956). Other presentations include breech (bottom first) (see Figure 8.3), shoulder (usually resulting from an oblique lie) and compound such as head and hand. Cephalic presentations include the vertex (the top of the head), face and brow.

Denominator: This is the name given to a specific part of each presentation which is used as a reference point for describing the fetal position in the pelvis.

In a cephalic presentation the denominator is the occiput.
In a breech presentation it is the sacrum.
In a face presentation it is the mentum (chin).

Position: This is determined by the relationship of the denominator to eight areas on the mother's pelvis (see Figure 8.4). These areas are:

Direct anterior
Right and left anterior
Right and left lateral
Right and left posterior
Direct posterior

The fetal position is given as, for example, left occipito anterior (LOA) or right sacro posterior (RSP). Where the fetus is lying with the occiput towards the lateral portion of the mother's pelvis, it is sometimes described as being in a transverse position as an indication of the direction of the sagittal suture.

Anterior positions of the fetus are more common; the fetal back and head are able

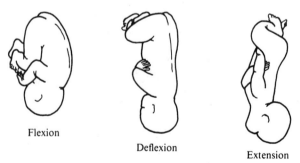

Flexion

Deflexion

Extension

Figure 8.2 Fetal attitudes.

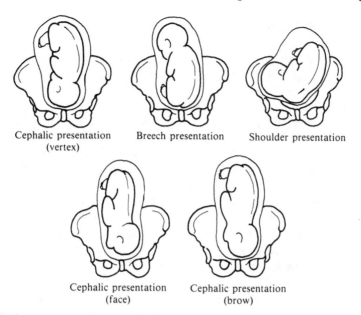

Figure 8.3 Fetal presentations.

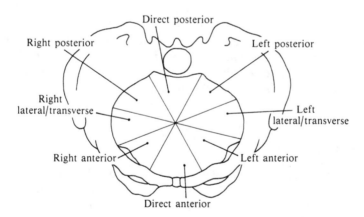

Figure 8.4 Areas of the pelvic brim which determine fetal positions.

to flex allowing smaller diameters to present at the pelvic brim. Where the fetal back is posterior, flexion of the fetal body may be impeded by its alignment with the maternal spine.

Engagement: Refers to the descent of the presenting part into the pelvis. It is easier to assess abdominally for cephalic presentations. The head is said to be engaged when its largest transverse diameter, i.e. the biparietal (9.5 cm) has passed through the pelvic brim.

Examination techniques

Before examining the pregnant woman it is important to ensure that she has had an opportunity to empty her bladder, is comfortable and relaxed, and to ascertain whether she feels at ease lying on her back (if not, a wedge should be inserted on one side under her lumbar region and pelvis to keep the weight of the uterus off the inferior vena cava and aorta). The woman is positioned on an examination couch with her head on one pillow and her shoulders flat upon the bed. It is traditional to perform all examinations and delivery with the midwife standing on the woman's right-hand side. The midwife must ensure that the examination room is private and that they will not be disturbed. A covering for the pregnant woman's legs is helpful to maintain her modesty, feeling of 'self' and personal dignity.

Inspection: The major features to be noted are the size and shape of the uterus. Through practice the midwife can learn to assess uterine size, although this may be difficult depending on the size of the mother. A very much larger than expected uterus may indicate multiple pregnancy or polyhydramnios; the diagnosis may be confirmed on palpation. Where the fetal lie is longitudinal the uterine shape is ovoid, this is most marked in primiparous women. Where the woman is multiparous or obese, the uterine shape may be less distinct and appear to protrude slightly at the sides. The side on which the fetal back is positioned may appear more prominent. Where the lie is transverse, the uterus may appear rather wide. If the fetus is lying in a posterior position a slight depression may be above the maternal umbilicus and fetal movements are more likely to be seen during inspection. Also of note are scars (which could indicate a previous uterine or abdominal examination) or any skin changes such as a pigmented linea nigra (which is common in brunettes) or striae gravidarum: these stretch marks may be pink if they have been caused in the present pregnancy or silvery if they are old.

Palpation

Whilst inspection, assessment of fundal height and auscultation occur throughout most of pregnancy, a full palpation is normally performed from 28–30 weeks onwards, being of most importance from 32–34 weeks after which, lie and presentation should have stabilised. The midwife should attempt to maintain in contact with the woman throughout the examination and to communicate all findings to her on its completion.

Fundal palpation

Whilst facing the mother and using the tips of the fingers the midwife gently but firmly examines the fundus of the uterus (see Figure 8.5). In the majority of cases the soft bulky breech of the fetus can be identified. To confirm this the breech can

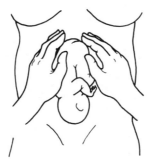

Figure 8.5 Fundal palpation.

be held between the fingers and thumb of one hand; if it attempts to 'wriggle' out of the way, it is not balottable. The uterine size can then be assessed.

Uterine size

Traditionally, uterine size was assessed by measuring in finger breadths the distance between the positions of the fundus and particular landmarks such as the umbilicus or xiphisternum.

Beazley and Kurjak (1973) showed that after 36 weeks gestation 20–25% of the predictions of birthweight were more than 500 g in error. The inaccuracy of this method is greatest for very small or very large babies, whose size is most crucial (Loeffler 1967). Difficulties in accuracy also arise where a number of observers conduct the examination, as there are variations in finger width between individuals, especially between men and women. Individual differences in height between women account for inaccuracies when comparing results; for a woman of small stature, her fundus may reach the xiphisternum at 34 weeks, whereas for a taller woman it may not touch this landmark for a further 3–4 weeks. Traditionally the following are approximate fundal heights by gestation although they should be treated only as a guideline (see Figure 8.6).

12 weeks:	Fundus just palpable above the pubic symphysis.
16–18 weeks:	Fundus midway between symphysis and umbilicus.
22–24 weeks:	Fundus at the umbilicus.
32 weeks:	Midway between umbilicus and xiphisternum.
36–38 weeks:	Fundus at xiphisternum.
38–40 weeks:	2–3 finger breadths below the xiphisternum due to lightening.

Lightening (the feeling of relief of pressure on the diaphragm caused by the descent of the fetus into the pelvis) occurs at about 38 weeks gestation. Under the influence of progesterone and relaxin, the joints and ligaments of the pelvis and

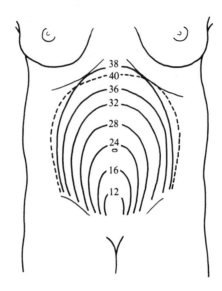

Figure 8.6 Traditional assessment of uterine growth in weeks of amennorhoea.

the pelvic floor are softened. There is more room in the pelvis for the presentation; in the primiparous woman firm abdominal muscles guide the presenting part downwards and engagement occurs; for the multiparous woman the uterus may be displaced anteriorly resulting in increased backache. Women are aware of lightening, since their breathing becomes easier due to a reduction of pressure from the fetus under the diaphragm.

It is now more usual for fundal height to be determined with the help of a tape measure, the distance between the top of the fundus and the upper border of the symphysis pubis being measured in centimetres. After 20 weeks, this recording accords with the weeks of pregnancy – fundal height increases by approximately 1 cm/week. This method has the advantage of allowing for the curvature of the uterus as well as its height. The measurements of fundal height can then be plotted on a centile chart and individual patterns of growth visualised. Calvert *et al.* (1982) found that this method detected 64% of babies who were found at birth to be small for gestational age. However Crosby and Engstrom (1989) demonstrated inaccuracies in the measurements of fundal height using this method, both between and within individuals. The level of accuracy was unrelated to the experience of the individual.

Lateral palpation

Still facing the mother, the midwife places her left hand on the right side of the uterus (i.e. the side nearest to her). Using this hand to steady the uterus whilst gently feeling down the other side with the right hand. The fetal back feels firm and smooth, fetal limbs rather irregular and if no fetal parts are adjacent to the uterine wall the area may just feel soft. To examine the other side the right hand is used to steady the uterus whilst the left feels for the fetal back. To confirm the suspicion as to the position of the fetus, the tips of the fingers of both hands can 'walk' across the abdomen at the level of the umbilicus. When the back is encountered, the abdomen should feel firm rather than soft or indistinct. The fetal back is smooth and firm and its boundaries can be determined (see Figure 8.7).

Pelvic palpation

Facing the woman's feet and using the ulnar border of the hands along the lower boundary of the uterus, the fingers can be placed alongside the presenting part. To ensure relaxation the mother is asked to breathe out whilst the midwife presses down firmly into the pelvis. The palmar surface of the fingers feels the presenting part and can assess how much has entered the pelvis (see Figure 8.8); Figure 8.9 presents a guide to the amount of head palpable. The head is said to be engaged when two-fifths or less is palpable abdominally; the head is normally engaged from 38 weeks in primiparous women. Bader (1936) noted however that the outcome was normal for a group of 499 primiparous women who began labour with a non-engaged fetal head. The head normally engages during labour in multiparous women. If the fingers of both hands can meet around the fetal head it is described as high and free (see Figure 8.10). If more head is felt at one side than the other this is helpful in indicating the degree of flexion. Where the head is well flexed, the midwife will feel the sinciput (forehead) on one side and on the other side, though she cannot feel the head, may well feel the shoulders. Practice is required in the interpretation of such findings.

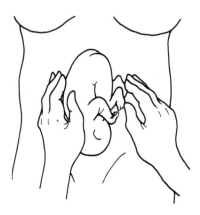

Figure 8.7 Lateral palpation.

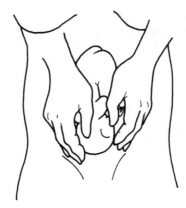

Figure 8.8 Deep pelvic palpation.

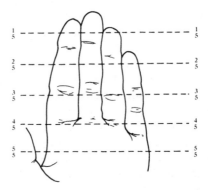

Figure 8.9 Using 'landmarks' on the palmar surface of the examiners hand to determine abdominal descent of the fetal head.

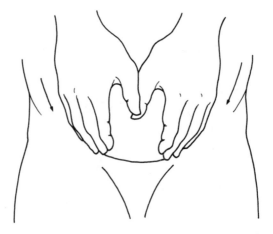

Figure 8.10 The examiner's fingers meeting around a high and free fetal head.

An alternative method of pelvic palpation is Pawlik's Grip; this is most useful when the head is not engaged. Using the right hand, the midwife holds the presenting part between fingers and thumb (see Figure 8.11). This manoeuvre can be very painful to the woman unless carefully performed. This gives information about head size, mobility and degree of flexion. The head can, if free, be balotted between the thumb and fingers. Unlike the breech the head will 'bounce' within the hand.

In addition to the above information the midwife will obtain an impression of fetal size and also of the quantity of liquor present by assessing the amount of free space within the uterus around the fetus. It is difficult to differentiate at times between oligohydramnios (too little liquor) which is an indication of fetal or placental pathology, and that which is on the lower borders of normality. Small degrees of reduction in liquor volume can be assessed by ultrasound and used as an indication of IUGR (Gohari *et al.* 1977). Chronic intrauterine hypoxia causes a reduction in amniotic fluid volume, as does an abnormality of the fetal kidneys or renal tract (Baskett 1989).

Auscultation

From 24–28 weeks gestation the midwife can listen to the fetal heart using the Pinard's stethoscope, although it is detectable using this method from 17 weeks (Jimenez *et al.* 1979). The area where the sound is clearest is usually through the fetal back at the level of the shoulder blade (the fetal heart can be heard with doppler apparatus such as a sonicaid from 10 weeks of pregnancy). The midwife should listen to the fetal heart for at least 1 minute assessing its rate and rhythm. Normal range is 120–160 beats/ minute. Mothers enjoy listening to their baby's heartbeat heard using the doppler apparatus.

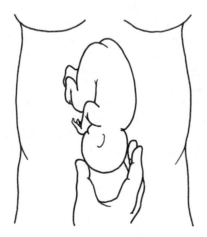

Figure 8.11 Pawlik's grip (to assess mobility of the fetal head).

The abdominal examination is not complete until the results have been documented and the mother informed of findings. Many mothers enjoy being taught how to palpate their own abdomen and identify fetal parts.

Fetal activity

Fetal activity is detectable by the mother from 18 weeks in primigravidae women and from 16 weeks in multiparous women, although there is great variability in these timings between individuals with a range of 15–20 weeks for primiparous women and 14–22 weeks amongst multiparae (O'Dowd and O'Dowd 1985). Activity reaches a maximum at 28–32 weeks decreasing gradually until delivery (Griffin 1984). It has been noted that in cases of fetal compromise, activity is reduced and it ceases 12–48 hours before fetal death (Sadovski and Yaffe 1973). Fetal activity tends to be greatest in the late evening and early morning, but there are large differences in maternal perception of fetal activity and in the levels of activity between fetuses (Ehrstrom 1984). In addition some mothers are unaware of even major fetal movements whereas other can mistake Braxton Hicks contractions for fetal activity (Biale and Mazor 1985). It must be remembered that fetuses have active and quiet periods (Timor-Tritsch et al. 1978) and that the period of testing must be long enough to allow for this.

One tested method of assessing fetal movements is to use the Cardiff 'count-to-ten' fetal activity chart (Pearson and Weaver 1976). The counting is commenced at 9 am using a chart, which is marked in half hour periods. When the woman has felt 10 fetal movements she records the time on the chart. It is expected that an active fetus will 'meet its quota' early on in the day whereas an at-risk fetus may not make 10 movements in the 12 hour-time scale of the chart (Pearson and Weaver 1976). Rayburn (1982) noted that fetal movement counts in a 12 hour period for the majority of babies fell within the range of 10–1000 movements. This is a useful, non-invasive test which can alert the woman at risk of placental insufficiency to contact her midwife or doctor for further investigation. It does not always predict impending problems (Pearson 1981). However it is demanding of the mother's time, is reliant on her perception and can give rise to anxiety (McIlwaine et al. 1980). Draper et al. (1986) found that 55% of women using the chart were reassured by it but 23% of them experienced anxiety at having to assess fetal movements. Shafi et al. (1989) have devised a pictorial chart which can be used for women who have a poor command of English or experience difficulties in reading. Fetal movement charts have been used, together with cardiotocography, in monitoring fetal condition where pregnancy is prolonged. A large-scale evaluation of the counting of fetal movements is under way.

Cardiotocography

The use of cardiotocography (CTGs) to assess fetal condition in the antenatal period is now commonplace for women with high risk pregnancies; it forms a part of the biophysical profile (Baskett 1989). The method currently favoured in the United Kingdom is that of the Non-Stress Test which aims to record changes in fetal heart rate produced by fetal movements or Braxton Hicks contractions (Hammacher 1969). The normal fetal heart rate is 120–160 bpm; there is a beat-to-beat variation of 5–10 bpm and there should be no decelerations or gross irregularities (Hon 1968). A healthy fetus will respond to movement with a small acceleration in heart rate, such a recording is described as 'reactive' (Spencer 1989). Any trace which has little or no beat-to-beat variation, shows decelerations or where no movements are felt during the 20 minutes of the test, should be reported to the medical staff (Spencer 1989).

Conducting a full abdominal examination prior to the procedure assures the midwife of fetal well-being and allows accurate positioning of the transducer. With the mother placed in a comfortable position (such as sitting upright), the ultrasound transducer is coated with a conductive gel and is placed on the position where the fetal heart was best heard. The tocograph (activity) monitor is placed on the uterine fundus and the trace commenced. Fetal activity is recorded using an electronic marker by the mother or the midwife. If, after 20 minutes of monitoring, the trace is reactive, the test is discontinued and the recording paper (carefully labelled) placed with the woman's records. Should the trace be 'flat' or there are no fetal movements, the trace should be continued for a further 20 minutes. If this has no effect, the test may be repeated in a few hours, after discussion with medical staff. Brown and Patrick (1981) have shown that only 1% of fetal heart traces remain unreactive after 120 minutes of recording. Attempting to 'rouse' the fetus by performing a palpation has not been shown to effect the fetal heart rate (Vissier et al. 1981).

Where the woman is considered to have a high-risk pregnancy, CTG recordings may be performed daily; for other women once or twice weekly may be sufficient to confirm well-being. In cases of diminished fetal movement, a reactive trace can put the minds of mothers and obstetricians at rest. CTG recordings are, however, of limited value in measuring beat-to-beat variation since it averages the fetal heart rate creating inaccuracy (Spencer 1989). The use of doppler also makes the quality of some of the recordings difficult to interpret (Spencer 1989). There is little evidence of the predictive value of CTGs or of the biophysical profile in detecting problems of fetal well-being (Mohide and Keirse 1989). Abnormal patterns are more common with preterm babies (Dawes et al. 1982).

It is now possible for midwives to conduct CTG recordings in the mother's own home, the results being signalled along a telephone line to a base station (Dawson et al. 1988). This has the advantage of reducing travelling times and disruption or of reducing the necessity of hospital admission (Steer and Carter 1989). In certain areas the mothers have been able to do the monitoring themselves and to gain confirmation from the distant hospital that all is well (Middlemiss 1987). Steer and Carter (1989) argue that home monitoring of CTGs should not be widely introduced until the value of antenatal CTGs in general have been evaluated.

Hormone assays

These have largely been superseded by direct assessment of fetal well-being. The aim of these tests was to measure maternal serum levels of hormones produced by the placenta and thus assess placental functioning. Serial recordings were necessary to assess the increase or decrease in hormone production, which varies greatly according to gestation. Hormones measured include oestrogens (oestriol, oestrone and oestradiol), human placental lactogen, pregnancy-associated plasma proteins A and B and placental protein 5.

Ultrasound

Obstetric ultrasound was developed in the 1950s and 1960s in Glasgow by Ian Donald utilising technology devised for the detection of submarines (Donald *et al.* 1958). The principle involves producing high-frequency sound waves which, when they reach a junction of one tissue with another, are partially reflected (Chudleigh and Pearce 1986). This echo is detected by the apparatus and converted into an image on a screen. The real-time scanners currently used are very sophisticated, producing a clear image on which fetal activity such as a beating heart can be seen (Chudleigh and Pearce 1986).

For many women ultrasound has become a routine part of their antenatal care, with medical staff using it to confirm findings from history or clinical investigation. The basis for the routine use of ultrasound is however as yet unproven (Neilson and Grant 1989). Whilst it is not directly harmful, long-term benefits and hazards have yet to be evaluated on a sufficiently large scale to detect any problems (Neilson and Grant 1989). For this reason, a degree of caution in its application is advisable. The ultrasound scan may be performed by a radiologist, an obstetrician or a midwife and many women find 'seeing' their baby to be of great reassurance (Reading and Platt 1985).

Findings on ultrasound scan:

- First trimester: Gestation sac visible from 5 weeks.
  Fetal heart beating from 6 weeks.
  Crown rump length (to assess gestation) from 6 weeks.
  Multiple pregnancy.
- Second trimester: Bi-parietal diameter (to assess gestation,
  very accurate until 18 weeks).
  Localisation of the placental site.
  Visualisation of fetal spine to exclude
  neural tube defect − 16 weeks.
  From 18–20 weeks the fetal kidneys, bladder
  and heart can be examined.

● Third trimester: Biparietal diameter ⎫
                      Trunk circumference ⎬ to assess fetal growth
                                           ⎭
                      Placental localisation and condition.
                      Bloodflow in umbilical/fetal vessels.
                      Confirmation of fetal position and
                      presentation (Chudleigh and Pearce 1986).

For an early ultrasound examination to be performed, a full bladder facilitates visualisation; this is not required after 16 weeks gestation when the uterus is easily accessible within the abdomen (Chudleigh and Pearce 1986). Assessment of gestation is most accurate in the first 20 weeks and of limited value thereafter because of the reduced accuracy of the recordings. Although third-trimester serial measurements of biparietal diameters are performed to detect IUGR, they are of limited use; where placental functioning is compromised the last area to suffer is the fetal brain. For this reason many authorities recommend measuring trunk circumference to detect body wasting, a much earlier sign (Chudleigh and Pearce 1986).There are two types of growth retardation detectable using ultrasound:

1. Growth retardation. This is where the fetus is small but in proportion; it results from an early insult such as infection or chromosomal anomaly. The fetal head and brain are small, cells have been lost permanently and there is no facility for catch-up growth (Cunningham *et al.* 1989).
2. Small for gestational age. Growth was satisfactory in early pregnancy but poor placental circulation, due to structural anomalies, has resulted in a deficiency of nutrients. The fetus compensates by allocating the scarce resources to its most sensitive area, the brain, as a result of which the body becomes wasted long before there is a reduction in the rate of head growth. To detect such a condition serial scans are advised at 7–10 day intervals (Chudleigh and Pearce 1986).

   Doppler ultrasound is also employed to assess the uteroplacental and fetoplacental circulations as a guide to the functioning of the fetoplacental unit. There are as yet no completed studies to demonstrate the value or otherwise of this specific test (Redman 1989).

References

Altman D G and Hytten F E (1989) 'Assessment of fetal size and fetal growth' in I Chalmers, M Enkin and M J N C Keirse (eds) *Effective Care in Pregnancy and Childbirth* Ch 26 411–18 Oxford Medical: Oxford

Bader A (1936) 'The significance of the unengaged head in primiparous labour' *Ber ges Gynak u Geburtsh* (Abstract) 31: 395

Baskett T F (1989) 'The fetal biophysical profile' in J Studd (ed) *Progress in Obstetrics and Gynaecology Vol 7* Ch 9 145–59 Churchill Livingstone: Edinburgh

Beazley J M and Kurjak A (1973) 'Prediction of foetal maturity and birthweight by abdominal palpation' *Nursing Times* 14 June 763–5

Beischer N A, Abell D A and Drew J H (1984) 'Intrauterine growth retardation' in J Studd (ed) *Progress in Obstetrics and Gynaecology Vol 4* Ch 6 82–91 Churchill Livingstone: Edinburgh

Biale Y and Mazor M (1985) 'Absence of fetal movements and normal infants' *European Journal of Obstetrics, Gynaecology and Reproductive Biology* 19: 133–6

Brown R and Patrick J (1981) 'The non-stress test. How long is long enough?' *American Journal of Obstetrics and Gynecology* 141: 646–51

Calvert J P, Crean E E, Newcombe R G and Pearson J F (1982) 'Antenatal screening by measurement of symphysis-fundal height' *British Medical Journal* 285: 846–9

Chudleigh P and Pearce M J (1986) *Obstetric Ultrasound: How, Why and When?* Churchill Livingstone: Edinburgh

Crosby M E and Engstrom J L (1989) 'Inter-examiner reliability in fundal height measurement' *Midwives Chronicle* Aug: 254–6

Cunningham F G, MacDonald P C and Gant N F (1989) *Williams' Obstetrics* (18th edn) Prentice Hall: London

Dawes G S, Houghton C R S, Redman C W G and Visser G H A (1982) 'Pattern of the normal fetal heart rate' *British Journal of Obstetrics and Gynaecology* 89: 276–84

Dawson A J, Middlemiss C, Jones E M and Gough N A J (1988) 'Fetal heart rate monitoring by telephone. 1. Development of an integrated system in Cardiff' *British Journal of Obstetrics and Gynaecology* 95(10): 1018–23

Donald I M, MacVicar J and Brown T G (1958) 'Investigations of abdominal masses by pulsed ultrasound' *Lancet* i: 1188–94

Draper J, Field S, Thomas H and Hare M J (1986) 'Women's views on keeping fetal movement charts' *British Journal of Obstetrics and Gynaecology* 93: 334–8

Ehrstrom C (1984) 'Circadian rhythm of fetal movements' *Acta Obstetrica and Gynaecologica Scandanavica* 63: 539–41

Gohari P, Berkowitz R L and Hobbins J C (1977) 'Prediction of intrauterine growth retardation by determination of total intrauterine volume' *American Journal of Obstetrics and Gynecology* 127: 255

Griffin D (1984) 'Fetal activity' in J Studd (ed) *Progress in Obstetrics and Gynaecology Vol 4* Ch 7 92–117 Churchill Livingstone: Edinburgh

Hall M H, Chng P K and MacGillivray I (1980) 'Is routine antenatal care worthwhile?' *Lancet* ii: 78–9

Hammacher K (1969) 'The clinical significance of cardiotocography' in P S Huntingford, E A Huter and E Saling (eds) *Perinatal Medicine* 80–93 Academic Press: New York

Hon E H (1968) *An Atlas of Fetal Heart Rate Patterns* Harty Press: New Haven, Connecticut

Jimenez J M, Tyson J E, Santos-Ramos R and Duenhoelter J H (1979) 'Comparison of obstetric and pediatric assessment of gestational age' *Pediatric Research* 13: 498

Kitchen W H (1968) 'The relationship between birthweight and gestational age in an Australian hospital population' *Australian Paediatric Journal* 4: 29–37

Loeffler F E (1967) 'Clinical foetal weight prediction' *Journal of Obstetrics of the British Commonwealth* 74: 675–7

McFadyen I R (1985) 'Fetal growth' in J Studd (ed) *Progress in Obstetrics and Gynaecology Vol 5* Ch 4 58–77 Churchill Livingstone: Edinburgh

McIlwaine G M, Howat R C L, Dunn F H and MacNaughton M C (1980) 'Perinatal practise and compensation for handicap' *British Medical Journal* 281: 1067

Middlemiss C (1987) 'Fetal cardiotocography by telemetry' *Midwives Chronicle* July: 190–1

Mohide P and Keirse M J N C (1989) 'Biophysical assessment of fetal wellbeing' in I Chalmers, M Enkin and M J N C Keirse (eds) *Effective Care in Pregnancy and Childbirth* Ch 30 477–92 Oxford Medical: Oxford

Neilson J and Grant A (1989) 'Ultrasound in pregnancy' in I Chalmers, M Enkin and M J N C Keirse (eds) *Effective Care in Pregnancy and Childbirth* Ch 27 419–39 Oxford Medical: Oxford

O'Dowd, M J and O'Dowd T M (1985) 'Quickening – a re-evaluation' *British Journal of Obstetrics and Gynaecology* 192: 1037–9

Pearson J F (1981) 'The value of antenatal fetal monitoring' in J Studd (ed) *Progress in Obstetrics and Gynaecology Vol 1* Ch 9 105–124 Churchill Livingstone: Edinburgh

Pearson J F and Weaver J B (1976) 'Fetal activity and fetal wellbeing – an evaluation' *British Medical Journal* 1: 1305

Rayburn W F (1982) 'Antepartum fetal assessment: fetal activity monitoring' *Clinics in Perinatology* 9: 231–52

Reading A E and Platt L D (1985) 'Impact of fetal testing on maternal anxiety' *Journal of Reproductive Behaviour* 30: 907–10

Redman C W G (1989) 'Examination of the placental circulation by Doppler ultrasound' *British Medical Journal* 298: 621–2

Robinson S (1989) 'Caring for childbearing women: the interrelationship between midwifery and medical responsibilities' in S Robinson and A M Thomson (eds) *Midwives, Research and Childbirth Vol 1* Ch 2 8–41 Chapman and Hall: London

Sadovski E and Yaffe H (1973) 'Daily fetal movement recordings and fetal prognosis' *Obstetrics and Gynecology* 41: 845

Scheer K and Nubar J (1976) 'Variation of fetal presentation with gestational age' *American Journal of Obstetrics and Gynecology* 125: 269

Shafi M I, Dover M S, Dyer C A, Byrne P, Constantine G, and Luesley D M (1989) 'Pictorial fetal movement charts in a multiracial antenatal clinic' *British Medical Journal* 298: 1688

Spencer J D (1989) 'Fetal heart rate variability' in J Studd (ed) *Progress in Obstetrics and Gynaecology Vol 7* Ch 7 103–22 Churchill Livingstone: Edinburgh

Steer P J and Carter M C (1989) 'Cardiotocographs at a distance' *British Medical Journal* 299: 933–4

Timor-Tritsch I E, Dierker L J, Hertz R H, Deagan N C and Rosen M G (1978) 'Studies of antepartum behavioural state of the human fetus at term' *American Journal of Obstetrics and Gynecology* 132: 524–8

Vissier G H, Dawes G S and Redman C W G (1981) 'Numerical analysis of the normal human antenatal fetal heart rate' *British Journal of Obstetrics and Gynaecology* 88: 792–802

Wallis S M and Harvey D (1986) 'Fetal growth, intrauterine growth retardation and small for dates babies' in N R C Roberton (ed) *Textbook of Neonatology* Ch 8 119–128 Churchill Livingstone: Edinburgh

White A J (1956) 'Spontaneous cephalic version in the later weeks of pregnancy and its significance in the management of breech presentation' *British Journal of Obstetrics and Gynaecology* 63: 706

9 Parent education

'The prepared childbirth movement provides the mother and father with the means to participate knowledgeably and actively in the birth process.' (Kuczynski 1984, p. 188)

This is the rationale behind the provision of parent education, which has not been proven by research to any significant extent. This chapter will review the issues surrounding parent education and the place of exercise in pregnancy, and suggest how the birth plan can be used as a basis for discussion in teaching sessions.

Parent education classes

Parent education is of importance in assisting a couple in their transition from adults to parents (Perkins 1980a). As childbirth becomes an increasingly rare event and family size reduces, new parents have fewer opportunities to observe at first hand the demands placed upon and the skills required by parents (Simkin and Enkin 1989). The need for a specific educational programme has evolved as the processes of childbirth have been removed from everyday life into an institutional setting. Such provision has to meet these new needs, as well as being a substitute for the loss of shared experiences amongst women (Simkin and Enkin 1989).

The effectiveness of parent education classes is difficult to assess (Clark 1983; Bulger 1988). The measurement of concepts such as confidence, ease, and feeling of being in control is notoriously complex. Most studies have concentrated on the more immediate effects of the education, such as the use of pain relief in labour (Simkin and Enkin 1989) rather than more long-term aspects such as ease of parenting. Studies have shown that education programmes can reduce the need for analgesia in labour (Enkin *et al.* 1972; Kuczynski 1984) although it is hard to determine whether the cause is increased understanding and/or a reduction in anxiety and stress. Hayward (1975) demonstrated that giving information to pre-operative patients reduced the need for post-operative analgesia and the time spent in hospital; this may provide a partial explanation. A study by Enkin *et al.* (1972) controlled for the effects of the mother's motivation by using as a control group women who wished to attend classes but were unable to do so because the classes were oversubscribed. Because of the lack of randomisation between experimental and control groups, it could be argued that those mothers who requested to attend classes early enough to obtain a place differed significantly from those who were too late. The experimental group required significantly less analgesia than those in the control group (Enkin *et al.* 1972). Hibbard *et al.* (1979) showed that, although antenatal education did increase knowledge and reduce anxiety, the extent to which this was achieved was not significant.

The traditional approach to parent education in the United Kingdom (previously known as 'mothercraft' was one of 'chalk and talk' (Perkins 1980a). The content of this was often determined by the philosophy of those giving the information and could be somewhat 'middle-class' in origin (Perkins 1979). Theories surrounding parent education today suggest that it is important to involve both partners, to determine what they wish to gain from the exercise and then to meet these needs (Perkins 1980a; Murphy-Black and Faulkner 1988). The subject areas included in the birth plan can be used as the basis for individual discussion. By teaching individual couples or small groups of like-minded individuals, the midwife is more able to meet their varying demands (Perkins 1980a). Whilst much teaching today is informal around a loose framework of knowledge, there is still a place for a more formal approach to cope with the large numbers who attend evening sessions at some district general hospitals. For some activities, the audience can be subdivided into smaller groups where a more individual approach can be adopted (Murphy-Black and Faulkner 1988). There is an increased frequency of provision of specialist groups for those who previously did not attend or whose needs were not being met. These include sessions for young mothers, especially those without a stable partner, who might be intimidated by being with couples (Todd 1988), groups with specific language or cultural needs and classes for would-be adoptive parents (Fraser 1987).

Since their introduction 'mothercraft' and 'preparation for parenthood' classes have attracted far more educated women from better-off social groups (Perkins 1980b). Whilst most mothers are invited to attend sessions (the Royal College of Midwives in 1966 found that 95% were invited but only 55% attended), women from lower socio-economic groups are far less likely to accept this invitation (Rathbone 1973; Cartwright 1979). McIntosh (1988) speculates that the cause is the lack of perceived value of the classes. This is further compounded by the fact that the usefulness of the sessions is not usually apparent until after the birth itself (McIntyre 1981). Those middle-class women who do attend are usually articulate, motivated and well able to find information for themselves from the media. It could be argued that they would suffer very little if classes were no longer provided.

Although much information-giving occurs at scheduled sessions midwives should not fail to utilise any opportunity to answer questions, give information and provide clarification of points (Simkin and Enkin 1989). There are many occasions on which it is possible for the midwife to give an introduction to parent education in early pregnancy. These could include visits to the general practitioner's surgery, in the antenatal clinic during the initial visit, or best of all, in the woman's own home while taking the woman's history. Although in the United Kingdom there is usually provision in large hospitals for parent education, there may also be sessions organised by the community midwife in local health centres or even in the woman's own home. These last two have the advantages that local mothers can get to know one another and establish links which can continue for many years whilst reducing any travelling time (Perkins 1980a). Mothers in an antenatal ward provide a bored and to some extent captive audience for preparation for parenthood teaching. The disadvantage of this is that their partners are rarely present and cannot take part.

In most centres, the classes (6–8 in number) follow a similar pattern, with one session in early pregnancy and weekly meetings from 28 weeks onwards (Perkins 1979, 1980a). It must be questioned whether this type of provision is appropriate or adequate. As Perkins (1980a) comments, these classes are arranged at times to suit the service and not specifically to meet the needs of clients. For example, preparation-for-labour classes which welcome the attendance of fathers are unlikely to be attended by many if they are scheduled during the day. By the time most programmes begin (usually after 28 weeks) many women will have ceased work. It is helpful if women can start the course whenever it is convenient (although the sessions on labour are best taken together), as this increases the woman's chances of being able to attend all the sessions before she delivers. It must be remembered that most couples although motivated to attend will be apprehensive about what will be involved and about the knowledge of other couples (Rogers 1971). Sensitive 'ice breaking' activities at the start of each session together with a non-authoritarian attitude by the teacher can help to put people at ease (Murphy-Black and Faulkner 1988). Thought should be given to the seating arrangements with chairs placed in a circle being less threatening than formal rows with their associated memories of school attendance (Murphy-Black and Faulkner 1988).

The midwife must be sure of her material and be well prepared so that she inspires confidence but not pretending if she is unable to answer specific queries (Perkins 1980a). Each session should ideally be organised around a core topic which is briefly explained at a level appropriate to the audience (Murphy-Black and Faulkner 1988). Plenty of time should then be allocated to further questions by which the group can express their individual needs. It may also be helpful when describing the next session to seek any areas to which the group would like to give particular attention.

When deciding on the content of the session, it is also necessary to consider the expertise available (Perkins 1980a). Whilst a hospital could call upon the services of an obstetric physiotherapist, a dietitian or an anaesthetist, it is unlikely that such people would be available in the community. For classes provided locally the advantages of local contacts can be increased by utilising for example, a general practitioner, a health visitor and local mothers to provide some of the input. Throughout, however, the midwife is the central facilitator of the sessions; the other speakers are there to complement her contributions. However it must be remembered that midwives require specific preparation for this teaching role (which may be part of their formal education), something which has not always occurred (Brammer 1977).

Changes in the education programme for health visitors in the UK may alter their role in antenatal education. Although they receive teaching in health education, Hyde (1982) commented that it was not advisable for health visitors without a midwifery qualification to teach about pregnancy, labour and early child care. This will become increasingly relevant, since potential health visitors now require no formal experience of maternity care.

Parent education curriculum

The following is an outline of a traditional education programme (adapted from Gillett 1985; Bulger 1988; Clements 1989). It should be remembered that it is helpful to introduce the key points before covering them in detail and finally to sum up. This is necessary to help parents remember (Rogers 1971).

These are purely descriptive studies, containing no evaluation. Comments on the content by Perkins (1980a) from her evaluation of antenatal education are included.

14–18 weeks   Physiology of pregnancy including minor disorders. Fetal growth. Exercise in pregnancy. Diet. Dental health. Sexual activity in pregnancy. (It is most important that this session together with information about how the maternity services work and what to buy for the new baby should be as early as possible to allow maximum benefit for the couple (Perkins 1980a).)

1. Relaxation I. Exercises for childbirth.
2. Relaxation II. Breathing exercises. Squatting and position for birth.
3. Physiology of labour. Management. Positions. Normal, forceps and operative. Delivery.
4. Pain relief. Tour of labour suite.
5. The postnatal period in hospital and at home.
6. Care of the neonate, with a demonstration baby bath. Perkins (1980a) suggests that since these topics are taught

after the birth the time would be more usefully spent in a discussion of more general issues about parenting.

7. Infant feeding.
8. Childcare. Immunisation. Weaning.

This last session is usually given by a health visitor and it may possibly be viewed by mothers as the most important in the long term. It can be delayed until after the birth. The baby bath (session 6) is usually demonstrated using a slightly older baby (which is preferable to using a doll (Perkins 1980a)). The mother can be asked by the audience how she has adapted to motherhood. The infant feeding session should include both breast and bottle feeding. If a breast-feeding mother can come with her baby to this session, this can be a useful role model, which can help those unsure of feeding methods to decide (Coombes 1979). Depending on the wishes of the audience, alternative medical techniques such as homeopathy in pregnancy, acupressure in labour, and baby massage may be covered.

One key criticism of the content of the classes by Perkins (1980a) was that they did little to widen the women's choice or to foster variation in practices.

Whilst the above refers to classes provided within the NHS there are other individuals and organisations who offer such a service. They include independent midwives and the National Childbirth Trust.

Exercise in pregnancy

There are three main areas of exercise which are undertaken in pregnancy. These are general exercise, relaxation and exercises specifically devised to help in labour and at the time of delivery. The principle regarding general exercise is that if the mother has been exercising prior to pregnancy, there is no reason why it should not continue. It has been shown that women who take regular exercise during pregnancy have a lower frequency of delivery by caesarean section (Hall and Kaufman 1987). However, it is not advisable for women unused to strenuous physical exercise to begin this for the first time in pregnancy (American College of Obstetricians and Gynecologists 1986). Regular exercise of whatever type encourages muscle tone, improves posture and stimulates the circulation (Shepherd 1985). It is also enjoyable (Barr 1985). As pregnancy progresses, the woman may find her chosen form of exercise becoming increasingly difficult. She can be assured that walking is good exercise and also that swimming, with its added buoyancy, facilitates easy muscle movement. In some areas there are specific water exercise classes for pregnant women. The use of these has not been evaluated. Other types of exercise described by Balaskas and Gordon (1987) include stretching, strengthening, aerobic and centring exercises.

There are many different types of relaxation exercises used in pregnancy; many involve consciously relaxing particular muscle groups and/or specific patterns of breathing. These can be used both in pregnancy to assist sleeping and in labour to reduce pain and tension. By every woman becoming aware of her own natural rhythms of breathing, she can develop those techniques which are of most assistance (Balaskas and Gordon 1987). It is usually advised that breathing should become shallower and lighter as labour progresses (Mackay 1984). Shallow breathing prevents any further increase in intra-abdominal pressure, thus preventing more pain. At all times breathing should be natural and not forced (Mackay 1984). In transition (at the end of the first stage) or during delivery, it can be helpful to use breathing to prevent pushing (Mackay 1984). A short quick breath out (like blowing a crumb off the back of your hand) which relaxes the diaphragm, is helpful at this time to control delivery. Another pattern is to follow three such quick breaths, with a fourth which is much slower and more akin to extinguishing a candle.

Exercises which will assist with the birth include those involving the practice of postures which may be used in labour. The positions available for labour and birth vary from country to country depending on local preference and the skill of the midwives. One of the more common alternative positions for birth is squatting. Because women in the West are unused to squatting for long periods, practice in this position is required (Kitzinger 1989). At the start, support can be used, such as resting the buttocks on a small pile of books (telephone directories are good) or leaning against a wall. Squatting can also be practised with support from a partner, especially if this position will be used for delivery. Other positions helpful in labour include resting on 'all fours' and kneeling while leaning forward onto a chair or low table to reduce backache. For a full description of appropriate exercises see Balaskas (1983) and Balaskas and Gordon (1987).

Birth plans

A birth plan is a written statement of the wishes of the woman and her partner regarding the conduct of their labour and delivery. It should be prepared prior to the labour by the couple and, if they will be accompanied by a known midwife, in consultation with her. The contents of the birth plan can be used as the basis for topic selection is preparation-for-labour classes or as a stimulus for discussion. The birth plan covers a number of areas of care and it is meant to be permissive rather than an inflexible; however conflicts may arise in their use where the clinical judgement of the midwife differs from the wishes of the mother. Birth plans are of great help where the midwife caring for the woman is unknown to her. It can be difficult for a woman in labour to articulate clearly her wishes or to make rational decisions whilst in pain. The plan must be based on discussion of the issues involved. It is not a list of prohibitions, nor should it be so restrictive that the woman feels a failure if its contents are not adhered to. It is part of the process of preparing for and contributing to the birth.

Areas which are usually included are:

1. Choice of birth companion(s) (including other children).
2. Preferred birth attendant (for example, she may wish to be cared for solely

by women or not by a medical student). This should be a realistic decision depending on the place of birth.

3. Admission procedures. Although perineal shaving and bowel preparation are no longer routine procedures in labour some women request to have them or that they never be used.
4. Clothing during labour. Many women prefer to wear their own nightdress or their partner's shirt rather than the one provided by the hospital.
5. Mobility in labour, including the use of the bath or shower.
6. Diet in labour.
7. Fetal monitoring – intermittent, continuous, telemetry.
8. Rupturing the membranes.
9. Augmentation of labour.
10. Pain relief.
11. Position for delivery.
12. Parental involvement, for example, partner cutting the cord.
13. Baby delivered onto mother's abdomen.
14. Use of an episiotomy.
15. If an instrumental or operative delivery, presence of partner?
16. Active management of the third stage.
17. Breast/bottle feeding after delivery.

(Adapted from Jackson 1986; Kitzinger 1987; Crooke and Smith 1988.

Depending on circumstances, a free choice may not be available in all areas. For example, where the woman has had a previous postpartum haemorrhage, the midwife might advise her to use active management of the third stage. The plan should be completed after full discussion with the woman, her partner and (if possible) the midwife. It is usually completed at about 34 – 36 weeks gestation. It may be preferable after discussion for the woman to take the plan away to think about it further. One copy of the plan is filed in the notes and the woman retains the other.

References

American College of Obstetricians and Gynecologists (1986) *Women and Exercise* Technical Bulletin No 87 (Sept)

Balaskas J (1983) *Active Birth* Unwin: London

Balaskas J and Gordon G (1987) *The Encyclopaedia of Pregnancy and Birth* Macdonald Orbis: London

Barr C (1985) 'The relationship of physical activity to mental health' *Public Health Reports* 100(2): 195–202

Brammer A C (1977) *An Enquiry into the Classes Provided by the Maternity Services In England in 1975* Maws Educational Research Scholarship 1974/5 Royal College of Midwives: London

Bulger D (1988) 'Perinatal education' in T W Hudson, M A Reinhart, S D Rose and G K Stewart (eds) *Clinical Preventive Medicine* Ch 7 43–8 Little, Brown: Boston, Massachussetts

Cartwright A (1979) *The Dignity of Labour* Tavistock: London

Clark J (1983) 'Evaluating health visiting practice' *Health Visitor* 56: 205–8

Clements J (1989) 'Antenatal education' *Nursing Standard* 4(1): 51–4

Coombes S (1979) 'Breast feeding: a problem conquered' *Nursing Times Community Outlook* 7S: 387–9

Crooke L I and Smith V A (1988) 'Birth plans' *Maternal and Child Health* 13 (5): 116–21

Enkin M W, Smith S L, Dermer S W and Emmett J O (1972) ' An adequately controlled study of the effectiveness of PPM training' in N Morris (ed) *Psychosomatic Medicine in Obstetrics and Gynecology* 62–7 Karger: Basle

Fraser J (1987) 'Parenthood education for adoptive parents' *Midwives Chronicle* (Sept) i: 276–8

Gillett J (1985) 'A childbirth preparation course' *Senior Nurse* 3(3): 12–15

Hall D C and Kaufman D A (1987) 'Effects of aerobic and strength conditioning on pregnancy outcomes' *American Journal of Obstetrics and Gynecology* 157: 1199

Hayward J (1975) *Information – A Prescription Against Pain* Royal College of Nursing: London

Hibbard B M, Robinson J O, Pearson J F, Rosen M and Taylor A (1979) 'Effectiveness of antenatal education' *Health Education Journal* 38(2): 39–46

Hyde B I (1982) 'Curriculum planning for antenatal health education' *Nurse Education Today* 1(6): 6–10

Jackson P (1986) 'The Huddersfield birthplan' *Maternal and Child Health* 11(1): 14–17

Kitzinger S (1987) *Freedom and Choice in Childbirth* Penguin: Harmondsworth

Kitzinger S (1989) 'Childbirth and society' in I Chalmers, M Enkin and M J N C Keirse (eds) *Effective Care in Pregnancy and Childbirth* Ch 6 99–109 Oxford Medical: Oxford

Kuczynski H J (1984) 'Benefits of childbirth education' *Midwives Chronicle* June: 188–92

Mackay D (1984) *Relaxation with Breathing* National Childbirth Trust, Mid Cheshire Branch

McIntosh J (1988) 'A consumer view of birth preparation classes' *Midwives Chronicle* Jan: 8–9

McIntyre S (1981) *Expectations and Experiences of First Pregnancy* Occ. Paper No. 5 Institute of Medical Sociology: Aberdeen

Murphy-Black T and Faulkner A (1988) *Antenatal Group Skills Training* Wiley: Chichester

Perkins E R (1979) 'Defining need: An analysis of varying teaching goals in antenatal classes' *International Journal of Nursing Studies* 16: 275–82

Perkins E R (1980a) *Education for Childbirth and Parenthood* Croom-Helm: London

Perkins E R (1980b) 'The pattern of women's attendance at antenatal classes: Is it good enough?' *Health Education Journal* 39: 3–9

Rathbone B (1973) *Focus on New Mothers* Royal College of Nursing: London

Rogers J (1971) *Adults Learning* Penguin: Harmonsdworth

Royal College of Midwives (1966) *Preparation for Parenthood* RCM: London

Shepherd R (1985) 'The value of physical fitness in preventive medicine' in D Evered and J Whelan (eds) *The Value of Physical Fitness* CIBA Foundation Symposium No 110 Pitman Medical: London

Simkin P and Enkin M (1989) 'Antenatal classes' in I Chalmers, M Enkin and M J N C Keirse (eds) *Effective Care in Pregnancy and Childbirth* Ch 20 318–34 Oxford Medical: Oxford

Todd J E (1988) 'Teenage club at the Royal Berkshire' *Midwives Chronicle* Aug: 238

10   Early teenage pregnancy

This chapter concentrates upon the subject of early teenage pregnancy, that is, conception occurring to women aged 16 and younger. It is amongst this group of young women that pregnancy has its most major effects physically, socially and emotionally (Russell 1988). Russell (1988) comments that for teenagers aged 17 years and older the advent of a pregnancy need not be so traumatic. Marriage is permitted, basic education is complete and reproduction is at its most 'efficient'. Birch (1989) notes that age-specific maternal mortality rates show that teenagers aged 16–19 had rates lower than the national average, whereas for those aged less than 16 years the figure was 3–4 times the mean. Both Fogel (1984) and Birch (1989) point out that adverse outcomes are usually related to multiple deprivations, late booking, poor antenatal care and restricted diet.

Numbers of early teenage pregnancies

The number of babies born to schoolgirls (of all ages) in the United Kingdom has stayed fairly constant at about 1050/year (Birch 1989). The abortion rate for those aged under 16 years has increased greatly, doubling between 1977 and 1983 to 4000/year (Black 1986) and increasing to 5240 in 1985 (Office of Population Census and Surveys 1985). However, because the proportion of under 16 year olds in the population has fallen, the trend in the fertility rate is upwards. Despite the levelling off of the number of pregnancies in all those aged under 16, there has been a marked rise in pregnancies occurring amongst the under 14s which accounted for 4% of schoolgirl pregnancies in 1978 but 6% by 1983 (Office of Population Census and Surveys 1983).

The situation in the United Kingdom seems minor in comparison with the one million pregnancies occurring annually to teenagers in the United States (Fogel 1984). These form 20% of all births and are the most common reason for young women to end their education prematurely (Kuczynski 1988). This in an educational system where it is more usual than in the United Kingdom to continue full-time schooling until at least 18 years of age and where graduation from high school is the minimum requirement for all but the very lowest paid jobs.

Much thought has been given as to the reasons why pregnancy in those aged under 14 is becoming more common. Until the mid 1950s the figures were very low. A slow increase occurred until the early 1960s when the numbers increased rapidly (Russell 1982). A partial explanation could be the reduction of the age of menarche in the developed world from 17 at the turn of the century to 12–13 years at the end of the 1980s (British Broadcasting Corporation 1990). This has lead to physical maturity occurring long before the necessary psychological maturity (Short 1978). The introduction of the 1967 Abortion Act resulted in a stabilisation in the number of births but an escalating proportion of therapeutic abortions (Russell 1988).

Birch (1986) in her study has shown that young pregnant teenagers were very unlikely to have received any sex education in the home. Only 64% received any instruction in school, often becoming pregnant before the sessions started or being absent as a result of truancy. This is contrary to some opinion that sex education only encourages promiscuity (Birch 1989). In the study, most young women had stable relationships, three-quarters having known the baby's father for at least 6 months at the time of conception, with two-thirds of the women becoming pregnant during their first sexual relationship (Birch 1986).

Both knowledge and availability of contraception to the under 16s is limited (Miller 1984). This has been complicated in the United Kingdom by the Gillick Ruling where professionals were prevented from giving advice to anyone under the age of 16 without their parent's permission. Although the House of Lords overruled this case, there is still confusion amongst teenagers as to their rights. It takes a very brave and motivated schoolgirl to request contraception from such an establishment figure as her family doctor. In addition, many teenagers say that using contraception removes spontaneity and implies promiscuity (Birch 1989). The use of contraception is also connected with the adolescent developing an awareness and an acceptance of their own sexuality (Kuczynski 1988).

This chapter will consider the obstetric aspects of early teenage pregnancy before discussing financial provision, housing, education, prevention of further pregnancies and social consequences.

Obstetric aspects

One of the major differences between pregnancy in young teenagers and those in other women is the delay in recognising and reporting the pregnancy (Russell 1982). The younger the girl, the longer it takes for her to recognise and acknowledge the significance of symptoms such as amenorrhoea (Birch 1986). The awareness that they are pregnant is very difficult to deal with, so much so that teenagers are more likely to do nothing than to tell someone, most notably their parents (Birch 1989). Birch (1986) noted that some young women either dropped hints to family members or left clues such as antenatal clinic cards lying around.

When considering seeking professional help, 27% of 533 teenagers sampled in one study visited their doctors for the first time during the second trimester. When questioned 45% stated that the delay was not deliberate but due to not knowing that they were pregnant (Simms and Smith 1984). In the same survey, nearly 38% of under 17s did not attend a hospital antenatal clinic until after 20 weeks gestation. Because approximately 3 pregnancies are terminated for each one which continues amongst 15 year olds, this has implications for maternal safety, whether the pregnancy continues or is terminated. The risks of therapeutic abortion are necessarily increased because safety falls with increasing gestation (Russell 1988). In addition, the younger the woman, the more likely she is to have physical complications such as cervical lacerations following the termination of pregnancy; these occurred in 5.4% of women aged 16 and under, but only 1.4% of older teenagers (Russell 1982). Such young women require considerable counselling and support while deciding whether or not to continue with the pregnancy. This is not a decision which can be made for them. Amongst teenagers in one survey, those who had the pregnancy terminated without it being their idea were likely to be pregnant again soon afterwards (Birch 1986).

It is important to give the objective facts about all outcomes. Having the baby adopted is no longer a popular choice (Birch 1989). Where the pregnancy continues, the young teenager is at more risk of pregnancy complications than older women. Whether this is a simple aspect of age is disputed (Russell 1982; Fogel 1984; Birch 1989). Risks are especially high where the young woman has not completed her physical development, including the adolescent growth spurt and full pelvic development (Fogel 1984). It appears that outcome is related to a combination of factors including poverty, age, race, socio-economic status, nutrition and standard of antenatal care, the last two of which are of major importance (Fogel 1984). The chaotic lifestyle of some teenagers, where high-risk activities, such as smoking, drinking alcohol, solvent and drug abuse occur, will further increase the risks (Fogel 1984).

The major obstetrical complications experienced by pregnant teenagers are hypertensive disease, anaemia and antepartum haemorrhage. Most of these are related to low socioeconomic status and poor antenatal care (Fogel 1984). Anaemia in teenagers is very much related to diet and income, regardless of whether or not the woman is pregnant (Birch 1989). Antenatal care can only hope to detect and ameliorate these conditions if the young women are attending. Since they are more likely both to book late and to default from care (Simms and Smith 1984), those most in need of care are least likely to receive it (Birch 1989).

There is no evidence that delivery complications and caesarean section rates are raised in young teenagers (Russell 1982). It is, however, agreed that there is an increase in the proportion of low-birthweight babies, mainly as a result of preterm birth, especially where related to premature rupture of the membranes (Russell 1982; Fogel 1984). Midwives should pay particular attention to informing teenagers of the signs and symptoms of preterm labour to ensure prompt attendance at the hospital. In the United States, some teenage antenatal clinics give their clients a simple algorithm to follow which permits them to assess the normality or otherwise of their symptoms and the actions which should be taken (Silverton, unpublished data). Perinatal mortality is highest amongst babies born to women aged less than 20, although it is difficult to separate age from all the other contributing factors such as socio-economic status.

Although we have considered the obstetric outcome of early teenage pregnancy, what these young women often lack is educational and psychological support. They may suffer acute embarrassment at having to attend clinics with older, married women (Simms and Smith 1984). Many schemes have been established to assist these young women in their transition to motherhood. Black (1986) suggests that such special antenatal clinics are only feasible in large cities. Whilst this is probably true, there is nothing to prevent individual midwives both in hospitals and the community providing alternative or additional services for such young women. Todd (1988) and Lapthorn (1988) describe one such scheme to provide parent education on an informal basis for teenagers; unfortunately they do not give any evaluation of their programme. Such specific provision allows the women to share their common experiences and feelings while gaining and giving support. In the United States, where the need is greater than in the United Kingdom, teenage antenatal clinics have been established where care and teaching can be given. The service is provided free to those without personal or state medical insurance (Silverton, unpublished data). These services are funded by local government or charities such as the March of Dimes.

When giving advice to pregnant teenagers, for example on diet, it is important to remember that whilst the teenager may know what she should eat and why, she may be lacking the specific motivation, finance or ability to change her behaviour, especially where this conflicts with the beliefs of her peer group. The most one can do is to state the facts clearly, describe the effects of following particular decisions and demonstrate an awareness of the individual's culture and social values.

Finance

Money is a problem for most teenage mothers, but especially to those under the age of 16 who are still their parents' responsibility. In the United Kingdom, these women are only able to claim child benefit and the additional single parent benefit on behalf of their baby. They have no other entitlement. Since they are already exempt (on account of age) from prescription and dental charges they receive no further benefit from this provision. When the teenager's mother claims child benefit on behalf of her grandchild, single parent benefit cannot be claimed.

Changes in United Kingdom social security regulations since 1988 mean that teenagers between 16 and 18 years old are not eligible for long-term income support unless they undertake government-sponsored training schemes for which they receive a training allowance. Since pregnant teenagers are already from less stable backgrounds with poor achievement and high rates of school truancy, such schemes are unpopular. After delivery, the mother is eligible for benefit on behalf of herself and her baby. Williams *et al.* (1987) have highlighted the extent of poverty amongst single teenage mothers in their survey in Glasgow. They conclude by asking whether inequalities in health will continue and be perpetuated, as poverty has an influence on both maternal and child health (Jennings and Sheldon 1985).

Housing

Money and the provision of housing for teenage mothers are very closely linked. Whilst most young teenagers are living in the parental home (or in local authority care) at the time of conception, some may leave or be expelled by their parents when the pregnancy becomes known. For the under 16s the local authority has a duty to house such young women, usually in foster care rather than childrens' homes. Some youngsters may, however, leave home and move to the big cities in search of work. This is hard to find especially given the shortage of suitable affordable accommodation. When forced to sleep rough the risks of violence, prostitution and drug abuse increase, creating a spiral of worsening problems.

Whilst the majority of young teenagers remain with their families, conditions may be far from ideal – overcrowding is a big problem (Birch 1986). This is, however, usually the only option. Mother and baby homes are often run in conjunction with religious organisations, but are now becoming rare. They do, however, allow the mother some breathing space so she can sort out her priorities. Local authority housing is limited, with many areas having long waiting lists. It is unusual for a teenager to obtain accommodation before the birth. Following delivery she may be given a place in bed and breakfast accommodation until a more permanent solution can be found, although such accommodation has been associated with adverse effects for both mother and baby. Such provision usually applies to teenagers over the age of 18 years as those younger are not of the legal age of majority and cannot be 'key holders' or hold a lease. For those who are younger, the social worker attached to the case may act as guarantor to the landlord until the woman is of age. Where tenancies are awarded, they tend to be in less desirable areas which can later reduce her chances of finding employment. Some teenagers are sufficiently mature to care for themselves, but others without experience can become isolated, further increasing their deprivation.

Choosing to marry does not ease the accommodation problem but it does widen the options (the couple may live with the father's or mother's family, which may itself not be ideal) but it can reduce the sense of isolation. The effects of early marriage will be discussed later.

Education

It is in the area of education, and the limitations that this disruption places on future prospects, that early teenage pregnancy has some of its major effects (Fogel 1984). Employment and future financial security depend very much on scholastic achievement, with basic numeracy and literacy being of prime importance (Joint Working Party 1979). Teenagers from unstable backgrounds with poor school attendance records may find that an early pregnancy hinders their future chances (Russell 1983). Not only does pregnancy curtail education but to some extent psychological development and personal choice are limited (Kuczynski 1988).

The 1979 report of the Joint Working Party on Pregnant Schoolgirls and Schoolgirl Mothers, which carried out in-depth interviews with 30 pregnant schoolgirls showed that 22% had left school by the end of the first trimester and 74% by the end of the fifth month. Of the teenagers in their survey, 61% received no education between leaving school and the birth of their baby. After the birth, 53% of those still below the statutory leaving age did not return to school (Joint Working Party 1979). These are youngsters who have a legal requirement to attend school. Local educational authorities can, within certain constraints, provide alternatives where it is impractical for the student to continue in regular education (Joint Working Party 1979).

There is no evidence that continuing in school is detrimental to the teenager with a normal pregnancy (Tyrrell 1984); indeed it has the advantage of not isolating the girl from her networks of social support. Staff will need to make allowances for clinic attendance and the restriction on some physical activities (Kuczynski 1988). There may be a perceived conflict between the welfare of the pregnant individual and the interests of other pupils. Indeed it could be argued that a real-life portrayal of the reality of the situation could well prove an effective deterrent. Parental support for continuing in education is vital to improve chances of success, especially after delivery. If suitable childcare arrangements can be made, there is nothing to prevent the mother returning to school after the birth (Kuczynski 1988). To assist this, it is helpful if contact can be maintained during the break in education (Russell 1983). By keeping in touch, the staff will improve the young woman's chances of completing her education with all the attendant advantages for future job prospects (Kuczynski 1988).

Home tuition, although theoretically available, depends on local provision (Joint Working Party 1979). Although it does not help with social isolation, some teenagers benefit greatly from the intensive individual attention. In some areas, home tuition is only given to those undertaking examinations, which discriminates further against the non-academic student with the previous poor performance record (Joint Working Party 1979). In other areas, special educational units have been established for schoolgirl mothers (Joint Working Party 1979). These have the advantage of reducing stigma and embarrassment, but may isolate the young women from the educational mainstream. Such provision has had success with teenagers who were poor school attenders previously. Individualised teaching concentrating on basic mathematics and English, together with subjects such as childcare, sewing and office skills can be of great help (Silverton 1988). Antenatal and postnatal care can be given by visiting midwives and health visitors. A social worker may be attached to the unit. Return to regular schooling may be made more difficult, due to the prolonged period away and the difference in aim and content of educational programmes (Joint Working Party 1979).

Social aspects

'Why must they [teenagers] wait until they pass through an illegitimate birth before having access to contraceptives?' (Kuczynski 1988, p 236).

It is vital that good contraceptive advice is made available from an early age. Access to contraception has not been shown to increase promiscuity. Since today's teenagers mature physically before they do emotionally (Short 1978), it is necessary to be more explicit about the consequences of unprotected sexual intercourse and to emphasise that contraceptive use implies responsibility rather than promiscuity. To the emotionally immature adolescent, a baby of their own who they can love may seem an attractive proposition (Birch 1986; British Broadcasting Corporation 1990). Pregnant schoolgirls are, on the whole, unable to comprehend the duties and responsibilities of motherhood or the restrictions that this will place on their own development (Birch 1989). Perhaps teenage mothers could be encouraged themselves to highlight the less attractive aspects of their situations?

Where the teenage mother remains with her family, this can have a significant effect on its stability. Russell (1982) demonstrated an increase in breakdown of parental marriages following an early pregnancy in the family. Even where the baby is accepted, it may further exacerbate problems of overcrowding and finance (Birch 1986). In some circumstances the baby is raised by its grandparents as its mother's 'sister'. This can produce psychological problems and intergenerational tensions. It does, however, allow the young mother a greater chance to develop her own life.

Campbell (1968) wrote that the young teenage mother who keeps her baby has 90% of her 'life script' written for her. She drops out of school, is unable to find employment that pays sufficient to care for herself or her child and she has few choices for the future. If she chooses to marry, this may cause further problems. Breakdowns occur most commonly where one or both of the partners is aged under 20 at the time of the marriage (Dominian 1979). Pregnancy before the marriage increases the risk of future divorce (Thornes and Collard 1979). It seems that the worst outcomes occur for women from lower socio-economic groups who are more likely to continue with the pregnancy, not give the baby up for adoption and to have housing, money and marriage problems (Russell 1982).

The future for children from one-parent families depends very much on social and economic circumstances. Poorer families have more health problems, the children have delayed physical and developmental milestones and more referrals to hospital and social service departments (Jennings and Sheldon 1985; Parker and Ness 1986). Midwives have a vital role to play in educating youngsters of all ages about the effects of early parenthood and the necessity of taking responsibility for one's own future. Once a pregnancy does occur, the midwife's role is one of support, encouragement and education. This is not easy, as the teenager concerned may be working through the developmental processes of adolescence. The midwife must be prepared to continue with her non-judgemental and non-directional approach, despite possible displays of bad temper and antisocial behaviour from the teenager (Silverton 1988). It may seem to be a thankless task, but any gains will be hard won and all the more important when viewed against the blight that an early pregnancy can have on the life of the young women.

References

Birch D (1986) Schoolgirl Pregnancy in Camberwell Unpublished MD Thesis University of London

Birch D (1989) 'Schoolgirl pregnancies' in J Studd (ed) *Progress in Obstetrics and Gynaecology VII* Ch 8 75–90 Churchill Livingstone: Edinburgh

Black D (1986) 'Schoolgirl mothers' *British Medical Journal* 293: 1047

British Broadcasting Corporation (1990) *The Child Mothers* Horizon Originally screened 5/6/90

Campbell A (1968) 'The role of family planning in the reduction of poverty' *Journal of Marriage and the Family* 30: 236–40

Dominian J (1979) 'Social factors and marital pathology' *British Medical Journal* 2: 531–2

Fogel C I (1984) 'The adolescent mother: special problems' in M J Houston (ed) *Maternal and Infant Health Care* Ch 5 92–121 Churchill Livingstone: Ediburgh

Jennings A J and Sheldon M G (1985) 'Review of the health of children in one parent families' *Journal of the Royal College of General Practitioners* 35: 478–83

Joint Working Party on Pregnant Schoolgirls and Schoolgirl Mothers (1979) *Pregnant at School* National Council for One Parent Families and the Community Development Trust: London

Kuczynski H J (1988) 'An approach to preventing adolescent pregnancy' *Midwives Chronicle* Aug: 234–37

Lapthorn J (1988) 'The midwife's account' *Midwives Chronicle* Aug: 239–41

Miller S H (1984) 'Childbearing and childrearing among the very young' *Children Today* May/June: 26–9

Office of Population Censuses and Surveys (1983) *Birth Statistics England and Wales 1983* HMSO: London

Office of Population Censuses and Surveys (1985) *Birth Statistics England and Wales 1985* HMSO: London

Parker M and Ness M (1986) 'Supporting city mothers' *Nursing Times Community Outlook* Oct: 18–23

Russell J K (1982) *Early Teenage Pregnancy* Churchill Livingstone: Edinburgh

Russell J K (1983) 'School pregnancies—medical, social and educational considerations' *British Journal of Hospital Medicine* 29: 159–66

Russell J K (1988) 'Early teenage pregnancy' *Maternal and Child Health* 13(2): 43–6

Short R V (1978) 'Fertility in adolescence' *Journal of Biosocial Science* 5: (Suppl) 255–6

Silverton L I (1988) *Midwifery Education in the USA* School of Social Studies: University College of Swansea

Simms M and Smith C (1984) 'Teenage mothers: late attenders at medical and antenatal care' *Midwife, Health Visitor and Community Nurse* 20(6): 192–200

Thornes B and Collard J (1979) *Who Divorces?* Routledge and Keegan Paul: London
Todd J E (1988) 'Teenage club at the Royal Berkshire' *Midwives Chronicle* Aug: 238
Tyrrell S (1984) 'Schoolgirl mothers' *Nursing Times* 80(23 May): 29–31
Williams S, Forbes J F, McIlwaine G M, and Rosenberg K (1987) 'Poverty and teenage pregnancy' *British Medical Journal* 294: 20–1

Suggestions for further reading

Bury, J (1984) *Teenage Pregnancy in Britain* Birth Control Trust: London
Coyne, A M (1986) *Schoolgirl Mothers* Health Education Council (Research Report No 2): London

11   Bleeding in early pregnancy

Vaginal bleeding at any stage of pregnancy is a frightening experience for a woman (Moulder 1990). The resulting anxiety and uncertainty can blight the remainder of the pregnancy. In early pregnancy (that is before 20 weeks of amenorrhoea), fear of spontaneous abortion (miscarriage) is paramount (Moulder 1990). Vaginal bleeding in early pregnancy is experienced by 16% of women (South and Naldrett 1973). This chapter focuses on the causes of bleeding in early pregnancy, their management (by medical and midwifery/nursing staff) and the effects on the parents. The topic of bereavement in relation to childbirth is discussed at greater length in Chapter 31. The final part of this chapter concerns the area of therapeutic abortion, legislation, practice and outcomes.

Abortion is still one of the leading causes of maternal mortality world-wide, although it only led to five deaths in England and Wales between 1985 and 1987 (Department of Health 1991). Of the eleven deaths in England and Wales between 1982 and 1984, four followed spontaneous abortion and the remainder legally induced abortion (Department of Health 1989).

The majority of women who experience bleeding in the early stages of pregnancy remain at home (Moulder 1990). Many do not seek specialist help whilst others are cared for by their GP (Everett *et al*. 1987). A woman admitted to hospital may, according to local policy and gestation, be cared for in gynaecology or antenatal wards (Moulder 1990). The community midwife (especially in rural areas) may be the first person to be called. A knowledge of the causes of bleeding and their management is needed to complete the theoretical basis of midwifery practice.

Estimates of the number of women who experience bleeding in early pregnancy vary greatly due to differences and inaccuracies in reporting (Cunningham *et al.* 1989). Early fetal loss before pregnancy has been confirmed or before the woman has sought professional help is rarely reported. Edmonds *et al.* (1982) suggest that up to 50–60% of fertilised ova fail to progress beyond 12 weeks gestation, the vast majority of which (up to 90%) are lost very early (before 6–8 weeks after the last menstrual period) and are unrecognised by the mother (Edmonds *et al.* 1982).

Causes of bleeding

1. Implantation bleeding.
2. 'Breakthrough' bleeding.
3. Cervical lesions:
   (a) erosions,
   (b) polyps,
   (c) carcinoma.
4. Ectopic gestation.
5. Abortion.
6. Hydatidiform mole.

Implantation bleeding

Implantation or decidual bleeding occurs approximately 10 days after conception (or 4 days prior to the expected menstrual period) (Speert and Guttmacher 1954). As the developing trophoblast erodes the uterine decidua during implantation of the blastocyst, a small quantity of blood is lost from the eroded vessels and sinuses in the uterine lining. In some cases this can be confused with the expected period in calculating the period of gestation.

'Breakthrough' bleeding

'Breakthrough' bleeding is less common than implantation bleeding, occurring where the corpus luteum is not producing sufficient hormones to prevent shedding of the decidua at the time of the expected period. Where hormone levels are very low, the whole of the uterine lining can be lost (together with the blastocyst). Small amounts of bleeding can however occur as the pregnancy continues. Where a woman conceives whilst taking oral contraception she may experience some blood loss after completing the course of tablets and may not be alerted to the existence of the pregnancy.

Cervical lesions

Erosions

Erosions are very common in pregnancy when overgrowth of cells at the squamo-columnar junction of the cervix occurs (Hibbard 1988). The dividing line between the two layers of cells is often visible on speculum examination on the outside of the cervix. The overgrowth (which is entirely normal) accounts for the significant number of women whose cervical smears taken in early pregnancy show atypical results. The advice given is to repeat the test at the woman's postnatal examination (Hibbard 1988). Where any bleeding is present, it is very important to confirm that no malignancy is present (Cunningham *et al.* 1989).

Polyps

Cervical polyps should not cause any more than a small amount of blood-stained discharge. Again, further investigation is necessary to exclude the presence of malignancy.

Carcinoma

Vaginal blood loss may be the first indication of the presence of cervical cancer. Pregnancy accelerates the growth rate of some types of malignant tissue (Hacker *et al.* 1982). Depending on the gestation at the time of diagnosis, curtailment of the pregnancy by therapeutic abortion or elective preterm delivery is usually advised to allow treatment to begin (Hacker *et al.* 1982).

Ectopic gestation

Ectopic gestation is a dangerous condition which can be difficult to diagnose (Kadar 1983). The most common form of this disorder occurs where the fertilised ovum develops and attempts to implant into the fallopian tube (Myerscough 1982). Eventually the tube will rupture giving rise to a variety of symptoms which can include lower abdominal pain and vaginal blood loss (Kadar 1983). If this is severe, the woman may collapse from pain, blood loss and the presence of blood in the Pouch of Douglas (Myerscough 1982). Diagnosis is by laparoscopy, with ultrasound assisting in demonstrating an empty uterine cavity (Kadar 1983). Risk factors for ectopic gestation include increasing maternal age, previous pelvic infection, use of an intrauterine contraceptive device and a history of surgery to correct tubal damage (Kadar 1983). Treatment involves admission to hospital and surgical removal of all or part of the affected fallopian tube (Kadar 1983).

Hydatidiform mole

Hydatidiform mole is a rare but serious complication of pregnancy. Its frequency in the United Kingdom is approximately 1.5 cases per 1000 live births (Bagshawe *et al*. 1986). In this condition, development of the placenta is altered resulting in the formation of large grape-like vesicles from the chorionic villi (Myerscough 1982). The vesicles are filled with blood and in most cases there is no sign of the embryo or fetus (Myerscough 1982). Detection of hydatidiform mole relies on the presence of specific signs and symptoms, together with the use of ultrasound scanning and urinary hCG assay (Myerscough 1982). The first symptom apparent may be the presence of a pale pink or brown vaginal loss resulting from the rupture of vesicles containing fresh or old blood. The woman may complain of severe vomiting (hyperemesis gravidarum) which is more acute than the usual morning sickness and persists after 13–14 weeks gestation (Schlaerth *et al*. 1988). This may be caused by very high levels of hCG produced by the mole. On examination, the uterus may appear larger than the period of gestation feeling soft and dough-like with no palpable fetal parts (Myerscough 1982). The fetal heart is not detectable. Another highly suggestive sign is the development of pregnancy-induced hypertension with proteinuria before the twentieth week of pregnancy (Schlaerth *et al*. 1988).

Confirmation of the diagnosis is by measurement of urinary hCG levels. These will be strongly positive at dilutions in excess of 1:1000. On ultrasound examination, there is a characteristic speckling or 'snowstorm' appearance in the uterus due to the presence of fluid-filled vesicles (Chudleigh and Pearce 1986). Although hydatidiform mole is itself a benign condition, it can become malignant and develop into a choriocarcinoma (Cunningham *et al*. 1989). For this reason scrupulous follow-up is necessary (Bagshawe *et al*. 1986).

To treat the condition, it is necessary to empty the uterus of all products of conception. This is far from straightforward, however, since the myometrium is often paper-thin and therefore liable to perforation (Myerscough 1982). Usually, with the woman under general anaesthesia, the partly open cervix, which occurs with this condition, allows for digital exploration or suction curettage of the uterus (Myerscough 1982). An alternative is to use high doses of an oxytocin infusion to encourage the uterus to empty itself of the products of conception. The uterus is not particularly sensitive to oxytocin in early pregnancy.

Rigorous follow-up producedures are instituted to detect the development of any malignancy (Bagshawe *et al*. 1986; Crawford and Pettit 1986). This is achieved by testing of the urine for the level and presence of hCG. Three centres in the United Kingdom (Charing Cross Hospital, London, Ninewells Hospital, Dundee and Royal Hallamshire, Sheffield) undertake this testing for hormone levels and maintain a register of cases for statistical purposes (Bagshawe *et al*. 1986). Samples are tested as follows:

1. Weekly until negative (usually 6–10 weeks).
2. Monthly for 6 months.

3. Bimonthly for 6 months.
4. Four monthly for a year (Bagshawe *et al*. 1986).

If the tests remain negative at the end of this period, the woman is regarded as being clear of risk. If the hCG assay fails to become negative or becomes positive again, an endometrial biopsy is performed to look for choriocarcinoma (Myerscough 1982). If the diagnosis is confirmed, the cytotoxic drug methotrexate is given. This has a success rate of 90% (Crawford and Pettit 1986). Pregnancy is not advised during the 2 year follow-up period, although all cases require individual consideration (Myerscough 1982).

The midwife's role in caring for the woman is one of explanation and support. It is a difficult condition for the woman and her partner to comprehend, especially since its causation is unclear. There is also the added uncertainty over the period of supervision and the future of pregnancies.

Abortion

For many women this is an emotive word reserved only for medical termination of pregnancy or illegal abortion (Moulder 1990). Lay people tend to use the word miscarriage when referring to all types of spontaneous abortion. It is important to explain the use of the word abortion to avoid causing further distress to women for whom the midwife is giving care.

Definition of abortion

The accepted United Kingdom definition of abortion is the interruption of pregnancy prior to 28 completed weeks of gestation; this has not altered following recent changes in legislation which reduced the time limit after which a termination of pregnancy on 'social' grounds is no longer permitted from 28 to 24 weeks. It does not solve the problem which occurs where a baby born before 24 weeks survives whereas one born dead at the same gestation is classified as an abortion, whose birth is not registered. Where the fetus shows any signs of life at delivery in the United Kingdom, it is registered as a live birth. Should the fetus be born dead, it is classified as an abortion prior to 24 weeks gestation (not requiring any legal registration) or as a stillbirth after this gestation. After 24 weeks gestation, the birth (whether live or still) has to be registered and the baby can be named; the parents can also arrange their own funeral should they so wish (see Chapter 31).

In 1977 the World Health Organization put forward its definition of abortion:

'the expulsion or extraction from its mother of a fetus or embryo weighing 500 gms or less, or an otherwise product of gestation of any weight and specifically designated, irrespective of gestational age and whether or not there is evidence of life' (World Health Organization 1977).

A 500 g fetus is approximately 20–22 weeks gestation. The type of 'specifically designated' product of gestation would include for example, hydatidiform mole. The adoption of such a definition in the United Kingdom would simplify the work of labour ward staff and paediatricians who currently follow local guidelines on the conduct of delivery and gestation. It would also permit the parents to have legal acknowledgement of a delivery occurring after this time. Although the basis of certain statistical indices of health (such as perinatal mortality) would be altered, the data collected could be more accurate than at present, where it is difficult to confirm the gestation of the fetus.

Classification

The frequency of spontaneous abortion is approximately 15–20% of diagnosed pregnancies, although this excludes early fetal loss where professional help is not sought (World Health Organization 1970; Regan *et al.* 1989). Dewhurst (1981) estimated that 50% of pregnancies do not progress beyond the second trimester. Abortions are classified according to whether they are spontaneous or induced (Myerscough 1982) (see Figure 11.1).

Any suspected spontaneous abortion is treated as 'threatened' until proved otherwise (Myerscough 1982). The bleeding may cease and the pregnancy progress to term. An abortion is termed inevitable when the cervical os is seen on speculum examination to be dilated (open) (Hibbard 1988). The terms 'complete' and 'incomplete' indicate whether all the products of conception have been passed spontaneously or whether there is a need to perform an evacuation of products of conception from the uterus under general anaesthesia. A missed abortion occurs where the embryo/fetus has died but the pregnancy has not been aborted (Myerscough 1982). (In some cases layers of blood or calcium can be laid down around the dead embryo/fetus, these are called a blood or carneous mole, respectively (Myerscough 1982). A similar condition is one of blighted ovum where the embryo has failed to develop and the gestation sac appears to be empty on ultrasound examination (Donald *et al.* 1972). The most common cause of blighted ovum is chromosomal abnormality. In cases of missed abortion, there may be no

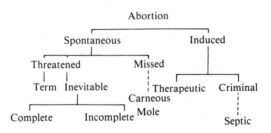

Figure 11.1 Classification of abortion.

vaginal blood loss, the uterus will stop growing and may feel small for the period of gestation, and the test to assay human chorionic gonadotrophin (hCG) will become less strongly positive (Myerscough 1982).

Diagnosis

Confirmation of the diagnosis of spontaneous abortion is by ultrasound scan and measurement of urinary hCG levels (Drumm 1981). For the latter, hCG will remain positive for as long as active placental tissue and a functioning corpus luteum are present (Kadar 1983). By diluting an early morning urine sample, laboratory staff can determine the extent to which the sample is positive. Plasma levels of hCG provide a more reliable indicator to the prognosis of pregnancy (Nygren *et al.* 1973). The development of ultrasound scanning has revolutionised the diagnosis of bleeding in early pregnancy (Drumm 1981). A gestation sac can be seen from as early as 5 weeks of amenorrhoea (3 weeks after conception), fetal echoes can be seen as early as 6–7 weeks after the last menstrual period (LMP) and the fetal heart can be seen beating from 7 weeks (Chudleigh and Pearce 1986). Ultrasound can demonstrate an empty gestation sac, retained products of conception and an open cervical os, indicating that the abortion is inevitable (Chudleigh and Pearce 1986).

Causation

The causes of spontaneous abortion are complex, with a number of predisposing factors playing a part (Cunningham *et al.* 1989). Since the cause of all abortions is not investigated (usually only after the second or third), definitive information is hard to come by. The most frequently detectable conditions are abnormalities of maternal anatomy (Heinonen *et al.* 1982) and fetal chromosomal aberrations (Poland *et al.* 1981). The following are some of the other major predisposing factors:

- Specific gene defects such as phenylketonuria may not be apparent until after birth, since the maternal placenta protects the fetus from toxicity. However other inborn errors of metabolism may be incompatible with intrauterine survival (Stein *et al.* 1980; Cunningham *et al.* 1989).
- Maternal starvation. At marginal levels of nutrition, amenorrhoea, infertility and early pregnancy loss are common (Stein *et al.* 1975).
- Smoking increases the risk of spontaneous abortion (Kline *et al.* 1980).
- Irradiation of the mother (Hibbard 1988).
- Presence of an intrauterine contraceptive device (Cunningham *et al.* 1989).
- Parents with abnormal chromosomal karyotypes (Sant-Cassia 1985).
- Uterine anomalies (Heinonen *et al.* 1982).
- Intrauterine adhesions (Bergquist *et al.* 1981).
- Endocrine disturbances, such as defects of the corpus luteum (Jones 1976).

- Infections, including toxoplasmosis, salmonella, influenza, syphilis, measles and cytomegalovirus (Sant-Cassia 1985).
- Following amniocentesis or chorion villus sampling.
- Trauma to the cervix or cervical incompetence, following cone biopsy or surgery, can give rise to cervical incompetence, especially in the second trimester (Myerscough 1982).

Signs and symptoms

The woman may complain of hypogastric or low back pain (Cunningham *et al.* 1989). The pain may feel similar to cramps experienced during a menstrual period. Vaginal bleeding of some degree is usually present, although the amount is variable (Cunningham *et al.* 1989).

Management

Where blood loss is slight and the gestation early, the GP may advise bed rest (except for visits to the toilet) and keep the woman under periodic observation at home (Everett *et al.* 1987). Admission to hospital is common and the nurse/midwife caring for the woman must not underestimate the anxiety this can cause (Moulder 1990). Not only does the woman worry about the future of her pregnancy, but she is in strange surroundings with the added concerns about her family at home (Rosen 1976).

On admission, a full assessment of the woman's condition is necessary in case she requires some form of resuscitation (Hibbard 1988). The diagnosis requires confirmation by medical staff. The initial investigation is usually observation of the state of the cervix on speculum examination (Myerscough 1982). Sometimes products of conception are visible in the cervical os. Their removal with sponge-holding forceps can do much to improve the woman's condition (Myerscough 1982). If the abortion is thought to be inevitable, the woman may require an evacuation of the uterus. In preparation for this, she fasts for approximately 4 hours depending upon when and what she last ate. An intravenous line is usually established to allow for fluids to be given to correct any dehydration.

Where the abortion is still regarded as threatened, the woman remains on bed rest (except for toileting purposes) until a definite diagnosis is arrived at or until 24 hours after the bleeding has stopped. This was recommended by 90% of GPs in a study by Everett *et al.* (1987). This is despite the fact that bed rest has not been shown to improve outcome (Diddle *et al.* 1953). In all cases there is a need to give the woman comfort, support and full explanations, especially where the outcome is uncertain. Analgesia may be needed (Smith *et al.* 1979). It is important to obtain a sample of maternal blood to determine the woman's rhesus status. If she is rhesus-negative, anti-D is given as a prophylactic measure to prevent development of any antibodies. The aborted fetus is assumed to be rhesus-positive.

Habitual abortion

Habitual abortion is a term which is used where a woman has experienced three or more spontaneous abortions (Cunningham *et al.* 1989). It is a most distressing condition for the couple, who may find that their lives are blighted by their inability to maintain a pregnancy (Borg and Lasker 1981). The most common causes (where one is found) are parental or fetal chromosomal anomalies and uterine abnormalities (Sant-Cassia 1985). Successful pregnancies have been achieved where natural hCG levels are low, by giving a supplement between 8 and 16 weeks gestation until the pregnancy is fully established (Sant-Cassia 1985). Another treatment, which has had some success, involves manipulating the immunological changes which occur during pregnancy. Normally, to prevent the mother rejecting the fetus (which is made up of 50% foreign genetic material), a plasma-blocking factor is produced, but this is lacking in some women who experience recurrent abortion (Rocklin *et al.* 1976). Where the parents have a similar genetic makeup there may be insufficient stimulation to produce this factor and the fetus is rejected as being genetically foreign (Mowbray *et al.* 1985). Inoculating a woman with a purified suspension of her partner's lymphocytes has increased the rate of successful pregnancies (Mowbray *et al.* 1985).

Effects of early fetal loss on parents

Whilst this topic is covered in more detail in Chapter 31, there are some important areas specific to fetal loss in early pregnancy. It was thought previously that the loss of a fetus early in pregnancy had only a transient effect upon the mother. More recent studies have demonstrated that mothers experience a degree of guilt, anxiety and depression following a spontaneous abortion. Taylor and Emery (1986) comment on the variety of emotions experienced by any one woman on confirmation of her pregnancy. Women are individuals and it is hardly surprising that they react differently to fetal loss. Peppers and Knapp (1980) performed a comparative study of the grief reactions of mothers following spontaneous abortion, stillbirth and neonatal death. They found that there were no significant differences between the three groups, although mothers following stillbirth and neonatal death did receive follow-up care and counselling. Why not the other group? The birth of another child also had similar effects on women in all categories (Peppers and Knapp 1980). In another study it was noted that severe depression occurred, not after the abortion itself, but at the time of the expected confinement (Hayton 1988). The author suggests that alerting the woman to the possibility of psychological disturbances could do much to improve her ability to cope.

The lack of follow-up after spontaneous abortion has been commented upon (Moore 1985; Oakley *et al.* 1984; Arber 1985). Even advice regarding physical symptoms such as blood loss and the use of tampons or the production of milk is often lacking (Oakley *et al.* 1984). Arber (1985) suggests that there is a need to offer a visit by a community midwife to aid the woman in adjusting to her loss and to give general health advice. This idea has been under discussion by both professional and lay groups such as the Royal College of Midwives, the National Childbirth Trust and the Miscarriage Association. There are also books designed to help the grieving parents, including those written by Borg and Lasker (1981), Oakley *et al.* (1984) and by Moulder (1990).

Therapeutic abortion

Therapeutic abortion has been legal in England, Wales and Scotland since the passing of the 1967 Abortion Act. This lays down specific grounds under which a termination of pregnancy can be performed (Munday *et al.* 1989). The decision must be made in 'good faith' by two medical practitioners, who are obliged to inform their local district medical officer. The abortion can only be performed on premises licensed for that purpose, such as hospitals and nursing homes. Prior to the passing of the Act, large numbers of illegal abortions were performed, with resulting tragedies of maternal mortality and morbidity (Munday *et al.* 1989). It is not within the remit of this text to discuss in detail the ethical issues involved with termination of pregnancy, which include the issues of the sanctity of life and the age of fetal viability. A bibliography on this topic is included at the end of this chapter.

The grounds for performing a therapeutic abortion under the 1967 Act are that continuation of the pregnancy would involve risk:

- to the life of the woman greater than if the pregnancy were terminated,
- of injury to the physical or mental health of the woman greater than if the pregnancy were terminated,
- of injury to the physical or mental health of existing children of the family greater than if the pregnancy were terminated,
- there is a substantial risk that, if the child were born, it would suffer from such physical or mental abnormalities as to be seriously handicapped,
- to save the life of the pregnant woman,
- to prevent grave permanent injury to the physical or mental health of the pregnant woman.

The grounds are far from specific and therefore interpretation can vary between medical practitioners. The Act does not specify any time limit after which abortion is illegal, relying on the 1929 Infant Life Preservation Act which makes 'wilful destruction ... of a child capable of being born alive' a criminal offence. The 1991 Human Fertilisation and Embryology Act has removed this anomaly by placing a 24 week limit on abortion, except where there is a risk of severe fetal handicap or where the physical or mental health of the woman is at risk (Carlisle 1990). In practical terms, therapeutic abortions are rare after 24 weeks gestation, with the majority being performed before 16–18 weeks gestation (Munday *et al.* 1989). The exceptions involve women awaiting the results of amniocentesis which cannot be performed until 16 weeks. Bureaucratic delays, mistaken symptoms of menopause, failure of contraception, the very young and the mentally handicapped account for many of those pregnancies which are far advanced before termination is sought (British Birth Control Campaign 1980). In 1988 of 183 798 abortions performed in England and Wales 80% were before the end of the twelfth week of gestation, only 2% were after the twentieth week, and in many of these cases the woman was not normally resident in the United Kingdom (Office of Population Census and Surveys 1989). Two hundred took place between 20 and 22 weeks and only 23 abortions occurred after 24 weeks (Office of Population Censuses and Surveys 1989).

Methods

Early termination of pregnancy (prior to 8 weeks of amenorrhoea) can be performed under local anaesthetic as an out-patient procedure. It is more usual to carry out the termination of pregnancy as a 'day case' or as an in-patient.

1. Menstrual evacuation can be performed until 6 weeks after the last menstrual period (LMP) using a suction aspirator. It is easier to perform on multiparous women, in whom the cervix would not be so tightly closed (Cunningham *et al.* 1989).
2. Suction aspiration/curettage can be used under local anaesthesia until 10 weeks after the LMP and under general anaesthesia until 14 weeks (Munday *et al.* 1989).
3. Dilatation and curettage is performed under general anaesthesia up until 14 weeks after the LMP. It is associated with the rare complications of perforation of the uterus and cervical damage (Cunningham *et al.* 1989).
4. Dilatation and fetal extraction is rarely performed, as it involves a large degree of cervical dilatation and extraction of the fetus piecemeal.
5. Extra-amniotic prostaglandins can be used from 14 weeks gestation. A Foley catheter is inserted through the cervical os and a solution of prostaglandins given, using a pump (MacKenzie 1990). Large doses of intravenous oxytocin may also be used. The whole procedure can take up to 24 hours and it is extremely painful and distressing for the woman. Psychological support and analgesia are important. In about 10% of cases an evacuation of uterus is required to remove retained products of conception (Cunningham *et al.* 1989)
6. Intra-amniotic prostaglandin is sometimes preferred to extra-amniotic, especially with more advanced gestation (MacKenzie 1990).
7. Trials are continuing with the French abortion pill RU486. It is a steroid which acts by blocking progesterone receptors in the decidua. It is claimed to have no significant side-effects if used up until 8 weeks after the LMP (Cameron and Baird 1988). It will induce abortion in 3 days in 80% of women. The remainder require surgical removal of the pregnancy, since there is a risk of teratogenesis.

Morbidity following therapeutic abortion

A collaborative study by members of the Royal Colleges of General Practitioners and Obstetricians and Gynaecologists (1985) followed up 6105 women referred for therapeutic abortion. The cohort excluded woman who bypassed their GPs and went directly to the private sector.

The survey found an overall morbidity rate of 16.9%, with 4% of women experiencing some degree of haemorrhage, 3.6% an episode of associated infection, 0.6% operative trauma (cervical lacerations or uterine perforations), 0.5% thromboembolic conditions and 2.4% requiring psychiatric admission. For this last complication, women with a previous history of depression were 2.6 times more likely to have this condition post-operatively than those with no such history. Women referred to the NHS for treatment were more likely (27%) than those in the private sector (14%) to spend at least 3 weeks between the initial consultation and the operation. NHS operations were less likely to be performed prior to the end of the first trimester and also less likely to be treated using prostaglandins. Morbidity was raised amongst all women having NHS treatment, although some of this difference was accounted for by the method chosen, the length of gestation and characteristics of the women (smoking and age) (Royal Colleges of General Practitioners and Obstetricians and Gynaecologists 1985).

As with spontaneous abortion, the psychological effects of termination of pregnancy have been understated. Feelings of guilt, regret, self-reproach and mild depression have been reported (Gibbons 1984). Some aspects remain unresolved until the birth of a later child. Pre- and post-abortion counselling can aid women in coming to terms with complex psychological adjustments (Cooper 1983; Broome 1984). For women having an abortion due to fetal abnormality, there are a number of conflicting issues:

1. Waiting time before the results are confirmed. By this time the pregnancy may be visible and fetal movements detectable.
2. The relief at sparing themselves and the child from the trauma of handicap.
3. Guilt at denying their child a life.
4. Mourning for the normal child they were originally expecting.
5. Concern as to future pregnancies.

These complex emotions may require specialist help in their resolution but every midwife can help by simply listening and allowing the woman and her partner to voice their feelings.

References

Arber S (1985) 'Aftercare following miscarriage' *Midwife, Health Visitor and Community Nurse* 21(12): 432–6

Bagshawe K D, Dent J and Webb J (1986) 'Hydatidiform mole in England and Wales 1973–83' *Lancet* ii: 673–7

Bergquist C A, Rock J A and Jones H W (1981) 'Pregnancy outcome following treatment of intrauterine adhesions' *International Journal of Fertility* 26: 107–11

Borg S and Lasker J (1981) *When the Pregnancy Fails* Beacon Press: Boston

British Birth Control Campaign (1980) *Why Late Abortions* British Birth Control Campaign: London

Broome A (1984) 'Abortion counselling' *Nursing Mirror* 158(20): 19–26

Cameron I T and Baird D T (1988) 'Early pregnancy termination: a comparison between vacuum aspiration and medical abortion using prostaglandin or the antiprogesterone RU 486' *British Journal of Obstetrics and Gynaecology* 95: 271

Carlisle D (1990) 'New limits' *Nursing Times* 86(19): 22–3

Chudleigh P and Pearce J M (1986) *Obstetric Ultrasound* Churchill Livingstone: Edinburgh

Cooper G (1983) 'Post abortion counselling' *Nursing Mirror* 24 Aug: supplement: viii

Crawford M and Pettit D (1986) 'Treatment schedules for hydatidiform mole and choriocarcinoma' *Nursing Times* 82(10 Dec): 40–2

Cunningham F G, MacDonald P C and Gant N F (1989) *William's Obstetrics (18th edn)* Prentice Hall: London

Department of Health (1989) *Report on Confidential Enquiries into Maternal Deaths in England and Wales 1982–4* HMSO: London

Department of Health (1991) *Report on Confidential Enquiries into Maternal Deaths in the United Kingdom 1985–7* HMSO: London

Dewhurst J (1981) *Integrated Obstetrics and Gynaecology for Post Graduates* 205 Blackwell: Oxford

Diddle A W, O'Connor K A, Jack R and Pearce R L (1953) 'Evaluation of bed rest in threatened abortion' *Obstetrics and Gynecology* 2: 63–7

Donald I, Morley P and Barnett E (1972) 'The diagnosis of blighted ovum by sonar' *British Journal of Obstetrics and Gynaecology* 70: 305

Drumm J E (1981) 'The value of ultrasonography in the management of first-trimester haemorrhage' in J Studd (ed) *Progress in Obstetrics and Gynaecology Vol I* 30–8 Churchill Livingstone: Edinburgh

Edmonds D K, Lindsay K S, Miller J F, Williamson E and Wood P J (1982) 'Early embryonic mortality in women' *Fertility and Sterility* 38: 447–57

Everett C, Ashurst A and Chalmers I (1987) 'Reported management of threatened miscarriage by general practitioners in Wessex' *British Medical Journal* 295: 583–6

Gibbons M (1984) 'Psychiatric sequelae of induced abortion' *Journal of the Royal College of General Practitioners* 34(3): 146–50

Hacker N F, Berek J S, Lagasse L D, Charles E H and Moore J G (1982) 'Carcinoma of the cervix associated with pregnancy' *Obstetrics and Gynecology* 59: 735

Hayton A (1988) 'Miscarriage and delayed depression' *Lancet* i: 834

Heinonen P E, Saarikoski S and Pystynen P (1982) 'Reproductive performance of woman with uterine anomalies: an evaluation of 182 cases' *Acta Obstetrica et Gynaecologica Scandanavica* 61: 157–62

Hibbard B M (1988) *Principles of Obstetrics* Butterworths: London

Jones G S (1976) 'The luteal phase defects' *Fertility and Sterility* 27: 351–6

Kadar N (1983) 'Ectopic pregnancy: a reappraisal of aetiology, diagnosis and treatment' in J Studd (ed) *Progress in Obstetrics and Gynaecology Vol III* 305–23 Churchill Livingstone: Edinburgh

Kline J, Stein Z A, Susser M and Warbuton D (1980) 'Environmental influences on early reproductive loss in a current New York City Study' in I H Porter and E B Hook (eds) *Human Embryonic and Fetal Death* 225 Academic Press: New York

MacKenzie I Z (1990) 'The therapeutic use of prostaglandins in obstetrics' in J Studd (ed) *Progress in Obstetrics and Gynaecology Vol VIII* 149–73 Churchill Livingstone: Edinburgh

Moore J (1985) 'A common tragedy' *Nursing Times, Community Outlook* 81(June): 210

Moulder C (1990) *Miscarriage. Women's experiences and needs* Pandora: London

Mowbray J F, Gibbings C, Liddell F, Reginald P W, Underwood J L and Beard A W (1985) 'A controlled trial of recurrent spontaneous abortion by immunisation with paternal cells' *Lancet* i: 941

Munday D, Francome C and Savage W (1989) 'Twenty one years of legal abortion' *British Medical Journal* 298: 1231–4

Myerscough P R (1982) *Munro Kerr's Operative Obstetrics (10th edn)* Balliere Tindall: London

Nygren K G, Johansson E D B and Wide L (1973) 'Evaluation of the progress of threatened abortion from the peripheral plasma levels of progesterone, estradiol and human chorionic gonadotrophin' *American Journal of Obstetrics and Gynecology* 116: 916–22

Oakley A, McPherson A and Roberts H (1984) *Miscarriage* Fontana: London

Office of Population Censuses and Surveys (1989) *Legal Abortions* 1988 OPCS Monitor

Peppers L G and Knapp R M (1980) 'Maternal reaction to involuntary fetal death' *Psychiatry* 43(2): 155–9

Poland B J, Miller J R, Harris M and Livingston J (1981) 'Spontaneous abortion. A study of 1961 women and their abortuses' *Acta Obstetrica et Gynaecologica Scandanavica* 102(Suppl): 1

Regan L, Braude P R and Trembath P L (1989) 'Influence of past reproductive performance on risk of spontaneous abortion' *British Medical Journal* 299: 541–5

Rocklin R E, Kitzmiller J H, Carpenter C B and David J R (1976) 'Maternal–fetal relation; absence of an immunological blocking factor in women chronic abortions' *New England Journal of Medicine* 295: 1209–13

Rosen E L (1976) 'Concerns of an obstetric patient experiencing long-term hospitalisation' *Journal of Obstetrical, Gynecological and Neonatal Nursing* 4: 15–19

Royal College Of General Practitioners/Royal College Of Obstetricians and Gynaecologists Joint Working Party (1985) 'Induced abortion operations and their early sequelae' *Journal of the Royal College Of General Practitioners* 35(4): 175–80

Sant-Cassia L J (1985) 'Recurrent abortion' in J Studd (ed) *Progress in Obstetrics and Gynaecology Vol V* 248–58 Churchill Livingstone: Edinburgh

Schlaerth J B, Morrow C P, Montz F and d'Ablaing G (1988) 'Initial management of hydatidiform mole' *American Journal of Obstetrics and Gynecology* 158: 1299

Smith G M, Stubblefield P G, Chirchirillo L and McCarthy M J (1979) 'Pain of first trimester abortion' *American Journal of Obstetrics and Gynecology* 133: 489–98

South J and Naldrett J (1973) 'The effect of vaginal bleeding on the infant born after 28 weeks of pregnancy' *British Journal of Obstetrics and Gynaecology* 80: 236

Speert H and Guttmacher A F (1954) 'Frequency and significance of bleeding in early pregnancy' *Journal of the American Medical Association* 155: 172

Stein Z, Susser M, Saenger G and Marolla F (1975) *Famine and Human Development* Oxford University Press: Oxford

Stein Z, Kline J, Susser E, Shrout P, Warburton D and Susser D (1980) 'Maternal age and spontaneous abortion' in I H Porter and E B Hook (eds) *Human Embryonic and Fetal Death* 129 Academic Press: New York

Taylor E M and Emery S (1986) 'Early fetal loss: effects on parents and professionals' *Maternal and Child Health* 11(5): 141–4

World Health Organization (1970) *Spontaneous and Induced Abortion* WHO Technical Report Series No 41: Geneva

World Health Organization (1977) *International Classification of Diseases* WHO: Geneva

Further reading

Reading on the legal and ethical aspects of therapeutic abortion.

Bart S (1981) 'Seizing the means of reproduction: an illegal feminist abortion collective – how and why it worked' in H Roberts (ed) *Women, Health and Reproduction* Ch 5 109–28 Routledge and Kegan Paul: London

Brewer C (1988) 'The fatal flaw' *Nursing Times* 84(17): 25

Bromwich P (1987) 'Late abortion' *British Medical Journal* 294: 527–8

Dunn P (1985) 'Age of fetal viability' *Maternal and Child Health* 10(4): 102–4

Dyer C (1987) 'Father fails in attempt to stop girl friend's abortion' *British Medical Journal* 294: 631–2

Francome C (1986) *Abortion Practice in Britain and the United States* Allen and Unwin: London

Horan F (1984) 'Abortion who decides?' *Nursing Times* 80(7 March): 16–17

Kenny M (1986) *Abortion. The Whole Story* Quartet: London

Mason J K and McCall Smith R A (1987) *Law and Medical Ethics (2nd edn)* Butterworth: London

Pollack Petchesky R (1985) 'Abortion in the 1980's: feminist morality and women's health' in E Lewin and V Oleson (eds) *Women's Health and Healing* Ch 6 139–73 Tavistock: London

Smith A (1988) 'Late abortions and the law' *British Medical Journal* 296: 446–7

12   Hypertensive disorders in pregnancy

Hypertension is the commonest complication of pregnancy. In the United Kingdom it was amongst the leading causes of death in the 1985–87 Confidential Inquiry into Maternal Deaths (Department of Health 1991), being responsible for 27 maternal deaths.

Blood pressure

Blood pressure can be described as the force exerted upon the walls of blood vessels by the blood within them. Since blood enters the arterial system before the capillaries and venous system (i.e. there is a delay), the pressure in the arteries is higher than in the veins. Systolic blood pressure is produced when the left ventricle of the heart contracts, pushing blood into an already full aorta (Hankins 1986). Diastolic blood pressure refers to pressure within the arteries when the left ventricle is relaxed (Detweiler 1972).

The levels for systolic and diastolic blood pressures vary between individuals. They are affected by time of day, posture (especially in pregnancy), age and gender (MacGillivray *et al.* 1969). Measurement of blood pressure using a sphygmomanometer is altered by the size of the cuff used (Maxwell *et al.* 1982) and the relative position of the upper arm with respect to the heart, in addition to any observer error (Webster *et al.* 1984).

Maintenance of blood pressure

The following factors are involved in the maintenance of blood pressure:

1. Stroke volume: This is the amount of blood expelled from the heart by each contraction of the ventricles.
2. Heart rate: The number of times the heart beats per minute. The cardiac output (minute volume) can be calculated by multiplying the stroke volume by the heart rate.
3. Blood volume: To maintain normal blood pressure, a sufficient amount of blood must be circulating. In cases of reduced blood volume, such as haemorrhage, blood pressure falls (Detweiler 1972).
4. Peripheral resistance: The walls of peripheral vessels are made of smooth muscle, which is stimulated by nervous impulses to maintain tone. Increasing stimulation of the sympathetic nervous system leads to vasoconstriction and a rise in blood pressure. A reduction in nervous stimulation produces blood pooling and a drop in blood pressure (Detweiler 1972; Wallenburg 1988).
5. Arterial wall elasticity: In order to adjust to changing blood volumes, the walls of arteries are elastic, allowing them to distend, then recoil to continue blood flow. Diastolic blood pressure is maintained through this elasticity.
6. Venous return: The heart relies on blood being returned to it through forces other than that of the left ventricle, which is unable to push blood through both arterial and venous systems unaided. Venous return is assisted in three ways: when upright gravity assists venous return from the upper body; during respiration, when inspiration produces a negative pressure in the thorax which serves to pull blood toward the heart; and by muscular contractions which put pressure on the veins and thus squeeze blood towards the heart (Detweiler 1972). Backflow is prevented by a series of valves in the veins (Detweiler 1972).

Receptors in the body, such as the Baro receptors, record stretch in the walls of the aortic arch and carotid sinus. These assist the body in maintaining a balance of the constituent parts which produce blood pressure. An alteration in any one component can be compensated for by changes in the others. The maintenance of the equilibrium is assisted by adrenaline and angiotensin. Adrenaline dilates central vessels, including those in the heart. This increases heart rate and cardiac output, thus increasing blood pressure. Where blood volume is low, angiotensin, a powerful vasoconstrictor, is produced. This stimulates the adrenal cortex to produce aldosterone, resulting in retention of sodium (and with it water) in the kidneys. Antidiuretic hormone from the posterior pituitary also assists in maintaining normal blood volume (Ganong 1973).

Blood pressure in pregnancy

Blood pressure falls at the beginning of pregnancy, reaching its lowest level at 16–20 weeks gestation, before rising slowly to pre-pregnant levels by term (MacGillivray *et al.* 1969). Diastolic blood pressure can fall by up to 15 mmHg from its prepregnant level (Friedman and Neff 1977). This occurs together with an increasing cardiac output and a fall in peripheral resistance.

In the last trimester, some women are very intolerant of lying supine (Stewart 1985). This can result in compression of the vena cava, reduced cardiac output and hypotension. The woman may feel faint and if placental perfusion is affected the fetus can become hypoxic (Stewart 1985).

The diagnosis of hypertension in pregnancy is far from simple. The dividing line between normality and abnormality is usually placed at a systolic pressure of over 140 mmHg and a diastolic pressure of over 90 mmHg (Nelson 1955). Care should be taken to avoid too rigid a definition which does not take account of either labile hypertension or the woman with a normally low prepregnant blood pressure, such as 100/60 mmHg. Although Adams and MacGillivray (1961) stated that it is the actual level of blood pressure reached in late pregnancy which is important rather than the rise during pregnancy. Some obstetricians disagree with this and would include a rise in diastolic pressure of 15–20 mmHg from prepregnant levels as part of their criteria for pregnancy hypertension (Hibbard 1988). It has been noted (MacGillivray 1983) that late pregnancy hypertension alone carries no increased perinatal risks, whilst the presence of accompanying proteinuria leads to reduced birthweight and an increase in perinatal mortality.

Hypertensive disease in pregnancy

The terminology used in the classification of hypertensive disease in pregnancy can be somewhat confusing. Davey and MacGillivray (1988) reported the terminology and definitions recommended by the International Society for the Study of Hypertension in Pregnancy:

(a) Gestational hypertension or proteinuria. Hypertension or proteinuria developing after 20 weeks gestation in a woman who prior to pregnancy had no hypertension or proteinuria.

(b) Gestational proteinuric hypertension. Hypertension and proteinuria developing after 20 weeks gestation in a woman who previously had no hypertension or proteinuria. (This was previously known as pre-eclampsia.)

(c) Chronic hypertension or renal disease. Hypertension and/or proteinuria in pregnancy in a woman who has had chronic hypertension or renal disease diagnosed before, during or persisting after pregnancy.

(d) Chronic hypertension with superimposed gestational proteinuric hypertension. Proteinuria developing for the first time in pregnancy in a woman with chronic hypertension.

(e) Unclassified hypertension and/or proteinuria. Hypertension and/or proteinuria found at the first antenatal examination after 20 weeks gestation which may be classified after delivery.

(f) Eclampsia. Generalised convulsions occurring during pregnancy, labour or within 7 days of delivery which are not caused by epilepsy or other convulsive disorders. (Davey and MacGillivray 1988)

Chronic renal disease is discussed in Chapter 13.

Gestational proteinuric hypertension

This is a condition which is peculiar to pregnancy. It is characterised by hypertension and proteinuria, which usually develop after 20 weeks gestation (Davey and MacGillivray 1988). Renal biopsy of affected women has shown characteristic glomerular lesions not present in uncomplicated hypertension, indicating kidney damage (Sheehan and Lynch 1973). Gestational proteinuric hypertension is mainly a disease of the primigravida (Chesley 1978) (a previous abortion gives some protection against it), although a change in partner can produce the condition in a previously unaffected multipara (Ikedife 1980). It is more common in the very young (under 17 years), in women over 35 years, in women with diabetes or with a multiple pregnancy (MacGillivray 1985b). Gestational proteinuric hypertension can also occur before 20 weeks gestation in cases of hydatidiform mole (MacGillivray 1985b).

Much research has been carried out to determine the cause of gestational proteinuric hypertension, which is believed to be multifactorial in origin (Petrucco 1981; MacGillivray 1985b). Possible contributory factors include dietary deficiencies although the picture is far from clear (Green 1989), excess hormonal alterations (MacGillivray 1983), changes in the renin–angiotension–aldosterone system, prostaglandins, familial predisposition (Chesley et al. 1968) and immunological disturbances (Petrucco 1981). The last factor is in keeping with the prevalence of pre-eclampsia in first pregnancies where a faulty maternal immune response to the fetus (which is half foreign tissue) may lead to the body's attempt at rejection (Petrucco 1981). Murphy et al. (1986) found a relationship between the haemoglobin level in early pregnancy and the occurrence of hypertension in 54 000 women. Only 7% of those whose early haemoglobin level was below 10.5 g/dl developed hypertension, compared with 42% of those with a haemoglobin level of more than 14.5 g/dl. A similar and more useful association has been noted in late pregnancy (Hytten, personal communication).

MacGillivray (1985a) has described gestational proteinuric hypertension as a 'disease of cascades'. One alteration in the equilibrium of body systems results in disturbance of other processes, making discovery of the cause virtually impossible. The systems most commonly affected are the renal system (producing raised serum uric acid and proteinuria (MacGillivray 1983)) and the blood coagulation mechanism (Bonnar 1977). Disseminated intravascular coagulation may occur, an early sign of which is falling platelet levels (Redman *et al.* 1978). The earlier in pregnancy the rise in blood pressure, the worse the outlook for the mother and fetus (Page and Christianson 1976). Increasing proteinuria is a sign of a worsening condition.

Oedema is no longer considered to be part of the diagnosis as it occurs normally in 80% of pregnant women (Robertson 1971). Hall *et al.* (1985) advise that all primiparae should be screened for gestational proteinuric hypertension from 26 weeks onwards, whilst multiparous women (with their lower risk) do not require testing until 30 weeks. Earlier testing is not effective in terms of increasing the rate of additional correct diagnoses.

The only effective treatment for gestational proteinuric hypertension is to remove the cause, that is, to deliver the baby (MacGillivray 1983). It is therefore much better to detect the disorder early and minimise its effects (MacGillivray 1983). Blood pressure should return to normal within 48 hours of delivery unless the gestational proteinuric hypertension was superimposed on essential hypertension.

Eclampsia can be seen as the end result of untreated severe gestational proteinuric hypertension, but it can occur without previous warning (Worley 1984). Forty-one per cent of women having eclamptic fits have had little or no proteinuria prior to their occurrence (Porapakkham 1979). Eclampsia occurs in approximately 1–3:1000 pregnancies in large obstetric centres (Worley 1984). The term 'imminent' or 'impending' eclampsia is used to describe the transition stage where symptoms occur. The woman usually complains of at least one of the following: headache, visual disturbance, epigastric pain (due to hepatic oedema) and vomiting (Worley 1984). Oliguria (of less than 400 ml in 24 hours) may be present. This state can occur antenatally, during labour or within 48 hours of delivery (MacGillivray 1983). Grand mal convulsions may occur, which can be repeated. If the woman has not delivered, spontaneous labour often occurs following the fits (Pritchard 1980). Eclampsia is an obstetric emergency requiring intensive care facilities (MacGillivray 1983). The fetal outlook is poor as severe intrauterine hypoxia occurs (Pritchard 1980). Maternal hazards include cerebral haemorrhage, liver damage, renal failure and renal cortical necrosis (Sheehan and Lynch 1973). Maternal injury can occur during convulsions. Pipkin (1986) has noted that eclampsia is less common in the developed world, due to early detection of pre-eclampsia, but it can have a devastating effect in poorer areas of the world.

Gestational hypertension

Chesley (1980) argued for a further type of hypertension: the woman with an inherited tendency to hypertension which manifests itself in pregnancy. This he called gestational hypertension. It occurs in primiparae but is more common in the multiparous woman (Nelson 1955). The condition gets worse with succeeding pregnancies and there is an increased risk of developing essential hypertension in later life (Adams and MacGillivray 1961). This type of hypertension is not complicated by proteinuria (Altchek 1964).

Effects of hypertension

The maternal risks of hypertension are no different in pregnancy than at any other times. They are cerebral haemorrhage, renal impairment, heart disease and eye damage (Moore and Redman 1987). The effects on the placenta and thus the fetus are obviously specific. The fetus is totally dependent on the placenta for its supply of nutrients, oxygen and excretion of waste products. Blood flow in the maternal sinuses in the decidua is reduced in hypertension (Johnson and Clayton 1957). The spiral arterioles become less elastic, instead of being dilated and funnel-shaped (Brosens 1977). The spiral arteriole is therefore not able to expand to permit the necessary increase in blood flow (Fox 1991). Whether these vascular changes are the cause or the effect of the hypertension is not known, but their end result is premature ageing of the placenta (MacGillivray 1983) and intrauterine growth retardation of the fetus, which is especially severe in the presence of proteinuria (Lunell et al. 1982). This results in an increase in the number of stillbirths and a reduction in weight for gestational age (Friedman and Neff 1977).

Management

Prevention of any condition is always preferable to attempting a cure (the only cure for pre-eclampsia being delivery) (MacGillivray 1985a). Early attendance at antenatal clinics is encouraged to obtain a baseline blood pressure recording and to detect any proteinuria (usually due to infection or renal disease). Because the fall in blood pressure occurs early in the first trimester (MacGillivray et al. 1969), one must question the value of the recordings made between 10 and 14 weeks. Urinalysis (of an uncontaminated sample) is performed at each antenatal visit from 26 weeks onwards to detect proteinuria. Dipsticks used to detect the presence of protein in urine have a 25% false-positive rate for a trace of protein and a 6% false positive rate for one + (Shaw et al. 1983). Weight gain, an unreliable sign of fetal well-being, may be of little use in pregnancy-induced hypertension where physiological oedema can further complicate the picture (Hytten 1990).

Stirratt (1985) comments that when considering treating hypertension in pregnancy one must ask three questions:

1. Will the treatment result in fewer maternal complications?
2. Will the perinatal mortality and morbidity be reduced?
3. Are there any long-term effects of the treatment for either mother or baby?

The management of hypertensive disease in pregnancy will be considered in two parts: mild and severe hypertension.

Attendance at the antenatal clinic can produce labile hypertension in some women, especially if the journey was difficult and the waiting time long (de Sweit 1980). Resting the woman for 15 minutes before remeasuring the blood pressure may prevent unnecessary action being taken (Davey and MacGillivray 1988).

Admission to hospital in cases of mild hypertension (a diastolic of 90–95 mmHg and no proteinuria) is less common now, although it is still advocated by some authorities (MacGillivray 1985b). It has been recognised that worrying about being away from home and family is not helpful in lowering blood pressure (Rosen 1976). Bed rest has not been shown to have great benefits, but the woman should not undertake strenuous physical activity (Mathews *et al.* 1982).

Part of the role of the community midwife is visiting women with mild hypertension at home. This is usually at the request of the obstetrician; visits can occur daily, saving the woman the strain of a hospital visit. Full antenatal care can be given at home if requested, but usually all that is involved are a blood pressure recording and urinalysis for proteinuria to assess maternal condition between clinic visits. To assess fetal well-being, cardiotocography may be performed at home, at the local health centre or on an out-patient basis at the maternity hospital. If the blood pressure rises or proteinuria occurs, the midwife refers back to the hospital for further instructions. Weekly or fortnightly ultrasound scans may be performed to assess fetal growth. If the fetal condition and the hypertension are satisfactory the woman is usually left until term, when labour is induced (MacGillivray 1985b).

Where a woman is on long-term therapy for pre-existing hypertension, treatment is continued, although the drug used may be changed to methyldopa or labetalol, which have been used for some time in pregnancy (Redman *et al.* 1976a; Walker *et al.* 1982). Trials are ongoing with calcium-blocking drugs.

Severe hypertension (a diastolic of 95–100 mmHg and over) or hypertension with proteinuria (more than a trace of protein on urinalysis) usually requires admission of the woman to hospital. Hypotensive drugs are rarely given unless diastolic pressure rises above 110 mmHg. Where there is no obvious cause for the hypertension, tests for rarer aetiologies such as phaeochromocytoma may be performed (Redman 1984). Management falls into three categories:

1. Prevention and assessment of maternal complications.
2. Prevention and detection of eclampsia.
3. Assessment of fetal well-being (this is discussed in Chapter 7).

Maternal observations

These take the form of four-hourly blood pressure recordings (taking account of diurnal variations), daily urinalysis for protein and a full daily antenatal examination. In a normotensive pregnancy, the blood pressure follows a circadian rhythm similar to that of non-pregnant women. The blood pressure is at its highest midmorning, followed by a slow fall to the lowest reading at approximately 3 a.m. before rising again. In pregnant women with gestational hypertension, the pattern is disrupted, with the peak blood pressure recordings occurring at midnight (Ruff *et al.* 1982). Twenty-four hour urine collection may be obtained to measure creatinine clearance, an assessment of renal function (Moore and Redman 1987), and a fluid balance chart may be kept to observe for signs of oliguria, a precursor of eclampsia. Some obstetricians prefer to rely on serum urate levels as a more sensitive marker (Redman *et al.* 1976b). Blood platelet levels may be obtained to check for the occurrence of any intravascular coagulation, another sign of worsening condition and possible impending eclampsia (Redman *et al.* 1977).

The woman will be anxious about her own condition and about her partner and family. Full explanations should be given at all times, to allow her to do some forward planning; flexibility of visiting times may help prevent feelings of isolation. Boredom can be a problem – each ward should have a selection of books, magazines, puzzles, etc., to help the woman pass the time. Should she wish, she could attend parent education sessions or watch television.

Prevention and detection of eclampsia

The midwife caring for the woman with hypertension should always be alert to the onset of symptoms. Attention should be paid to maternal complaints of headache or feelings of nausea. Should the blood pressure begin to rise, it may be controlled using a slow intravenous infusion of hydrallazine or labetalol. This requires very close observation of blood pressure, preferably using an automatic pressure recorder (Knuppel and Drukker 1986). If one is not available, 5 minute recordings should be taken for 15 minutes and thereafter every 15 minutes and charted to detect rebound hypotension, which can further reduce placental perfusion.

There are many varied protocols for the care of women with impending or actual eclampsia, none of which has been evaluated in a controlled trial (Moore and Redman 1987). If the woman begins to show signs of imminent eclampsia, she may be given anticonvulsive therapy to prevent convulsions (Worley 1984). The drugs most commonly used are diazepam or chlormethiazole by slow intravenous infusion, titrated against the woman's condition to keep her drowsy (Worley 1984). Her level of consciousness is determined by assessment of her reflexes and her neurological condition. Diazepam should not be given for too long, as the baby when born may be hypotonic (Berkowitz *et al.* 1981). The paediatricians should be alerted that the mother has received diazepam due to the increased risk of neonatal jaundice.

Urinary output should be closely observed to assess renal function; this is best achieved by using an indwelling foley catheter, measuring and testing output hourly with a urometer to minimise disturbance (Rafferty and Berkowitz 1980). Oliguria is a poor prognostic sign. Diuretics should not be given as they are of no value and they can complicate the hypovolaemia of severe pre-eclampsia (Palomaki and Lindheimer 1970). A central venous pressure line may be set up to ensure an adequate circulating fluid volume. The woman is examined for the development of pulmonary oedema, which is a sign of a deteriorating condition.

Fetal well-being must be closely observed either using a doptone or cardiotocograph. It is important that the mother in danger of developing eclampsia is cared for in a safe environment where she will not suffer any physical damage should a fit occur (Knuppel and Drukker 1986). An airway and suction apparatus should be at hand while the woman is cared for in a bed with padded cot sides. Any worsening of maternal or fetal condition must be noted and reported immediately to the medical staff. Should the woman have a fit she should not be left. The principles of care are give below:

1. Ensure an adequate airway. A padded tongue depressor may be used with care to aid insertion of the airway. Suction apparatus should be used to clear excess secretions.
2. Place the woman in the recovery position.
3. Administer oxygen (to assist maternal and fetal oxygenation).
4. Prevent maternal injury.
5. When the convulsion has ceased, the maternal and fetal condition can be assessed and the findings documented.

An eclamptic fit has four stages:

1. A premonitory stage lasting 10–20 seconds. The woman is restless with altered awareness; she may show rapid eye movements.
2. A tonic stage lasting 20–30 seconds with spasm of muscle groups, arching of the back. Her teeth may be clenched and cyanosis can develop.
3. A clonic phase lasting 1–2 minutes of generalised grand mal convulsions. The woman is unconscious and her breathing may be noisy.
4. Coma. The recovery period lasting a variable length of time. Breathing may be irregular and noisy.

Labour and delivery

For the woman with mild hypertension, labour, whether spontaneous or induced, can proceed as normal. An epidural, if available and acceptable to the mother, is helpful to avoid further rises in blood pressure (Willocks and Moir 1968). Should the blood pressure rise during labour, forceps may be used in the second stage of labour to avoid maternal exertion. Ergometrine should not be given for the management of the third stage, as this can produce a sudden rise in blood pressure (Forman and Sullivan 1952).

For the woman with severe hypertension, the obstetrician has to decide when (given the risk of prematurity) and how to deliver. If the latter, continuous fetal monitoring is essential (MacGillivray 1985b), preferably using a scalp electrode to obtain ECG recordings. Labour will be monitored as normal, with additional observations of blood pressure, urinary output and level of consciousness. An epidural can be the analgesic method of choice (Worley 1984) although it can affect the circulating fluid volume (Pritchard and Pritchard 1975). The severe hypertensive woman in labour should never be left alone by the midwife, whether or not the woman's partner is present (Knuppel and Drukker 1986). If there is any deviation from accepted limits in fetal or maternal condition, a caesarean section may be ordered (MacGillivray 1985b). If a vaginal delivery is to occur, forceps are usually used with syntocinon to assist management of the third stage.

Postnatal eclampsia

Close observations on all women with pregnancy hypertension must be maintained for the first 48 hours after delivery, while there is still a risk of eclampsia. The woman with severe hypertension will continue to be given intensive care on the delivery unit. If she remains not fully conscious, actions must be taken to avoid deep venous thrombosis or chest infection. The woman's partner must be kept informed of all developments and given free access to both mother and baby. As soon as the mother feels able, her baby (unless it is in poor condition in the Special Care Baby Unit) should be brought to see her. If the woman wishes to breast feed, either the baby could be put to the breast or the breasts expressed to stimulate lactation; this may be dependent on the type of medication given to the mother.

After an initial slow recovery period of about 36–48 hours, the mother usually makes a rapid return to normal puerperal state. Her memory may be somewhat hazy, due to drowsiness and temporary amnesia which occurs during convulsions; any questions should therefore receive frank answers.

Where the hypertension was mild, four-hourly blood pressure recordings and daily urinalysis should be sufficient to assess her return to normality and signs of developing eclampsia. A 6 week postnatal examination at the hospital is advisable to ascertain that blood pressure and renal function have returned to normal. If they have not, the woman will be referred to a physician for further investigation. In cases of pre-eclampsia, if the blood pressure is normal, the obstetrician can reassure the couple that the chances of recurrence in subsequent pregnancies are small.

References

Adams E M and MacGillivray I (1961) 'Long term effect of pre-eclampsia on blood pressure' *Lancet ii*: 1373–5

Altchek A (1964) 'Renal biopsy and its clinical correlation in toxaemia of pregnancy' *Circulation* 29(30(Suppl II)): 43–51

Berkowitz R L, Coustan D R and Mochizuki T K (1981) *Handbook for Prescribing Medications During Pregnancy* Little Brown: Boston

Bonnar J (1977) 'Acute and chronic coagulation problems in pregnancy' in L Poller (ed) *Recent Advances in Blood Coagulation Vol 2* 363–77 Churchill Livingstone: Edinburgh

Brosens I A (1977) 'Morphological changes in the utero-placental bed in pregnancy hypertension' *Clinics in Obstetrics and Gynaecology* 4: 573–93

Chesley L C (1978) *Hypertensive Disorders of Pregnancy* Appleton-Century-Crofts: New York

Chesley L C (1980) 'Hypertension in pregnancy' *Kidney International* 18: 234–40

Chesley L C, Annito J E and Cosgrove R A (1968) 'The familial factor in toxemia of pregnancy' *Obstetrics and Gynecology* 32: 303

Davey D W and MacGillivray I (1988) 'The classification and definition of hypertensive disorders in pregnancy' *American Journal of Obstetrics and Gynecology* 158: 892–8

Department of Health (1991) *Report on Confidential Enquiry into Maternal Deaths in the United Kingdom 1985–87* HMSO: London de Sweit M (1980) 'The cardiovascular system' in F E Hytten and G Chamberlain (eds) *Clinical Physiology in Obstetrics* 3–42 Blackwell Scientific: Oxford

Detweiler D K (1972) 'Circulation' in J R Brobeck (ed) *Best and Taylor's Physiological Basis of Medical Practice (9th edn)* Section C Williams and Willens: New York

Forman J B and Sullivan R L (1952) 'Effects of intravenous injections of ergonovine and methergine on the post partum patient' *American Journal of Obstetrics and Gynecology* 63: 640–4

Fox H (1991) 'A contemporary view of the human placenta' *Midwifery* 7: 31–9

Friedman E A and Neff R K (1977) *Pregnancy Hypertension* PSG Littleton: Massachusetts

Ganong W F (1973) *Medical Physiology (6th edn)* Lange: Los Altos

Green J (1989) 'Diet and the prevention of pre-eclampsia' in I Chalmers, M Enkin and M J N C Keirse (eds) *Effective Care in Pregnancy and Childbirth* Chapter 18 281–300 Oxford Medical: Oxford

Hall M, McIntyre S and Porter M (1985) *Antenatal Care Assessed* Aberdeen University Press: Aberdeen

Hankins G D V (1986) 'Principles of invasive hemodynamic monitoring' *Clinics in Perinatology* 13: 765

Hibbard B M (1988) *Principles of Obstetrics* Butterworth: London

Hytten F E (1990) 'Is it important or even useful to measure weight gain in pregnancy?' *Midwifery* 6(1): 28–32

Ikedife D (1980) 'Eclampsia in multipara' *British Medical Journal* 1: 985–6

Johnson T and Clayton C G (1957) 'Diffusion of radioactive sodium in normotensive and pre-eclamptic pregnancies' *British Medical Journal* 1: 312–4

Knuppel R A and Drukker J E (1986) 'Hypertension in pregnancy' in R A Knuppel and J E Drukker (eds) *High Risk Pregnancy: A team approach* Chapter 20 362–98 W B Saunders: Philadelphia

Lunell N O, Nylund L E, Lewander R, Sarby B and Thornstrom S (1982) 'Uteroplacental blood flow in pre-eclampsia measurements with indium-113 m and a computer linked gamma camera' *Clinical and Experimental Hypertension* B1: 105–17

MacGillivray I (1983) *Pre-eclampsia: Hypertensive disease in pregnancy* W B Saunders: London

MacGillivray I (1985a) 'Aetiology of pre-eclampsia' in G Chamberlain (ed) *Contemporary Obstetrics* 64–74 Butterworth: London

MacGillivray I (1985b) 'Pre-eclampsia' *Midwifery* 1(1): 12–18

MacGillivray I, Rose G A and Rowe B (1969) 'Blood pressure survey in pregnancy' *Clinical Science* 37: 395–407

Mathews D D, Agarwal V and Shuttleworth T P (1982) 'A randomised controlled trial of complete bed rest versus ambulation in the management of proteinuric hypertension during pregnancy' *British Journal of Obstetrics and Gynaecology* 89: 128–31

Maxwell M H, Waks A U, Schroth P C, Karam M and Dornfield L P (1982) 'Error in blood pressure measurement due to incorrect cuff size in patients' *Lancet* ii: 33–5

Moore M P and Redman C W G (1987) 'Hypertension in pregnancy' in J Bonnar (ed) *Recent Advances in Obstetrics and Gynaecology Vol XV* 3–31 Churchill Livingstone: Edinburgh

Murphy J F, O'Riordan J, Newcombe R G, Coles E C and Pearson J F (1986) 'Relation of haemoglobin levels in the first and second trimesters to outcome of pregnancy' *Lancet* i: 992–4

Nelson T R (1955) 'A clinical study of pre-eclampsia' *Journal of Obstetrics and Gynaecology of the British Empire* 62: 48–57

Page E W and Christianson R (1976) 'The impact of mean arterial blood pressure in the middle trimester upon the outcome of pregnancy' *American Journal of Obstetrics and Gynecology* 125: 740–6

Palomaki J F and Lindheimer M D (1970) 'Sodium depletion stimulating deterioration in a toxemic pregnancy' *New England Journal of Medicine* 282: 88–9

Petrucco O (1981) 'Aetiology of pre-eclampsia' in J Studd (ed) *Progress in Obstetrics and Gynaecology Vol 1* Ch 5 51–69 Churchill Livingstone: Edinburgh

Pipkin F B (1986) 'Hypertension of pregnancy' *Cardiology in Practice* March: 15–20

Porapakkham S (1979) 'An epidemiologic study of eclampsia' *Obstetrics and Gynecology* 54: 26–30

Pritchard J A (1980) 'Management of pre-eclampsia and eclampsia' *Kidney International* 18: 259

Pritchard J A and Pritchard R A (1975) 'Standardized treatment in 154 cases of eclampsia' *American Journal of Obstetrics and Gynecology* 123: 543

Rafferty T D and Berkowitz R L (1980) 'Hemodynamics in patients with severe toxemia during labor and delivery' *American Journal of Obstetrics and Gynecology* 138: 263

Redman C W G (1984) 'Hypertension in pregnancy' in M de Sweit (ed) *Medical Disorders in Obstetric Practice* Ch 6 149–91 Blackwell Scientific: Oxford

Redman C W G, Beilin L J, Bonnar J and Ounstead M K (1976a) 'Fetal outcome in a trial of antihypertensive treatment in pregnancy' *Lancet* ii: 753–6

Redman C W G, Beilin L J and Bonnar J (1976b) 'Renal function in pre-eclampsia' *Journal of Clinical Pathology* 29(Suppl 10): 91–4

Redman C W G, Denson K W E, Beilin L J, Bolton F G and Stirrat G M (1977) 'Factor VIII consumption in pre-eclampsia' *Lancet* ii: 1249–52

Redman C W G, Bonnar J and Beilin L J (1978) 'Early platelet consumption in preeclampsia' *British Medical Journal* i: 467–9

Robertson E G (1971) 'The natural history of oedema during pregnancy' *Journal of Obstetrics and Gynaecology of the British Commonwealth* 78: 520–9

Rosen E L (1976) 'Concerns of an obstetric patient experiencing long-term hospitalisation' *Journal of Obstetrical, Gynecological and Neonatal Nursing* 4: 15–19

Ruff S C, Mitchell R H and Murnaghan G A (1982) 'Long-term variations of blood pressure rhythms in normotensive pregnancy and preeclampsia' in M B Sanmour, E M Symonds, T F Zuspan and A el-Tomi (eds) *Pregnancy Hypertension* 129–33 Ain Shams University Press: Cairo

Shaw A B, Risdon P and Lewis-Jackson J D (1983) 'Protein creatinine index and Albustix in assessment of proteinuria' *British Medical Journal* 287: 929–32

Sheehan B L and Lynch J B (1973) *Pathology of Toxaemia of Pregnancy* 211–5 Churchill Livingstone: Edinburgh

Stewart M (1985) 'An updated view of the physiology of pregnancy' in G N Marsh (ed) *Modern Obstetrics in General Practice* 69–84 Oxford Medical: Oxford

Stirratt G M (1985) 'Management of hypertension' in G Chamberlain (ed) *Contemporary Obstetrics* 84–92 Butterworth: London

Walker J J, Belch J J F, Erwin L, McLaren M, Lang G, Forbes C D, Prentice C R M and Calder A A (1982) 'Labetalol and platelet function in pre-eclampsia' *Lancet* ii: 279

Wallenburg H C S (1988) 'Haemodynamics in hypertensive pregnancy' in P Rubin (ed) *Handbook of Hypertension Vol 10 Hypertension in Pregnancy* 66–101 Elsevier: Amsterdam

Webster J, Newnham D, Petrie J C and Lovell H G (1984) 'Influence of arm position in measurement of blood pressure' *British Medical Journal* 288: 1574–5

Willocks J and Moir D (1968) 'Epidural analgesia in the management of hypertension in labour' *Journal of Obstetrics and Gynaecology of the British Commonwealth* 75: 225–8

Worley R J (1984) 'Eclampsia' in J Studd (ed) *Progress in Obstetrics and Gynaecology Vol 4* Ch 13 183–96 Churchill Livingstone: Edinburgh

13 Medical disorders and childbirth

This chapter considers the effects of pre-existing medical diseases on pregnancy, labour and the puerperium. The disorders described are diabetes mellitus, cardiac disease, renal disease, epilepsy and cystic fibrosis (essential hypertension is considered in Chapter 24).

The role of the midwife

The presence of a medical disorder results in the woman's progress from preconception care to the puerperium being closely observed by physician and obstetrician. This can create a medicalised and pathological approach to the supervision and care which is given (Merkatz *et al.* 1978). There may be little maternal choice in the selection of place of confinement. The woman will usually be booked for delivery at a consultant unit or possibly a regional referral centre. The role of the midwife in the care of such women is to seek to emphasise those aspects of the pregnancy, labour and the puerperium which are normal. These include parent education and the psychological aspects of childbirth. This is important to assist the parents to establish a satisfactory relation with their new baby (McDonald 1968). Depending on the severity of the disease, having a baby could be the first time that the woman has felt any similarity with other healthy women (Merkatz *et al.* 1978).

Psychologically, childbirth puts a strain on the woman with a pre-existing medical disorder (Johnson and Murphy 1986). She may worry whether the decision to embark upon the pregnancy was correct, what effect the disease will have on the baby and what deterioration will occur in her condition as a result of the processes of childbirth (Johnson and Murphy 1986). The woman must be kept fully informed about the progress of the pregnancy and of her disease. The couple may require much information about normal pregnancy and childbirth against which to assess their own progress (Browne and Dixon 1978).

Diabetes mellitus

Diabetes is a condition of the cells of the pancreas, where there is a deficiency in the production of insulin (Strong and Baird 1971). This produces alterations in the metabolism of protein, fat and carbohydrate resulting in hyperglycaemia and associated glycosuria (Strong and Baird 1971). Prior to the discovery of insulin, pregnancy was rare amongst diabetics; if it did occur, mortality rates were high (Donald 1979). Although maternal outcome is much improved, Coustan and Felig (1988) report perinatal death rates in the USA of 30–50/1000 total births. Some British centres quote mortality rates in the range 16–20/1000 (Vaughan 1987). This is considerably higher than amongst the general population. One of the major problems still to be solved is the high rate of congenital abnormality amongst the infant of the diabetic mother (IDM) (Pederson 1977). Most pre-existing diabetics receive preconception advice before embarking on a pregnancy and, once pregnant, have joint care from obstetricians and physicians (Steel *et al.* 1982).

There are four main types of diabetic as described by Lind (1980).

1. The known clinical diabetic who is usually managed with insulin. They have the symptoms of diabetes with an abnormal glucose tolerance test (GTT), i.e. serum glucose estimation and urinalysis following a measured oral dose of glucose taken after a 12 hour fast.
2. The asymptomatic diabetic whose only sign is an abnormal response to the GTT.
3. The latent diabetic who at times of stress (such as pregnancy or obesity) has an abnormal GTT; this group were previously referred to as gestational diabetics.
4. The final group are those people who are at risk of diabetes in the future, due to family history of diabetes in a close relative or a previous birth (live or still) of a baby weighing more than 4.5 kg. (Lind 1980). Pyke (1962) showed that, whereas 1.5% of all newborn babies weigh over 4.5 kg, the frequency of such births is 4–31% where the mother subsequently develops diabetes.

The effect of pregnancy on diabetes

The midwife is unlikely during antenatal care to detect an unknown clinical diabetic but by history-taking, she may well suspect the presence of a latent or potential diabetic. Pregnancy itself is diabetogenic (West 1983). The resistance of tissues to insulin increases during pregnancy, necessitating a rise in insulin production to move glucose from the blood stream to the tissues (Kuhl 1975). Women whose insulin production is only just sufficient when they are not pregnant will be unable to increase secretion to the levels required (Abell and Beischer 1975).

The demand for insulin rises as pregnancy continues (Kalkhoff et al. 1979). If insulin production is insufficient, hyperglycaemia may result and if severe, it will be accompanied by intracellular dehydration (Kalkhoff et al. 1979). When serum glucose levels exceed the ability of the renal tubules to reabsorb the glucose, glycosuria occurs. This is a useful test in non-pregnant women, since glycosuria does not occur until serum glucose exceeds 10 mmol/l. Unfortunately, in pregnancy the renal threshold for glucose is reduced. Glycosuria can occur at serum levels of 8.4 mmol/l, well within the normal response range for a GTT (Strong and Baird 1971). For this reason, glycosuria in pregnancy should only be used as a screening test for diabetes rather than as diagnostic. Where a woman has shown more than a trace of glucose on urinalysis on at least one occasion she is usually sent for a GTT (Jowett and Nicol 1986). Some obstetricians favour performing a random blood sugar analysis on all women as a screening test (Lind and Anderson 1984). This can be dependent upon when and what the woman last ate.

When insulin level is low in a normal person, serum glucose level is also low and the tissues are short of available energy. This results in the breakdown of protein and fats to produce more glucose (Kalkhoff et al. 1979). However, when this happens in a diabetic whose low insulin levels are not related to low blood sugar but to deficient insulin production, high serum glucose levels are further boosted (Kalkhoff et al. 1979). Glucose is unavailable to the tissues due to an absence of insulin to facilitate its passage out of the blood stream. Oxidation of free fatty acids produced by fat breakdown results in the production of ketones, which can give rise to acidosis (Kalkhoff et al. 1979). Even normal women are likely to develop ketosis in pregnancy especially following an overnight fast (Coustan and Felig 1988). Pederson (1977) has shown that, due to the instability of diabetes in pregnancy, there is an increased risk of diabetic complications (such as retinopathy) occurring.

Effects of diabetes on pregnancy

Poor control of diabetes from conception onwards results in increased rates of spontaneous abortion and congenital abnormalities (Coustan and Felig 1988). There is also an increased risk of intrauterine death, which is greatly reduced with good diabetic control. Complications such as gestational proteinuric hypertension and polyhydramnios are higher in diabetic mothers, being worst amongst those with poor metabolic control (Coustan and Felig 1988). There is also an increased risk of infection in pregnancy and the puerperium. Laurini et al. (1984) have reported changes in the morphology of the placentae of diabetic mothers. This differential rate of maturation has been demonstrated in women with good diabetic control.

Fetal effects of maternal diabetes are those of macrosomia (Dandona *et al.* 1984), hyperinsulinaemia (West 1983) and delayed lung maturity (Speidal 1983). Unlike congenital anomalies, these can also occur in the infant of the latent (gestational) diabetic. Increased production of growth factors results in the infant being born large for gestational age. The fetus becomes accustomed to high circulating glucose levels. To compensate, fetal insulin production is stimulated and excess calories are stored as fat (Dandona *et al.* 1984). After delivery, when the placental supply of glucose ceases, high insulin levels cause neonatal hypoglycaemia. This excess insulin production resolves itself within 48 hours after birth. Neonatal blood sugar levels require careful observation (Lewis and Steyger 1985).

High insulin levels (which can occur where the mother is receiving insulin therapy) delay lung maturation, causing a fivefold increase in the occurrence of respiratory distress syndrome (Speidal 1983). The lecithin:sphyngomyelin ratio in amniotic fluid is unreliable as a determinant of lung maturity in the infant of the diabetic mother (Farnell *et al.* 1984). Respiratory support may be required for such infants (see Chapter 37).

Management of pregnancy

The known diabetic is usually cared for in joint antenatal and diabetic clinics (Steel *et al.* 1982). This prevents excessive journeys to hospital. To detect fetal abnormality, which is more common in the infant of the diabetic mother, an early ultrasound scan should be performed. Modern diabetic management with accurate home blood glucose estimation and modern insulins has superseded the earlier practice of admitting women to achieve diabetic control (Murphy *et al.* 1984). This minimises disruption to the woman and her family. The aim of diabetic care during pregnancy is to achieve a state of normoglycaemia. This is usually achieved by giving a twice daily combination of short- and long-acting insulins (Gilmer 1983). These can be supplemented where necessary with small multiple injections via, for example, the Novopen. Blood glucose levels are determined using Boehringer-Mannheim (BM) sticks, which remain accurate after use and can be examined on hospital visits. Blood profiles are usually taken four to six times daily two or three times weekly (Gilmer 1983).

Modern theories about diet include having 40–45% of calories as carbohydrate (preferably complex and starchy rather than simple and sugary) and a high fibre intake (Vaughan 1987). Fibre delays glucose absorption, thus reducing peak blood sugar levels after a meal (Jenkins 1981). Fat restriction is encouraged because of the risk of arterial disease amongst diabetics.

An assessment of the degree of diabetic control over the previous 3 months is achieved by measurement of glycosylated haemoglobin, HbA1 (Saunders *et al.* 1980). High levels are seen where control is poor (Gonen *et al.* 1977). Normal HbA1 levels are 5–6% of the total haemoglobin. The diabetic mother should also have examinations for the onset or worsening of diabetic complications (Coustan and

Felig 1988). The progress of pregnancy is assessed by frequent tests of fetal well-being, including cardiotocography and serial ultrasound scans. Blood pressure recordings and urinalysis for protein should be carefully performed to detect early signs of gestational proteinuric hypertension. Measurements of abdominal height and girth will be made to detect onset of polyhydramnios (West 1983).

A major diabetic complication in pregnancy is ketoacidosis. This must be rapidly treated as there is a high risk of fetal death (Brumfield and Huddleston 1984). Diabetics should have glucose close at hand at all times. This is especially important in the early hours of the morning if insufficient carbohydrate was eaten prior to retiring.

Apparently normal women who show glucose on urinalysis will usually be given a GTT (Jowett and Nicol 1986). In pregnancy, this is often amended to involve 4 blood tests only, a fasting level and at 1, 2 and possibly 3 hours after the carbohydrate dose. If the test is abnormal, the woman is treated as a latent (gestational) diabetic. Diet alone may be sufficient to control blood glucose levels, if not, insulin therapy will be required. Obstetric and diabetic surveillance depend upon the severity of the condition (Oats and Beischer 1987).

Provided diabetic control is good and there are no obstetric complications, the diabetic mother is usually allowed to reach at least 38 weeks gestation before delivery is considered (West 1983). Where the diabetes is well controlled and fetal growth is normal, the mother may be left to go into spontaneous labour at term (Brudenell 1989). Where the cervix is favourable, induction of labour is preferable to elective caesarean section (Essex *et al.* 1973). Prior to induction the woman fasts overnight. In the morning, an infusion of 5–10% of dextrose is established (Brudenell 1989). Soluble insulin is given subcutaneously or via a small infusion pump. One- or two-hourly blood glucose estimations are performed (Crichton and Silverton 1985). Induction proceeds as normal, using intravenous oxytocin. It is important to provide sufficient glucose to meet the energy needs of the contracting uterus.

Where an elective caesarean section is to be performed, the woman is starved on the day of operation and her insulin dose omitted (Crichton and Silverton 1985). Dextrose 5% intravenously is commenced and soluble insulin given as appropriate. This infusion is continued after delivery until a normal diet is resumed (West 1983).

Immediately after delivery the need for insulin reduces. By 48 hours prepregnant demands are usually restored (West 1983). Lactation can be established with due allowance being made for increased energy needs. Blood glucose levels and urinalysis are necessary to observe for hypoglycaemia (Lewis and Steyger 1985). The mother should be encouraged to care for her baby as normal. Should the baby require admission to the Special Care Baby Unit, the mother should visit as soon as possible. Neonatal glucose levels should be explained, to prevent unnecessary anxiety over what she would think are very low levels (see Chapter 37 for the care of the baby).

The latent diabetic should be referred to the diabetic physician for a GTT at 6 weeks after delivery to assess her response to glucose (Oats and Beischer 1987).

Cardiac disease

In normal pregnancy, there is an approximate 40% increase in cardiac output from 3.5 to 6 l/min (de Swiet 1980). This increase is brought about by a rise in both the heart rate and the stroke volume (de Swiet 1980). Blood pressure is kept low by a fall in peripheral resistance. Any condition in which the heart is unable to increase cardiac output, such as significant mitral stenosis and Eisenmenger's syndrome, will worsen in pregnancy (de Swiet 1986). de Swiet and Fidler (1981) estimate the occurrence of cardiac disease in pregnancy as between 0.5 and 1.8% of women, depending on the socio-economic status of the community. It is apparent that whilst the overall incidence of cardiac disease is relatively static, there has been a reduction in rheumatic heart disease and an increase in congenital abnormalities, some of which have been surgically corrected (McAnulty et al. 1988). Cardiac disease is still a significant non-obstetric cause of maternal death (Department of Health 1989, 1991).

Diagnosis of cardiac disease for the first time in pregnancy is complicated by the presence of breathlessness or an ejection-systolic murmur caused by physiological changes (de Swiet 1984a). In addition, there are other changes in heart sounds during pregnancy which require careful identification.

Rheumatic heart disease

One of the major defects resulting from rheumatic disease is mitral stenosis (de Swiet 1984a). This produces an increase in pressure in the left atrium to push blood through the stenosed valve (de Swiet 1984a). If the atrium is unable to cope with the blood flow, pressure rises in the pulmonary circulation, resulting in pulmonary oedema or heart failure (de Swiet 1984a). In pregnancy the woman's condition can worsen rapidly, especially if sudden changes occur in the distribution of her blood volume (McAnulty et al. 1988). In contrast, women with either aortic or mitral valve regurgitation (incompetence) tolerate pregnancy well and they may even experience some improvement in their condition (McAnulty et al. 1988). Antibiotic cover in labour is advised as prophylaxis against bacterial endocarditis (McAnulty et al. 1988).

Congenital heart disease

Increasing numbers of women with congenital heart disease (CHD) are reaching child-bearing age. Some have minor degrees, whereas others have had total or partial surgical repair of the defect. Depending on each abnormality, the response to pregnancy can be different. The woman may carry an increased risk of maternal mortality or morbidity or of fetal growth retardation or death (McAnulty et al. 1988). It must also be remembered that there is an increased risk of the child developing CHD, depending on the balance of genetic and environmental factors (McAnulty et al. 1988).

The most common disorders of CHD, atrial septal defect, patent ductus arteriosus and ventricular septal defect, are usually repaired by surgery if severe (McAnulty *et al.* 1988). Despite surgery, a small degree of deficit may remain. This would tend to cause shunting of blood from the left to the right side of the heart (McAnulty *et al.* 1988). Unless pulmonary vascular disease occurs, the relative resistances of systemic and pulmonary circulations remain similar and therefore no deterioration occurs in the condition (Metcalfe and Ueland 1974). Should gestational proteinuric hypertension occur, pulmonary vascular resistance rises and a left-to-right shunt with cyanosis and a right ventricular hypertrophy can result (McAnulty *et al.* 1988). Intrauterine growth retardation and fetal death can occur, depending on the severity of the condition (Batson 1974).

More serious are the (thankfully) rarer defects such as Eisenmenger's syndrome (a large ventricular septal defect with a reverse (right-to-left) shunt) and Fallot's tetralogy (a large subaortic ventricular septal defect, stenosis of the pulmonary valve and pulmonary artery, and hypoplasia of the infundibulum below the pulmonary valve) which result in permanent cyanosis (de Swiet 1984b). They carry a high maternal mortality (especially Eisenmenger's syndrome). Early termination of pregnancy may be advised (Gleicher *et al.* 1979).

Care in pregnancy

Each woman must be assessed as an individual to determine the effects of pregnancy on her condition and vice versa (McAnulty *et al.* 1988). Joint care between physician and obstetrician is advised, as this reduces travelling time (de Swiet 1984a). Where cardiac disease is suspected or diagnosed for the first time in pregnancy the woman should be seen by a physician who will order diagnostic tests such as chest X-Ray and ECG (X-Ray will be used with caution in early pregnancy) before confirming the diagnosis (de Swiet 1984a). Some conditions are completely asymptomatic and require no follow-up, although de Swiet (1984b) recommends antibiotic cover in labour.

Medical management is aimed at removing those factors which predispose to heart failure, meanwhile observing the mother so that should failure occur, it is actively managed (McAnulty *et al.* 1988). Risk factors for heart failure include:

- Infections – urinary tract and upper respiratory tract.
- Anaemia.
- Hypertension – pregnancy associated hypertension and pre-existing hypertension.
- Obesity.
- Multiple pregnancy – due to the larger increase in cardiac output.
- Smoking (de Swiet 1984a).

The amount of rest required depends on the individual. For some, admission to hospital may be necessitated, with all the attendant physical and emotional disruption

(McAnulty *et al*. 1988). For others, rest at home or simply taking sick leave from employment may be sufficient. (After 28 weeks in the United Kingdom, if eligible, the woman will be on maternity leave.) De Swiet (1984a) comments that it is hard to determine who may gain more from rest, the mother or the fetus. Should heart failure develop admission to hospital is necessary.

The mother should be screened carefully for the presence of infections, especially those of the urinary tract (McAnulty *et al*. 1988). Prophylactic iron therapy may be given to prevent anaemia. Fetal well-being needs close assessment, especially given the risk of intrauterine growth retardation. Parent education should be provided for the woman and her partner either at home or in hospital (if she is an in-patient). It may not be advisable for her to attend normal classes. Specific information regarding the conduct of labour and childcare could be particularly useful (Johnson and Murphy 1986).

Ideally the woman will go into spontaneous labour (McAnulty *et al*. 1988). In certain cases, induction at term using prostaglandin pessaries is advised to plan labour and delivery for a time when expert medical care is at hand (de Swiet 1984a). Where the woman is taking drugs which react with prostaglandins, giving rise to pulmonary oedema, prostaglandin pessaries should not be used. Care must be taken to not overtransfuse with fluid, nor to permit the woman to be on her back, causing supine hypotension (de Swiet 1984b). Women with cardiac disease, especially if receiving digoxin, do labour quickly and easily (Weaver and Pearson 1973). Epidural anaesthesia (which decreases cardiac output) is advisable, except where there is out-flow obstruction (as in Eisenmenger's syndrome and hypertrophic cardiomyopathy) (James 1989). During labour, careful observation of cardiac function should be maintained. This may include an ECG monitor with 15 minute recordings of pulse, respiration and fetal heart rate and half-hourly blood pressure and maternal colour. Any deviation from normal, such as tachypnoea, should be reported. Undue maternal effort is contra-indicated in the second stage, with forceps being used where the mother cannot deliver the baby easily (de Swiet 1984a).

Antibiotic prophylaxis may be prescribed during labour and for 48 hours afterwards to prevent bacterial endocarditis, although there have been no randomised controlled trials to demonstrate its efficacy (de Swiet 1984a). In addition, heparin may be given as an anticoagulant to prevent thrombi developing. It is usually prescribed for women with artificial heart valves. It should be used with caution to avoid causing antepartum or postpartum haemorrhage (de Swiet 1984a).

Ergometrine is not advisable for management of the third stage, since it causes a non-physiological tonic contraction of the uterus, with an increase of about 500 ml in blood volume (de Swiet 1984a).

Syntocinon is usually sufficient to prevent haemorrhage. A diuretic such as frusemide may also be given to reduce the risk of pulmonary oedema; this is possibly the only indication for the use of diuretics in pregnancy (Hytten, personal communication).

Careful monitoring during the first 48 hours after birth is necessary until the circulating blood volume and cardiac output return to prepregnant levels (McAnulty *et al*. 1988). The mother must also be closely observed for any signs of her developing an infection. Care in the puerperium can proceed as normal, although the mother may require extra rest and support in the home. The baby should be carefully examined for signs of congenital heart disease. Breast feeding is advisable (except where maternal medications contra-indicate it), since the mother gets a rest whilst she feeds the baby. Contraception should be discussed, together with the need for pregnancy spacing. Where the family is complete, sterilisation (male or female) is usually delayed until 3 months after the delivery.

Chronic renal disease

During pregnancy, the kidney increases in length by 1 cm and there is dilation in the calyces, renal pelves and in the ureters. These changes predispose to urinary stasis and infection, especially acute pyelonephritis (Davison 1984). Increases of up to 50% in the glomerular filtration rate (GFR) alter the parameters used to assess renal function (Davison 1984). Plasma creatinine levels in pregnancy should not exceed 75 mmol/l (non-pregnant range 70–130 mmol/l) and plasma urea a maximum of 4.5 mmol/l (non-pregnant level 2.5–6.6 mmol/l) (Davison 1984).

Women with pre-existing renal disease should receive prepregnancy advice about the advisability of childbirth. Where there is no obvious renal insufficiency or significant hypertension prior to conception, the pregnancy will usually end success-fully (Davison and Lindheimer 1984). There is no evidence that pregnancy causes deterioration in renal disease over and above the effects of time (de Swiet 1986).

Antenatal care involves visits to see the obstetrician and the physician every 2 weeks until 32 weeks and weekly thereafter (Davison 1984). The care is aimed at preventing and detecting hypertension, assessment of renal function (by measurement of protein excretion and creatinine clearance in 24 hour samples), nutritional assessment (especially where proteinuria is marked), screening for asymptomatic bacteruria and urinary tract infections and measurements of fetal well-being (intrauterine growth retardation is common) (Davison 1984). Any deterioration in maternal or fetal condition would necessitate admission to hospital.

For women on haemodialysis, amenorrhoea is common and conception is rare, although it can occur (de Swiet 1986). Since accidental pregnancy can occur, where it is not desired or it is unadvisable for medical reasons, good contraceptive advice is necessary. Where pregnancy does occur, there is a high rate of fetal loss from both spontaneous and therapeutic abortions (Davison 1984). If the pregnancy continues, dialysis times need to be increased by up to 50% to cope with the excretory demands of the fetus (Kobayashi et al. 1981).

In women who have received a renal transplant, their fertility is greatly improved, with many successful pregnancies now being reported (Davison 1987). Prepregnancy assessment is important to highlight both short- and long-term prospects. Davison et al. (1976) give the following guidelines for a successful outcome:

1. Good general health for 2 years after transplantation.
2. Stature compatible with good obstetric outcome.

3. No proteinuria.
4. No significant hypertension.
5. No evidence of graft rejection.
6. No evidence of pelvic distention on a recent excretory urogram.
7. Plasma creatinine 180 mmol/l or less.
8. During therapy: prednisolone 15 mg/day or less and azathioprine 2 mg/kg/day or less. (Davison and Lindheimer 1984)

Long-term issues include consideration of the survival time of both the recipient and the graft. Since the technique is only 25 years old, improvements in survival are occurring as management is developing. The chance for a normal life with parenthood often outweighs worries about the mother's own survival (Davison 1987).

The organisation and provision of care is similar to that for mothers with pre-existing renal disease. In addition, the function and acceptance of the graft must be kept under constant surveillance (Davison 1987). Problems in pregnancy include the occurrence of gestational proteinuric hypertension in 30% of pregnancies, which is difficult to differentiate from the other forms of hypertension which can also affect renal functioning (Davison 1987). The woman should be carefully observed for the presence of any infection to which she is vulnerable due to immunosuppression. Urinary tract infections occur in as many as 40% of women with a transplant whose renal failure was as a result of chronic pyelonephritis (Davison 1987). Other risks to mother and baby include viral infections such as herpes simplex, hepatitis B and cytomegalovirus (CMV) (Davison 1984).

The timing of delivery is dependent on the progress of the mother, the pregnancy and the fetus. Spontaneous or induced preterm delivery is common (Davison 1987). Labour usually proceeds as normal with the addition of extra steroid cover for the stress of labour. Maternal fluid balance, cardiovascular well-being and temperature need close observation (Davison 1987). The woman is prone to infection, so strict asepsis is required. Prophylactic antibiotics may be prescribed (Davison 1987). Operative delivery is used for obstetric reasons only.

The neonate is often both preterm and small for gestational age. The baby needs screening for viral infections (including CMV and hepatitis) which are more common amongst people who have undergone renal dialysis. It appears that the small doses of maternal immunosuppressents used do not cause significant congenital abnormalities (Ferris 1988). More research is needed to assess the effects of small gaps in the chromosomes of lymphocytes which are seen in early infancy (Davison 1987). Breast feeding is still not advisable, due to a lack of information on the effects of azathioprine and its metabolites which are excreted in breast milk (Davison and Lindheimer 1984).

In the puerperium, the mother requires careful assessment of her renal function. Although pregnancy appears to have no effect on graft functioning or survival, 10% of mothers die within 7 years of the birth of their child (Davison 1987). The choice of method of contraception is difficult, since combined hormonal oral contraception increases the risk of hypertension and thromboembolism, whilst intrauterine contraceptive devices predispose to pelvic infection in immunosuppressed women (Davison 1987).

Epilepsy

Epilepsy occurs in 0.5% of pregnant women (James 1989). For known epileptics, prepregnancy counselling is necessary to explore the implications of childbirth. Pregnancy is not advisable in women whose epilepsy is poorly controlled (Royal College of Midwives 1988). Ramsey *et al.* (1978), in a study of known epileptics during pregnancy, found that 45% experienced more seizures, 12% fewer and in 43% of women there was no change. Epilepsy may appear for the first time during pregnancy, but this is a chance event. The pregnancy does not cause the epilepsy (Hopkins 1984).

The parent's concerns are usually related to the risks of transmitting epilepsy genetically, the effects of anticonvulsive therapy and the effect of a fit, should it occur. Most types of epilepsy are not hereditary. Espir (1986) states an overall increased risk of epilepsy in a child where one parent is affected of between 3 and 6%. Some of the anticonvulsant drugs are known to be teratogenic. For example, phenytoin therapy is associated with a threefold increase in congenital anomalies such as cleft lip and palate (Espir 1986). However, the risk of a fit is far more dangerous to the fetus than the risk of abnormality, with at least 80% of children being normal (de Swiet 1986). In some cases, the drugs may need to be changed prior to pregnancy and in others, the woman may find that her treatment can be reduced or discontinued. Those taking anticonvulsants are usually advised to have folate supplementation throughout pregnancy to reduce the risk of megaloblastic anaemia (de Swiet 1986). Serum levels of anticonvulsants should be measured, since changes in blood volume and hormonal effects can alter the therapeutic dose (Hopkins 1984).

Midwifery care involves careful listening and giving advice about safety (Royal College of Midwives 1988). Most existing epileptics will be well aware of the need for safety in the home. It is advisable that during pregnancy the woman should not bathe or shower alone in case a seizure occurs. While she is in hospital, a member of staff should be informed so that they can maintain 'discrete supervision' (Royal College of Midwives 1988). Should a seizure occur during pregnancy, the woman should contact her midwife or her doctor so that the fetal heart rate can be checked (Royal College of Midwives 1988). Should a seizure occur when the midwife is with the woman, the following steps should be taken:

(a) Place something soft under her head.
(b) Carefully loosen any tight clothing around her neck.
(c) Do not stop any body movements. Wait until these movements stop and the first deep breath is taken.
(d) Turn the person onto one side into the recovery position.
(e) Stay with the mother until she recovers fully.

(f) Do not restrain her or try to 'bring her round'.

(g) Do not give her anything by mouth until you are certain she is fully recovered.

(h) Tell the woman what has been happening.

(i) Medical staff **must** be kept informed.

(j) Appropriate records must be made. (Royal College of Midwives 1988, pp. 8 and 9)

During labour, care should be taken that anticonvulsive treatment continues; intravenous administration may be required to counteract the poor absorption of oral therapy. In later pregnancy, labour and the puerperium, it is sometimes difficult to differentiate epileptic from eclamptic fits (Hopkins 1984). Eclamptic fits rarely occur later than 48 hours after delivery and nor do they occur in the absence of hypertension or proteinuria (Hopkins 1984). It is important to try to make the labour and delivery of this mother as normal as possible (Royal College of Midwives 1988). Delivery on mattresses on the floor has certain advantages, should a seizure occur. It must be remembered that stress and tiredness both increase the risk of fits. The mother should be cared for during labour and the puerperium in an area where she can come to no harm. In labour this may mean having a midwife in constant attendance (Royal College of Midwives 1988) in the puerperium; cot-sides may need to be attached to the bed.

In the puerperium, the mother should learn to care for her baby in such a way that it is placed at the minimum of risk should a seizure occur. This may include changing and bathing the baby on the floor. In fact, feeding can be carried out whilst sitting on the floor supported by pillow or cushions (Royal College of Midwives 1988). Breast feeding is not contra-indicated, except for mothers receiving phenobarbitone medication. If she wishes to breast feed, her therapy should be changed before or during pregnancy (Hopkins 1984).

Cystic fibrosis

Cystic fibrosis is an autosomal recessive condition whose gene is carried by 1:20 caucasians (British Medical Journal 1979). The incidence of cystic fibrosis is approximately 1:2000 live births (British Medical Journal 1979). The disease affects the exocrine glands of the body, resulting in pancreatic disease and lung disease, both obstructive and restrictive (Weinberger and Weiss 1988). The condition is managed using a programme of intensive antibiotic therapy and frequent physiotherapy, with postural drainage and dietary supplementation of protein and sodium (de Swiet 1984c).

As people with cystic fibrosis are now living longer, they are reaching the reproductive years. Most males are sterile; women are fertile, but less than the general population (Weinberger and Weiss 1988). This is possibly due to the presence of thick cervical mucus which is resistant to penetration by sperm (Weinberger and Weiss 1988). Surveys of some of the pregnancies which have occurred have shown a geater rate of low maternal weight gain (41%) and congestive cardiac failure (13%) (Cohen *et al*. 1980). There were also increased frequencies of preterm delivery and perinatal death (Cohen *et al*. 1980). Maternal mortality in the 2 years following delivery was 18%, but this was not more than would be expected for non-pregnant women of the same age with cystic fibrosis (Cohen *et al*. 1980).

It is important to assess lung function in early pregnancy. If the vital capacity is less than 50% of normal, then termination of pregnancy is recommended (Mayberry *et al*. 1986). Prior to pregnancy, antibiotic therapy may need to be changed to a form safe for use in pregnancy, such as penicillin. During pregnancy, maternal rest is helpful to reduce energy expenditure. Dietary supplementation, including the use of pancreatic enzymes, is necessary to ensure maternal and fetal growth. Induction of labour is only necessary should a deterioration occur in the mother's condition (Mayberry *et al*. 1986). The risk of the child being born with cystic fibrosis is 2.5%, although all will carry one affected gene (Weinberger and Weiss 1988). Preconception screening of the partner can help decide whether gene typing of the fetus will be required.

References

Abell D A and Beischer N A (1975) 'Evaluation of the 3-hour oral glucose tolerance test in detection of significant hyperglycaemia and hypoglycaemia in pregnancy' *Diabetes* 24: 874–80

Batson G A (1974) 'Cyanotic congenital heart disease and pregnancy' *British Journal of Obstetrics and Gynaecology* 81: 549–53

British Medical Journal (1979) 'Editorial: Cystic fibrosis in adults' *British Medical Journal* 2: 626

Browne J C M and Dixon G (1978) *Browne's Antenatal care* Churchill Livingstone: Edinburgh

Brudenell M (1989) 'Diabetic pregnancy' in A Turnbull and G Chamberlain (eds) *Obstetrics* 585–603 Churchill Livingstone: Edinburgh

Brumfield C G and Huddleston J F (1984) 'The management of diabetic ketoacidosis in pregnancy' *Clinical Obstetrics and Gynecology* 27: 50–9

Cohen, L F, di Sant' Agnese P A and Friedlander J (1980) 'Cystic fibrosis and pregnancy' *Lancet* ii: 842

Coustan, D R and Felig P (1988) 'Diabetes mellitus' in G N Burrow, and T F Ferris (eds) *Medical Complications During Pregnancy (3rd edn)* Ch 2 34–64 W B Saunders: Philadelphia

Crichton M A and Silverton L I (1985) 'The sweeter side of life: a review of diabetes in pregnancy' *Midwifery* 1(4): 195–206

Dandona P, Besterman H S and Freedman D B (1984) 'Macrosomia despite well controlled diabetic pregnancy' *Lancet* i: 737

Davison J M (1984) 'Renal disease' in M de Swiet (ed) *Medical Disorders in Obstetric Practice* Ch 7 192–259 Blackwell Scientific: Oxford

Davison J M (1987) 'Pregnancy and motherhood following renal transplantation' *Midwifery* 3(3): 125–32

Davison J M and Lindheimer M D (1984) 'Pregnancy and renal disease' in J Studd (ed) *Progress in Obstetrics and Gynaecology Vol IV* Ch ll 151–65 Churchill Livingstone: Edinburgh

Davison J M, Lind T and Uldall P R (1976) 'Planned pregnancy in a renal transplant recipient' *British Journal of Obstetrics and Gynaecology* 83: 518–27

Department of Health (1989) *Report on the Confidential Enquiries into Maternal Deaths in England and Wales 1982–4* HMSO: London

Department of Health (1991) *Report on Confidential Enquiries into Maternal Deaths in the United Kingdom 1985–7* HMSO: London

de Swiet M (1980) 'The cardio vascular system' in F Hytten and G Chamberlain (eds) *Clinical Physiology in Obstetrics* Ch 1 3 Blackwell Scientific : Oxford

de Swiet M (1984a) 'Heart disease in pregnancy' in M de Swiet (ed) *Medical Disorders in Obstetric Practice* Ch 5 116–48 Blackwell Scientific: Oxford

de Swiet M (1984b) 'Heart disease in pregnancy' in J Studd (ed) *Progress in Obstetrics and Gynaecology Vol IV* Ch 12 166–82 Churchill Livingstone: Edinburgh

de Swiet M (1984c) 'Diseases of the respiratory system' in M de Swiet (ed) *Medical Disorders in Obstetric Practice* Ch 1 1–34 Blackwell Scientific: Oxford

de Swiet M (1986) 'Pre existing medical diseases' in G Chamberlain and J Lumley (eds) *Pre pregnancy Care: A Manual for Practice* Ch 5 69–111 John Wiley: Chichester

de Swiet M and Fidler J (1981) 'Heart disease in pregnancy: some controversies' *Journal of the Royal College of Physicians* 15: 183–6

Donald I (1979) *Practical Obstetric Problems (5th edn)* Lloyd Luke: London Ch 6 181–97

Espir M L E (1986) 'Epilepsy and pregnancy' *Update* 15 April: 703–8

Essex M L, Pyke D A, Watkins P J, Brudenell J M and Gamsu H R (1973) 'Diabetic pregnancy' *British Medical Journal* iv: 89–93

Farnell P, Engle M, Curet L, Perelman R and Morrison J (1984) 'Saturated phospholipids in amniotic fluid of normal and diabetic pregnancies' *Obstetrics and Gynecology* 64: 77–85

Ferris T F (1988) 'Renal diseases' in G N Burrows and T F Ferris (ed) *Medical Complications During Pregnancy (3rd edn)* Ch 12 277–302 W B Saunders: Philadelphia

Gilmer M (1983) 'Diabetes in pregnancy' *Medicine International* 1(35): 1639–40

Gleicher N, Midwall J, Hochberger D and Jaffin H (1979) 'Eisenmenger's syndrome and pregnancy' *Obstetrical and Gynecological Survey* 34: 721–41

Gonen B, Rubenstein A H, Rochma H, Tanega S P and Horowitz D L (1977) 'Haemoglobin A: an indicator of metabolic control of diabetic patients' *Lancet* ii: 734–9

Hopkins A (1984) 'Neurological disorders' in M de Swiet (ed) *Medical Disorders in Obstetric Practice* Ch 14 456–82 Blackwell Scientific: Oxford

James D (1989) 'High risk pregnancies' in J Studd (ed) *Progress in Obstetrics and Gynaecology Vol VII* Ch 4 53–74 Churchill Livingstone: Edinburgh

Jenkins D J P (1981) 'Can diabetes mellitus be treated with dietary fibre?' in I M Baird and M H Ornstein (eds) *Dietary Fibre: Progress Towards the Future* 36–44 Kellogg UK: Manchester

Johnson T M and Murphy J M (1986) 'Psychosocial implications of high risk pregnancy' in R A Knuppel and J E Drukker (eds) *High Risk Pregnancy: a team approach* Ch 9 173–86 W B Saunders: Philadelphia

Jowett N I and Nicol S G (1986) 'Gestational diabetes – are the right women being screened?' *Midwifery* 2(2): 98–100

Kalkhoff R K, Kissebah A H and Kim H J (1979) 'Carbohydrate and lipid metabolism during normal pregnancy' in K R Merkatz and P A J Adam (eds) *The Diabetic Pregnancy* 3–21 Grune and Stratton: New York

Kobayashi H, Matsumoto Y, Otsubo O and Naito T (1981) 'Successful pregnancy in a patient undergoing chronic haemodialysis' *Obstetrics and Gynecology* 57: 382–6

Kuhl C (1975) 'Glucose metabolism during and after pregnancy in normal and gestational diabetic women' *Acta Endocrinologica* 79: 709–19

Laurini R N, Visser G A H and van Ballegooie E (1984) 'Morphological feto-placental abnormalities despite well controlled diabetic pregnancy' *Lancet* i: 800

Lewis P and Steyger J (1985) 'Caring for the infant of a diabetic mother' *Midwifery* 1(4): 207–12

Lind T (1980) 'Carbohydrate metabolism' in F Hytten and G Chamberlain (eds) *Clinical Physiology in Obstetrics* Ch 8 234–56 Blackwell Scientific: Oxford

Lind T and Anderson J (1984) 'Does random blood glucose sampling outdate testing for glycosuria in the detection of diabetes during pregnancy?' *British Medical Journal* 289: 1569–71

Mayberry J F, Bond A P and Morris J S (1986) *Medical Problems in Pregnancy* Edward Arnold: London

McAnulty J H, Metcalfe J and Ueland K (1988) 'Cardio vascular disease' in G N Burrows and T F Ferris (eds) *Medical Complications During Pregnancy (3rd edn)* Ch 7 180–203 W B Saunders: Philadelphia

McDonald R L (1968) 'The role of emotional factors in obstetric complications: a review' *Psychosomatic Medicine* 30: 222

Metcalfe J and Ueland K (1974) 'Maternal cardiovascular adjustments to pregnancy' *Progress in Cardiovascular Disease* 16: 363

Merkatz R B, Budd K and Merkatz I R (1978) 'Psychologic and social implications of scientific care for pregnant diabetic women' *Seminars in Perinatology* 2: 373

Murphy J, Peters J, Hayes T M and Pearson J F (1984) 'Conservative management of pregnancy in diabetic women' *British Medical Journal* 288: 1203–8

Oats J N and Beischer N A (1987) 'Gestational diabetes' in J Studd (ed) *Progress in Obstetrics and Gynaecology Vol VI* Ch 5 101–117 Churchill Livingstone: Edinburgh

Pederson J (1977) *The Pregnant Diabetic and Her Newborn* Munksgaard: Copenhagen

Pyke D A (1962) 'Pre-diabetes' in D A Pyke (ed) *Disorders of Carbohydrate Metabolism* Pitman: London

Ramsey R E, Strauss G, Wilder J and Willmore M J (1978) 'Status epilepticus in pregnancy' *Neurology* 28: 85–9

Royal College of Midwives (1988) *Midwives. The Care of Mothers with Epilepsy* RCM: London

Saunders J, Baron M D, Shenouda F S and Sonkson P H (1980) 'Measuring glycosylated haemoglobin concentrations in a diabetic clinic' *British Medical Journal* 281: 1394–5

Speidal B (1983) 'Infant of the diabetic mother' *Medicine International* 1(35): 1641–2

Steel J M, Johnstone F D, Smith A and Dincan I J P (1982) 'Five years experience of a pre-pregnancy clinic for diabetics' *British Medical Journal* 285: 353–6

Strong J A and Baird J D (1971) 'Diabetes mellitus' in S Davidson and J Macleod (eds) *Principles and Practice of Medicine (10th edn)* Ch 'Diabetes Mellitus' 786–827 Churchill Livingstone: Edinburgh

Vaughan N J A (1987) 'Treatment of diabetes in pregnancy' *British Medical Journal* 294: 558–60

Weaver J B and Pearson J F (1973) 'Influence on time of onset and duration of labour in women with cardiac disease' *British Medical Journal* 2: 519–20

Weinberger S E and Weiss S T (1988) 'Pulmonary diseases' in G N Burrows and T F Ferris (eds) *Medical Complications During Pregnancy (3rd edn)* Ch 19 448–84 W B Saunders: Philadelphia

West T E T (1983) 'Diabetic pregnancy' *Update* 26(4): 633–42

14   Antepartum haemorrhage

Antepartum haemorrhage (APH) is defined in the United Kingdom as any bleeding from the genital tract after the twenty-eighth week of pregnancy and prior to the onset of labour (Hibbard 1988). It is a common complication, occurring in approximately 3% of pregnancies (Paintin 1962). Donald (1979) comments that APH is an unusual condition in that it

> 'very often has to be managed before it can be diagnosed' (p. 420).

The severity and effects of an APH are variable; blood loss may be slight but it could be catastrophic, resulting in the death of the fetus and/or the mother (Fraser and Watson 1989). In the 1982–1984 Confidential Enquiry into Maternal Deaths there were four deaths from APH, two following placenta praevia and two from abruptio placentae (Department of Health 1989). Whatever the severity of the APH, it causes severe anxiety in the woman, her partner and other family members.

Maternal and fetal blood loss

The blood loss can be of maternal or fetal origin. If maternal, bleeding can occur from the placental site, from local causes in the cervix or vagina and due to clotting disorders (Hibbard 1988). In a significant number of cases the site of bleeding is not identified (Watson 1982).

Fetal blood loss occurs where blood vessels in the umbilical cord are inserted into the membranes rather than into the placenta (velamentous insertion of the cord) (Robinson *et al.* 1983). If these vessels pass in front of the presenting part (vasa praevia), there is a risk of spontaneous rupture during labour or as a result of an intervention such as artificial rupture of the membranes (Kouyoumdjian 1980). This is a rare cause of APH (less than 1% of the total), although the consequences for the fetus can be catastrophic (Myerscough 1982). To determine whether blood loss is of fetal origin an Apt Test may be performed, but in most cases the presence of severe fetal distress necessitates immediate delivery by forceps (if the cervix is fully dilated) or by caesarean section. The Apt Test (Apt and Downey 1955) to differentiate between blood of fetal or maternal origin is performed as follows: using maternal blood as a control, 4–6 drops of the APH blood and the mother's blood are each added to a test tube containing 10 ml of water. To each tube is added 2 ml of sodium hydroxide. The tubes are shaken and observed for a rapid colour change; they are watched for a further 2 minutes. The control blood will rapidly change to a green/brown which remains. If the APH blood is of fetal origin the sample will remain red/pink for the 2 minutes, turning green/brown after 10–20 minutes.

Diagnosis is usually made during or after delivery. Messer *et al.* (1987), in their survey of university and community obstetric units, found that only 15% of obstetricians routinely tested for the presence of fetal blood in cases of late pregnancy bleeding, although the effect of this on subsequent management is unclear. Bleeding in the case of vasa praevia results in profound asphyxia and/or perinatal death (Kouyoumdjian 1980).

The majority of cases of APH in which a cause is demonstrated occur due to bleeding from the placental site. These can be divided into two main groups:

1. Haemorrhage due to the partial separation of a placenta normally situated in the corpus or fundus of the uterus (i.e. in the upper segment) (Egley and Cefalo 1985). Such bleeding is referred to as abruptio placentae; in older texts it may still be called accidental haemorrhage.
2. Haemorrhage due to the partial separation of a placenta abnormally sited wholly or partially in the lower segment of the uterus (Fraser and Watson 1989). This is called placenta praevia (placenta first) and may also be described as an unavoidable haemorrhage. Due to changes in the lower segment during the later weeks of pregnancy and labour, haemorrhage is inevitable as labour progresses (Gabert 1971; Myerscough 1982).

For the sake of completeness, bleeding from any other recognised cause may be referred to as incidental.

Abruptio placentae

This is the most frequent cause of APH; in Hibbard's 1988 study it accounted for

31% of cases. It occurs where the placenta becomes separated from its uterine attachment (Myerscough 1982). With the large supply of maternal blood to the placental site, blood escapes from open sinuses into the space behind the membranes caused by the separation (Egley and Cefalo 1985). This blood can either work its way down between the decidual lining and the membranes to escape at the cervix, a revealed haemorrhage; or, it can be contained behind the placenta and seep into the myometrium, a concealed haemorrhage (Egley and Cefalo 1985). In the latter case, the mother's degree of shock and other symptoms can be out of all proportion to the amount of any visible blood loss (Myerscough 1982). In some cases, a concealed haemorrhage can become revealed. The quantity of bleeding can range from the presence of a small retroplacental clot seen at delivery to an amount sufficient to separate a significant portion of the placenta causing fetal death in utero (Knab 1978).

In some cases of concealed haemorrhage, blood under pressure penetrates into the myometrium and between the layers of the broad ligament (Knab 1978). Some blood may pass through the uterine wall, and the presence of blood-stained serous fluid in the peritoneal cavity has been reported at caesarean section. Free blood in the myometrium causes the muscle to go into spasm (Myerscough 1982). The uterus is tense or even 'board like' (couvelaire uterus) and very painful; fetal asphyxia occurs due to severe diminution of placenta blood flow (Egley and Cefalo 1985). In some cases, disseminated intravascular coagulation (DIC) can occur due to the large amount of bleeding and the entry of tissue thromboplastins into the general circulation (Boulton and Letsky 1985). This is discussed in Chapter 27.

The causes of placental abruption are in many cases far from clear (Fraser and Watson 1989), although there are certain contributory factors which increase the risk:

1. Parity. Abruption is more common in women of high parity (para 5 and over) (Hibbard and Hibbard 1963).
2. Hypertension (the presence of chronic or acute gestational hypertension is related to abruption (Egley and Cefalo 1985), but Naeye *et al.* (1977) suggest that abruption occurs before the hypertension). It is thought that uterine vasospasm caused by the hypertension can be followed by venous engorgement and subsequent rupture of the arterioles (Egley and Cefalo 1985). It must of course be remembered that the vast majority of pregnant women with hypertension do not have a placental abruption.
3. Trauma. Bleeding can occur following a blow to the abdomen, for example, following a road traffic accident, particularly where a seat belt is worn (Crosby and Costiloe 1971), although placental attachment is remarkably durable. Traction on a short cord or external cephalic version has been shown in some cases to result in placental separation (Hibbard and Hibbard 1963).
4. Previous history of abruption. It is possible that there is some genetic or constitutional predisposition. The recurrence rate in subsequent pregnancies has been reported as being 5.6% (Paterson 1979) or even as high as 17.3% (Hibbard and Jeffcoate 1966).

5. Nutritional deficiencies, notably a lack of folic acid during the period of placental development, have been suggested as a contributory factor, but this has not been substantiated by research (de Valera 1968).
6. Sudden release of polyhydramnios with rapid reduction in uterine size and limited accommodation of the placenta to the changes in area of placental attachment (Hibbard and Hibbard 1963).
7. Cigarette smoking is a very important risk factor. Naeye (1978) noted that the frequency of placental abnormalities such as necrosis of the decidua basalis or large recent infarct (lesions associated with abruption) increases with the number of cigarettes smoked per day. Smoking may cause spasm of the spiral arterioles which can rupture on relaxation (Goujard et al. 1975).

Naeye (1978) thought that recent coitus could be a contributory factor, but this has not been shown by other workers.

Signs and symptoms

A characteristic of abruptio placentae is pain which can be severe and accompanied by shock out of all proportion to visible blood loss (Myerscough 1982). Shock is caused by the presence of blood in the myometrium (similar to shock caused by a 'crush' injury), stretching of the perimetrium (peritoneum overlying the uterus) and by hypovolaemia (Hurd et al. 1983).

Revealed haemorrhage (where vaginal blood loss is present)

The uterus will feel tender over the site of placental attachment (Myerscough 1982). Depending on the extent of placental separation there may be fetal distress or death; in minor cases the fetus can be unaffected (Myerscough 1982). Labour may ensue and progress normally. If the mother is primiparous, the presenting part may be engaged and this can assist in the making the differential diagnosis from placenta praevia.

Concealed (where there is no visible blood loss)

Severe constant abdominal pain with a hard, 'woody' uterus may occur. The uterus is globular in shape and, due to the amount of blood loss, may be larger than expected for the gestation (Myerscough 1982). The uterine spasm is known as a couvelaire uterus (Naeye et al. 1977); it is extremely tender. Contraction and retraction of the myometrium cannot be detected, fetal outlines may be indistinguishable on palpation and the fetal heart (even if present) is rarely heard. Shock is often present with a low blood pressure, although, if the blood loss is small, the mother may simply report feeling faint or nauseous. Differential diagnoses should exclude placenta praevia, ruptured uterus, advanced ectopic gestation and acute polyhydramnios.

The prognosis in cases of abruptio placenta is dependent on the degree of shock and its duration (Hibbard 1988). This in turn reflects the amount and location of the blood loss. In some cases, the labour may commence and uterine contractions become established (Hurd *et al*. 1983), often accompanied by an increase in external bleeding, despite an overall improvement in the maternal condition (Donald 1979). Bleeding will not be arrested properly until the uterus has been emptied, following either vaginal or operative delivery (Myerscough 1982). Fetal/neonatal prognosis is poor in cases of severe concealed haemorrhage, where mortality from asphyxia and prematurity can be as high as 70% (Egley and Cefalo 1985).

Management

In all cases of APH, the woman should be admitted to hospital; if her condition is poor an obstetric flying squad should be summoned to stabilise the situation before transfer (Hibbard 1988). A vaginal examination should not be performed (Myerscough 1982). In all cases the woman and her relatives will be very anxious; although the midwife is unable to offer much reassurance, she can prepare the woman for some of the procedures which will occur following admission. Depending on the gestation, fears regarding prematurity, for example, can be lessened by talking about facilities for neonatal care. Great tact and a sympathetic approach are required in the absence of a detectable fetal heart prior to confirmation of fetal death.

Treatment of a woman with a revealed haemorrhage depends on its severity. Where bleeding is slight and fetal and maternal conditions are good, the situation is usually managed conservatively (Myerscough 1982). Bed rest until the bleeding has subsided is advised while tests are undertaken to localise the placenta and confirm the cause of the bleeding (Myerscough 1982). This is usually achieved using ultrasound scanning (Egley and Cefalo 1985); fetal well-being is assessed using cardiotocography. The midwife has a clear role to play in the care of the woman. In addition to physical care, she can prepare the woman for future events and discuss with her the procedures which are being carried out. If the bleeding resolves, the pregnancy is left to continue to term; fetal well-being will be assessed before deciding whether a reduction in placental function necessitates induction of labour at/or following term (Myerscough 1982).

In cases of severe revealed bleeding, the mother may require resuscitation to reverse the effects of shock (Fraser and Watson 1989). If labour ensues and placenta praevia has been excluded, it is allowed to continue, especially if the fetus is already dead (Myerscough 1982). Bleeding will not cease until the uterus is empty, so faced with a worsening maternal condition or where the fetus is still alive, a caesarean section may be considered (Golditch and Boyce 1970). However, as the obstetrician does not know for certain whether there has been any DIC, he or she has to obtain clotting screen results prior to operating (Boulton and Letsky 1985). The paediatricians should be alerted to expect an asphyxiated and/or preterm infant. Preparing the mother for operative delivery in such cases can be a balancing act of trying to restore her blood volume to acceptable levels whilst blood loss is continuing. The operation will be performed under general anaesthesia, as hypovolaemia is a contra-indication to the use of an epidural.

Depending on maternal condition, the mother may remain in the delivery unit for some considerable time following delivery until her condition is properly stabilised as regards blood clotting and an adequate circulating fluid volume.

Where the haemorrhage is concealed, the situation can be very serious. The woman may be in a state of collapse from blood loss and pain (Myerscough 1982). Expert emergency action to treat the shock is required (Fraser and Watson 1989). To treat the pain, a powerful analgesic such as morphine 15 mg intramuscularly would be given (Egley and Cefalo 1985). In some cases this action brings about an immediate improvement in maternal condition. To correct the hypovolaemia, blood, plasma or a plasma expander may be given. As it is difficult to assess the amount of blood lost, the establishment of a central venous pressure line will assist in ensuring an adequate circulating fluid volume (O'Driscoll and McCarthy 1966; Muldoon 1969).

Close observation of the maternal condition will be made, with frequent recordings of pulse, blood pressure and fetal heart rate (if present). Meticulous record-keeping by the midwife is essential to assist the medical staff in deciding their management. Decisions as to future treatment must await the results of the coagulation screen on blood taken at the time of setting up the intravenous infusion. Although the woman may be drowsy following analgesia, the midwife must still inform her of what is happening (such as the giving of injections or being repositioned), as it is difficult to determine the woman's level of consciousness.

Once the shock has been corrected, labour may ensue, especially if the woman is parous (Fraser and Watson 1989). Should the baby be alive and the coagulation profiles satisfactory, a caesarean section will be performed (Myerscough 1982). Otherwise, once the maternal condition is stable, the membranes will be ruptured and oxytocin used if required to stimulate labour (Myerscough 1982). The midwife has an important role to play in preparing the couple for the delivery of a stillborn baby (see Chapter 31). Even after the delivery, the situation is far from resolved; there is a risk of postpartum haemorrhage and a close watch needs to be maintained to observe for signs of heart, renal or liver failure (Egley and Cefalo 1985). The mother must not be left until her pulse and blood pressure are fully stabilised.

Placenta praevia

Placenta praevia occurs when all or part of the placenta is situated in the lower segment of the uterus. There are four types or degrees of placenta praevia (see Figure 14.1):

> *Type 1* Also known as lateral placenta praevia. The lower margin of the placenta dips down into the lower uterine segment. The major portion of the placenta is normally attached to the upper uterine segment (Myerscough 1982).

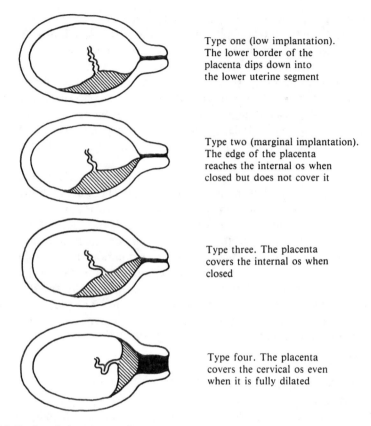

Type one (low implantation).
The lower border of the
placenta dips down into
the lower uterine segment

Type two (marginal implantation).
The edge of the placenta
reaches the internal os when
closed but does not cover it

Type three. The placenta
covers the internal os when
closed

Type four. The placenta
covers the cervical os even
when it is fully dilated

Figure 14.1 Grades of placenta praevia.

Type 2 Marginal placenta praevia. The placenta reaches the internal os when
it is closed, but does not cover it (Myerscough 1982).
Type 3 Partial placenta praevia. The placenta covers the closed internal os,
but does not do so when the os is fully dilated (Myerscough 1982).
Type 4 Complete placenta praevia. The placenta covers the os, even when the
cervix is fully dilated.

The amount of bleeding from placenta praevia is usually in proportion to the area
of placental separation (Fraser and Watson 1989). Even damage to a single large
blood vessel can produce torrential blood loss. The first episode of bleeding is
seldom severe (Myerscough 1982), although Morgan (1965) found that, in 1 in 6
cases in his study, there was no warning bleeding before the onset of labour.

Placenta praevia occurs in approximately 1:200 pregnancies and it is more
common in multiparous than primiparous women (Fraser and Watson 1989). The
cause is unclear, although it is known that many placentae seen to be low lying in
early pregnancy are correctly positioned in later pregnancy following growth of the

upper uterine segment (King 1973). Large placental size, which occurs in multiple pregnancy, increases the risks of placenta praevia (Green-Thompson 1982). Singh *et al*. (1981) in their survey showed that woman who had undergone a caesarean section had a 3.9% incidence of placenta praevia in a later pregnancy and postulated that this was related to the presence of the scar on the lower uterine segment. Eastman and Hellman (1964) found that the risk of placenta praevia increased with age, whereas other workers suggest that parity, independent of age, is a more important factor (Clark *et al*. 1985). There is also an association of placenta praevia with cigarette smoking although this is not as significant as for placental abruption (Naeye 1980).

The placenta may separate slightly during pregnancy especially from 28 weeks with the formation of the lower segment (Gabert 1971). This is, however, minor compared to the severe bleeding which occurs during prelabour and labour, which is related to effacement and dilation of the cervix (Myerscough 1982). Unless the placenta is damaged or torn the blood loss is usually of maternal origin. However, Naeye (1978) suggests that fetal bleeding is more common than is appreciated. In support of this McShane *et al*. (1985) have demonstrated a statistically significant correlation between the level of maternal blood loss antenatally and the occurrence of anaemia requiring neonatal blood transfusion. The fetal condition is compromised, due to the reduction of placental attachment for nutrient exchange and the deterioration in maternal condition (Naeye 1978).

Signs and symptoms

Some women with placenta praevia experience a number of small episodes of painless bleeding (Cotton *et al*. 1980). These may be unprovoked but they can follow exercise or sexual intercourse. In fewer than 20% of cases is there no warning bleeding (Morgan 1965). Severe bleeding may occur while the woman is at rest at home, but is more usual as labour progresses or following obstetrical interference such as a vaginal examination (Myerscough 1982). The main clinical feature of placenta praevia is the absence of pain. Unless blood loss is severe, the woman feels well. For these reasons, women reporting vaginal bleeding should be dissuaded from visiting their doctor's surgery or local hospital, but should remain at rest at home until transfer to hospital can be arranged (Hibbard 1988). In this way, there is more likelihood of preventing a torrential blood loss before arrival in hospital.

Diagnosis must take account of the woman's history before a clinical examination is made. When a mother contacts her midwife to report any bleeding, it is important that she is advised to keep any soiled clothes or linen so that the extent of the loss can be assessed (Hibbard 1988). On clinical examination, the presenting part is usually not engaged and is frequently mobile (Fraser and Watson 1989). The lie of the fetus may be oblique rather than longitudinal (Cotton *et al*. 1980). Breech presentations are more common because, due to lack of space in the pelvis, the fetus finds more room for its relatively large head in the fundus. The uterus feels soft and relaxed, there is no tenderness and the fetal heart (if present) is distinctly heard (Hibbard 1988). A vaginal examination should never be performed, unless in theatre, with the woman prepared for caesarean section in case of torrential bleeding (Myerscough 1982). Once the blood loss has subsided, a gentle speculum examination to exclude cervical causes of bleeding may be performed by the obstetrician (Hibbard 1988). To confirm the diagnosis, placental localisation is performed using diagnostic ultrasound (Donald and Abdulla 1968).

Although bleeding from placenta praevia in its early stages is not immediately life-threatening to mother and fetus, without prompt attention the situation can quickly deteriorate (Myerscough 1982). Risks to the mother include shock from hypovalaemia, although this is less common, since small bleeding episodes are rigorously investigated. The prognosis for the fetus is far from good where the area of placental separation is significant (Myerscough 1982). Hypoxia occurs due to diminution of placenta blood flow from maternal hypotension and anaemia, in addition to a reduction in the area of attachment. With advances in neonatal care, prematurity is no longer a major cause of neonatal death following placenta praevia (Myerscough 1982).

Management

The woman should be admitted to hospital. If blood loss is slight she can use an ordinary ambulance, preferably with a midwife in attendance. Where haemorrhage is moderate or severe an obstetric flying squad may be required to stabilise the woman's condition before transfer is attempted (Hibbard 1988). All blood loss should be saved. On arrival the mother with a slight haemorrhage will be placed on bed rest while careful monitoring of maternal and fetal well-being is carried out (Myerscough 1982). Placental localisation tests will be ordered. If the diagnosis of placenta praevia is confirmed and the bleeding settles, the woman will be kept under observation in hospital until the fetus is sufficiently mature to stand the best chance of survival (Macafee 1945). Delivery will be by elective caesarean section.

Mothers get very bored just sitting around in hospital; they do not feel ill and apart from the assessment of fetal well-being (usually using a cardiotocograph) do not receive any active treatment. The midwife has an important duty to explain to the woman exactly why it would be dangerous for her to return home. The risk of a large haemorrhage is ever present (D'Angelo and Irwin 1984). Any deterioration in the situation will be treated vigorously (Hibbard 1988).

Where blood loss is severe or becomes so, the preferred treatment is caesarean section (Myerscough 1982). It is important for the obstetrician to exclude abruptio placentae as the cause of the haemorrhage and, should there be any doubt, a coagulation screen is advisable before performing surgery. Where the woman is shocked this should of course be corrected before the operation is performed (Hibbard 1988). Bleeding can be severe during the caesarean section, since the lower uterine segment into which the placenta has implanted and through which the incision is made is not normally so vascular (Myerscough 1982). In addition, following delivery, the lower segment does not contract as efficiently as the upper, increasing the risk of postpartum haemorrhage (Williamson and Greeley 1945).

If placental localisation cannot be determined and the blood loss is not severe, especially where the woman seems to be in early labour, an examination under anaesthesia may be performed (Fraser and Watson 1989). General anaesthesia can be used, but epidurals are being used with increasing frequency. With all facilities prepared for a caesarean section, a vaginal examination is performed in the operating theatre (Hibbard 1988). Should the diagnosis of placenta praevia be confirmed or further bleeding be provoked, an immediate operative delivery can be performed (Myerscough 1982). If, however, there is no sign of the placenta on examination, an artificial rupture of the membranes is carried out and labour induced or allowed to progress. This examination has its advantages where there were doubts over the diagnosis, especially with a type 1 placenta praevia where vaginal delivery is possible since the risks of maternal mortality and morbidity are considerably less for a vaginal than for an operative delivery (Department of Health 1989).

References

Apt L and Downey W S (1955) 'Melena neonatorum. The swallowed blood syndrome. A simple test for differentiation of adult and fetal hemoglobin in bloody stools' *Journal of Pediatrics* 47: 6–12

Boulton F E and Letsky E A (1985) 'Obstetric haemorrhage: Causes and management' *Clinics in Heamatology* 14(3): 683–728

Clark S L, Koonings P P and Phelan J P (1985) 'Placenta previa/accreta and prior cesarean section' *Obstetrics and Gynecology* 86: 846–8

Cotton D B, Read J A, Paul R H and Quilligan E J (1980) 'The conservative aggressive management of placenta previa' *American Journal of Obstetrics and Gynecology* 137: 687–95

Crosby W M and Costiloe J P (1971) 'Safety of lap belt restraint for pregnant victims of automobile collisions' *New England Journal of Medicine* 284: 632–6

D'Angelo L J and Irwin L F (1984) 'Conservative management of placenta previa: a cost benefit analysis' *American Journal of Obstetrics and Gynecology* 149: 320–3

Department of Health (1989) *Report on Confidential Enquiries into Maternal Deaths in England and Wales 1982–4* HMSO: London

de Valera E (1968) 'Abruptio placentae' *American Journal of Obstetrics and Gynecology* 100: 599–606

Donald I (1979) *Practical Obstetric Problems (5th edn)* Lloyd Luke: London

Donald I and Abdulla U J (1968) 'Placentography by sonar' *Journal of Obstetrics and Gynaecology of the British Commonwealth* 75: 1193–2006

Eastman J N and Hellman L M (1964) *Williams Obstetrics (13th edn)* Appleton-Century-Crofts: New York

Egley C and Cefalo R C (1985) 'Abruptio placentae' in J Studd (ed) *Progress in Obstetrics and Gynaecology Vol 5* Ch 7 108–20 Churchill Livingstone: Edinburgh

Fraser R and Watson R (1989) 'Bleeding during the latter half of pregnancy' in I Chalmers, M Enkin and M J N C Keirse (eds) *Effective Care in Pregnancy and Childbirth* Ch 37 594–611 Oxford Medical: Oxford

Gabert H A (1971) 'Placenta previa and fetal growth' *Obstetrics and Gynecology* 38: 403–6

Golditch J A and Boyce N E (1970) 'Management of abruptio placentae' *Journal of the American Medical Association* 212: 288–93

Goujard J, Rumeau C and Schwartz D (1975) 'Smoking during pregnancy, stillbirth and abruptio placentae' *Biomedicine* 23: 20–2

Green-Thompson R W (1982) 'Antepartum haemorrhage' *Clinics in Obstetrics and Gynaecology* 9: 479–515

Hibbard B M (1988) *Principles of Obstetrics* Butterworth: London

Hibbard B M and Hibbard E D (1963) 'Aetiological factors in abruptio placentae' *British Medical Journal* 2: 1430–6

Hibbard B M and Jeffcoate T N A (1966) 'Abruptio placentae' *Obstetrics and Gynaecology* 27: 155–67

Hurd W W, Miodovnik M and Hertzbert V (1983) 'Selective management of abruptio placentae: a prospective study' *Obstetrics and Gynecology* 61: 467–73

King D L (1973) 'Placental migration demonstrated by ultrasonography' *Radiology* 109: 167–70

Knab D R (1978) 'Abruptio placenta: An assessment of the time and method of delivery' *Obstetrics and Gynecology* 52: 625–9

Kouyoumdjian A (1980) 'Velamentous insertion of the umbilical cord' *Obstetrics and Gynecology* 56: 737

Macafee C H G (1945) 'Placenta praevia–study of 174 cases' *Journal of Obstetrics and Gynaecology of the British Empire* 52: 313–24

McShane P M, Heys P S and Epstein M F (1985) 'Maternal and perinatal mortality resulting from placenta previa' *Obstetrics and Gynecology* 65: 176–82

Messer R H, Gomez A R and Yamboa T J (1987) 'Antenatal testing for vasa previa: Current standard of care' *American Journal of Obstetrics and Gynecology* 156: 1459

Morgan J (1965) 'Placenta praevia: report on a series of 538 cases' *Journal of Obstetrics and Gynaecology of the British Commonwealth* 72: 700–5

Muldoon M J (1969) 'The use of central venous pressure monitoring in abruptio placentae' *Journal of Obstetrics and Gynaecology of the British Commonwealth* 76: 225–8

Myerscough P R (1982) *Munro Kerr's Operative Obstetrics (10th edn)* Balliere Tindall: London

Naeye R L (1978) 'Placenta previa. Predisposing factors and effects on the fetus and surviving infants' *Obstetrics and Gynaecology* 52: 521–5

Naeye R L (1980) 'Abruptio placentae and placenta praevia , perinatal mortality and cigarette smoking' *Obstetrics and Gynecology* 55: 70–4

Naeye R L, Harkness W I and Utts J (1977) 'Abruptio placentae and perinatal death: A prospective study' *American Journal of Obstetrics and Gynecology* 128: 740–6

O'Driscoll K and McCarthy J R (1966) 'Abruptio placentae and central venous pressures' *Journal of Obstetrics and Gynaecology of the British Commonwealth* 73: 932–9

Paintin D B (1962) 'The epidemiology of ante-partum haemorrhage: A study of all births in a community' *Journal of Obstetrics and Gynaecology of the British Commonwealth* 69: 614–23

Paterson M E L (1979) 'The aetiology and outcome of abruptio placentae' *Acta Obstetrica and Gynaecologica Scandanavica* 58: 31–5

Robinson L K, Jones K L and Benirschke K (1983) 'The nature and structural defects associated with velamentous and marginal insertion of the umbilical cord' *American Journal of Obstetrics and Gynecology* 146: 191

Singh P M, Rodrigues C and Gupta A N (1981) 'Placent previa and previous cesarean section' *Acta Obstetrica and Gynaecologica Scandanavica* 292: 371–2

Watson R (1982) 'Antepartum Haemorrhage of uncertian origin' *British Journal of Clinical Practice* 36: 222–6

Williamson H C and Greeley A V (1945) 'Management of placenta previa: 12 year study' *American Journal of Obstetrics and Gynecology* 50: 398–406

15　Anaemia in pregnancy

Physiological changes in blood composition

During pregnancy there is a rise in plasma volume, the maximum rate of increase being between 12 and 16 weeks gestation (Hytten and Paintin 1963) with most of the change having occurred by 34 weeks (Pirani *et al*. 1973). There is a relation between the increase in plasma volume and the size of the baby at birth (Hytten and Leitch 1971); where the fetus experiences intrauterine growth retardation, there is only a small rise in volume (Gibson 1973). Plasma volume rises from a prepregnant average of 2500 ml to a level of 3750 ml in primigravidae and 4000 ml in multiparous women, an increase of 1250–1500 ml (Hytten and Leitch 1971). Even larger increases have been recorded in multiple pregnancies; 1960 ml for twins and 2400 in the case of triplets (Rovinsky and Jaffin 1965). The rise in plasma volume is required to supply the increased circulatory demands of the kidneys (for excretion) and the skin (for temperature control) (de Swiet 1980).

Like plasma volume, red cell mass rises throughout pregnancy from a prepregnant level of 1400–1750 ml in late pregnancy (Letsky 1980). Where the woman has received iron supplementation, a mean increase in red cell mass of 400 ml has been reported, compared with 240 ml for a woman not receiving iron (Hytten and Leitch 1971). As the increase in plasma volume is proportionately higher than the rise in the red cell mass, there is a progressive haemodilution (Letsky 1984). The increase in red cell mass is required for the increase in the transportation of oxygen around the body (de Swiet 1980). Mahomed and Hytten (1989) suggest that since the rationales behind the increases in plasma volume and red cell mass are different, there is no reason why they should increase by a similar percentage.

There is considerable argument as to what level of haemoglobin could be regarded as signifying anaemia in pregnancy (Mahomed and Hytten 1989). The World Health Organization (1972) regards ll g/100 ml as being the lowest acceptable limit, whilst Chanarin (1986) states that haemoglobin may be as low as l0.5 g/100 ml at 32 weeks in a healthy pregnancy. Mahomed and Hytten (1989) are critical of the application of an absolute cut-off point between normality and the diagnosis of anaemia. They argue that this is neither philosophically nor physiologically sound, since the assay of haemoglobin level is only one factor in the diagnosis of anaemia. No account is taken of the level of iron stores or the altitude at which the woman is living. It is the size of the fetus which determines the rise in plasma volume and the associated fall in haemoglobin level.

Causes of anaemia in pregnancy

This chapter will consider anaemia in pregnancy caused by iron and folate deficiency before describing further causes such as sickle cell disease and thalassaemia. The dangers of anaemia in pregnancy, especially where it occurs amongst a predominantly well-fed and affluent group, are hard to demonstrate (Mahomed and Hytten 1989). Indeed Garn et al. (1981) have noted that some of the worst outcomes have been amongst groups of women with haemoglobin levels above 13 g/100 ml. In confirmation of this opinion, Murphy et al. (1986) demonstrated that both high (above 13.2 g/100 ml) and low (below 10.4 g/100 ml) haemoglobin levels in early pregnancy are associated with the worst outcomes. In their review of 54 000 women they showed that the incidence of gestational proteinuric hypertension increased from 7%, with first and early second trimester haemoglobin levels below 10.5 g/100 ml to 42% at concentrations above 14.5 g/100 ml (Murphy et al. 1986). Mahomed and Hytten (1989) argue that a low haemoglobin level in a well-nourished woman may be an advantage, since it shows that she has experienced a large rise in her plasma volume. Where haemoglobin remains high, this may indicate that the required increase in plasma volume has not occurred. Pregnancy anaemia in less-developed countries is a problem and still gives rise to considerable maternal mortality (World Health Organization 1978).

Iron deficiency anaemia

This is the commonest anaemia in pregnancy (Letsky 1987), being due to a combination of increased utilisation, dietary deficiency and poor absorption of dietary iron (Letsky 1984). Iron is required in pregnancy for the increased red cell mass, for the placenta and for the fetal haemoglobin and iron stores (Letsky 1984).

The fetus obtains its iron by active transport across the placenta, especially from 36 weeks onwards while it is laying down iron stores for the first 3 months of life (Fletcher *et al.* 1971). The total extra dietary iron required during pregnancy (excluding lactation) has been calculated at 900 mg less 120 mg 'saved' by amenorrhoea (Letsky 1980). More iron is required in the last trimester, the amount needed being 6–7 mg/day (Letsky 1980, 1987). Iron is poorly absorbed from the diet, an absorption rate of 5–10% being suggested (Bull and Buss 1980). It is known that absorption rates increase when anaemia is present. Although 'average' western diets contain approximately 14 mg of iron per day (Letsky 1987), Barber *et al.* (1985), surveying non-pregnant women aged between 15 and 25, found intakes far below this amount. Whilst iron absorption is improved in cases of iron deficiency (Svanberg 1975), such women may well come to pregnancy with normal haemoglobin levels but low iron stores, especially where menstrual loss is heavy or pregnancies occur close together (Bentley 1985).

Iron occurs in foods of both animal and vegetable origin. Iron in meat, which is derived from the animal's haemoglobin and myoglobin, is readily available for absorption (Letsky 1984). Iron in vegetables, being in the 'ferric' state rather than the usable 'ferrous' condition, requires conversion before it can be absorbed (Letsky 1987). This process is aided by the presence of haem iron in the diet (Letsky 1987). Women who eat little or no animal protein should plan their diet to maximise iron intake. Vitamin C is necessary for the absorption of iron and care should be taken that the woman is not impairing her iron intake by the liberal use of antacids. The midwife has a role to play in discussing diet and offering advice, which may include the minimising of side-effects of treatment. Iron absorption rates increase during pregnancy in women not receiving iron supplementation (Svanberg 1975).

Maternal haemoglobin levels should be assessed at least at the initial antenatal visit and again at 28–30 and 34–36 weeks gestation (Hall 1974). As pregnant women rarely show the classic signs of iron deficiency (Mahomed and Hytten 1989), it is hard to decide whether any tiredness is due to the strains of late pregnancy or to anaemia. Letsky (1987) suggests that any woman with a haemoglobin level below 10.5 g/100 ml in the second or third trimesters requires further investigation. This would include examination of the cells themselves, which may appear small (microcytic), indicating iron deficiency anaemia. This can be confusing as red cell size does increase slightly in pregnancy (Letsky 1987) and larger increases in size have been noted where the woman is taking supplemental iron (Taylor and Lind 1976). Mean cell haemoglobin can be reduced (Letsky 1987). Some authorities recommend assessing plasma ferritin levels in the first trimester as a guide to the level of iron stores, the normal range being 15–300 µg/l (Jacobs *et al.* 1972). Bentley (1985) recommends giving iron supplementation to any woman with serum ferritin level below 50 µg/l regardless of her haemoglobin level.

The treatment of iron deficiency anaemia is dependent upon the severity of the condition and the proximity of its occurrence to delivery (Letsky 1987). Iron therapy is not recommended before 16 weeks of pregnancy, as it is potentially teratogenic (Nelson and Forfar 1971). Until 32–34 weeks oral therapy is usually sufficient (Letsky 1987). Both oral and parenteral iron will increase haemoglobin by about

0.8 g/100 ml/week, although the initial response to oral iron may be slower (Letsky 1987). Once a satisfactory level has been achieved, Hall (1974) recommends continuing treatment for a further 3 months to replenish iron stores. Side-effects (such as gastric disturbances) occurring with oral iron therapy account for some women failing to take the tablets. Reducing the dose can be of assistance, but the use of slow-release compounds is not recommended, as much of the iron is excreted unabsorbed (Letsky 1987).

For women in whom oral iron therapy has been ineffective, a course of intramuscular iron sorbital (Jectofer) may be given (Letsky 1984). The injections are painful and can result in black staining of the injection site if tracking occurs, which may take some years to fade (Letsky 1987). An occasional alternative treatment is the intravenous use of iron dextrans (imferon) given in normal saline as a slow infusion (Hall 1974). Oral iron should not be given simultaneously, as the body's iron binding capacity can become overloaded (Hall 1974). The dose is calculated according to haemoglobin level and body weight. When commencing treatment, the infusion should run slowly and frequent observations be made of maternal vital signs, due to the risk of anaphylactic shock (Mahomed and Hytten 1989). In addition to toxic reactions, the woman may complain of headache, nausea and vomiting (Scott 1963). In rare cases with severe anaemia presenting in late pregnancy, blood transfusion may be performed, although this is to be avoided if at all possible (Letsky 1987).

Much discussion has occurred over the need for prophylactic iron therapy (Mahomed and Hytten 1989). Even where the obstetrician does not recommend supplementation, the woman may obtain iron pills from her general practitioner or purchase them alone or with multivitamins. What should be considered is that, although the woman may not be anaemic, she may end pregnancy with low iron stores which will take a considerable time to replenish if she has a diet low in iron (Bentley 1985). Perhaps a better solution would be to provide sound dietary advice prior to pregnancy and to assess iron stores (via serum ferritin estimation) at the antenatal visit, before giving prophylactic oral iron to those women at particular risk (Bentley 1985). The use of routine supplemental iron in the developed world has not been shown to have proven benefits as regards outcome (Hemminki and Starfield 1978; Mahomed and Hytten 1989). Iron supplementation is however vital for undernourished women from developing countries who are also subjected to tropical diseases such as malaria, which of themselves cause anaemia (Fleming et al. 1986).

Folic acid deficiency

Folic acid, a constituent of all human tissues, is required in increasing amounts, especially where there is a multiple pregnancy (Chanarin 1979). Deficiency is common in Third World countries, where there may be frequent pregnancies and dietary intake is low (Mahomed and Hytten 1989). Folate is present in many foods, but is extremely sensitive to heat (Letsky 1987). Green leafy vegetables such as spinach, brussels sprouts and broccoli are a good source, but much of the folate is lost in cooking (Letsky 1987). Even if the food is eaten raw, absorption of folate is poor.

Folic acid deficiency is usually suspected when a woman treated for anaemia, assumed to be caused by iron deficiency, fails to respond to treatment (Chanarin 1985). Chanarin (1979) gives the frequency of folic acid deficiency as 1 in 80 single pregnancies raising to 1 in 11 with twins. Many more women than this may show changes in the bone marrow not apparent on examination of a blood film (Chanarin 1985). The characteristic megaloblastic picture of folic acid deficiency, seen on examination of the blood, is complicated in pregnancy; although large immature cells may be seen, due to the normal increase in red cell size in pregnancy, interpretation may be difficult and bone marrow examination necessary (Letsky 1987).

Treatment of megaloblastic anaemia in pregnancy (almost never due to vitamin B12 deficiency which causes infertility) is with oral folate supplementation usually combined with iron. Chanarin (1979) suggests a divided daily dose of 5–15 mg of folic acid in cases of proven deficiency. As with oral iron prophylaxis, a similar argument is going on concerning routine folic acid supplementation (Mahomed and Hytten 1989). Letsky (1987) suggests that such a course of action is warranted in countries where megaloblastic anaemia is common, but is more sceptical about its use in a well-nourished population. Researchers have suggested that folate deficiency as a contributory factor in the cause of fetal abnormalities such as neural tube defects (Smithells *et al.* 1983)

There seem to be few adverse effects from folate supplementation in pregnancy (Mahomed and Hytten 1989). As a prophylactic measure for both iron and folate deficiency Chanarin and Rothman (1971) recommend 200 μg of folate combined with 30 mg of iron as a daily dose, which is considerably less than the content of many popular preparations.

Haemoglobinopathies

These are inherited variants of haemoglobin where the globin is incorrectly synthesised (thalassaemia) or is structurally abnormal (sickle cell anaemia and other variants) (Letsky 1987). Many of these disorders occur amongst people originating from specific geographical areas (Lehmann and Ager 1960). Increasing international mobility has resulted in their spread to previously unaffected locations (Letsky 1987).

Thalassaemias

Adult haemoglobin (HbA) contains 4 globin chains which in the vast majority of cases are 2 alpha and 2 beta chains (Letsky 1987). Fetal haemoglobin (HbF) consists mainly of 2 alpha and 2 delta chains; the change over to HbA is complete by about 6 months of age (Letsky 1987). Beta thalassaemia occurs due to an inherited defective gene for the beta globin chain; the resulting red cells have a much reduced haemoglobin content (Letsky 1987). If only one gene is affected, i.e. the heterozygous state known as thalassaemia minor, the sufferer presents with chronic anaemia. Thalassaemia major is a much more serious homozygous condition where all the haemoglobin is affected (Letsky 1987). Prior to the availability of blood transfusion, death would occur in early childhood from severe anaemia and congestive cardiac failure (Letsky 1987). Although survival is now possible into the early 20s pregnancy is rare. Iron overloading from frequent transfusions is an intractable problem, so any parenteral iron supplementation should be avoided if pregnancy should occur (Letsky 1984). Thalassaemia minor is treated with oral iron and folate therapy or blood transfusion to ensure an adequate haemoglobin at delivery (Letsky 1984).

Beta thalassaemia was initially found in people of Mediterranean origin, although it is now known to exist across a geographical strip from the Mediterranean to the Far East (Lehmann and Ager 1960).

Alpha thalassaemia is only seen as the heterozygous condition, being due to an absent gene coding for the alpha chain (Letsky 1987). The fetus would be affected by the total absence of alpha chains if the homozygous state exists, producing profound anaemia, hydrops and ultimately fetal death in utero. Alpha thalassaemia minor, which is most common in South-East Asia, is treated during pregnancy in the same way as beta thalassaemia minor. Given the changing ethnicity of women for whom midwives provide care, it is important to ask women in high-risk groups about a personal or family history of such conditions.

Sickle cell disease

There are many variations on haemoglobin, the most common of which is sickle cell disease. This exists in both heterozygous (sickle cell trait) and homozygous (sickle cell anaemia) states (Davies and Hewitt 1984). It is an inherited autosomal recessive condition, the gene for which is carried by up to 1 in 3 people of Central and West African origins (Davies and Hewitt 1984), although the frequency amongst Afro-Caribbeans in the United Kingdom is approximately 12% (Horn et al. 1986). In the heterozygous state (HbAS), where only half the haemoglobin is affected, there is protection against infection with malaria. Health problems are few and difficulties only occur with severe hypoxia or dehydration (Letsky 1984). Carriers of the gene may be unaware of the fact and, because of this, at-risk groups are establishing screening centres to help reduce the incidence of the homozygous state (World Health Organization 1972). If 2 carriers have children there is a 1:4 chance of any baby having sickle cell disease (Davies and Hewitt 1984). Screening should be offered to all at-risk groups as a preconceptual service giving the couple the freedom of choice whether to embark upon a pregnancy. The midwife has an educational role in alerting prospective parents to the risks of sickle cell disease. The topic can be discussed in family planning clinics, preconception or antenatal clinics, in addition to generalised health education campaigns.

In sickle cell anaemia there is a defect in the haemoglobin molecule which reduces its solubility when oxygen levels are low (Tuck and White 1981). In times of hypoxia or stress, crystals form, which cause the red cell to be distorted into a sickle shape (Pauling *et al.* 1949). When oxygenation returns to normal, the cells regain their previous shape, but their capacity to do this is limited (Davies and Hewitt 1984). Sickle cells become lodged in small capillaries, causing disruption to blood flow and anoxia in areas beyond the blockage. Such episodes are extremely painful. They are often referred to as sickle cell crises. Sickle cells have a shorter than average life cycle and are constantly being removed from the circulation, resulting in a haemolytic anaemia (Davies and Hewitt 1984). Children suffer particularly severely, with both increased morbidity and mortality (Davies and Hewitt 1984). For a woman with sickle cell anaemia, pregnancy can be extremely dangerous, carrying a high risk for both mother and fetus, including pulmonary embolism, gestational proteinuric hypertension, stillbirth and intrauterine growth retardation (Tuck and White 1981).

If a woman attending the antenatal clinic is found to be carrying the sickle cell gene, she should receive sympathetic advice from the midwife. This would include suggesting that her partner have a blood test to determine whether or not he carries the gene (Davies and Hewitt 1984). If he does not, there is no risk of the baby having sickle cell anaemia. Should the partner have sickle cell trait, the couple require counselling as to the next steps to be undertaken. In order to assess whether the fetus is affected, fetal blood must be obtained via fetoscopy. Parents should be aware of the severity of the disease and the lack of curative treatment; should the fetus be affected a termination of pregnancy would be offered.

References

Barber S A, Bull N L and Buss D H (1985) 'Low iron intakes amongst young women in Britain' *British Medical Journal* 290: 743–5

Bentley D P (1985) 'Iron metablism and anaemia in pregnancy' *Clinics in Haematology* 14(3): 613–28

Bull S A and Buss D H (1980) 'Haem and non-haem iron in British household diets' *Journal of Human Nutrition* 34: 141–5

Chanarin I (1979) 'Megaloblastic anaemias of pregnancy' in I Chanarin (ed) *The Megaloblastic Anaemias (2nd edn)* Blackwell Scientific: Oxford

Chanarin I (1985) 'Folate and cobalamin' *Clinics in Haematology* 14: 629–41

Chanarin I (1986) 'The importance of iron and folate in pregnancy' *Update* 1st Feb: 163–5

Chanarin I and Rothman D (1971) 'Further observations on the relationship between iron and folate status in pregnancy' *British Medical Journal* 2: 81–4

Davies S C and Hewitt P E (1984) 'Sickle cell disease' *British Journal of Hospital Medicine* June: 440–4

de Swiet M (1980) 'The respiratory system' in F E Hytten and G V P Chamberlain (eds) *Clinical Physiology in Obstetrics* 79–100 Blackwell Scientific: Oxford

Fleming A F, Ghatoura G B S, Harrison K A, Briggs O D and Dunn D T (1986) 'The prevention of anaemia in pregnancy in primigravidae in the Guinea Savanna of Nigeria' *Annals of Tropical Medicine and Parasitology* 80: 211–33

Fletcher J, Gurr A, Fellingham F R, Pranker T A J, Brant H A and Menzies D N (1971) 'The value of folic acid supplements in pregnancy' *Journal of Obstetrics and Gynaecology of the British Commonwealth* 75: 781–5

Garn S M, Ridella S A, Petzold A S and Falkner F (1981) 'Maternal haematological levels and pregnancy outcome' *Seminars in Perinatology* 5: 155–62

Gibson H M (1973) 'Plasma volume and glomerular filtration rate in pregnancy and their relations to differences in fetal growth' *Journal of Obstetrics and Gynaecology of the British Commonwealth* 80: 1067–74

Hall M H (1974) 'Pregnancy anaemia' *British Medical Journal* 2: 661–3

Hemminki E and Starfield B (1978) 'Routine administration of iron and vitamins during pregnancy: review of controlled trials' *British Journal of Obstetrics and Gynaecology* 85: 404–10

Horn M E C, Dick M C, Frost B, Davis L R, Bellingham A J, Stroud C E and Studd J E (1986) 'Neonatal screening for sickle cell disease in Camberwell' *British Medical Journal* 292: 737–40

Hytten F E and Leitch I (1971) 'The volume and composition of the blood' in F E Hytten and I Leitch (eds) *The Physiology of Human Pregnancy (2nd edn)* 1–68 Blackwell Scientific: Oxford

Hytten F E and Paintin D B (1963) 'Increase in plasma volume during normal pregnancy' *Journal of Obstetrics and Gynaecology of the British Commonwealth* 70: 402–7

Jacobs A, Miller F, Worwood M, Beamish M R and Wardrop C A (1972) 'Ferritin in the serum of normal subjects and patients with iron deficiency and iron overload' *British Medical Journal* 4: 206–8

Lehmann H and Ager J A M (1960) 'The hemoglobinopathies and thalassemia' in J B Stanbury, J B Wyngaarden and D S Frederichson (eds) *The Metabolic Basis of Inherited Disease* McGraw-Hill: New York

Letsky E A (1980) 'The haematological system' in F E Hytten and G V P Chamberlain (eds) *Clinical Physiology in Obstetrics* 43–78 Blackwell Scientific: Oxford

Letsky E A (1984) 'Blood volume, haematinics, anaemia' in M de Swiet (ed) *Medical Disorders in Obstetric Practice* Ch 2 35–69 Blackwell Scientific: Oxford

Letsky E A (1987) 'Anaemia in obstetrics' in J Studd (ed) *Progress in Obstetrics and Gynaecology Vol 6* Ch 2 23–58 Churchill Livingstone: Edinburgh

Mahomed K and Hytten FE (1989) 'Iron and folate supplementation in pregnancy' in I Chalmers, M Enkin and M J N C Keirse (eds) *Effective Care in Pregnancy and Childbirth* Ch 19 300–17 Oxford Medical: Oxford

Murphy J F, O'Riordan J, Newcombe R G, Coles E C and Pearson J F (1986) 'Relation of haemoglobin levels in first and second trimesters to the outcome of pregnancy' *Lancet* i: 992–4

Nelson M M and Forfar J O (1971) 'Associations between drugs administered during pregnancy and congenital abnormalitites of the fetus' *British Medical Journal* 1: 523–7

Pauling L, Itano H A and Singer S T (1949) 'Sickle cell anaemia, a molecular disease' *Science* 110: 543

Pirani B B K, Campbell D M and MacGillivray I (1973) 'Plasma volume in normal first pregnancy' *Journal of Obstetrics and Gynaecology of the British Commonwealth* 80: 884–7

Rovinsky J J and Jaffin H (1965) 'Cardio vascular haemodynamics in pregnancy 1' *American Journal of Obstetrics and Gynecology* 93: 1–13

Scott J M (1963) 'Iron sorbitol citrate in pregnancy and anaemia' *British Medical Journal* 2: 354–7

Smithells R W, Nevin N C, Seller N J, Shepherd S, Harris R, Read A P, Fielding D W, Walker S, Schorah C J and Wild J (1983) 'Further experiences of vitamin supplementation for prevention of neural tube defect recurrences' *Lancet* i: 1027–31

Svanberg B (1975) 'Absorption of iron in pregnancy' *Acta Obstetrican et Gynaecologica Scandanavica* 48(Suppl): 7–108

Taylor D H and Lind T (1976) 'Haematological changes during normal pregnancy: Iron induced macrocytosis' *British Journal of Obstetrics and Gynaecology* 83: 760–7

Tuck S and White J M (1981) 'Sickle cell disease' in J Studd (ed) *Progress in Obstetrics and Gynaecology Vol 1* Ch 6 70–8 Churchill Livingstone: Edinburgh

World Health Organization (1972) *Nutritional Anaemias* Report Series No. 503 WHO: Geneva

World Health Organization (1978) *The Prevalence of Nutritional Anaemia in Women in Developing Countries* WHO: Geneva

16   Multiple pregnancy

Incidence

A multiple pregnancy occurs where more than one fetus is present in the uterus at the same time. In the United Kingdom twins occur in approximately 1 : 100 spontaneous pregnancies and triplets in 1 : 1400 (Botting *et al.* 1987). Assisted reproduction increases the incidence of twins and higher-order births (Botting *et al.* 1990). The incidence of twinning varies world-wide, being highest amongst the Yoruba of South-West Nigeria (4.5 : 100) and lowest amongst the Japanese and other Far Eastern races (2–5 : 1000). The world-wide occurrence rate of monozygotic (identical) twins is fairly constant. The differences are therefore in the rates of dizygotic (non-identical) twins (Leroy 1981a). The incidence of dizygotic twins increases with age (up until 40 years) and independently of age, with increasing parity (Waterhouse 1950). This chapter will concentrate upon the more commonly seen twin pregnancies rather than 'super twins' (triplets and above) which have particular problems of increased perinatal mortality and morbidity, together with more stress for the parents. Caring for such babies can be a full-time occupation for at least two care givers, further increasing the physical strain and expense (Botting *et al.* 1990).

Society's attitude to twins is variable. In mythological times twin gods such as Apollo and Diana were much revered; Rome was said to have been founded by the abandoned twins Romulus and Remus (Leroy 1981a). Amongst certain cultures, wishing the birth of twins upon a woman was a bad curse–it was considered that one child was fathered by the husband and the other welcomed by a god or an evil spirit (Leroy 1981a). In wandering tribes, multiple births could be a great burden, whereas twins were welcomed by agricultural peoples (Leroy 1981a).

Causes of twin pregnancy

Dizygotic, binovular or non-identical twins occur with the fertilisation of two separate ova (Bryan 1986a). The resulting children are no more alike than siblings, except that they are the same age (Scerbo *et al.* 1986). Each fetus has its own placenta and set of fetal membranes (2 amnions and 2 chorions). However the placentae may be fused and appear as one; careful examination of the membranes is required after delivery (Bryan 1986a). The use of drugs to stimulate ovulation (such as clomiphene or gonadotrophins) can result in this type of multiple birth. The incidence of twin pregnancy following administration of clomiphene has been reported as being 8.4% (Hack *et al.* 1981). Due to the difficulty with the small margin for error between the achievement of single ovulation and overstimulation of the ovary, the use of gonadotrophins (most commonly perganol) is associated with an incidence of multiple pregnancy of 20–40% (Jewelewicz and Vande Wiele 1975). Dizygotic twinning has a familial incidence; women who are themselves a dizygotic twin have twice the incidence of dizygotic twins (White and Wyshak 1964).

Monozygotic, uniovular or identical twins are the result when one ovum which has been fertilised by one sperm splits into two (Bryan 1986a). As only one set of genetic material is involved, the babies will be of the same sex (very rarely, mosaicism can give rise to 'identical' twins of different sex), genetically identical and of similar physical appearance. Physical differences may occur due to environmental factors, such as inequalities in placental bloodflow (Naeye 1965). These can persist into adult life (Babson and Phillips 1973). The most common time for the division to occur is at the end of the first week after fertilisation, when the inner cell mass splits to produce two embryonic primordia (MacGillivray 1976). Each embryo has its own amniotic sac, but due to the timing of the cleavage they share the same chorion. There is a common placenta with possible anastamoses of placental blood vessels. Blood supply to the fetuses is usually in balance.

Very early division of the embryonic cells can produce monozygotic twins with 2 amnions, 2 chorions and 2 placentae which may not be fused; this occurs in 18–36% of cases (MacGillivray 1976). Later division of the genetic material can result in 2 embryos within the same amniotic sac. There is a severe risk of cord entanglement which accounts for the high frequency of intrauterine death (over 50%) amongst such monoamniotic twins (Benirschke 1983). Should the embryonic disc fail to divide completely, the resulting fetuses will be attached to each other and may share some organs (Potter and Craig 1976). The outlook for such 'Siamese' twins is dependent upon the extent and area of the attachment, which can vary from skin tags to a common heart (Potter and Craig 1976). Surgical separation may be attempted in the neonatal period, but it can sometimes result in the death of one or both of the twins (Douglas 1989).

Triplet pregnancy may be due to one embryo which splits into three (very rare), to one embryo which splits into two and another fertilised ovum or to three separate fertilised ova (Daw 1987).

Diagnosis of multiple pregnancy

Despite the introduction of new technologies, clinical examination and history-taking are still important diagnostic tools. While taking the woman's reproductive history, the midwife always enquires about a family history of twinning, especially where the mother is herself a twin (White and Wyshak 1964). Information is also obtained concerning any treatment for subfertility such as the administration of drugs to stimulate ovulation. Such a history should alert the midwife to the possibility of multiple pregnancy (Scerbo et al. 1986).

Later in her pregnancy the woman with a multiple gestation may complain of increased minor disorders such as morning sickness or urinary frequency (Spillman 1987c). On inspection of her abdomen, it may appear larger than it should in the period of gestation (especially if polyhydramnios is present). On examination, the uterus may feel larger than expected (Cunningham et al. 1989). This, though, is not diagnostic, as the woman could be mistaken in her dates; there could be fibroids present, a hydatidiform mole, or if in early pregnancy the woman may have a full bladder (Cunningham et al. 1989). Other signs include the presence of three fetal poles (either heads or buttocks—however, a hard fibroid can feel like a fetal pole), which appear small in relation to the size of the uterus. A multiplicity of limbs may also be felt and should be differentiated from the findings where a single fetus is lying in an occipito-posterior position. Listening with two portable Doptone devices may detect two fetal hearts but can be an inaccurate procedure. Some multiple pregnancies are suspected when routine serum alpha feto protein determination shows a high level (Garoff and Seppala 1973).

Ultrasound scanning is the method of choice for diagnosing or confirming the diagnosis of multiple pregnancy. Multiple gestation sacs can be seen as early as 8 weeks after the last period (Chudleigh and Pearce 1986). There are numerous documented cases of 'the disappearing twin' where 1 fetus has died and been absorbed without any other signs (Robinson and Caines 1977). Jarvis (1979) reports that a fifth of women with a twin pregnancy had an ultrasound report showing a single pregnancy on at least one occasion. Cases of undiagnosed twins or an undiagnosed triplet can still occur in labour, although one study showed that following the introduction of routine ultrasound scanning at 17 weeks gestation, 98% of multiple pregnancies were diagnosed (Persson et al. 1979). Prior to the widespread use of scanning, up to 50% of multiple pregnancies were unrecognised prior to labour (Barter et al. 1965). Where twins are expected, an X-ray examination may be performed after 34 weeks to exclude the risk of triplets (Itzkowic 1979). Due to the risk to the developing fetus, such an examination would not be advocated at an earlier stage, but it does allow the obstetrician to disentangle a multiplicity of fetal parts to determine the number of fetuses present and their presentations (Cunningham *et al*. 1989).

The reaction of parents to the diagnosis of a multiple pregnancy is mixed, especially where the pregnancy was unplanned (Spillman 1987c). Apart from concern as to the progress of the pregnancy and the conduct of delivery, there are numerous logistical problems which can give rise to distress or anxiety (Spillman 1987c; Bryan 1990). Twins can be a great financial burden, with increased costs for food and clothing. Housing may already be overcrowded, travelling with twins is more difficult, as for the woman to return to work (Bryan 1990). It may be harder to find baby-sitters or relatives willing to undertake childminding when two babies are involved. The midwife should encourage the parents to talk through their concerns, while giving advice such as suggesting they contact their local twins club. Such organisations offer support and information, providing a market for second-hand items of baby equipment, such as double prams and buggies (Bryan 1988).

Pregnancy complications

Minor disorders of pregnancy are more frequent and in some cases worsened in multiple pregnancy (Scerbo *et al*. 1986). The larger-than-usual uterus worsens varicose veins and backache; tiredness is an intractable problem, especially as pregnancy advances (Bryan 1990). Sleeping may be difficult due to heartburn and cramps and since there are two fetuses who may be active just when the mother is wanting to sleep.

Spontaneous abortion is more common in multiple than in single pregnancies (MacGillivray 1984). It has been postulated that the cause is related to the fact that fetal abnormality is more common in multiple pregnancy (Corney *et al*. 1982; MacGillivray 1984). As few multiple pregnancies have been diagnosed at such an early stage of pregnancy, much of this is speculation. There are however well-documented cases of a disappearing twin or of a woman having a spontaneous abortion and still being pregnant (Robinson and Caines 1977). At later stages in pregnancy, one fetus may die and be reabsorbed, sometimes the remnants of this fetus can be seen within the membranes as a fetus papyraceous (Cunningham *et al*. 1989).

Gestational proteinuric hypertension is more common especially if the woman is primiparous (MacGillivray 1983). Whilst the hypertension may be mild, if severe or combined with proteinuria it may necessitate preterm delivery, with all its attendant effects on perinatal mortality and morbidity (MacGillivray 1984).

Preterm labour occurs more frequently than in single pregnancies, especially if polyhydramnios is present. MacGillivray (1982) reports an incidence of preterm births as high as 20% in all multiple births, being more common in monozygotic than dizygotic twins. The cause of onset of labour was evenly distributed between spontaneous rupture of membranes and spontaneous onset of contractions (MacGillivray 1982). It used to be policy to admit women with a twin pregnancy to hospital at 30 weeks gestation for bed rest, to encourage fetal growth, and to prevent preterm labour (Powers 1973). This is now out of favour as it is very disruptive to family life, has a high financial cost and is of little benefit (Weeks *et al.* 1977). It may indeed predispose the woman to complications (Saunders *et al.* 1985). Should preterm labour occur, tocolytics may be used, but prophylactic use of tocolytics in multiple pregnancy is not associated with an improvement in fetal outcome (O'Connor *et al.* 1979).

Polyhydramnios is also more common. Acute onset is usually confined to monozygotic twins whereas both types can experience chronic polyhydramnios (MacGillivray 1984). The causes are unclear, but they may be related to the increased incidence of fetal abnormality. One effect of polyhydramnios, especially if the onset is acute, is the increased risk of spontaneous mid-trimester abortion or premature rupture of the membranes with cord prolapse.

Due to the larger than normal increase in plasma volume of about 2000 ml, even more haemodilution than usual occurs, causing anaemia (Campbell and MacGillivray 1972). There are also two fetuses requiring to build iron stores in addition to their increased use of folic acid. Most obstetricians recommend iron and folic acid supplements if anaemia is demonstrated (MacGillivray 1984; Weaver 1990).

Intrauterine growth retardation is more common in multiple pregnancies where the babies weigh on average 500 g less than single births of an equivalent gestation (Bryan 1986b). Various explanations have been advanced for this, including intrauterine overcrowding which prevents placental development, insufficient uterine blood supply (Leroy 1981b) and an earlier than usual deceleration in fetal growth (Bryan 1986b). Where monochorionic twins share the placental circulation there may be a disproportionate allocation of blood, resulting in one anaemic growth retarded fetus and one plethoric polycythaemic large fetus, both of whom are at risk (Scerbo *et al.* 1986). This fetal transfusion syndrome can result in babies of disparate size whose physical differences may persist into adult life (Babson and Phillips 1973).

Antenatal care

A woman with a multiple pregnancy should receive her antenatal care and be delivered in a hospital consultant unit. Should this be distant, antenatal care may be arranged locally by the midwife or general practitioner. Careful supervision is necessary to detect the onset of complications. The midwife can also offer advice on diet and exercise. She can put the parents in touch with twins clubs who can advise on baby clothes and equipment. Parent education on a one-to-one basis can be beneficial, especially where the couple have no other children (Spillman 1987c). Specialist advice and preparation concerning the conduct of labour can help to allay the woman's fears and allow her to discuss how she would like labour to be managed (Spillman 1987c).

Labour

In cases of particular concern for fetal or maternal well-being or where there is a poor obstetric history, it may be decided to deliver the babies by caesarean section (Crawford 1987). This may also be the decision with certain combinations of fetal presentation. The following is the frequency of fetal presentations in decreasing order of their occurrence:

Vertex	Vertex	38.6%
Vertex	Breech	25.5%
Breech	Cephalic	13.1%
Breech	Breech	9.2%
Vertex	Transverse	8.0%
Breech	Transverse	3.9%
Transverse	Transverse	0.6%
Transverse	Cephalic	0.6%
Transverse	Breech	0.6%

(Thompson *et al.* 1987, p. 328)

The first stage of labour is managed in the same way as any labour, with the mother being encouraged to be mobile (should she so wish) and analgesia being given as required. The obstetrician, paediatrician and obstetric anaesthetist require to be informed that a woman expecting twins is in labour, should their services be required later (Crawford 1987). Should continuous fetal monitoring be required, this can be achieved by using an internal electrode for the first twin and an external detector for the second (Weaver 1990). However such an arrangement will severely curtail the mother's mobility. The midwife should support the woman, who may be nervous and apprehensive about the delivery and anxious about the well-being of her babies (Spillman 1987c). Where there have been antenatal complications such as hypertensive disease, the labour will be managed accordingly. Slow progress or fetal distress may be dealt with more aggressively than for a single pregnancy, because of the increased risk with two babies (Weaver 1990).

All the equipment for delivery should be assembled in plenty of time. This includes having at least one warmed cot prepared, resuscitation apparatus on hand if required and extra instruments or two delivery packs. These include an amnihook to rupture the second set of membranes, an extra cord clamp and another set of marked Spencer Wells forceps to clamp the second umbilical cord. These are important for identifying which cord belongs to which baby to facilitate the taking of cord blood.

Once the woman is in the second stage of labour, the medical staff should be standing by (not necessarily in the room) in case they are needed. Two midwives are usual for the delivery; it is preferable if both are known to the parents, as this can encourage mutual trust. The first baby is delivered as normal (according to its presentation) and in accordance with the mother's wishes. The cord is clamped and cut and the baby identified as twin one. (If necessary, resuscitation is performed.)

The baby is then dried, wrapped in warmed drapes and handed to the mother. It is now that any difficulties are more likely to occur; these are uterine inertia, abnormal lie of the second twin, cord prolapse and premature separation of the placenta (Cunningham *et al.* 1989).

After clamping and cutting the first twin's cord, the lie and presentation of the second twin are determined; if longitudinal and cephalic, the second set of membranes are ruptured. (Where the second twin has an oblique or transverse lie, the obstetrician may attempt version (either internal or external) to a longitudinal lie or he/she may decide to perform a caesarean section (Weaver 1990).) The midwife should then listen to the fetal heart of twin two. She should ensure that no umbilical cord is palpable before or after the procedure. The fetal heart is then auscultated and recorded.

Should contractions fail to recommence, the first baby may be put to the mother's breast, and if she intends to breast feed, encouraged to suckle to stimulate contractions. If this is not successful, medical assistance should be sought and an intravenous infusion of syntocinon commenced (Weaver 1990). The maximum safe interval between the deliveries of the twins was said to be 15–30 minutes, although Rayburn *et al.* (1984) have argued that with continuous fetal monitoring, longer intervals are not harmful in the absence of fetal distress. Once the second twin has been delivered, resuscitated and identified, its cord is then clamped and cut using the marked Spencer Wells forceps. The baby is warmly wrapped and handed to his/her parents. It is the midwife's decision for each delivery as to whether she deems it necessary to perform an episiotomy.

Intramuscular syntometrine should be given to the mother on delivery of the anterior shoulder of the second twin to aid expulsion of the placenta and the control of bleeding (Weaver 1990). Controlled cord traction can be performed as normal, although the midwife should hold both cords together. Once the third stage is completed the uterus should be well contracted to control bleeding from the extra large placental site (Cunningham *et al.* 1989). If labour has been prolonged or if there was uterine inertia between the two deliveries, extra vigilance is needed to observe for signs of haemorrhage from an atonic uterus (Weaver 1990). The woman's perineum is examined for its integrity, to determine whether suturing is required.

After assessing that the mother's condition is satisfactory, the midwife must examine the placenta and membranes for completeness and to try to determine the zygosity of the twins (Bryan 1986a). This last is only necessary where the twins are of the same sex. The presence of 1 chorion is diagnostic of monozygosity, whereas if there are 2 chorions this suggests but does not confirm dizygosity. Confirmation could be obtained by chromosome studies or by awaiting the development of physical characteristics (Bryan 1986a). The 2 babies should be examined carefully by the midwife for physical abnormalities, which are more common amongst multiple births (Corney *et al.* 1982). A paediatrician will carry out a further more extensive examination within the first 24 hours.

If at any stage in the labour the midwife decides that events are deviating from the normal, she should summon the appropriate medical aid before documenting her findings and her actions. If one baby is delivered by forceps or as an assisted breech, this is no reason why the midwife should not deliver the next baby if the conditions are correct. If possible, the parents should be allowed time to get to know both their babies (Spillman 1987a). Should it be necessary for one baby to be admitted to the Special Care Baby Unit, it is preferable that the two babies are kept together (Klaus and Kennell 1982) or for them to be cared for at the mother's bedside in a transitional care unit.

Postpartum care

This is similar to the care given to any mother after delivery but there are a few differences. The mother may feel absolutely exhausted after labour, especially if she has had difficulty sleeping for the last few weeks of pregnancy (Spillman 1987c). In addition she is required to care for two babies (Spillman 1987c; Bryan 1990). Due to the large placental site there may be an increase in lochia as well as a predisposition to infection. The midwife should be vigilant to this as involution can appear slow, due to the greater-than-normal size of the uterus at delivery. Afterpains may be troublesome, particularly when breast feeding. Breast feeding, however, allows both babies to feed together and although sometimes complex to master as regards positioning the babies, is less time-consuming in the long term (Bryan 1990). The mother may well require continued assistance after the first day (Bryan 1990). Helping the mother to slow down and relax when feeding can be of help (Stables 1980). Danger periods for stopping feeding are at the time of transfer home from hospital and when the midwife passes over her care of the mother and babies to the health visitor, especially if this latter coincides with a growth spurt. It is now that antenatal education and the support of another mother who has successfully fed twins can pay dividends. When helping the mother with her babies, the midwife should be wary of 'taking over', only giving help when requested or when the mother accepts an offer of assistance (Spillman 1987c).

Getting into a routine at home is even more difficult with twins (Spillman 1987b; Bryan 1990). The mother should take advantage of any help which is offered, even though it may not last for long. Where there are siblings there may be problems of rivalry and the parents should try to spend time alone with the older child(ren). Trips out could involve one child and one baby, for example (Spillman 1987a). The current thinking on raising twins is to encourage them to be as individual as possible through different clothes (or at least different colours), changes in hairstyle, having their own toys and the choice of different sounding names (Bryan 1984). Milestone such as the start of talking may be delayed as twins can devise their own methods of communication which exclude adults (Bryan 1984).

Psychological problems

Bonding difficulties may occur where one baby remains in the Special Care Baby

Unit and the other goes home (Klaus and Kennell 1982). Parents may seek to protect their emotions from harm by distancing themselves from an ill twin, in case he/she does not recover (Evans *et al*. 1972). Where there is much difference in size between the babies, the parents may find themselves preferring one baby to the other, usually the one which is easier to feed (Spillman 1987b). Should one baby die either before or after birth or be severely handicapped, the parents may suffer emotional trauma (Lewis and Bryan 1988). This can be severe if the mother has had a dead baby and a living fetus in the uterus together. Not only do the parents have to make time to mourn for their dead baby (a hard enough task) but they also have the continuing demands of the living baby (Lewis and Bryan 1988). Later celebrations of birthdays bring reminders of the earlier death (Bryan 1986b). Expert counselling may be required, but the midwife can give much support by encouraging the parents to talk about and name their dead baby whilst cherishing the one who remains (Lewis and Bryan 1988). 'Survivor guilt' may be experienced by the living twin and persist into adult life; personality development can be affected (Lewis and Bryan 1988).

References

Babson S G and Phillips D S (1973) 'Growth and development of twins dissimilar in size at birth' *New England Journal of Medicine* 289: 937

Barter R H, Hsu I and Ekkenbach R V (1965) 'The prevention of prematurity in multiple pregnancy' *American Journal of Obstetrics and Gynecology* 91: 787

Benirschke K (1983) Personal communication. Cited by F G Cunningham, P C MacDonald and N F Gant (1989) in *William's Obstetrics (18th edn)* 639 Prentice Hall: London.

Botting B J, Macdonald Davies I and Macfarlane A J (1987) 'Recent trends in the incidence of multiple births and associated mortality' *Archives of Disease in Childhood* 62: 941–50

Botting B J, Macfarlane A J and Price F V (1990) *Three, Four and More: A Study of Triplet and Higher Order Births* HMSO: London

Bryan E M (1984) 'The development of twins' *Maternal and Child Health* 9(10): 307–10

Bryan E M (1986a) 'Are they identical? The importance of determining zygosity in twins' *Maternal and Child Health* 11(5): 171–6

Bryan E M (1986b) 'The intrauterine hazard of twins' *Archives of Disease in Childhood* 61: 1044–5

Bryan E M (1988) 'The multiple births foundation' *Midwife, Health Visitor and Community Nurse* 24(12): 513–5

Bryan E M (1990) 'Twins in the family.' *Midwives Chronicle* March: 66–9

Campbell D M and MacGillivray I (1972) 'Comparisons of maternal response to first and second pregnancies in relation to baby weight' *Journal of Obstetrics and Gynaecology of the British Commonwealth* 79: 684

Chudleigh P and Pearce J M (1986) *Obstetric Ultrasound* Churchill Livingstone: Edinburgh

Corney G, MacGillivray I, Campbell D M, Thompson B and Little J (1982) 'Congenital anomalies in twins in Aberdeen and North East Scotland' *Acta Geneticae et Gemellologiae* 32: 31

Crawford J S (1987) 'A prospective study of 200 consecutive twin pregnancies' *Anaesthesia* 42: 33

Cunningham F G, MacDonald P C and Gant N F (1989) *William's Obstetrics (18th edn)* Prentice Hall: London

Daw E (1987) 'Triplet pregnancy' in J Studd (ed) *Progress in Obstetrics and Gynaecology Vol 6* Ch 6 119–31 Churchill Livingstone: Edinburgh

Douglas J (1989) 'Double miracle' *Nursing Times* 85(32): 16–17

Evans S, Rheinhart J B and Succop R A (1972) 'A study of 45 children and their families' *Journal of the American Academy of Child Psychiatry* 11: 440

Garoff L and Seppala M (1973) 'Alpha feto protein and human placental lactogen in maternal serum in multiple pregnancies' *Journal of Obstetrics and Gynaecology of the British Commonwealth* 80: 695

Hack M, British M and Serr D M (1981) 'Outcome of pregnancy after induced ovulation' *Journal of the American Medical Association* 220: 1329

Itzkowic D (1979) 'A survey of 59 triplet pregnancies' *British Journal of Obstetrics and Gynaecology* 86: 23–8

Jarvis G J (1979) 'Diagnosis of multiple pregnancy' *British Medical Journal* 2: 593–4

Jewelewicz R and Vande Wiele R L (1975) 'Management of multifetal gestation' *Contemporary Obstetrics and Gynecology* 6: 59

Klaus M H and Kennell J H (1982) *Parent Infant Bonding (2nd edn)* C V Mosby: St Louis

Leroy F (1981a) 'The cultural and biological significance of twins' *Midwife Health Visitor and Community Nurse* 17(6): 226–30

Leroy F (1981b) 'The hazards and management of twin pregnancies' *Midwife Health Visitor and Community Nurse* 17(7): 173–5

Lewis E and Bryan E M (1988) 'Management of the perinatal loss of one twin' *British Medical Journal* 297: 1321–3

MacGillivray I (1976) 'Twin pregnancies' in R M Wynn (ed) *Obstetrics and Gynecology Annual* 135 Appleton: New York

MacGillivray I (1982) 'Complications of twin pregnancies' *European Journal of Obstetrics, Gynaecology and Reproductive Biology* 15: 263

MacGillivray I (1983) 'Pre-eclampsia in twin pregnancies' in I MacGillivray (ed) *Pre-eclampsia: the Hypertensive Disease of Pregnancy* Holt-Saunders: Eastbourne

MacGillivray I (1984) 'Maternal response to twin pregnancy' in J Studd (ed) *Progress in Obstetrics and Gynaecology Vol 4* Ch 10 139–50 Churchill Livingstone: Edinburgh

Naeye R L (1965) 'Organ abnormalities in a human parabiotic syndrome' *American Journal of Pathology* 46: 829

O'Connor M C, Arias E and Royston J P (1979) 'The merits of special antenatal care for twin pregnancies' *British Journal of Obstetrics and Gynaecology* 86: 706

Persson P H, Grennert L and Gennser G (1979) 'On improved outcome in twin pregnancies' *Acta Obstetrica et Gynaecologica Scandanavica* 58: 3

Potter E L and Craig J M (1976) 'Multiple pregnancies and conjoined twins' *Pathology of the Fetus and Infant (3rd edn)* Ch 13 Lloyd Luke: London

Powers W F (1973) 'Bedrest in twin pregnancy: identification of a critical period' *Obstetrics and Gynecology* 42: 795

Rayburn W F, Lavin J P, Miodovnik M and Varner M W (1984) 'Multiple gestation: Time interval between delivery of first and second twins' *Obstetrics and Gynecology* 63: 502

Robinson H P and Caines J S (1977) 'Sonar evidence of early pregnancy failure in patients with twin conceptions' *British Journal of Obstetrics and Gynaecology* 84: 22

Saunders M C, Dick J S, Brown I M, McPherson K and Chalmers I (1985) 'The effects of hospital admission for bed rest on the duration of twin pregnancy' *Lancet* ii: 793–5

Scerbo J C, Rattan P and Drukker J E (1986) 'Twins and other multiple gestations' in R A Knuppel and J E Drukker (eds) *High Risk Pregnancy: A team approach* Ch 19 335–61 W B Saunders: Philadelphia

Spillman J R (1987a) 'Emotional aspects of experiencing multiple birth' *Midwife Health Visitor and Community Nurse* 23(2): 54–8

Spillman J R (1987b) 'Double exposure–coping with newborn twins at home' *Midwife Health Visitor and Community Nurse* 23(3): 92–4

Spillman J R (1987c) 'The emotional impact of multiple pregnancy – the midwife's role in support of the family' *Midwives Chronicle* March: 58–62

Stables J (1980) 'Breast feeding twins' *Nursing Times* 21 Aug: 1493–4

Thompson S A, Lyons T L and Makowski E L (1987) 'Outcome of twin gestations at the University of Colorado Health Sciences Center 1973–83' *Journal of Reproductive Medicine* 32: 328

Waterhouse J A H (1950) 'Twinning and twin pedigrees' *British Journal of Social Medicine* 4: 197

Weaver J B (1990) 'The management of twin pregnancy' *Progress in Obstetrics and Gynaecology Vol 8* Ch 7 97–105 Churchill Livingstone: Edinburgh

Weeks A R L, Menzies D N and de Boer C H (1977) 'The relative efficacy of bedrest, cervical suture and no treatment in the management of twin pregnancy' *British Journal of Obstetrics and Gynaecology* 84: 161–4

White C and Wyshak G (1964) 'Inheritance in human dizygotic twinning' *New England Journal of Medicine* 271: 1003

17 Infectious disease in pregnancy

This chapter concentrates on some of the infections which can cause problems to the pregnant woman or her growing fetus. None of these is particular to childbirth, but each has a specific impact on the course and outcome of pregnancy and labour for both mother and child; their impact upon the child will be described in more detail in Chapter 37. For the most part, these infections are acquired by sexual intercourse (syphilis, herpes simplex, human immuno deficiency virus–HIV) (Lee 1988), from infected blood (HIV, hepatitis) or by vertical transmission from mother to fetus (HIV, hepatitis and syphilis).

The area of cervical cytology, carcinoma and precancerous changes in the cervix, is also included. Although the cause of this is still unconfirmed, in many cases human papillomavirus (similar to that which causes genital warts) has been isolated from the cervix, demonstrating a link with sexual activity. Before describing infections of the genital tract, it is necessary to discuss the functions and properties of normal vaginal secretions. The more common infections causing vaginal discharge will be considered before hepatitis, HIV and cervical cytology.

Normal vaginal secretions

Vaginal secretions consist of a mixture of fluids which come from various sources, including cervical mucus, vulval secretions from sebaceous glands, and transudates from Bartholin's and Skene's glands (Emens 1983). The quantity of fluid varies through a woman's lifetime and with each phase of the menstrual cycle (Emens 1983). During the reproductive years, vaginal secretions are acid, with a pH as low as 3.8–4.2 (Emens 1983). There is a high level of lactic acid (up to 2–3%) produced by the action of commensal organisms (Doderlein's bacilli) on glycogen contained in desquamed vaginal epithelial cells. The amount of glycogen present is dependent on hormone levels, being lowest during the immediate premenstrual phase and after the menopause (Emens 1983). Vaginal acidity is one of the main defences against genital infection (Emens 1983).

The normal production of vaginal secretion varies considerably between individuals; an important point to bear in mind when differentiating physiological from pathological discharges. A reported increase in vaginal secretions is common during pregnancy and is known as leucorrhoea. In one study, fewer than 1% of pregnant women complained of this discharge, although a further third when questioned directly admitted to having leucorrheoa (Thin and Michael 1970). It is necessary to eliminate the possibility of infection by microscopic examination of the discharge/ secretion and determination of its level of acidity, before giving any reassurance. Vulval irritation can be due to infection, but a common cause is the use of bath preparations, scented soaps or a change in detergents (Blackwell 1987a). Careful questioning can often elicit a benign and easily remedied cause (Blackwell 1987a).

Bacterial discharges

Gardnerella vaginalis (previously called *Haemophilus vaginalis*) is an organism found to be present in the vaginal secretions of most women suffering from non-specific (anaerobic) vaginitis (NSV) (Kelsey *et al.* 1987). Whether *Gardnerella* is the sole causative organism in NSV is open to question (Emens 1983). The organism is known to be present in asymptomatic women (West *et al.* 1988) and may only be pathological in large numbers or in the presence of other anaerobes.

Gardnerella vaginalis was first isolated by Gardner and Dukes (1955). It is a gram-negative bacillus which is difficult to culture. For this reason and because of its unusual properties, there has been much discussion about placing it in its correct genus (hence the changes in its name). The signs and symptoms of infection include a grey, frothy and malodorous discharge, the presence of 'clue' cells and a vaginal pH (obtained by testing secretions in the posterior cervical fornix) of between 5.0 and 6.0 (Blackwell 1987b). 'Clue' cells were first described in 1955 (Gardner and Dukes) as large cells of the vaginal epithelium which appeared granular and with indistinct outlines due to the excessive number of *Gardnerella* organisms attached to the surface. NSV, unlike other infections, rarely presents with symptoms of vaginal irritation (Emens 1983).

Since male partners are usually asymptomatic reservoirs of infection, it is preferable to treat both partners (Emens 1983). Metronidazole 200 mg, 3 times daily for 7 days is the treatment required (Blackwell 1987b).

Gonococcal vaginitis is caused by the gram-negative diplococcus *Neisseria gonorrhoea*. Infections with this bacteria are reported (anonymously) to the Sexually Transmitted Disease Surveillance Unit, which maintains statistics. Gonorrhoea is prevalent throughout the world. In less-developed countries, it is a significant contributor to infertility (Lee 1988). Although primarily a sexually transmitted microorganism, it can provoke premature rupture of the membranes (Faro and Pastorek 1986) and be transmitted to the fetus at delivery (Fong 1987). The resulting conjunctivitis (ophthalmia neonatorum) which occurs within 24 hours of delivery was, prior to the discovery of penicillin, a major cause of blindness (Pearce and Roberton 1986). The advent of penicillin-resistant gonococcus has necessitated recourse to alternative treatments, such as tetracycline eye drops (Fong 1987).

The signs and symptoms of infection are variable, with most women being asymptomatic (Emens 1983). Where symptoms are present, they include a green purulent discharge and vulval oedema appearing 2–7 days after the initial infection (Emens 1983). On examination, the genital mucus membranes are oedematous. Dysuria may be reported as a result of the urethritis (Lee 1988). Most cases come to light following detection of the infected male partner who is more commonly symptomatic than the female (Fong 1987). Diagnosis is confirmed by obtaining a sample of the secretions, performing a gram stain and looking for the diplococcus under the microscope. It is important to rule out the presence of multiple infections with other microorganisms (Blackwell 1987b).

Treatment utilises procaine penicillin, 2.4 Mu intramuscularly into each buttock (4.8 Mu in total) and 1 g of probenicid orally (Emens 1983). Where there is an allergy to penicillin, a 7 day course of tetracycline (contra-indicated in pregnancy) or erythromycin will be prescribed. For penicillin-resistant strains of gonorrhoea, the newer cephalosporins are normally used. When infections are confirmed, it is important to instigate contact tracing of partners to prevent spread of infection or reinfection from occurring (Fong 1987).

Syphilis is caused by the spirochaete, *Treponema pallidum*. This bacteria moves in a characteristic pattern of undulations and corkscrew rotations along its long axis (Faro and Pastorek 1986). The spirochaete gains entry to the body through mucus membranes or via abrasions in surface tissues (Lee 1988). The initial result is an ulcer at the point of entry, which appears 10–90 days following infection. This ulcer is known as a chancre; it contains multitudes of spirochaetes, making the person highly infectious (Lee 1988). Diagnosis is by microscopy of fluid from the ulcer to look for the presence of spirochaetes. This is known as primary syphilis (Faro and Pastorek 1986). Vaginal discharge is rare in cases of syphilis (Blackwell 1987b).

Because the chancre is painless, many cases in women go unnoticed. If the chancre is missed, about 8–10 weeks later spirochaetes will have entered the general circulation, causing the more diverse secondary syphilis (Lee 1988). Any body organ can be affected; there may be systemic symptoms resembling a viral infection and lymphadenopathy. More usually detected are the wide range of skin rashes and eruptions which can occur (Lee 1988). These clinical signs will disappear, although serological changes remain. The person is in a non-infective latent stage which can persist for many years. Tertiary syphilis then occurs which can affect the cardiovascular and central nervous systems (Faro and Pastorek 1986).

Syphilis is very dangerous in pregnancy as the organism crosses the placenta and spreads throughout the fetal body (Holder and Knox 1972). This usually occurs in the second half of pregnancy. Faro and Pastorek (1986) state that 25% of affected fetuses die in utero and 30% in the early neonatal period. Of the survivors 40% are affected with congenital syphilis where symptoms include failure to thrive, syphilitic pemphigus (skin rash), saddle nose (giving noisy breathing), jaundice, periostitis, anaemia, Hutchinson's teeth (pointed), nephritis, hydrocephalus, deafness and mental retardation (Speck *et al.* 1986).

Because of the risks in pregnancy all pregnant women in the UK have their blood screened at the first antenatal visit for antibodies to *Treponema pallidum* (Wang and Smaill 1989). The Venereal Disease Research Laboratory Test is the one usually employed. False positive results can occur amongst women from tropical countries such as the West Indies who have antibodies to the endemic infection Yaws, another Treponema organism (Parker 1989). In such cases, more specific serological tests such as the *Treponema pallidum* haemaglutination test should be employed to confirm the diagnosis (Wang and Smaill 1989). Treatment is usually by intramuscular injection of procaine penicillin 0.6–0.9 mega units daily for 14–21 days (Fong 1987). In cases of penicillin allergy, erythromycin can be employed (Fong 1987).

Fungal infections

In 80% of genital yeast infections, the causative microorganism is *Candida albicans* (Emens 1983). Candida has been isolated from asymptomatic women and can therefore be regarded as part of the normal vaginal flora (Blackwell 1987b). When the vaginal environment and physiology are disturbed, for example during pregnancy, following antibiotic therapy or in the presence of other infections, *Candida* can become pathogenic (Emens 1983). In addition, current fashions in undergarments, such as the use of man-made fibres, prevent free circulation of air and can predispose to infection (Emens 1983). The signs and symptoms of *Candida* are quite characteristic. The woman usually complains of severe vulval itching, which is often worse during the night and there is a thick creamy discharge (Emens 1983). On examination, erythema is a common sign, usually on the labia, perineum and perianal regions. Diagnosis is by microscopic examination of vaginal secretions which have been mixed with a 10% solution of potassium hydroxide. This dissolves blood and vaginal epithelial cells, leaving the characteristic mycelia (Emens 1983).

Where the attack is mild, a change in bathing behaviour (using unscented soap and no bath additives), wearing loose-fitting underwear of natural materials such as cotton (Emens 1983) and the use of live natural yogurt impregnated-tampons which are inserted into the vagina, may be of help. For more severe conditions, medication using antifungal pessaries and creams (containing nystatin or imidazole or triazole antifungal agents) will need to be prescribed (Wang and Smaill 1989). The woman must be warned that nystatin can stain her underwear and that she should wear a protective pad. Oral antifungals such as butoconazole and econazole have been developed, but these have not as yet been shown to be safe in pregnancy (Wang and Smaill 1989). For women who experience repeated attacks of Candidiasis, the treatment for mild infection can be utilised with recourse to topical use of natural yogurt at the first sign of infection.

Parasitic infections

Chlamydia trachomatis is an intracellular parasite with many of the characteristics of bacteria, including a sensitivity to broad spectrum antibiotics (Emens 1983). Infection is primarily by sexual contact, although it has been found in a small percentage of asymptomatic women attending Well Woman clinics (Munday 1983). *Chlamydia* is known as the major cause of non-specific (non-gonococcal) urethritis in men (Saunders 1988). Partners of these men have a high risk of infection with the parasite (Dunlop 1985). Because there is a significant rate of spontaneous recovery and some infections are asymptomatic, it is difficult to define the pathogenicity of chlamydia (Emens 1983).

Chlamydia can cause infections of the Bartholin's glands, cervicitis, salpingitis, pelvic inflammatory disease, spontaneous abortion and infertility (Munday 1983). In the neonate it has been shown to cause severe conjunctivitis (Saunders 1988). In areas where chlamydia is endemic, antenatal screening of mothers would be cost effective in preventing infection and the resultant corneal adhesions. In tropical countries, infection with *chlamydia* causes trachoma, which affects approximately 400 million people, many of whom are partially sighted or blind.

Diagnosis involves inoculating cervical secretions into a tissue culture such as a monolayer of irradiated McCoy cells (Emens 1983). If infection is present, microscopic examination after 24 hours will demonstrate inclusion bodies (Emens 1983). Treatment in the adult is with oral tetracycline, although in pregnancy erythromycin must be substituted (Munday 1983). The neonate is usually treated with oral erythromycin and topical tetracycline ointment (Rees *et al.* 1981).

Trichomonas is a five-tailed mobile protozoa transmitted by sexual intercourse. As with many organisms, asymptomatic infections can occur. The signs and symptoms when present include acute vaginitis and the presence of a copious foul smelling discharge (Blackwell 1987b). Blackwell (1987b) comments that the odour is probably caused by the presence of co-existent anaerobic bacteria. The textbook descriptions of a green frothy discharge are questioned by Emens (1983), who says that these characteristics are rare. Diagnosis is by microscopic examination of a wet smear of the discharge to demonstrate the mobile protozoa. Staining of smears has the advantage of detecting non-viable *trichomonas* (Wasley 1988). In addition, the pH of any secretions will be above 5.5–6.0 (Blackwell 1987b).

Treatment is with oral metronidazole 200 mg three times daily for 7 days (Wang and Smaill 1989). This will also treat any anaerobic bacteria which may be present. Metronidazole is contra-indicated in the first trimester (Chow and Jewesson 1985) and its use in breast feeding mothers is controversial. In these cases clotrimazole pessaries and creams (where use may increase vaginal and vulval discomfort) are the only suitable treatment. Since the male partner can be an asymptomatic reservoir of infection, it is important that he also receives treatment to prevent reinfection (Lossick 1982).

Viral infections

Herpes simplex, herpes simplex type II is also known as herpes genitalis; the type I virus, causes the familiar cold sore (Grossman 1980). Infection with herpes has been known throughout history, with Hippocrates describing it. Its name comes from the Greek verb meaning 'to creep'. Herpes simplex is part of a larger group of viruses including those which cause chickenpox (*varicella zoster*), glandular fever (Epstein-Barr) and cytomegalo virus (CMV). Transmission is by sexual intercourse and the virus occurs worldwide. The whole virus group shares a particular characteristic, that of remaining dormant in the host after the initial attack, being reactivated (often at times of stress or debility) to cause recurrent but usually less severe symptoms (Baker 1983).

The primary infection is usually the most severe and is accompanied by systemic effects, including low grade pyrexia, a general feeling of malaise and enlargement of inguinal lymph nodes (Baker 1983). Painful lesions can occur singly or in clusters on any area of the genitalia, including the vulva, cervix and perineum (Baker 1983). They ulcerate, form a scab and heal within 3 weeks. Successive cropping of lesions can occur. Severe vulval discomfort and dysuria can occur; in severe cases retention of urine requiring hospital admission and catheterisation may be present (Blackwell 1987b). Subsequent attacks occur when viruses in the sacral ganglia are reactivated (Lee 1988). Recurrences are usually far less severe than the initial attack (Baker 1983). In some cases, successive infection occurs with little or no break between attacks (Emens 1983).

Since serological tests are unable to differentiate between active and latent infections, active infection can only be confirmed by virus isolation or identification (Emens 1983). Since this is a lengthy procedure, diagnosis usually relies on clinical signs (Blackwell 1987b). Attempts at treatment have not been particularly successful although a 5 day course of acyclovir (blocking DNA synthesis) has reduced the duration of lesions and viral shedding in initial attacks (Faro and Pastorek 1986).

Herpes infection of the neonate carries a high mortality rate of up to 50% (Faro and Pastorek 1986). Kelly (1988) states that the rate of transmission between mother and infant or fetus is 40% in primary infections, but as low as 3% in recurrent attacks. It has been the practice to deliver by caesarean section where active infection is present, although there have been no randomised trials of this management (Wang and Smaill 1989). However, as Kelly (1988) comments, the virus can be shed from apparently asymptomatic women. He suggests that where the woman in labour reports evidence of a recent infection, careful examination of the external genitalia, vagina and cervix should be made to detect the presence of any lesions. If present, operative delivery should be performed. If the lesion is seen prior to labour, swabs can be taken to confirm the diagnosis. The neonate should be screened for infection and, if necessary, treated with acyclovir (Kelly 1988).

Condylomata acuminata (genital warts) result from infection with specific strains of HPV. The virus is transmitted by sexual intercourse from an infected partner. On rare occasions, the virus can be transmitted to the neonate at birth (McMillan 1987). Vulval warts occur singly or in clusters on the labia, perineum or at the fourchette. Pregnancy and immunosuppression cause the warts to increase in size and number. Other manifestations of this infection are changes in the epithelium (usually of the vagina and cervix), including opacity (causing the tissue to appear white) and cellular changes (McMillan 1987).

Treatment of the warts is by local destructive therapy using laser, diathermy or cryotherapy with liquid nitrogen. For small lesions in the non-pregnant woman, topical podophyllin may be employed with repeated applications being required (Bunney 1986). Recurrence is fairly common, since the virus may be found in apparently normal (and therefore untreated) tissue (McMillan 1987). In addition, the woman's sexual partner can act as a reservoir of infection and should also be screened and treated to improve effectiveness of treatment (Emens 1983). In cases where the warts are extremely large, it may be necessary to affect delivery by caesarean section, since the warts are very vascular and bleed easily (Faro and Pastorek 1986). The clusters greatly reduce in size after delivery. HPV viruses have been implicated as a cause of cervical cancer. This will be discussed later in the chapter.

Hepatitis

There are three viruses which can cause acute viral hepatitis. There are hepatitis A or so-called infectious hepatitis, hepatitis B, also known as serum hepatitis and non-A, non-B hepatitis (now sometimes called hepatitis C). Hepatitis B is a major concern to all who care for pregnant women and neonates. The reason for this concern is the virus's high level of infectiveness, its routes of transmission via infected blood, maternal/fetal/neonatal vertical transmission, the existence of asymptomatic carrier states and the hardiness of the virus, for example in splashes of infected blood. In some areas of the world, hepatitis B is endemic; its survival is assured by transfer from mother to baby with the risk in later life of developing primary hepatocarcinoma (Boxall 1983b).

Initial infection with the blood-borne hepatitis B virus can occur in pregnancy. The incubation period is 2–6 months (Dulfer 1987; Boxall 1983a). Symptoms of infection with all three hepatitis viruses are similar, differential diagnosis relying on the presence of particular antibodies. The symptoms include malaise, fever, headache, nausea, vomiting and anorexia. The liver and spleen can be enlarged and jaundice may develop. However many people are subclinically infected and therefore show few adverse symptoms (Fallon 1988). In many cases, infection with hepatitis B is self-limiting with development of immunity, but a significant number of people will develop carrier states where they can unwittingly infect others (Faro and Pastorek 1986). They also are at risk of developing chronic hepatitis, cirrhosis and hepatoma (Dulfer 1987).

When taking a woman's history, it is important to enquire about the presence of risk factors such as a previous history of hepatitis or jaundice, intravenous drug abuse or residence in countries with endemic hepatitis (e.g. South-East Asia (Polakoff 1983)). In this way the woman can be screened for the presence of specific antigens including the Australian antigen, (HbsAg), which is contained on the surface of the virus and indicates that the person is still infectious (Dulfer 1987). It is conceivable that in the future all pregnant women will be screened, since with our ethnically mixed society, it is unethical to pinpoint certain national groups (Boxall 1983b). In areas where hepatitis is endemic, such as the Far East and West Africa, it would be more effective and economic to vaccinate all babies at birth in order to deplete the reservoir of infection (Dulfer 1987). Where the mother is a carrier of hepatitis B, strict precautions must be taken when dealing with all body fluids. Local guidelines relating to the disposal of soiled articles, labelling of laboratory specimens and the conduct of the birth should be adhered to. It is important to protect midwifery staff from the risk of infection. In some areas, employers are providing active immunisation with hepatitis B vaccine to all their midwifery staff. This is an intramuscular injection of 1 ml of vaccine which is repeated at 1 and 6 months followed by a check of antibody status (Campbell 1987). When conducting the delivery, eye covering (usually with goggles), gloves, gowns and protective footwear are usually advised. The room should be scrupulously cleaned and disinfected after use, since the virus can persist in dried secretions.

The mother and baby should be nursed together in a single room with its own toilet and bathing facilities. Boxall (1983b) does not advise against breast feeding, as it only plays a small role in virus transmission. To prevent the neonate becoming a chronic carrier it is usually vaccinated soon after birth. This can be achieved in three different ways: with hepatitis B immunoglobulin 2 ml intramuscularly given as soon as possible after birth (no later than 24 hours), and repeated monthly until 6 months when active immunisation can occur; or using 0.5 ml intramuscularly of hepatitis B vaccine repeated after 1 and 6 months; or a combination of 2 ml of immunoglobulin with the course of three injections of vaccine (Campbell 1987). It is hoped that this last protocol will be more effective and reduce the number of injections from six to four (Campbell 1987).

Human immunodeficiency virus (HIV)

When considering infection with human immunodeficiency virus (HIV), the virus will first be described, then the mode of transmission discussed and its serological detection and manifestations of the infection described, before considering the implications for midwifery practice.

Human immunodeficiency virus (HIV) is a virus of low infectivity which is carried in the blood and other body fluids (Redfield and Burke 1988). Its action is to undermine the body's immune system progressively by attacking T-helper cells (also known as T4 cells, which are thymus-derived lymphocytes), which are part of the body's early response to infection (Redfield and Burke 1988). HIV is a retrovirus, which means that it acts upon cells by changing the genetic material in the cell's nucleus to reproduce the virus. The cells become full of new viruses which can infect other cells in turn (Beverley and Sattentau 1987). It is very difficult to fight such a virus, since killing the virus would also kill the host cell (Youle 1987).

The virus is carried in T-helper cells, which are present in many body fluids. What determines the degree of infectivity is the number of infected T-cells present (Weber and Weiss 1988). Although cells containing HIV have been found in saliva, they are in low concentration and therefore the risk of infection is low (Adler 1987a). Theoretically, however, infection could be spread by contact between infected saliva and skin or mucus membrane abrasions (Adler 1987a). The major modes of transmission are by penetrative sexual intercourse, the transmission of infected blood (usually via shared syringes used by intravenous drug abusers or prior to screening in blood products such as Factor VIII given to haemophiliacs) and from an infected mother to her baby before or during birth (Department of Health and Social Security 1988). All blood in the United Kingdom is screened for the presence of HIV antibodies and donors in high-risk groups (such as intravenous drug abusers) are dissuaded from donating blood (Department of Health and Social Security 1988).

Currently cheaper tests for the presence of HIV antigen (and therefore the virus itself) in the blood are being developed. The test currently employed is to detect HIV antibodies. It takes 4–12 weeks after infection for antibodies to be present in the blood (Melbye 1986). Up until this time, the person is capable of transmitting the infection whilst having negative blood tests (Redfield and Burke 1988). All this negative antibody result implies is that the person does not have antibodies present at the time the sample was taken. They could be present a day, a week or a month later. The process of antibody formation is known as seroconversion and it may be accompanied by a non-specific glandular fever-like illness (Adler 1987b). Symptoms include malaise, fever, lethargy, sore throat, enlarged lymph glands and sore muscles and joints (Adler 1987b).

HIV has a very long incubation period averaging 5 years before the individual becomes ill (Department of Health and Social Security 1988). For this reason, the estimates of the number of people infected with the virus have to be gained using figures of these with known manifestations of the infection. There are four main types of illness resulting from infection with HIV: persistent generalised lymphadenopathy (PGL), AIDS-related complex (ARC), acquired immune deficiency syndrome (AIDS) and HIV neurological disease.

Persistent generalised lymphadenopathy is characterised by the development of enlarged lymph nodes, especially in the axilla and groin (Adler 1987b). These persist for longer than 3 months and there is usually no other disease present. Those with this complaint may go on to develop AIDS (Adler 1987b).

AIDS-related complex includes an intermittent or continuous pyrexia of more than 38°C, a weight loss of more than 10%, PGL, persistent diarrhoea, fatigue and night sweats (Adler 1987b). This is a very debilitating manifestation of HIV, which is often a precursor to AIDS itself.

Acquired immune deficiency syndrome includes two main areas of symptoms, opportunistic infections and unusual tumours. The former include *pneumocystis carinii* pneumonia, *cyclospiridium* gastroenteritis, cytomegalovirus (CMV) which causes pneumonia, colitis, and retinal damage and *Candida albicans*. With the exception of CMV, the other organisms are present in most healthy human beings, where they do not give rise to symptoms (Adler 1987b). They are pathogenic only in the severely immune-suppressed individual. The tumours include Kaposi's sarcoma (usually seen in elderly men of Mediterranean origin), cerebral lymphoma and non-Hodgkin's lymphoma. Tumours account for about 20% of the cases of AIDS (Adler 1987b).

HIV neurological disease includes painful neuropathy, encephalitis, fits and progressive presenile dementia. Neurological disease can occur alone or be superimposed onto AIDS (Carne 1987).

There is no treatment for HIV infection. Experiments are progressing with antiviral agents, such as acyclovir, which have had limited success in prolonging the lives of people with AIDS. Because the virus mutates rapidly, the search for a vaccine may take some time. Since the numbers of people infected with HIV are not known, it is difficult to estimate how many will develop specific diseases or what the prognosis is for any individual (Adler 1987a).

When considering HIV infection and childbirth there are a number of major issues which need to be addressed. These are: should women be screened for HIV in the antenatal period; what is the effect of HIV on pregnancy and pregnancy on HIV; how is the fetus affected; and what changes in procedures are required? Few studies of HIV prevalence have been undertaken in the United Kingdom. The Department of Health has initiated anonymous screening of a sample of pregnant women (and also of other groups who come into contact with the health services) who form a 'captive,' sexually active, sample of the general population. The concept of informed consent could militate against generalisable results, since women would be free to refuse to take part. Since blood cannot be used without consent, women perceiving themselves to be at risk may withdraw and therefore bias any results (O'Sullivan *et al*. 1989). Anonymous testing of women attending the antenatal clinic at St Thomas's Hospital, London, showed an increase in HIV-positive results from 2 : 3760 in 1988 to 18 : 4106 in 1990. Because the seropositivity rate for hepatitis B did not rise during this time, the route of HIV transmission is assumed to be heterosexual (Banatavla *et al*. 1991). The question of testing 'high-risk' groups has been raised in many antenatal clinics, despite the fact that all pregnant women could be considered to be so by having had unprotected (without a condom) vaginal intercourse. If testing is requested, it is vital to offer the necessary pre- and post-test counselling which is required (Miller and Bor 1990). Since this may not be available in the antenatal clinic, the woman may be referred to a specialist genitourinary clinic where such a service is available.

For the mother who is known to be antibody-positive, it is far from clear that termination of pregnancy offers any advantages. Given the worsening prognosis with the increasing length of infection, it could be argued that if a woman wants a child it is better to have it sooner rather than later (Pinching 1987). Certainly, American research has shown that infant infection rates and morbidity increase with the length of maternal infection and the presence of symptoms (Scott *et al.* 1985). Questioning women may produce false replies or the woman may be unaware of certain aspects of her partner's behaviour (such as bisexuality or intravenous drug use). For these reasons, it is usually advisable to treat all women as 'at risk' and to take precautions accordingly (Roth and Brierley 1988). These include covering abrasions on the hands of medical and midwifery staff, safe use and disposal of syringes, needles and other sharps, the use of gloves whenever contact with blood, liquor or vaginal secretions can occur and protective clothing at delivery (Brierley 1987). It appears that the risk to health professionals of contracting HIV is far less than that of hepatitis B even after needlestick injury (McEvoy *et al.* 1987).

Since HIV is transmitted via semen, changes have had to occur in centres offering treatment for subfertility by artificial insemination by donor (AID). Donations are now frozen and kept for 3 months, at which time a blood sample from the donor is screened for the presence of HIV. If negative, the sperm can then be used in treatment.

In the early history of HIV, it was thought that pregnancy, with its effect on the maternal immune system, hastened the development of AIDs and other disorders (Scott *et al.* 1985). Later research has shown that morbidity is related to the length of time the woman has been infected with the virus and whether or not symptoms are present (Johnstone *et al.* 1988). Further studies are necessary before any concrete data can result; it is, however, important for the known HIV carrier to maintain good health and nutrition whilst trying to avoid and treat early any infections (Roth and Brierley 1988).

As with the effects of pregnancy on HIV, the research into the prognosis of the children of HIV-positive mothers continues. It is unclear whether infection occurs in utero or during labour and delivery, although caesarean section has not been shown to offer any protection (Grossman 1988). European data suggest that 25% of infants born to infected mothers will be affected (Mok *et al.* 1987), although all infants will be antibody-positive at birth due to the presence of maternal antibodies (Grossman 1988). By the end of the first year, 75% of these children no longer have antibodies (Mok *et al.* 1987). For infants who remain infected, few will show symptoms before 4 months of age (Grossman 1988). Symptoms include a slow down in growth and in weight gain, pyrexia, diarrhoea, thrush and an increased frequency of paediatric infections (Grossman 1988). Problems have occurred in the United States with antibody-positive, but not necessarily infected, infants being abandoned in maternity units. In some centres, a system of foster parents has been developed to avoid the children being isolated and forgotten in hospital.

Cervical cytology

The purpose of cervical screening is to detect precancerous changes which, if correctly diagnosed and treated, have a very high cure rate (British Medical Association 1986; Soutter 1986). Squamous cell carcinoma constitutes 95% of cervical cancers, the other 5% being adenocarcinomas (British Medical Association 1986). This type of cancer is diagnosed by examining cells from the junction between vaginal squamous and cervical columnar epithelia. Under the influence of oestrogen, this area becomes everted so that it can be seen on the surface of the cervix and is not hidden in the cervical canal. Such changes are common in women during puberty, pregnancy and when taking a combined oral contraceptive (Soutter 1989).

Precancerous changes in the cells are known as cervical intraepithelial neoplasia (CIN). Cellular changes are categorised as follows:

CIN I   mild dysplasia
CIN II   moderate dysplasia
CIN III severe dysplasia/carcinoma *in situ* (Harris 1985).

The cause of these changes has not been confirmed (Soutter 1989) but both CIN and cervical cancer have a higher incidence in certain groups, including those who had early onset of sexual activity, are of lower socio-economic status, have had (or their partners have had) multiple sexual partners and are of higher parity (Rotkin 1973). There is also evidence linking infection with herpes simplex II virus (Rawls *et al*. 1986) and human papillomavirus (especially the wart viruses, types 16 and 18) (Richart *et al*. 1984) with precancerous and cancerous changes. The long period of progression from CIN to cervical cancer had meant that the original screening programmes were aimed at women over the age of 35 years, the peak age group for cervical cancer. However screening is now designed to detect precancerous changes before they have opportunity to progress (Soutter 1986).

The modern diseases are appearing to be more virulent and younger women are becoming increasingly at risk (Soutter 1986). There has been speculation that this could be linked to the increasing prevalence of genital virus infections (Meisels 1981) or whether both factors are related to the unpopularity of barrier methods of contraception (Wright *et al*. 1978).

The British Medical Association (1986) recommends that cervical screening should be performed on all sexually active women every three years. There is, however, no adequate call and recall system yet operating nationally. Opportunistic screening of women at family planning, antenatal and postnatal clinics means that some women are being overexamined whilst others are not seen at all (British Medical Association 1986). Planned changes in the NHS may rectify this. International data have demonstrated the efficiency of blanket screening in reducing the incidence and mortality of cervical cancer (Boyes *et al*. 1981).

The test is performed simply by the passage of a vaginal speculum allowing the cervix to be visualised. An Ayres speculum is inserted into the cervical os and rotated through 360° to obtain a sample of cells from around the os. These scrapings are then smeared onto a labelled slide, which is covered with a fixative before being sent for examination (Chamberlain 1980). A newly introduced 'cytobrush' can be used as an alternative particularly where the squamocolumnar junction is further up in the cervical canal (Wolfendale *et al*. 1987). Unsatisfactory smears with insufficient cells or where these have been obtained from the wrong area (Singer 1986) account for many requests for repeat examinations.

Treatment for abnormal cervical smears depends on the nature of the findings. Inflammatory changes will be treated to remove the infection, followed by a repeat smear to confirm normality (Singer 1986). Where CIN II–III is found in small quantities, the smear is repeated in 4–6 months with colposcopic examination if still abnormal (Soutter 1989). The colposcope allows the cervix to be examined in detail and in a far less invasive manner than with a cone biopsy, which can have serious side-effects, especially in relation to a woman's obstetric future (Byrne *et al*. 1987; Soutter 1989). Treatment of early cell changes is usually by laser therapy or cryotherapy, with larger lesions requiring excision (Soutter 1986).

Health education has an important part to play in highlighting the necessity of regular cervical screening for all women. Mobile clinics which can visit geographically isolated or poor areas could help to improve uptake. Local initiatives have met with success in reaching previously unscreened women (Carr 1986). It is also necessary that the supportive infrastructure is present and functioning. This includes not only well-trained laboratory staff and quality control procedures, but also computer access to develop call and recall appointments, swift notification of results (both positive and negative) to the woman herself and adequate counselling services to explain the results if abnormal (Smith *et al*. 1989). None of these are without cost although, since deaths from cervical cancer are wholly preventable, it would certainly be money well spent.

References

Adler M W (1987a) 'Development of the epidemic' *British Medical Journal* 294: 1083–5
Adler M W (1987b) 'Range and natural history of infection' *British Medical Journal* 294: 1145–7
Baker D A (1983) 'Herpes genitalis' *Clinics in Obstetrics and Gynaecology* 10(1): 3–11
Banatavla J E, Chrystie I L, Palmer S J, Sumner D, Kennedy J and Kenney A (1991) 'HIV testing in pregnancy.' *Lancet* 337: 1218
Beverley P and Sattentau Q C (1987) 'Immunology of AIDS' *British Medical Journal* 194: 1536–8
Blackwell A L (1987a) 'Diagnosis and management of vaginal discharge' *Maternal and Child Health* 12(11): 336–40
Blackwell A L (1987b) 'Infectious causes of vaginal discharge' *Maternal and Child Health* 12(12): 368–75
Boxall E H (1983a) 'Hepatitis virus' *Midwives Chronicle* June: 203–6
Boxall E H (1983b) 'Hepatitis problems in the pregnant and nursing mother and the newborn' *Midwives Chronicle* July: 226–9
Boyes D A, Worth A J and Anderson G H (1981) 'Experience with cervical screening in British Columbia' *Gynecological Oncology* 12: S143–S155

Brierley J (1987) 'Human immunodeficiency virus: the challenge of a lifetime.' *Midwives Chronicle* Nov (Supp): x–xiii

British Medical Association (1986) *Cervical Cancer and Screening in Great Britain*. BMA: London

Bunney M H (1986) 'Viral warts: a new look at an old problem.' *British Medical Journal* 293: 1045–7

Byrne P, Nava G and Woodman C B J (1987) 'Premalignant lesions of the lower genital tract' in J Studd (ed) *Progress in Obstetrics and Gynaecology Vol 6* Ch 20 p 365–84. Churchill Livingstone: Edinburgh

Campbell A G M (1987) 'Immunisation-hepatitis' *Maternal and Child Health* 12(2): 50–1

Carne C A (1987) 'Neurological manifestations' *British Medical Journal* 294: 1399–1401

Carr P (1986) 'Limitations within the cervical cytology screening service' *Midwife, Health Visitor and Community Nurse* 22: 253–8

Chamberlain G (1980) 'How to take a cervical smear.' *British Journal of Hospital Medicine* Feb: 213–4

Chow A W and Jewesson P J (1985) 'Pharmokinetics and safety of antimicrobial agents during pregnancy.' *Reviews of Infectious Disease* 7: 287–313

Department of Health and Social Security (1988) *AIDS:- A Briefing Note*. DHSS AIDS Unit: London

Dunlop E M C (1985) 'Clinical aspects of chlamydia infection' *Update* 1 Dec: 339–45

Dulfers S C (1987) 'Hepatitis B and the newborn: a case for vaccination' *Maternal and Child Health* 12(7): 206–12

Emens M (1983) 'The diagnosis and treatment of vaginitis and vaginal discharge' in J Studd (ed) *Progress in Obstetrics and Gynaecology Vol 3* Ch 17 213–20. Churchill Livingstone: Edinburgh

Fallon H J (1988) 'Liver diseases.' in G N Burrow and T F Ferris (eds) *Medical Complications During Pregnancy* (3rd edn) Ch 14 318–44 W B Saunders: Philadelphia

Faro F and Pastorek J G (1986) 'Perinatal infections' in R A Knuppel and J E Drukker (eds) *High Risk Pregnancy: a team approach* Ch 5 74–111 W B Saunders: Philadelphia

Fong R (1987) 'Present trends in the treatment of gonorrhoea and syphilis' *Maternal and Child Health* 12(4): 103–7

Gardner G and Dukes C D (1955) 'Haemophilus vaginilas vaginitis' *American Journal of Obstetrics and Gynecology* 69: 962

Grossman J H (1980) 'Perinatal viral infections' *Clinics in Perinatology* 7(2): 257–71

Grossman M C (1988) 'Children with AIDS' *Infectious Disease Clinics of North America* 2(2): 533–41

Harris V G (1985) 'Management of the abnormal smear' *Maternal and Child Health* 10(10): 314–8

Holder W R and Knox J M (1972) 'Syphilis in pregnancy.' *Medical Clinics of North America* 56: 1151

Johnstone F D, MacCullum L and Brettle R (1988) 'Does infection with HIV affect the outcome of pregnancy?' *British Medical Journal* 196: 467

Kelly J C (1988) 'Genital herpes during pregnancy' *British Medical Journal* 197: 1146–7

Kelsey M C, Mann G K, Bangham G M and Milnthorpe J (1987) 'Non-specific (anaerobic) vaginitis'. *Journal of the Royal College of General Practitioners* 37: 56–8

Lee R V (1988) 'Sexually transmitted infections'. in G N Burrow and T F Ferris (eds) *Medical Complications During Pregnancy (3rd edn)* Ch 17 389–424 W B Saunders: Philadelphia

Lossick J G (1982) 'Treatment of Trichomonas vaginalis infections.' *Reviews of Infectious Disease* 4(Suppl): S801–18

McEvoy M, Porter K and Mortimer P (1987) 'Prospective study of clinical and laboratory staff with accidental exposures to blood or body fluids from patients infected with HIV' *British Medical Journal* 294: 1595–7

McMillan A (1987) 'Sexually transmissible viral diseases' *Update* 1 June: 1254–61

Meisels A, Roy M and Fortier M (1981) 'Human papilloma – virus infection of the cervix' *Acta Cytologica* 25: 7

Melbye M C (1986) 'The natural history of human T-lymphotropic virus-III infection: the cause of AIDS' *British Medical Journal* 292: 5–12

Miller R and Bor R (1990) 'Counselling for HIV screening in women' in J Studd (ed) *Progress in Obstetrics and Gynaecology Vol 8* Ch 2 17–29 Churchill Livingstone: Edinburgh

Mok J, De Rossi A and Ades A (1987) 'Infants born to mothers seropositive for HIV' *Lancet* i: 1164–8

Munday P E (1983) 'Chlamydial infections in women' in J Studd (ed) *Progress in Obstetrics and Gynaecology Vol 3* Ch 18 231–45 Churchill Livingstone: Edinburgh

O'Sullivan M J, Fajardo A, Ferron P, Efantis J, Senk C and Duthely M (1989) 'Seroprevalence in a pregnant multiethnic population' *5th International Conference on AIDS* Montreal Abstract No. MBP23

Parker J D (1989) 'Sexually transmitted disease and pregnancy' *Midwife, Health Visitor and Community Nurse* 25(5): 194–8

Pearce R G and Roberton N R C (1986) 'Infection in the newborn' in N R C Roberton (ed) *Textbook of Neonatology* Ch 28 725–81 Churchill Livingstone: Edinburgh

Pinching A J (1987) 'HIV, AIDS and pregnancy' *Maternal and Child Health* 12(5): 146–50

Polakoff S (1983) 'Transmission from mother to infant of Hepatitis B virus infection' *Midwives Chronicle* Jan: 4–5

Rawls W E, Tompkins W A F, Figueroa M E and Melnick J L (1986) 'Herpes simplex virus II, association with carcinoma of the cervix' *Science* 161: 1255–6

Redfield R R and Burke D S (1988) 'HIV infection: The clinical picture' *Scientific American* 259(4): 70–9

Rees E, Tait I A and Hobson D (1981) 'Persistence of chlamydial infection after treatment of neonatal conjunctivitis' *Archives of Diseases in Childhood* 56: 193–8

Richart R M, Ferenczy A and Meisels A (1984) 'Condyloma virus and cervical cancer – how strong a link?' *Contemporary Obstetrics and Gynecology* 23: 210–44

Roth J and Brierley J (1988) 'HIV and pregnancy' *Nursing Times* 84(46): 61–2

Rotkin E D (1973) 'A comparison view of key epidemiological studies in cervical cancer related to current searches for transmissible agents' *Cancer Research* 33: 1353–67

Saunders J (1988) 'Chlamydia infection' *Nursing Times* 84(49): 35

Scott G B, Fischl M and Klimas N (1985) 'Mothers of infants with AIDS' *Journal of the American Medical Association* 253: 363–6

Singer A (1986) 'The abnormal cervical smear' *British Medical Journal* 293: 1551–6

Smith A Elkind A and Eardley A (1989) 'Making cervical screening work.' *British Medical Journal* 298: 1662–4

Soutter W P (1986) 'Preventing cervical cancer' *Maternal and Child Health* 11(8): 271–6

Soutter W P (1989) 'A practical approach to colposcopy' in J Studd (ed) *Progress in Obstetrics and Gynaecology Vol 7* Ch 23 355–67 Churchill Livingstone: Edinburgh

Speck W T, Aronoff S C and Fanaroff A A (1986) 'Neonatal infections' in M H Klaus and A A Fanaroff (eds) *Care of the High Risk Neonate (3rd edn)* 262–85 W B Saunders: Philadelphia

Thin R N T and Michael A M (1970) 'Sexually transmitted disease in antenatal patients' *British Journal of Venereal Disease* 46: 126

Wang E and Smaill F (1989) 'Infection in pregnancy' in I Chalmers M Enkin and M J N C Keirse (eds) *Effective Care in Pregnancy and Childbirth* Ch 34 534–64 Oxford Medical: Oxford

Wasley G (1988) 'Detecting sexually transmitted diseases' *Nursing Times* 84(39): 59–61

Weber J N and Weiss R A (1988) 'HIV infection: The cellular picture' *Scientific American* 259(4): 80–7

West R R, O'Dowd T C and Smail J E (1988) 'Prevalence of Gardnerella vaginalis: an estimate' *British Medical Journal* 296: 1163–4

Wolfendale M R, Howe-Guest R, Usherwood M M and Draper G F (1987) 'Controlled trial of a new cervical spatula' *British Medical Journal* 294: 33–5

Wright N H, Vessey M P and Kenward B (1978) 'Neoplasia and dysplasia of the cervix uteri and contraception' *British Journal of Cancer* 38: 273

Youle M (1987) 'Current treatment and future prospects' *Maternal and Child Health* 12(8): 235–9

18   Risk in pregnancy

This chapter will consider some of the factors which may increase risk in pregnancy not considered elsewhere. These include demographic aspects, such as the age or parity of the mother, with special reference to the older primipara and the grande multipara. The problems surrounding the assessment of risk in pregnancy will be discussed, followed by a brief evaluation of the effects of paid employment on pregnancy. Finally complications of pregnancy, including the mother with rhesus antibodies, oligohydramnios, polyhydramnios and hyperemesis gravidarum will be considered.

The older mother

Increasing maternal age is associated with a higher rate of maternal mortality, especially for mothers over the age of 35 years (Department of Health 1989). Although older mothers are more likely than younger ones to be of high parity, both age and increasing parity (above para 3) independently increase the rate of maternal death. The safest birth is the second (Department of Health 1989).

In recent years, there has been a steady rise in the number of first pregnancies to women aged over 35 years, the so-called 'elderly primigravida' (Craig 1985). This rise is most marked in women who themselves or whose partners are categorised as belonging to social class II (the professional and managerial groups) (Craig 1985). The reasons for this increase are probably related to changing social attitudes to women's employment. Consistent evidence regarding the risks to these women and their babies is hard to find. One exception is the increase with age in the occurrence of chromosomal anomalies, which is well documented. Down's syndrome occurs in 1 : 1923 pregnancies at maternal age 20, 1 : 1205 at 25, 1 : 885 at 30, 1 : 365 at 35, 1 : 109 at 40 and 1 : 32 at 45 (Donnai 1988). In one study, there was no increase with age in the rates of preterm delivery or of the occurrence of low birth weight (Barkan and Bracken 1987). However Tuck et al. (1988) showed that preterm delivery was 4 times more common amongst primigravidae aged over 35 when compared with those aged 20–25.

Delaying pregnancy increases the woman's risk of involuntary infertility. This is said to affect 2% of couples where the woman is aged between 15–19 years rising to 16% at 40–44 years, excluding couples where one partner had been sterilised (Craig 1985). Couples embarking on a late pregnancy need careful counselling about the risks of fetal abnormality and the availability of diagnostic tests such as amniocentesis and chorion villus aspiration (Donnai 1988; Tuck 1989).

The pregnancy and labour of any woman over the age of 35 is classed as being of high risk, irrespective of parity, and she would not be considered suitable to give birth at home. The older primigravida, especially if well nourished and a non-smoker, can have an easy pregnancy, although she is at higher risk of spontaneous abortion, gestational proteinuric hypertension and placental abruption (James 1988). The woman and her partner will, however, need to make great adjustments to the way in which they order their lives (Kitzinger 1982). Especially where the couple has been together for some time, the arrival of a third person into the relationship and the change in the woman's role from career woman or wage earner to full or part-time mother can bring about many changes (Kitzinger 1982). During the antenatal period and in the early puerperium, the midwife can be instrumental in alerting the couple to some of the realities of childbearing and parenthood.

The older primigravida may experience prolonged labour, possibly due to reduced mobility of the pelvis and increased rigidity of the pelvic floor, lower vagina and perineum (Donald 1979). Tuck et al. (1988) showed that primigravidae aged over 35 were 6 times more likely to be delivered by caesarean section than the younger control group. Increased maternal anxiety can also delay progress (Naaktgeboren 1989).

The grande multipara

The term grande multipara is used to describe a woman who has had 4 or more pregnancies each of over 28 weeks duration (Caporto et al. 1987). In the United Kingdom grande multiparous women are more likely to be of lower socio-economic status. Such women have a higher risk of abnormal presentations, preterm delivery, placenta praevia and perinatal mortality (Caporto et al. 1987). Spellacy et al. (1986), in a survey comparing the outcome of pregnancy for mothers aged over 39 with those of women aged 20–30, found that risk was not related to age, but rather to maternal parity and obesity. The older mothers in this multiracial, deprived population were more likely to experience placenta praevia and to be delivered operatively (Spellacy *et al.* 1986). When the members of the two groups weighing less than 150 lbs (10 st 10 lbs) were compared, there was no increase in the occurrence of hypertension or stillbirth, which had been found in the earlier comparison. When women of equal parity in the two groups were compared, there was no difference in the occurrence of placenta praevia, showing that its frequency of occurrence was related not to age but to parity (Spellacy *et al.* 1986).

Unstable lie is a problem which can affect the grande multipara. This is defined as an alteration in the lie of the fetus between examinations where the pregnancy is of more than 36 weeks gestation. Causes include lax uterine or abdominal muscles in a multigravida, contracted pelvis, placenta praevia and polyhydramnios (Hibbard 1988). Because of the risk of spontaneous rupture of the membranes and cord prolapse, the woman is usually admitted to hospital at 37 weeks so she can remain under supervision (Hibbard 1988). Attempts are made by ultrasound scanning and X-rays to exclude uterine anomalies, placenta praevia or contracted pelvis as the cause (Hofmeyr 1989). If these are absent, the lie can be stabilised to the longitudinal with (for preference) a cephalic presentation (Edwards and Nicholson 1969). Labour is then induced using oxytocin. The membranes may be ruptured under controlled conditions and the mother is sat up to allow the baby's head to settle down into the pelvis (Phelan *et al.* 1985). Care is taken to observe for cord prolapse or signs of fetal distress. The lie and descent of the presenting part should be kept under observation. Contractions may be stimulated before the membranes are ruptured (Edwards and Nicholson 1969). This causes problems since the sensitivity of the uterus to oxytocin is greatly increased when the membranes are not intact, giving a risk of overstimulation and tonic contractions when the membranes rupture. If the lie cannot be stabilised, delivery will be by caesarean section (Phelan *et al.* 1986).

Risk assessment in pregnancy

Many attempts have been made to predict the outcome of pregnancy correctly (Alexander and Keirse 1989). These have fallen into two main approaches. The first and most successful has been the identification of those women who have a history of medical or obstetrical disorders (Howie 1986). The other method has been the development of scoring systems, in which specific factors or occurrences are given a weighted score. These are then added up and the total compared with an arbitrary scale allocating the women to the high-, medium- or low-risk categories (Alexander and Keirse 1989). Neither method is diagnostic, but they do indicate that the individual may have a higher risk of experiencing the designated outcome (Ledger 1980). Problems can occur if these methods are treated as diagnostic rather than screening tools.

Alexander and Keirse (1989) are critical of the lack of specificity of many of the scoring systems. Schemes identifying the risk of the occurrence of different outcomes may well employ the same criteria. Some of the schemes reviewed increased their 'effectiveness' by including women with pre-existing disorders such as chronic renal disease, which would be sufficient by themselves to warrant a high level of surveillence (Alexander and Keirse 1989). Other difficulties have been the problems in generalisability encountered when transferring the system from one institution to another. Alexander and Keirse (1989) conclude by highlighting the lack of any completed randomised controlled trials into formal risk scoring.

Employment and pregnancy

Historical evidence exists regarding the effects of employment on pregnancy outcomes. It was noted that birth weight was reduced and that there was an increase in preterm deliveries amongst women who continued to work throughout pregnancy (Saurel-Cubizolles and Kaminski 1986). Recent large studies have shown that being in paid employment brings a more favourable outcome than remaining at home. The working women were, however, of higher educational levels and social class than those at home, which could account for some of the differences, especially if those at home were involved in hard, physical domestic work (Joffe 1986).

Mamelle *et al.* (1984) described a scoring system to assess the degree of fatigue involved in employment. This takes account of the woman's posture, whether or not she works at a machine, her level of physical exertion, mental load, and environmental conditions such as heat and noise. There was a clear relation between the number of high indices and the occurrence of low birth weight and preterm delivery. Professional women (with the best outcomes) were least likely to be in an employment with high fatigue scores. In addition, there was an association between preterm deliveries and the number of hours worked per week (Mamelle *et al.* 1984).

Specific hazards at work and their effects on outcome have been known for some time. Joffe (1986) comments on the difficulties in proving cause and effect when one considers the wide range of hazards to which everyone is exposed in the environment. It is not known how much exposure is critical and at what stage (Joffe 1986). Some elements previously considered safe may have altered effects when combined with other substances. Apart from known risks, such as ionising radiation, advice has to be given to women on the basis of individual risk. For a review of this subject, see McCloy 1989. If the woman is the sole or major breadwinner, she may not be in a position to give up or change her employment without seriously undermining her family's financial position.

Antenatal care of rhesus-negative women

Where a rhesus-negative woman has no antibodies, the aim during pregnancy and the puerperium is to prevent her developing any (Cunningham *et al.* 1989). Blood samples will be taken and tested for the presence of antibodies at the first antenatal visit and again at 30 weeks gestation (Cunningham *et al.* 1989). The woman is advised of the importance of reporting any episodes of vaginal bleeding, to permit the administration of anti-D (Freda 1973). Following the birth, cord blood is tested to determine the baby's rhesus status. If rhesus positive, maternal blood will be tested for the presence of fetal cells (Kleihauer test). If positive, anti-D will be given within 48 hours of the birth to remove the rhesus-positive cells from the maternal circulation before antibodies are formed (Bowman 1985).

For the small number of isoimmunised women, careful antenatal management is required. Maternal antibody titres will be measured frequently, a rising titre indicating a worsening prognosis. The aim of care is to preserve the fetus in the best possible condition until a time at which it stands a good chance of surviving the complications of prematurity (Bowman 1986). The severity of fetal condition is assessed by measuring bilirubin levels in amniotic fluid obtained by amniocentesis (Liley 1961). This cannot be undertaken before 16 weeks gestation if there is insufficient liquor to permit sampling. The genotype of the father may be determined, because if he is homozygous rhesus-positive, all babies will be affected (Bowman 1986). Fetoscopy can be used to obtain a sample of fetal blood to determine its rhesus status (Nicolaides and Rodeck 1985). If the fetus is rhesus-negative no further action will be taken.

Treatment is aimed at either reducing the maternal antibody level (plasmaphoresis) or by correcting fetal anaemia (with intrauterine transfusions) (Cunningham *et al.* 1989). Plasmaphoresis is a technique by which whole blood is withdrawn from the mother, centrifuged and the red cells suspended in a normotonic solution, before transfusing them into the maternal circulation. The antibodies are contained in the discarded serum, thus reducing the titre. To have any lasting effect from the continual production of antibodies, this time-consuming procedure needs to be repeated on alternate days. Cunningham *et al.* (1989) comment that, from their experience, the benefits of this technique are far outweighed by its cost and level of risk.

Intrauterine tranfusion can be performed in two ways. They both utilise real-time ultrasound scanning to guide the procedure. The earlier technique is that of an injection of group O rhesus-negative blood into the fetal peritoneal cavity, from where it is slowly absorbed (Bowman 1978). The other technique is to use fetoscopy to catheterise an umbilical artery, allowing a direct slow infusion of cells to be administered (Nicolaides and Rodeck 1985). In one series of this procedure where treatment was begun before 25 weeks gestation, there was an 84% survival rate. The treated group included fetuses who were already developing hydrops fetalis (Rodeck and Nicolaides 1983). Delivery is planned for 32–34 weeks gestation, depending on fetal well being (Nicolaides and Rodeck 1985).

Abnormalities of liquor

The quantity of amniotic fluid increases as pregnancy progresses, reaching a maximum of 1 1 by 38 weeks gestation, although there are considerable individual variations (Fuchs 1966). There is then a slight reduction in quantity to term. Amniotic fluid is constantly produced by the amnion (and in early pregnancy it passes through the fetal skin) and absorbed, including being swallowed by the fetus, so that it is constantly changing (Lind *et al.* 1972). Polyhydramnios occurs when there is a clinically detectable excess of liquor; this makes the diagnosis somewhat inexact, but it is usually not detectable until it reaches 2000 ml (Cunningham *et al.* 1989). There are two types of polyhydramnios. Chronic polyhydramnios is the most common, with the liquor accumulating gradually usually after the thirtieth week of pregnancy. Acute-onset polyhydramnios is a rarer condition which can occur from as early as 20 weeks gestation. The onset can be over 2 or 3 days, producing dyspnoea, discomfort and a risk of preterm labour/spontaneous abortion (Hill *et al.* 1987). This type is commonly associated with homozygous twins (MacGillivray 1984).

Causes

1. Multiple pregnancy – especially uniovular twins (MacGillivray 1984).
2. Fetal anomaly – open neural tube defect, especially anencephaly. Oesophageal atresia where the fetus cannot swallow the liquor (Pritchard 1966).
3. Hydrops foetalis, as caused by rhesus isoimmunisation (Hibbard 1988).
4. Maternal diabetes mellitus.
5. A very rare cause is chorioangioma – a tumour of the placenta.

Clinical features

Especially with acute onset, the mother will complain that her abdomen feels large and tense (Hibbard 1988). It may even be painful. Pressure on the abdominal organs and diaphragm gives rise to dyspnoea, dyspepsia and heartburn (Hibbard 1988). Physical signs depend on the amount of liquor present. The uterus is very tolerant of extra fluid, provided it is accumulated gradually. On examination, the uterus will feel larger than expected for the period of gestation. It may appear globular in shape and the skin stretched and shiny. New striae gravidarum may be visible. On palpation it may be difficult to identify fetal parts, the fetal heart sound may be muffled or inaudible (Cunningham *et al.* 1989). In cases where the fluid is thought to be increasing, the abdominal girth can be measured. It is important to mark the position on the abdomen where the measurements are being taken to facilitate later recordings.

An ultrasound scan may be performed to check for signs of multiple pregnancy or fetal abnormality (Cunningham *et al.* 1989). The risks of polyhydramnios include unstable lie, malpresentation and cord presentation and prolapse, following premature rupture of the membranes (Hibbard 1988). A rapid reduction of liquor volume can cause not only a cord prolapse but also result in premature separation of the placenta and antepartum haemorrhage. Because of overstretching of the uterus, in the third stage of labour, contraction and retraction of the myometrium may be poor, giving a risk of postpartum haemorrhage.

After birth, the baby should be examined carefully by the paediatrician for the presence of abnormalities, particularly oesophageal atresia.

Oligohydramnios

This is a rare condition in which there is an abnormally small amount of liquor present. In most cases it is associated with an abnormality of the fetal kidneys, such as renal agenesis (Potter's syndrome) (Mercer and Brown 1986) or with severe degrees of placental insufficiency (Hibbard 1988). Compression deformities of the fetus including hypoplasia of the lungs, can occur due to lack of space within the uterus. This produces a characteristic squashed appearance of the face and underdevelopment of the jaw (micrognathia). Limb deformities such as talipes may also occur. Cord compression may result in fetal death in utero (Leveno et al. 1984).

Diagnosis relies on clinical examination which reveals a uterus small for the period of gestation. The fetus seems to fill the uterus, with little liquor being felt. An ultrasound scan will differentiate between growth retardation and oligohydramnios (Hibbard 1988). It can also assess the normality or otherwise of the renal tract. The mother may require admission to hospital for tests on fetal normality and placental function. If all is well, the pregnancy will be allowed to continue. If not, labour will be induced. A paediatrician should be present at delivery to resuscitate the baby if necessary and to examine for any abnormality.

Hyperemesis gravidarum

Vomiting is a common complication of pregnancy and can occur as a result of morning sickness, urinary tract infection or in the later stages of pregnancy due to pressure on the abdomen, which causes oesophageal reflux. Hyperemesis gravidarum is excessive vomiting, a condition which occurs in fewer than 1 : 1000 pregnancies (Donald 1979). The cause is unclear, but it is found in some cases of multiple pregnancy and hydatidiform mole. It is also found in women under psychological stress such as those who have a history of unsuccessful pregnancies, deliveries of babies of the (perceived) wrong sex, rejection of pregnancy or fear of unemployment.

If hyperemesis persists without treatment, it can lead to dehydration, hypovolaemia, electrolyte disturbances and vitamin deficiencies (Hibbard 1988). Death can occur from hyponatraemic shock (which affects the cardiac muscle), liver failure and renal necrosis (Hibbard 1988). The woman usually presents as being unable to retain food or fluid. She may well have weight loss and ketosis from metabolism of the fat store. She may show haemoconcentration and an unstable acid/alkaline balance (Cunningham *et al.* 1989).

The woman should be admitted to hospital for intensive investigation and support. It is important to exclude the presence of other diseases such as urinary tract infection, hiatus hernia, obstructive lesions of the gastrointestinal tract, abnormalities of the gall bladder or tumours of the central nervous system (Cunningham *et al.* 1989). A careful history must be taken to look for underlying psychological disturbances. The woman is usually cared for in a single room and she may be given mild sedation if agitated. The fluid and electrolyte balance should be restored with intravenous fluids to which vitamins can be added (Hibbard 1988). Specific anti-emetic drugs can be prescribed. This condition usually arises after the first trimester, so there is less risk of fetal abnormality resulting from the use of well-tested preparations. Small, attractively presented meals should be given to tempt the mother's appetite. Psychological treatment may be required, sometimes involving psychoanalysis or psychotherapy. Many women respond to counselling alone (Donald 1979).

Once the woman's condition is stabilised, she can return home. If the precipitating conditions persist, the condition may recur. It is very rarely impossible to improve the woman's condition and death can result unless the pregnancy is terminated (Hibbard 1988).

References

Alexander S and Keirse M J N C (1989) 'Formal risk scoring during pregnancy.' in I Chalmers, M Enkin and M J N C Keirse (eds) *Effective Care in Pregnancy and Childbirth* Ch 22 345–65 Oxford Medical: Oxford

Barkan S E and Bracken M B (1987) 'Delayed childbearing: no evidence for increased risk of low birthweight and preterm delivery' *American Journal of Epidemiology* 125(1): 101–9

Bowman J M (1978) 'The management of Rh-isoimmunisation' *Obstetrics and Gynecology* 52: 1

Bowman J M (1985) 'Controversies in Rh management: Who needs Rh immune globulin and when should it be given?' *American Journal of Obstetrics and Gynecology* 151: 289

Bowman J M (1986) 'Haemolytic disease of the newborn (Erythroblastosis foetalis)' in N R C Roberton (ed) *Textbook of Neonatology* 469–83 Churchill Livingstone: Edinburgh

Caporto A, Battarino O, Donatiello A and Giannatempo A (1987) 'The grand multipara: always an actual problem' *Surgery, Gynecology and Obstetrics* 165(10): 99–100

Craig G M (1985) 'The increased risk of childbirth with increasing maternal age' *Maternal and Child Health* (3): 88–94

Cunningham F G, MacDonald P C and Gant N F (1989) *William's Obstetrics (18th edn)* Prentice Hall: London

Department of Health (1989) *Report on Confidential Enquiries into Maternal Deaths in England and Wales 1982–4* HMSO: London

Donald I (1979) *Practical Obstetric Problems (5th edn)* Lloyd Luke: London

Donnai D (1988) 'Genetic risk' in D K James and G M Stirrat (eds) *Pregnancy and Risk* Ch 4 45–80 Wiley: Chichester

Edwards R L and Nicholson H O (1969) 'The management of unstable lie in late pregnancy' *Journal of Obstetrics and Gynaecology of the British Commonwealth* 76: 713–8

Freda V J (1973) 'Hemolytic disease' *Clinical Obstetrics and Gynecology* 16: 72

Fuchs F (1966) 'Volume of amniotic fluid at various stages in pregnancy' *Clinical Obstetrics and Gynecology* 9: 449

Hibbard E M (1988) *Principles of Obstetrics* Butterworth: London

Hill L M, Brekle R, Thomas M L and Fries J K (1987) 'Polyhydramnios: Ultrasonically detected prevalence and neonatal outcome' *Obstetrics and Gynecology* 69: 21

Hofmeyr G J (1989) 'Breech presentation and abnormal lie in late pregnancy' in I Chalmers, M Enkin and M J N C Keirse (eds) *Effective Care in Pregnancy and Childbirth* Ch 42 651–63 Oxford Medical: Oxford

Howie P W (1986) 'Past obstetrical performance' in G Chamberlain and J Lumley (eds) *Prepregnancy Care: A manual for practice* Ch 4 53–67 Wiley: Chichester

James D K (1988) 'Risk at the booking clinic' in D K James and D M Stirrat (eds) *Pregnancy and Risk: The basis for rationale management* 45–80 John Wiley: Chichester

Joffe M (1986) 'Women's work and pregnancy' in G Chamberlain and J Lumley (eds) *Prepregnancy Care: A manual for practice* Ch 12 245–61 Wiley: Chichester

Kitzinger S (1982) *Birth Over 30* Sheldon Press: London

Ledger W J (1980) 'Identification of the high risk mother and fetus – does it work?' *Clinics in Perinatology* 7(1): 125–34

Leveno K J, Quirk J G, Cunningham F G and Nelson S D (1984) 'Prolonged pregnancy: Observations concerning the cause of foetal distress' *American Journal of Obstetrics and Gynecology* 150: 465

Liley A W (1961) 'Liqour amnii analysis in management of pregnancy complicated by rhesus immunization' *American Journal of Obstetrics and Gynecology* 82: 1359–71

Lind R, Kendall A and Hytten F E (1972) 'The role of the fetus in the formation of amniotic fluid' *Journal of Obstetrics and Gynaecology of the British Commonwealth* 79: 289

MacGillivray I (1984) 'Maternal response to twin pregnancy' in J Studd (ed) *Progress in Obstetrics and Gynaecology* Vol 4 Ch 10 139–50 Churchill Livingstone: Edinburgh

Mamelle N, Laumon B and Lazar P (1984) 'Prematurity and occupational activity during pregnancy' *American Journal of Epidemiology* 119: 209–22

McCloy E C (1989) 'Work, environment and the fetus' *Midwifery* 5: 53–62

Mercer L J and Brown L B (1986) 'Fetal outcome with oligohydramnios in the second trimester' *Obstetrics and Gynecology* 67: 840

Naaktgeboren C (1989) 'The biology of childbirth' in I Chalmers, M Enkin and M J N Keirse (eds) *Effective Care in Pregnancy and Childbirth* Ch 48 765–804 Oxford University Press: Oxford

Nicolaides K H and Rodeck C H (1985) 'The role of fetoscopy in perinatal medicine' in M L Chiswick (ed) *Recent Advances in Perinatal Medicine Vol 2* 1–18 Churchill Livingstone: Edinburgh

Phelan J P, Stine L E, Edwards M B, Clark S L and Horenstein J (1985) 'The role of external cephalic version in the intrapartum management of transverse lie presentation' *American Journal of Obstetrics and Gynecology* 151: 724–6

Phelan J P, Boucher M, Mueller E, McCart D, Horenstein J and Clark S (1986) 'The nonlaboring transverse lie: a management dilemma' *Journal of Reproductive Medicine* 31: 184–6

Pritchard J A (1966) 'Fetal swallowing and amniotic fluid' *Obstetrics and Gynecology* 28: 606

Rodeck C H and Nicolaides K H (1983) 'Ultrasound guided invasive procedures in obstetrics' *Clinics in Obstetrics and Gynaecology* 10: 529–39

Saurel-Cubizolles M J and Kaminski M (1986) 'Work in pregnancy: its evolving relationship with perinatal outcome' *Social Science in Medicine* 22(4): 431–42

Spellacy I W, Miller S J and Winegar A (1986) 'Pregnancy after 40 years of age' *Obstetrics and Gynecology* 65: 442

Tuck S M (1989) 'Pregnancy risks in the older woman' *Maternal and Child Health* 14(4): 98–100

Tuck S M, Yudkin P L and Turnbull A C (1988) 'Pregnancy outcome in elderly primigravidae with and without history of infertility' *British Journal of Obstetrics and Gynaecology* 95: 230–7

19 Physiology of labour

Definition of labour

Labour is the term used to describe the process by which, after the twenty-eighth week of pregnancy, the fetus and placenta are expelled from the uterus. Labour can have a spontaneous onset (this is discussed later in this chapter) or it can be induced (see Chapter 22). The definition of normal labour is an area of controversy. Midwives and obstetricians differ in the way in which they classify labour as normal (Arney 1982; Tew 1990).

Midwifery classification – A labour is deemed to be normal if, following spontaneous onset after 37 completed weeks of pregnancy the condition of mother and fetus shows no abnormality and the progress of the labour is within acceptable limits.

Medical classification – A labour is deemed to be normal if following spontaneous onset and progression after 37 completed weeks of pregnancy, it ends in the delivery of a live infant (presenting by the vertex) and it is completed in no more than 24 hours in the absence of any complications (Baird 1952).

The major difference between the two definitions is that the medical one can only be applied in retrospect, whereas that of the midwife refers to the situation at that time. The midwifery definition allows for the labour to be regarded and managed as normal for as long as normality continues. If complications arise, treatment can be changed and the labour reclassified as abnormal (Robinson *et al.* 1983). It also permits those areas of the labour which are not affected by the complication(s) to be treated normally, such as pain relief in a labour where progress is very slow.

The medical definition is much more prescriptive, since until normality is confirmed (or otherwise) following birth, the woman's labour is regarded as being actually or potentially abnormal. Using this rationale, it has been easier to apply technologies devised for high-risk women to all (International Childbirth Education Association 1976). Examples of this include continuous electrical fetal monitoring and routine rupturing of the membranes (O'Driscoll *et al.* 1969; MacDonald *et al.* 1985).

Progress of labour

Stage of labour

Labour is divided into three stages, which are used to describe the activities occurring within them. To these can be added another two stages, one before and one after, the labour.

Prelabour: The time prior to the onset of labour when the uterus prepares for true labour (Hendricks *et al.* 1970). A primiparous woman can commence labour, having progressed some considerable way in the descent of the presenting part and the dilatation and effacement of the cervix.

First Stage: From the onset of regular uterine contractions until full dilatation of the cervical os. The latter part of the first stage is referred to as transition.

Second Stage: From full dilatation of the cervical os until the birth of the baby.

Third Stage: From the birth of the baby until expulsion of the placenta and membranes, any bleeding is fully controlled.

Fourth Stage: The early hour(s) following birth when the mother begins her recovery, initiates breast feeding and she and her partner begin to know their baby. For hospital births, this term is usually reserved for the time the mother spends on the labour ward following delivery until she is transferred to the postnatal area or for very early transfer home.

Duration of labour

To assess the average length of normal labour is a complex task. It depends very much upon which definition for the onset of the first stage is accepted, and also on the parity of the mother. O'Driscoll and Meagher (1980) consider that labour commences when the woman admits herself to the labour ward. They take no account of any labour occurring at home. They set maximum limits of 10 hours for the first stage of labour and for the second stage 2 hours for primiparous women and 1 hour for multiparous. There have been many who have argued against such an arbitrary time-scale (Studd 1973; Studd et al. 1975; Crawford 1985).

Approximate lengths for the various stages of labour should only be used as guidelines; it must be remembered that physiological processes vary between individuals and that these differences should be considered (Crowther et al. 1989). It is far from ideal to apply concepts of linear progression (regular progress, e.g. 1 cm dilatation per hour) to a physiological process where initial progress can be slow, with significant acceleration towards the end. Depending on one's definition of onset, the first stage should be completed by primiparous women in 16 hours and by multiparous in 10–12 hours (Friedman 1955; Studd 1973; O'Driscoll and Meagher 1980). Intervention may be required before these time periods have passed if progress is deemed to be unacceptably slow. Medical opinion states that the second stage is usually completed within 2 hours by a primiparous woman, of which no more than 1 hour is taken up by her actively pushing (Jeffcoate 1950; Duignan et al. 1975; Maresh et al. 1983). Friedman (1955) recorded a mean duration for the second stage of labour of 45 minutes. In multiparous women, because their lower genital tract and pelvic floor have been stretched previously, the second stage rarely lasts more than 30–60 minutes (Jeffcoate 1950). Duignan et al. (1975) recorded a range of 2–80 minutes.

The physiological third stage lasts on average 15 minutes (Prendiville et al. 1988), with 25% of third stages lasting longer than 30 minutes. When actively managed, the average length of the third stage was 5 minutes (Prendiville et al. 1988). To the above timings Hendricks (1983) would include the 4 weeks or so of prelabour prior to true labour when the uterus changes from an organ which contained and nurtured the pregnancy to one which expels it. Primiparous women who progress well in prelabour can commence true labour with cervical dilatations in excess of 4 cm, thus shortening the time required to complete the first stage of labour.

When describing the physiology and mechanism of labour, there are three aspects to consider. These are first the fetus, whose response to labour must be assessed and who also must adapt to labour and be moved through the pelvis in a process referred to as mechanism. Second, there are the pelvis, uterus, vagina and pelvic floor, the structure through or over which the fetus must pass. These also have to change during prelabour and true labour. Third is the action of the uterus, the contraction and retraction of the uterine muscles which bring about changes in the lower uterine segment together with effacement and dilatation of the cervical os. Before concentrating on the physiology of labour, it is necessary to consider first the anatomy of the gynaecoid (female type) pelvis and next the mechanism by which the fetus moves through it.

Mechanism of labour

The gynaecoid pelvis

The pelvis is a girdle of bones, joints and ligaments which supports, via the backbone, the weight of the upper part of the body and transmits this to the legs. It also forms a protective cage for the reproductive organs, the bladder and the rectum. Attached to and supported by the pelvis are the muscle groups which form the pelvic floor and give support to the pelvic organs. The pelvic floor is important in the maintenance of continence. As pregnancy progresses under the influence of various hormones including progesterone, the pelvic floor becomes less rigid and more relaxed. This is in preparation for the stretching which is required during the second stage of labour.

When the primitive human evolved from walking on all fours to walking upright, changes occurred in the spinal column and the pelvis. The spine became curved and the pelvis tilted, giving a curve to the birth canal. Woman is unusual amongst female mammals in that the passage taken by the fetus is not straight (Naaktgeboren 1989).

The pelvis consists of four bones: two innominate (see Figures 19.1 and 19.2), sacrum and coccyx.

Each innominate bone is made of three fused bones: the ilium, the ischium and the pubic bone (see Figure 19.1). The ilium is the upper expanded part of the innominate bone, at the top of which is the curved iliac crest; this ends at the front with the anterior superior iliac spine and at the rear with the posterior superior iliac spine. The anterior spines are easily palpated, whilst the posterior ones are marked by two dimples on either side of the spine. The concave inner surface of the ilium is known as the iliac fossa, below which there is a bony ridge, the iliopectineal line. The ilium forms the upper third of the acetabulum.

The ischium (plural: ischia) is the lower posterior thickened part of the innominate bone, which forms the side wall of the pelvic cavity. At its lower border, the ischium is a thick rounded mass, the ischial tuberosity. When sitting upright, the body rests upon these two tuberosities. On the inner surface of the ischium, a little

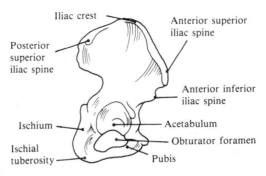

Figure 19.1 The right innominate bone, lateral view.

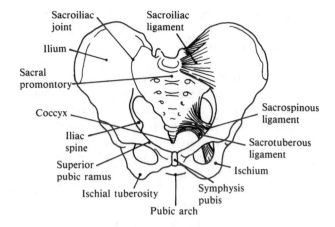

Figure 19.2 Bones, joints and some ligaments of the pelvis.

way above each tuberosity is an ischial spine, a small backward facing projection which if pronounced can reduce the size of the pelvic outlet and prevent passage of the fetus. The ischium forms third of the acetabulum.

The final constituent bone in each innominate bone is the pubic bone, which makes up the final third of the acetabulum. The pubic bone has an anterior flattened portion, which is connected via the symphysis pubis to the opposite pubic bone. From this pubic body there are two pubic rami (singular: ramus). The superior ramus attaches to the ilium and the iliopectineal eminence, forming the upper border of the obturator foramen. The inferior ramus joins the ischium just behind the tuberosities and makes the lower border of the obturator foramen. The two fused inferior rami and their joining pubic symphysis form the pubic arch, which in women should exceed 90°.

The sacrum is a triangular-shaped bone, formed of the five fused sacral vertebrae (see Figure 19.3) with four pairs of foramina which permit the passage of nerves into and out of the spinal cord. The anterior surface of the sacrum is smooth and

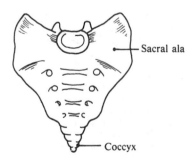

Figure 19.3 The sacrum and coccyx.

concave whilst the posterior is rough and convex. The upper inner surface of the first sacral vertebra has a promontory, known as the sacral promontory, on either side of which are the sacral alae (singular ala) or sacral wings. The final bone is the coccyx, a small wedge-shaped bone consisting of four fused rudimentary vertebrae.

There are four joints in the pelvis; two sacroiliac joints, which, due to the action of progesterone during pregnancy can become slightly mobile, giving rise to backache but also permitting an increase in pelvic diameters during birth; the symphysis pubis, which is composed of cartilage and softens in pregnancy, possibly causing discomfort in the third trimester; the sacrococcygeal joint, which acts like a hinge, allowing the coccyx to move posteriorly out of the way for the second stage of labour. There are various ligaments to reinforce the pelvic joints. The most important of these are the sacroiliac, which pass anteriorly and posteriorly to the sacroiliac joint, the sacrotuberous, from the ischial tuberosities to the sides of the sacrum, and the sacrospinous, from the ischial spines to the sides of the sacrum (see Figure 19.2).

The pelvis can be divided into two parts, the false pelvis which is the area above the pelvic brim and which plays no part in labour, and the true pelvis which lies below the pelvic brim. The brim is the first of three areas of the pelvis which have to be negotiated by the fetus, the others being the cavity and the outlet.

The pelvic brim

In females the pelvic brim is oval except for the projection of the sacral promontory (Caldwell *et al*. 1940). There are eight points or landmarks which can be described on the pelvic brim. These are as follows, commencing posteriorly (see Figure 19.4).

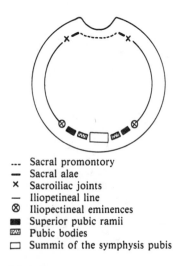

```
...  Sacral promontory
—    Sacral alae
×    Sacroiliac joints
—    Iliopetineal line
⊗    Iliopectineal eminences
▬    Superior pubic ramii
▨    Pubic bodies
☐    Summit of the symphysis pubis
```

Figure 19.4 Landmarks of the pelvic brim.

1. Sacral promontory.
2. Sacral ala.
3. Sacroiliac joint.
4. Iliopectineal line.
5. Iliopectineal eminence.
6. Superior pubic ramus.
7. Upper inner border of the pubic body.
8. Summit of the symphysis pubis.

These landmarks are used in measuring the diameter of the brim, through which the fetus must pass (see Figure 19.5).

Diameters of the pelvic brim

The antero-posterior diameter of the brim is taken from the midpoint of the sacral promontory to the upper inner border of the symphysis pubis. This diameter is also called the anatomical conjugate. This is the first obstacle which the fetal head must pass through and it measures on average 11.43 cm (Moir 1947). Not all of this space is available to the fetus and so the smaller obstetrical conjugate is normally preferred as a more accurate measurement of the space available for the fetus. This is measured from the midpoint of the sacral promontory to the midpoint of the inner surface of the symphysis pubis. It measures 11.2–11.8 cm (Moir 1947) (see Figure 19.6). Both the anatomical and obstetrical conjugates can be measured on X-ray pelvimetry. On vaginal examination, the measurement assessed is the diagonal conjugate; this is taken from the midpoint of the sacral promontory to the lower border of the symphysis pubis (see Chapter 24).

The transverse diameter of the pelvic brim is measured between the widest points on the iliopectineal line; it measures approximately 13 cm (12.6–12.9 cm) (Moir 1947). The oblique diameters, measured from each sacroiliac joint to the opposite iliopectineal eminence, are on average 12 cm. One final diameter which is important in certain malpositions (such as occipito posterior) is the sacrocotyloid, taken as the

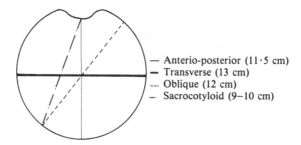

— Anterio-posterior (11·5 cm)
— Transverse (13 cm)
--- Oblique (12 cm)
— Sacrocotyloid (9–10 cm)

Figure 19.5 Diameters of the pelvic brim.

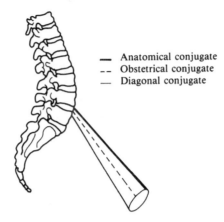

— Anatomical conjugate
-- Obstetrical conjugate
— Diagonal conjugate

Figure 19.6 Conjugates of the pelvic brim showing differences in calculating the antero-posterior diameter.

measurement from the sacral promontory to the iliopectineal eminence. It measures between 9 and 10 cm.

The pelvic cavity

The cavity is the part of the pelvis between the brim and the outlet. It is circular in shape, having straight side walls. Anteriorly are the inner surface of the pubic bones and the symphysis pubis. Posteriorly there is the curve of the sacrum. The side walls consist of the sacrospinous ligaments and the two ischia. The cavity is much deeper posteriorly than anteriorly, meaning that as the fetus passes through, it has to move in a curve. All measurements of the cavity of the gynaecoid pelvis are approximately 12 cm (range 11.14–12.86 cm) (Moir 1947).

The pelvic outlet

The pelvic outlet is the final bony obstacle to be negotiated by the fetus. It is diamond shaped. Like the brim, it has various landmarks, but there are two different outlets. The first is the anatomical outlet not all the space of which is available to the fetus as it passes through. The second is the obstetrical outlet, which gives a true picture of the area available to the fetus. The main differences occur because the coccyx is pushed posteriorly out of the way and also because the distance between the ischial spines is a smaller diameter than that between tuberosities.

The anatomical outlet (see Figure 19.7) has the following landmarks:

1. Coccyx.
2. Sacro-tuberous ligaments.

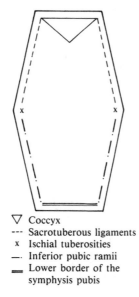

▽ Coccyx
--- Sacrotuberous ligaments
x Ischial tuberosities
—· Inferior pubic ramii
▬ Lower border of the
  symphysis pubis

Figure 19.7 Landmarks of the anatomical outlet.

3. Ischial tuberosities.
4. Inferior pubic rami.
5. Lower border of the pubic symphysis.

The obstetrical outlet has the following landmarks (see Figure 19.8):

1. The lower border of the sacrum.
2. Sacrospinous ligaments.
3. Ischial spines.
4. Inferior pubic rami.
5. Lower border of the pubic symphysis.

The diameters of the outlet are as follows (see Figure 19.9). The antero-posterior diameter is approximately 13 cm (range 12.1–13.8 cm); it is measured from the lower border of the sacrum to the lower border of the pubic symphysis (Moir 1947). The anatomical transverse diameter is measured between the two ischial tuberosities; it is known as the bituberous diameter and it averages 11 cm. Of more importance are the obstetrical transverse diameter and the bispinous diameter which is the distance between the two ischial spines. It measures approximately 10.5 cm (range 10.1–10.8 cm) (Moir 1947).

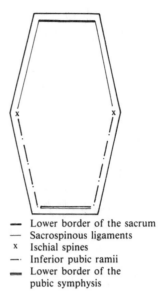

— Lower border of the sacrum
— Sacrospinous ligaments
x   Ischial spines
—· Inferior pubic ramii
▬ Lower border of the
    pubic symphysis

Figure 19.8 Landmarks of the obstetrical outlet.

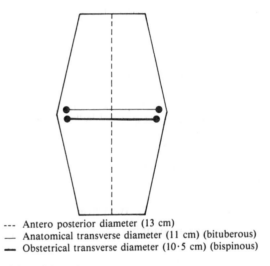

--- Antero posterior diameter (13 cm)
— Anatomical transverse diameter (11 cm) (bituberous)
▬ Obstetrical transverse diameter (10·5 cm) (bispinous)

Figure 19.9 Diameters of the pelvic outlet.

Inclination of the pelvis

Because of curves in the human spine, the pelvis is not horizontal, but at an angle. When standing erect, the plane (a term used for an imaginary flat surface) of the pelvic brim of a caucasian woman forms an angle of 55° to the horizontal (see Figure 19.10). The plane of the pelvic outlet is at only 15° from the horizontal. To determine the route through the pelvis through which the fetus is moved, an axis is drawn at 90° (right angles) to each plane (see Figure 10.11). When these axes are joined together, the pelvic curve can be clearly seen (see Figure 19.10). This is known as the Curve of Carus.

Onset of labour

As mentioned previously, labour is not a sudden event, but one for which the body has been in preparation for as long as 4 weeks (Hendricks *et al.* 1970). The factors involved in the initiation of labour are complex and not completely understood (Schwarz 1982; Sellers and Bernal 1985). Experiments on animals have demonstrated the importance of fetal hormones in initiating labour. Current theories involve an interrelationship of fetal hormones, such as cortisol and possibly androgen from the maturing adrenal glands together with an increase in maternal oestrogen and a fall in progesterone levels (Schwarz 1982). Liggins *et al.* (1977) have demonstrated the role of the fetal adrenal and pituitary glands in the initiation of labour in sheep, but no such clear association has been seen in humans. Of vital importance, however, are locally produced prostaglandins present in the decidua and the amnion, which are responsible for cervical ripening (the process by which the cervix becomes capable of effacement and dilatation) and for increasing uterine contractibility (Schwarz 1982). The prostaglandin precursor, arachidonic acid, is found in higher concentrations in the amniotic fluid of labouring women than in non-labouring ones and its concentration increases as labour progresses (MacDonald *et al.* 1974). Activation of this prostaglandin precursor occurs through the action of lysosomes in the fetal membranes. When the membranes are

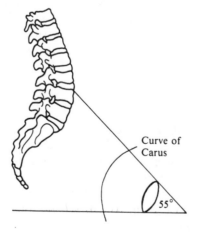

Figure 19.10 Lateral view to demonstrate the inclination of the pelvic brim and the Curve of Carus.

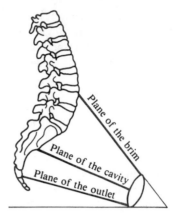

Figure 19.11 Planes of the pelvis.

disturbed (for example, due to dehydration, hypoxia or acidocis), the lysosomes become more fragile, resulting in the activation of arachidonic acid, production of prostaglandins and in the initiation of labour (Schwarz *et al.* 1980). This sequence of events may partly explain the onset of premature labour following premature spontaneous rupture of the membranes or intrauterine infection (Schwarz 1982). The fall in progesterone seen in some other mammals prior to the onset of labour has not been demonstrated in humans, although there is speculation that a local shortage of the hormone in the fetal membranes or kidneys could be of importance (Schwarz 1982).

Mechanical stimulation by stretching of the lower segment and cervix increases prostaglandin release, which may explain why preterm labour occurs in some cases of polyhydramnios. Sensitivity of the myometrium to oxytocin (from the posterior pituitary gland) increases throughout pregnancy. The relationship between prostaglandin and oxytocin in the production of uterine contractions and in the continuation of labour is far from clear.

Prelabour

During the 4 weeks or so prior to the onset of spontaneous labour, changes occur which alter the uterus from an organ which contained, protected and nurtured the developing fetus into one which will expel it into the outside world (Calder 1983). The uterine (Braxton Hicks) contractions, which have been occurring through most of the pregnancy are now coordinated and more easily felt by the mother (Caldeyro Barcia 1959). After 36 weeks gestation, the myometrium is much more sensitive to the effects of oxytocin (Fuchs 1973).

The most important changes are those in the cervix which changes from a rigid and unyielding body with a high collagen content to a soft and pliable structure

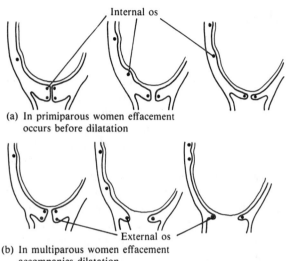

Internal os

(a) In primiparous women effacement
   occurs before dilatation

External os

(b) In multiparous women effacement
    accompanies dilatation
    • External cervical os
    • Internal cervical os
    • Retraction ring between upper and lower uterine segments

Figure 19.12 Formation of the lower uterine segment and effacement of the cervix in
(a) primiparous and (b) multiparous women.

which dilates easily in response to mechanical pressure (Bishop 1964; Anderson and
Turnbull 1969; Calder 1979). During the third trimester, the upper and lower uterine
segments become more clearly differentiated. When the upper segment contracts it
pulls on the lower, causing it to thin. This also pulls on the external cervical os,
which becomes incorporated into the lower segment; the cervix is now thinner. This
process is referred to as effacement (see Figure 19.12). The cervix may also start to
dilate in the week or so before labour. It is not unusual for a woman to begin
spontaneous labour with her cervical os already dilated by 3 or 4 cm (Hendricks *et
al.* 1970; Duignan *et al.* 1975). These changes are most noticeable in primiparous
women. Amongst multiparous women, effacement often occurs with dilatation
during labour. When cervical dilatation begins, the operculum (show) present in the
cervical canal can be shed. This is a mucus plug streaked with a little blood.
Although indicative of impending labour, it can be shed up to 1 week before
spontaneous labour begins (Hendricks *et al.* 1970).

The first stage of labour

This section will consider the physiology of the first stage of labour. Of major
importance are the uterine contractions and their effects on the upper and lower
uterine segments and upon the cervix. Next the function of amniotic fluid and of
the membranes will be considered, then the effects of labour on other body systems.

Uterine contractions

The muscles of the myometrium in the upper segment are unusual. Although like all muscles, they are capable of contracting, on relaxing they do not fully regain their normal length but become shorter and fatter. This process is known as retraction (see Figure 19.13). The effect of this process is that the upper uterine segment becomes shorter and thicker. An upwards pull on the lower segment (which is less muscular) is exerted, which stretches and thins this muscle. A ridge occurs between the active thickened upper segment and the passive thinned lower segment. This is known as the retraction ring. Normally this is not palpable abdominally, since the junction between the upper and lower uterine segments lies inside the bony pelvis; if the ridge is seen or can be palpated, this is indicative of obstructed labour, where the lower segment has become excessively thinned and uterine rupture is possible. Due to a reduced capacity in the upper segment, the fetus is forced downwards, putting pressure upon the cervix. Cervical dilatation occurs through a combination of pressure from above, exerted by the presenting part and also pulling on the lower segment as the upper segment becomes thicker. The cervix dilates to a maximum of 10 cm, depending on the size of the presenting part.

Spontaneous uterine contractions begin in the two cornua in the fundus. No specific pacemaker has been identified, but it is thought that the high concentration of myometrial cells in the fundus predispose to this fundal dominance (Sellers and Bernal 1985). The wave of contraction spreads outwards from the cornua and downwards to the lower segment. The peak of the contraction occurs simultaneously in all parts. As the contraction reduces, it does so in the opposite way to its build-up, lasting longest in the fundus.

Uterine contractility is controlled by the presence of free calcium ions; where the calcium is bound within the cells, relaxation occurs (Huszar 1981). Uterine contractions at the start of labour are of short duration and mild intensity. As labour progresses, both the duration and strength increase. In early labour, the mild contractions can occur quite frequently, e.g. once every 3 minutes, but as the intensity and length increase, they become less frequent. At the height of labour,

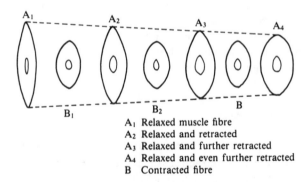

A₁ Relaxed muscle fibre
A₂ Relaxed and retracted
A₃ Relaxed and further retracted
A₄ Relaxed and even further retracted
B   Contracted fibre

Figure 19.13 Contraction and retraction of muscle fibres in the myometrium.

they again increase in frequency so that at their greatest, contractions lasting up to 60 seconds can occur every 2 minutes. In spontaneous labour, not all contractions are of identical length and intensity (Caldeyro Barcia *et al.* 1955). It is not unusual for a woman to experience a very severe contraction followed by one of lower intensity.

Intrauterine pressure during uterine relaxation averages 10 mmHg and during the active phase of labour 20–30 mmHg above the resting tone, rising to an increase of 50 mmHg in the later part of the first stage (Sellers and Bernal 1985). Pressure of the presenting part on the cervix maintains and stimulates the contractions by the release of prostaglandins from the cervix and nervous impulses relayed to the posterior pituitary gland which releases oxytocin (Gee 1980).

The amniotic fluid serves to equalise pressure within the uterus, protecting the fetus, umbilical cord and placenta from some of the extreme pressures which could be experienced at the fundus. As the cervix begins to dilate, a small area of chorion in front of the presenting part becomes detached from the decidua. This small bag of amniotic fluid is in direct contact with the cervix and protrudes through it (Myerscough 1982). When a contraction occurs, the presenting part is pushed against the cervix and seals off this bag of fluid (the forewaters) from the rest of the amniotic fluid behind the baby (the hindwaters). The membranes often remain intact throughout the first stage of labour. Schwartz *et al.* (1973) showed in his study of 517 mothers that 66% still had intact membranes at the end of the first stage of labour, 34% had spontaneous rupture at the time of full cervical dilatation, 20% ruptured during the second stage and 12% had intact membranes at delivery. If intact, the membranes reduce the intensity of pain experienced by the mother by cushioning the cervix against the presenting part (Schwartz *et al.* 1973). The formation of caput succedaneum (an oedematous swelling on the presenting part) is also reduced from 34% with early rupture to 5% following late rupture (Schwarz *et al.* 1973). Caldeyro Barcia *et al.* (1974) showed an increase in fetal heart rate abnormalities following early rupture of the membranes, but the methodology and findings of this study are disputed by Stewart *et al.* (1982), who showed no such variations.

When the woman's body is putting all its efforts into the actions of the uterus, other physiological functions are of lesser importance. These include digestion, which is slowed during labour, especially following the administration of narcotic analgesia (Holdsworth 1978). Many women can tolerate a light diet in the early stages of labour (Crawford 1978), but once in the more active phase (from 5 to 6 cm dilated onwards), wish only for fluids. The policy of the obstetric unit determines whether or not women are allowed to eat or drink during labour. Garcia *et al.* (1986) showed that in over a third of consultant units surveyed in England and Wales, no food or drink was permitted and in only 7% of units was the mother allowed to do as she wished.

Robson *et al.* (1987) showed that cardiac output increases during contractions; as labour progresses this increase becomes greater, on average from 6.99 l/min prior to labour to 7.88 l/min at rest at 8 cm dilated and 10.57 l/min during contractions. The vast majority of mothers are well equipped to cope with these changes, but care must be taken where there is any pre-existing cardiac disease.

Although not a physiological change but rather a mechanical one, the bladder changes during labour from being a pelvic organ to being an abdominal one (Myerscough 1982). As the presenting part descends into and through the pelvis, the bladder is displaced upwards. The urethra is stretched and it also may be compressed against the inner surface of the pubic symphysis by pressure from the presenting part.

The mechanism of normal labour

Mechanism describes the line through which the fetus is moved as it passes into and through the pelvis. The passive movements executed by the fetus begin in the later stages of pregnancy and continue throughout the first and second stages of labour. A knowledge of mechanism is vital for the midwife, so she can assess and understand progress in labour and to allow her to assist in the birth to the best advantage of both mother and baby. It is necessary for the fetus to follow a mechanism so that the best use can be made of the space available and also to allow for negotiation of the Curve of Carus. The fetal head enters the pelvic brim in the transverse diameter (its largest) and rotates to leave the outlet in its largest diameter, the antero-posterior. A knowledge of the fetal skull and its diameters is necessary for understanding mechanism (see Chapter 32). The mechanism being considered here is the normal one, that is, for a fetus presenting by the vertex, the most common presentation.

For a normal mechanism the following conditions must apply:

1. There must be a single fetus.
2. The lie must be longitudinal, that is, the longitudinal axis of the fetus (its spine) is parallel to the longitudinal axis of the mother (her spine).
3. The presentation is the vertex. This is the area of the fetal skull bounded by the two parietal eminences and by the anterior and posterior fontanelles. The engaging diameter is the sub-occipito bregmatic which measures 9.5 cm.
4. The fetal attitude is one of flexion.
5. The denominator is the occiput.
6. The position of the fetus with respect to the pelvic brim is right or left occipito lateral or anterior. (Beazley and Lobb 1983)

Descent

Descent occurs throughout the whole mechanism. Descent begins in the third trimester when engagement of the fetal head into the pelvis occurs. This is more common in primiparous women, where their firm abdominal muscles guide the fetal head into the pelvis. Amongst multiparous women, engagement usually occurs during labour. Bader (1936) noted that there was a normal outcome to labour for a group of 499 primiparous women who began labour with a non-engaged fetal head. In the course of labour the reduction in size of the uterine cavity forces the fetus downwards. In the second stage of labour, muscular forces are assisted by the mother's voluntary and involuntary efforts (see Figure 19.14).

Flexion

As labour progresses, the fetus becomes more compact. Pressure on the vertex further increases flexion ensuring that the smallest possible diameters pass through the pelvis.

Internal rotation of the head

The pelvic floor muscles are attached to the side wall of the pelvis and they slope forwards. This means that whatever meets the resistance of the pelvic floor first is rotated towards the front. A useful analogy is to imagine jumping on a small trampoline which is set at an angle. From whichever direction one jumps onto it, one will be bounced off towards the lowest edge. As the vertex meets the resistance of the pelvic floor, it rotates towards the front to lie directly anterior with the occiput behind the pubic arch (see Figure 19.15).

Crowning

Further descent allows the occiput to escape under the symphysis pubis. The widest transverse diameter transverse of the vertex (the biparietal, 9.5 cm) passes through

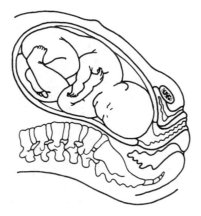

Figure 19.14 Commencement of labour. Fetal head engaged in the pelvis, position left occipito anterior.

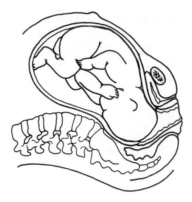

Figure 19.15 Descent of the presenting part has occurred. The occiput has hit the pelvic floor and rotated one-eighth of a circle to the front-internal rotation of the head.

the pelvic outlet. This results in the fetal head no longer receding between contractions (see Figure 19.16).

Extension of the head

To achieve the birth of the head with the smallest diameters distending the pelvic floor, it is necessary for extension to occur. The anterior fontanelle, forehead (sinciput), face and chin pass over the perineum and the head is born. The suboccipito-frontal diameter (10 cm) is the one which distends the perineum.

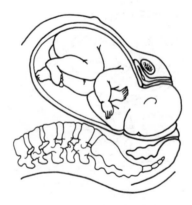

Figure 19.16 The head is crowned. The occiput has escaped under the symphysis pubis. The head is starting to extend allowing the sinciput, face and chin to sweep the perineum.

Restitution

At the time of internal rotation of the head, the shoulders remained at an oblique angle. The slight twist in the neck is straightened and the occiput now faces the mother's right or left thigh, the position it was in at the start of labour. This process is known as restitution (see Figure 19.17).

Internal rotation of the shoulders

The shoulder lying to the front of the mother's pelvis reaches the pelvic floor and is rotated forward to bring the shoulders into the antero-posterior diameter of the pelvic outlet. This movement is accompanied by external rotation of the already delivered head (see Figure 19.18).

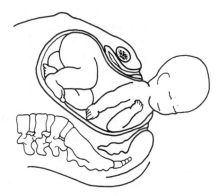

Figure 19.17 Restitution has occurred. The anterior shoulder is beginning to rotate one-eighth of a circle to the front.

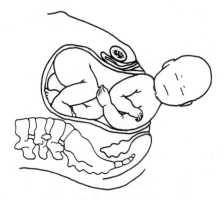

Figure 19.18 The shoulders are now in the antero-posterior diameter of the pelvic outlet. The anterior shoulder has escaped under the pubic symphyis and the posterior is beginning to sweep under the perineum. The trunk will then be delivered by lateral flexion.

Birth of the shoulders

The anterior shoulder escapes under the pubic arch before the posterior sweeps the perineum. The fetal trunk is then flexed sideways (lateral flexion) to follow the curve of the birth canal and the whole body is born.

The third stage of labour

The physiological changes in the third stage of labour include the separation and delivery of the placenta and the control of bleeding.

Separation of the placenta

During labour, the surface area of placental attachment reduces in size, as the upper segment of the uterus becomes smaller and thicker (Stander 1936). The placenta is normally able to cope with this decrease in surface area by becoming thicker. High intrauterine pressure keeps the placenta firmly pressed against the uterine wall, preventing premature separation (Stander 1936). In addition it has been suggested (Daels 1974) that since oxytocin selectively stimulates the outer layer of the myometrium during the first and second stages of labour, the placenta remains adherent until the inner muscle layer (comprising a third of the myometrium in the fundus) contracts in the third stage. For separation to occur, it is necessary that this inner layer contracts (Daels 1974).

Once the baby's body is born there is a great reduction in the size of the uterine cavity, causing the placenta with its inability to contract to become partially separated (Lavery 1987).

Contractions of the myometrium force some fetal blood back into the neonatal circulation. Maternal blood in the intervillous sinuses cannot pass through the contracted myometrium (Frankl 1919). These engorged vessels rupture and the blood (under pressure) forces its way between the placenta and the spongy layer of the uterine decidua (this process is also known as the formation of the retro-placental clot), completing the process of placental separation (Brandt 1933). The membranes are not contractile and are thrown into folds. When the separated placenta passes into the lower segment, the membranes follow. They are peeled off the uterine wall by contraction and retraction of the myometrium and by traction exerted by the separated placenta (Hendricks et al. 1962).

The placenta normally passes into the lower segment (see Figure 19.19) by its margin (Warnekros 1918) but, as it passes into the vagina, it emerges from the introitus by two different mechanisms. Most commonly, the fetal surface presents first with the maternal surface and membranes trailing behind like an inverted umbrella. Blood loss is contained behind the placenta. This method was first described by Schultze (1880) (see Figure 19.20). The alternative described by Duncan (1871) has the maternal surface of the placenta passing first through the introitus

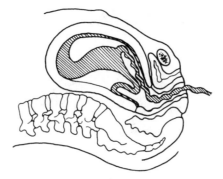

Figure 19.19 Separation of the placenta.

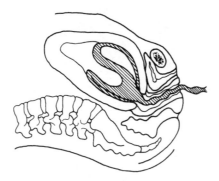

Figure 19.20 Schultz delivery of the placenta.

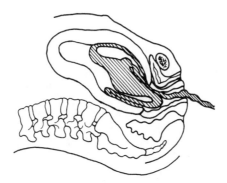

Figure 19.21 Mathews Duncan delivery of the placenta.

with a slight loss of blood (see Figure 19.21). The membranes and the rest of the placenta then follow. Retention of portions of the membranes is more common with the latter method of placental delivery (Lavery 1987).

Control of bleeding is achieved in the early stages after delivery of the placenta by contraction of the myometrium especially the cells in the oblique (figure-of-eight)

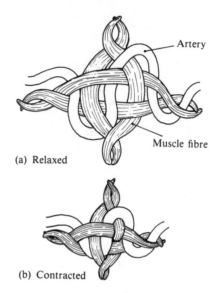

(a) Relaxed

(b) Contracted

Figure 19.22 'Living ligatures' in the myometrium (a) relaxed and (b) contracted.

layer of muscles (Harris 1966). These fibres are often called 'living ligatures'; they squeeze any blood vessels passing through this layer and prevent bleeding (see Figure 19.22). Later control of bleeding is achieved by blood clotting at the placental site and the sinuses of the decidua (Bonnar *et al*. 1969).

References

Anderson A B M and Turnbull A C (1969) 'Relationship between length of gestation and cervical dilatation, uterine contractility and other factors during pregnancy' *American Journal of Obstetrics and Gynecology* 105: 1207–45.

Arney W R (1982) *Power and the Profession of Obstetrics* University of Chicago Press: Chicago

Bader A (1936) 'The significance of the unengaged head in primiparous labour' *Ber ges Gynak u Geburtsh* (Abstract) 31: 395

Baird D (1952) 'The cause and prevention of difficult labour' *American Journal of Obstetrics and Gynecology* 63: 1200–12

Beazley J M and Lobb M O (1983) *Aspects of Care in Labour* Churchill Livingstone: Edinburgh.

Bishop E H (1964) 'Pelvic scoring for elective induction' *Obstetrics and Gynecology* 24: 266–8

Bonnar J, McNicol G P and Douglas A S (1969) 'Fibrinolytic enzyme system and pregnancy' *British Medical Journal* 3: 387

Brandt M L (1933) 'The mechanism and management of the third stage of labour' *American Journal of Obstetrics and Gynaecology* 23: 662–7

Calder A A (1979) 'Management of the unripe cervix' in M J N C Keirse, A B M Anderson and J Bennebroek Gravenhorst (eds), *Human Parturition* 201–17. Leiden University Press: Leiden

Calder A A (1983) 'Methods of inducing labour' in J Studd (ed) *Progress in Obstetrics and Gynaecology Vol 3* Ch 7 86–100 Churchill Livingstone: Edinburgh

Caldeyro Barcia R (1959) 'Uterine contractility in obstetrics' *Proceedings of the Second International Congress of Gynecology and Obstetrics* Montreal 1: 65–83.

Caldeyro Barcia R, Alvarez H and Poseiro J J (1955) 'Normal and abnormal uterine contractability in labour' *Triangle* 2: 41–52

Caldeyro Barcia R, Schwarz R, Belizan J M, Martell M, Nieto E, Sabatino H and Tenzer S M (1974) 'Adverse effects of early amniotomy during labour' in L Gluck (ed) *Modern Perinatal Medicine* 431–44. Year Book Medical Publishers: Chicago

Caldwell W E, Moloy H C and D'Esopo D A (1940) 'The more recent conceptions of pelvic architecture' *American Journal of Obstetrics and Gynecology* 40: 558

Crawford J S (1978) *Principles and Practice of Obstetric Anaesthesia (4th edn)* Blackwell Scientific: Oxford

Crawford J S (1985) 'The phases and stages of labour' *British Journal of Hospital Medicine* July: 32–6

Crowther C, Enkin M, Keirse M J N C and Brown I (1989) 'Monitoring the progress of labour' in I Chalmers, M Enkin and M J N C Keirse (eds) *Effective Care in Pregnancy and Childbirth* Ch 53 833–45 Oxford University Press: Oxford

Daels J (1974) 'Uterine contractility patterns of the outer and inner zones of the myometrium' *American Journal of Obstetrics and Gynecology* 44: 315–26

Duignan N M, Studd J and Hughes A O (1975) 'Characteristics of normal labour in different racial groups' *British Journal of Obstetrics and Gynaecology* 82(8): 593–601

Duncan J M (1871) 'On the mechanism of the expulsion of the placenta' *Edinburgh Medical Journal* 16: 899–903

Frankl H (1919) 'Ueber de normale Losung der Placenta' *Monatschrifft fur Geburtshuelfe und Gynaekologica* 50: 184–92

Friedman E A (1955) 'Primigravid labor – a graphicostatistical analysis' *Obstetrics and Gynecology* 6: 567–89

Fuchs F (1973) 'Initiation of labour – facts and fancies' in A Klopper and J Gardner (eds) *Endocrine Factors in Labour* 20: 1–24 Cambridge University Press: Cambridge.

Garcia J, Garforth S, and Ayers S (1986) 'Midwives confined? Labour ward policies and routines' *Research and the Midwife Conference Proceeding* Manchester 1985 2–30

Gee H (1980) 'Uterine Activity and Cervical Resistance Determining Cervical Change in Labour' MD Thesis Liverpool University

Harris J W and Ramsey E M (1966) 'The morphology of the human placental vasculature' *Contributions to Embryology* 38: 43–58

Hendricks C H (1983) 'Second thoughts on the induction of labour' in J Studd (ed) *Progress in Obstetrics and Gynaecology Vol 3* Ch 8 101–12 Churchill Livingstone: Edinburgh.

Hendricks C H, Brenner W E and Kraus G (1970) 'Normal cervical dilatation pattern in late pregnancy and labor' *American Journal of Obstetrics and Gynecology* 106: 1065–82

Hendricks C H, Eskea T K and Saameli K (1962) 'Uterine contractility at delivery and in the puerperium' *American Journal of Obstetrics and Gynecology* 83: 890–906

Holdsworth J D (1978) 'Relationship between stomach content and analgesia in labour' *British Journal of Anaesthesia* 50: 1145

Huszar G (1981) 'Biology and biochemistry of myometrial contractility and cervical maturation' *Seminars in Perinatology* 5: 216

International Childbirth Education Association (1976) 'International Childbirth Education Association replies to American College of Obstetricians and Gynecologists' *ICEA News* 15: 1

Jeffcoate T N A (1950) 'Delay in the second stage' *British Medical Journal* 1: 1359

Lavery B S (1987) 'The third stage' in J Lavery and M D Patrick (eds) *The Human Placenta* Ch 10 155–78 Aspen Publishers: Rockville Maryland

Liggins G C, Fairclough R J, Grieves S A, Foster K S and Knox B S (1977) 'Parturition in the sheep' in *The Fetus and Birth: Ciba Foundation Symposium* 47: 5

MacDonald D, Grant A, Sheriden-Pereira M, Boylan P and Chalmers I (1985) 'The Dublin randomised controlled trial of intrapartum fetal heart rate monitoring' *American Journal of Obstetrics and Gynecology* 152(5): 524–39

MacDonald P C, Schultz F M, Duenhoelter J H, Gant N F, Jiminez J M, Pritchard J A, Porter J C and Johnston J M (1974) 'Initiation of human parturition: 1 Mechanism of action of arachidonic acid' *Obstetrics and Gynecology* 44: 629

Maresh M, Foster C, Hackett G A and Beard R W (1983) 'The effects of an unlimited second stage on fetal wellbeing' *Journal of Obstetrics and Gynaecology* 4: 71

Moir J C (1947) 'The use of radiology in predicting difficult labour' *Journal of Obstetrics and Gynaecology of the British Empire* 54: 20–33

Myerscough P M (1982) *Munro Kerr's Operative Obstetrics (10th edn)* Balliere Tindall: London

Naaktgeboren C (1989) 'The biology of childbirth' in I Chalmers , M Enkin and M J N Keirse (eds) *Effective Care in Pregnancy and Childbirth* Ch 48 765–804 Oxford University Press: Oxford

O'Driscoll K and Meagher D (1980) *Active Management of Labour* W B Saunders: London.

O'Driscoll K, Jackson R J A and Gallagher J T (1969) 'Prevention of prolonged labour' *British Medical Journal* 2: 477–80

Prendiville W J, Harding J E, Elbourne D R and Stirrat G M (1988) 'The Bristol third stage trial: active versus physiological management of the third stage of labour' *British Medical Journal* 297: 1295–1300

Robinson S, Golden J and Bradley S (1983) *A Study of the Role and Responsibilities of the Midwife* NERU Report No 1 Chelsea College: University of London

Robson S C, Dunlop W, Boys R J and Hunter S (1987) 'Cardiac output during labour' *British Medical Journal* 295: 1169–72.

Schultze B S (1880) 'Ueber den Mechanismus der spontanen Ausscheidung der Nachgeburt und ueber den Credeschen und den Dubliner Handgriff' *Deutsche med Wochenschrifft* 6(Dec): 667–81, 689–92

Schwarz B E (1982) 'The onset of labour' in J Studd (ed) *Progress in Obstetrics and Gynaecology Vol 2* Ch 1 3–9 Churchill Livingstone: Edinburgh

Schwarz B E, MacDonald P C and Johnston J M (1980) 'Initiation of human parturition: X1 Lysosomal enzyme release in vitro from amnions obtained from laboring and non-laboring women' *American Journal of Obstetrics and Gynecology* 136: 21

Schwarz R, Althabe O, Caldyro Barcia R, Belitsky R, Lanchares J L, Alvarez R, Bedraguer P, Capurro H, Belizan J M, Sabatino J H and Abusleme C (1973) 'Fetal heart rate patterns in labors with intact and ruptured membranes' *Journal of Perinatal Medicine* 1: 153–65

Sellers S M and Bernal A L (1985) 'Physiology of labour' in J Studd J (ed) *Management of Labour* Ch 1 1–15 Blackwell Scientific: London

Stander H J (1936) *Williams Obstetrics (7th edn)* Ch 16 427–43 Appleton Century Crofts: New Jersey

Stewart P, Kennedy J H and Calder A A (1982) 'Spontaneous labour: When should the membranes be ruptured?' *British Journal of Obstetrics and Gynaecology* 89: 39–43

Studd J (1973) 'Patograms and normograms of cervical dilatation in the management of normal labour' *British Medical Journal* 4: 451–5

Studd J, Clegg D R, Saunders R R and Hughes A O (1975) 'Identification of high risk labours by labour normogram' *British Medical Journal* ii: 545–7

Tew M (1990) *Safer Childbirth? A critical history of maternity care* Chapman and Hall: London

Warnekros K (1918) 'Die Nachgeburtsperiode im Roentgenbilde' *Archives fur Gynaekologica* 109: 266–83

20 The first and second stages of labour

The aim of care in labour is to ensure the optimum level of maternal physical and mental well-being, fetal well-being and continued progress in labour, with the end result of a live, healthy mother and baby. Most care in labour is given by midwives, who have responsibility for the supervision of women having a normal labour and birth. Where complications occur, the midwife will follow the plan for care as determined by the medical staff. The principles of midwifery care are those of diligent observation, together with emotional and physical support.

Onset of labour

Defining the actual onset of labour is difficult. The start of coordinated uterine activity follows a period of prelabour; it is the onset of sustained progress which differentiates true from false labour (Hendricks et al. 1970). The onset of labour begins with the establishment of regular uterine contractions, which are usually perceived by the mother. In the early stages, the contractions cause discomfort and later, depending on the individual, pain (Hibbard 1988). Spontaneous rupture of the membranes, if not accompanied by uterine contractions, is not regarded as labour (Grant and Keirse 1989). The confirmation of labour is by vaginal examination, which should demonstrate effacement and dilatation of the cervix, together with formation of the bulging forewaters.

The mother's first contact with the midwife who will support her in labour whether at home or in hospital is vital, especially where the midwife is not already known to the mother. It can establish the relationship for the whole of labour, putting the mother at her ease or reinforcing her fears and apprehensions. Where the midwife is not already known to the mother, it is necessary that formal introductions are made. Especially in the situation of a first birth, the mother may be experiencing totally new sensations (Kitzinger 1987). These can include the often contradictory emotions of excitement, fear, anticipation and apprehension (Garforth and Garcia 1989). Regarding the labour itself, the mother may be surprised at the intensity of the contractions; she may be afraid of losing control of her own body and of how she will feel and behave in later labour (Cartwright 1979). These feelings are often accompanied by worries about the well-being and normality of the baby. For the mother who is booked for a hospital confinement, it may be her first ever admission to hospital. Being taken from familiar surroundings and people to a new environment can be very threatening. Those women (and their partners) who have had an opportunity to visit the delivery unit prior to labour may feel more at ease. Some women are fortunate in being accompanied on their journey to hospital by their midwife, as occurs with a DOMINO delivery which can be helpful (Keirse *et al.* 1989). This means that in addition to any companion, the woman has a friendly face who knows how to operate 'the system'. Flint (1991) found that women cared for in their 'Know Your Midwife' scheme appreciated having a midwife known to them giving care and required less analgesia in labour.

The second report of the Maternity Services Advisory Committee (1984, Maternity Care in Action II) advises that there should be a welcoming and friendly atmosphere to greet the woman on her arrival in the labour ward. Other recommendations include clear signposting of entrances to the maternity unit and delivery suite, a member of staff to be available to welcome mothers, that the mother's records should be readily available or the mother should carry her own casenotes (Maternity Services Advisory Committee 1984). Ideally each labouring woman should be allocated one midwife to care for her during the shift of duty; she should be introduced to the mother, as should any midwifery, nursing or medical students. The woman's permission should be obtained before the student enters the room if students are to contribute to her care (Maternity Services Advisory Committee 1984).

In some units mothers are asked if they wish to wear their own clothes in labour; this is appreciated as being more personal (Garforth and Garcia 1989). In addition there is a need for privacy in the admitting and labouring rooms with personnel knocking on the door and waiting to be admitted (Flint 1984; Garforth and Garcia 1989).

After greeting the woman in labour, it is important for the midwife to obtain a full history of recent events. If the woman's notes are available, records of past history and antenatal care should be read. If the notes are not at hand, the woman should be questioned for pertinent details regarding the history of this pregnancy, previous deliveries, pre-existing medical conditions, allergies and any complications. For the woman who meets her midwife in advanced labour, these formalities may be severely curtailed. The minimum information necessary is as follows:

History of contractions – since when? How often?
Membranes – ruptured or intact?
Show.
Pain – site and severity.
Has she been well in this pregnancy?
Recent contact with infections, e.g. chickenpox.
Previous deliveries – outcome, complications.
Pregnancy/medical complications.
Allergies/rhesus grouping.

It is recommended that this oral history is obtained whilst the mother is being examined. According to the mother's wishes, her partner or companion may be present during the admission procedure. Garforth and Garcia (1989), in their survey of mothers, found that most wished to have someone present, with only 3% wanting to be alone. At this stage, the midwife should ask the mother if she has any worries or concerns regarding the labour so that they can be discussed (Maternity Services Advisory Committee 1984). The following describes the initial examination of the mother. Depending on the stage reached in the labour, the order of observations may be altered. All recordings and the history should be clearly documented, signed and dated by the midwife.

1. Contractions – length, strength, frequency.
2. Maternal response to contractions.
3. Abdominal examination (The midwife must be firm but gentle when performing this palpation, as the mother's abdomen may be tender. The examination should not begin until the midwife is certain that the uterus is completely relaxed.):
   (a) inspection – this is to obtain an impression of uterine size (and therefore fetal size and number), scars which would indicate previous uterine or abdominal surgery; contractions may be seen if they are expulsive;
   (b) number of fetuses – if more than one, the labour is no longer considered normal;
   (c) lie – any lie other than longditudinal is considered abnormal;
   (d) presentation – only vertex presentations are considered normal;
   (e) position – posterior positions of the vertex affect the progress and management of labour;
   (f) level of the presenting part – to determine progress, the degree of flexion of the presenting part and the adequacy or otherwise of the pelvis;
   (g) fetal heart rate – between and following a contraction.

4. Vaginal loss – show, liquor, fresh blood. These can indicate the progress of the labour or, if meconium is present, possible fetal distress or the presence of a breech presentation.
5. Presence of varicose veins or oedema.
6. Pulse, blood pressure and temperature. These are usually recorded as a baseline for later measurements, although their value for women with a normal pregnancy and labour has not been demonstrated (Crowther *et al.* 1989).
7. Urinalysis for protein and ketones.

These readings will be used as the baseline for comparison with all other recordings in labour although, if labour is well advanced, their value may be limited. Confirmation of the onset of labour is by vaginal examination; this is discussed later in the section covering progress in labour.

A decision now has to be made whether the woman is actually in established labour or not. This is not as simple as it sounds, since many women experience one or more episodes of false labour before the actual event (Hendricks *et al.* 1970; O'Driscoll *et al.* 1973). Where the diagnosis is unclear, the woman is kept under observation for 1 or 2 hours, after which her progress or otherwise will be measured. During this period she is encouraged, if during the day, to be ambulant, helping the establishment of labour and is offered a light diet to prevent ketosis when labour actually begins.

Naaktgeboren (1989) has noted the way in which labouring animals cease their labour if moved or if strangers intervene. This alteration in physiology may well be similar to the common phenomenon, where the woman reports that her contractions reduce in intensity on admission to hospital.

Planning care in labour

To ensure a successful outcome of labour, a relationship of mutual trust between mother and midwife is of great importance (O'Driscoll and Meagher 1980). When planning care it is necessary to take account of the mother's wishes and also of the facilities available in the place of confinement, as this can limit choice (Chalmers *et al.* 1989). Birth plans can be very helpful, as they allow the woman (and her partner) to discuss the conduct of labour and delivery with the midwife before the actual event (Jackson 1986; Chalmers *et al.* 1989). They are especially useful where the mother is not accompanied in labour by her own midwife. Birth plans are discussed in greater detail in Chapter 9. Where there is no birth plan, the midwife should ask the couple if they have any specific wishes regarding the management of their care. In addition, fully explained choices (for example, regarding fetal monitoring) should be given where the situation allows this (for example, continuous monitoring is recommended for a woman with a complicated labour), although the parents can still refuse to have any treatment. Where a change in midwifery personnel occurs during labour, documentation and discussion of care with the new member of staff is vital to ensure continuity. The new midwife should be introduced to the couple, to help maintain the supportive environment (Garforth and Garcia 1989).

An atmosphere of mutual trust between mother and midwife, together with full, comprehensible explanations of procedures and progress, is the best way of assisting the woman's state of emotional well-being. It is also helpful in making the woman feel in control. A supportive companion, whether husband, partner, female relative or friend, can do much to give comfort and encouragement at this difficult time (Keirse *et al.* 1989). All information should be given in a way that is easily understood without being patronising. Questions should be encouraged and be answered in an open and friendly manner (Kirkham 1983). Great care must be taken that the midwife is not saying one thing whilst her body language is saying the opposite. For example, the midwife's statement that she is willing to answer questions would be contradicted by a closed posture with arms crossed. Women in labour are very perceptive and quickly notice inconsistencies in approach (Kirkham 1983). Midwives may develop techniques to avoid answering questions or giving information (Cartwright 1979; Kirkham 1983). This is despite the fact that 80% of mothers questioned in one survey wished to be involved in decisions regarding their care (Cartwright 1979). MacIntyre (1982) has described four stereotyped responses to questioning adopted by midwives as a means of restricting communication:

1. Lower-class women don't want information or explanation.
2. Women don't understand technical terms.
3. The best reply to questions is reassurance.
4. No news is good news (MacIntyre 1982).

Progress in labour

When assessing progress in labour it is important to remember that every woman is different and that physiology varies between individuals (Crowther *et al.* 1989). Time limits were originally placed on the various stages of labour to reduce maternal and fetal exhaustion (Baird 1952). This, however, was at a time when mortality rates were high, with infection and haemorrhage claiming many victims (Department of Health and Social Security 1969). The present situation with well-nourished and healthy women who are rarely debilitated from years of too-frequent childbearing, together with the development of potent antibiotics, oxytocics and blood transfusion services, has meant that a more conservative approach could be adopted. Despite these improvements, the length of labour is still restricted with 12 hours often being regarded as the upper limit of normal (O'Driscoll *et al.* 1984). Studd (1973) questioned the arbitrary application of rates of progress and time limits to labour, especially since there is confusion about the diagnosis of the onset of labour.

In addition, certain practices such as posture and lack of nourishment can themselves hinder progress (Flynn *et al.* 1978; Ludka 1987). There is no disagreement about the diligent observation of progress necessary when caring for women with complications such as gestational proteinuric hypertension, preterm labour or a trial of labour or trial of scar. Progress in labour is assessed using three main criteria:

1. The strength, length and frequency of contractions.
2. The descent and rotation of the presenting part.
3. The effacement and dilatation of the cervix and other changes. (Crowther *et al.* 1989)

In addition, one must take account of the woman's condition, her breathing and her assessment of progress (Hibbard 1988; Crowther *et al.* 1989).

It is very important to assess all criteria and not to rely on any one, for example, cervical dilatation, to the exclusion of the others. Progress is recorded graphically, using a record designed originally by Philpott (1972) for use in rural Africa as a method of detecting delay in labour early enough to facilitate transport to hospital while the mother and fetus were still in reasonable condition. These records based on the work of Friedman (1955) see Figure 20.1a, were amended by Studd (1973) for use in the United Kingdom. The graphs, known as the partogram, serve as a unified visual record of maternal progress and maternal and fetal well-being in labour (Figure 20.1b). The partogram is used to assess the progress of labour in 89% of UK maternity hospitals (Garcia *et al.* 1986). The contractions are recorded every half hour by assessing the number occurring in a 10 minute period and using a method of shading to record their relative strength (see Figure 20.1c). Each unit has its own preferred symbols for recording strength, relating to the density of shading used. Cervical dilatation and descent of the presenting part are recorded on the same graph, usually using different colours of pen (see Figure 20.2). Maternal well-being is recorded, including temperature, pulse, blood pressure, urine volume and urinalysis and response to pain (see Figure 20.3).

Any drugs given, such as oxytocin, analgesia or intravenous therapy, are also noted. Foetal well-being is assessed and charted by fetal heart recordings, colour of liquor, presence of caput or moulding on the presenting part and fetal blood-sampling results (if performed) (Hibbard 1988).

Assessment of satisfactory progress in labour is dependent upon the woman's parity, her gestation and the size and position of the fetus (Studd *et al.* 1982). It

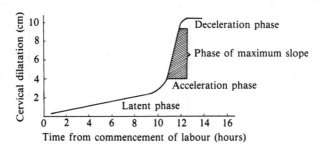

Figure 20.1a Friedman's (1955) curve showing phase of maximum slope of cervical dilatation.

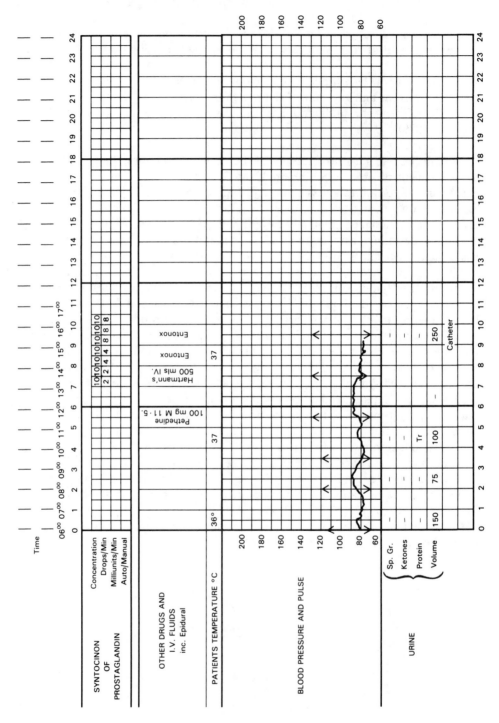

Figure 20.1b The partogram.

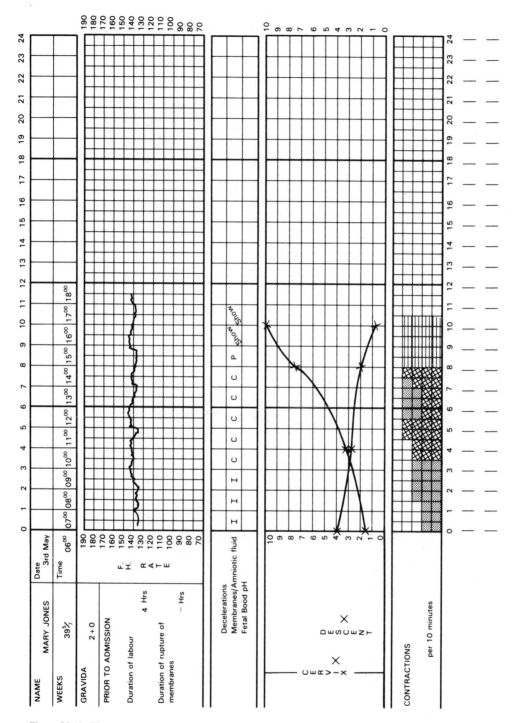

Figure 20.1b The partogram *cont*.

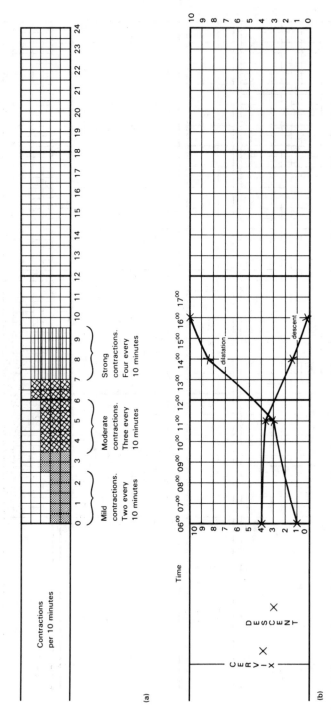

Figure 20.2 (a) One method of recording contraction frequency and strength on the partogram (b) Progress in labour – cervical dilatation and descent of the presenting part.

DELIVERY UNIT RECORD	Surname		Case No.

SPECIAL INSTRUCTIONS ON ADMISSION

First Names		Date of Birth
Address		Age
Post Code		

	Time	Date	
Admitted at			Temperature _____
Membranes Ruptures at			Pulse _____
			B.P. _____

Details of labour
before admission_____

_____   Urinalysis _____
_____   Sp.Gr. _____
General Examination _____   Ketones _____
_____   Glucose _____
_____   Protein _____
Abdominal Examination_____

INDUCTION OF LABOUR

Date .... Time .... hrs

Indications _____

Procedure _____

Fetal heart at end of procedure _____ Signature _____

INSTRUCTIONS FOR LABOUR

HMR 155(W) [WMF 7701]

Figure 20.3 Delivery unit record.

is now accepted that the diagnosis of the onset of a labour is not an absolute but rather a continuum from prelabour in the weeks prior to true labour up to the establishment of established, active labour (Hendricks *et al.* 1970; Crowther *et al.* 1989). In the first stage, it is now accepted that there is a latent phase (Friedman 1955) up until 3 or 4 cm of cervical dilatation when progress, especially in a primigravida, can be rather slow. This is followed by a rapid acceleration in progress lasting until 8 or 9 cm when, during the transition phase, descent and rotation are of more importance than the slowed rate of dilatation (Friedman 1955) (see Figure 20.1a).

Whilst an overall rate of progress of 1 cm of cervical dilatation per hour may be achieved this obscures individual differences, for example:

> ---3 cm   Time taken 5 hours
> 3–8.5 cm   Time taken 3 hours
> 8.5–10 cm   Time taken 2 hours (see Figure 20.3)
> Total time – 10 hours

For primiparous women, it may take 15 hours to reach full dilatation (Crowther *et al.* 1989). Misdiagnosis of the onset of labour accounts for some cases of 'tardy' progress (Cardoza and Studd 1985; Crowther *et al.* 1989).

Similarly, the second stage of labour can be divided into a latent resting phase of full dilatation with further descent and rotation of the presenting part, followed by an active pushing phase when the mother experiences the urge to push and there is thinning of the perineum and pelvic floor (Stewart 1984; Maresh 1987). An understanding of this can assist in preventing the woman becoming exhausted before she is ready to push. Stewart (1984) in his study, recorded the average time spent pushing as being 39 minutes for primiparous women and 15 minutes for multiparous. Mothers became exhausted after 45 minutes of active pushing (Wood *et al.* 1973). Maresh (1987) argues that where maternal and fetal conditions are both satisfactory, active pushing by the mother can be safely delayed. The second stage may be as long as 2 hours for primiparous women, especially where an epidural is *in situ*, to allow for further descent and rotation of the presenting part (Maresh *et al.* 1983; Kadar 1985).

During the first stage of labour, the length, strength and frequency of contractions should be assessed every 30 minutes, with the results charted on the partogram. It must be remembered that an individual's clinical assessment of uterine action is not particularly accurate (unless assessed mechanically) being subject to both intraobserver and interobserver error (Miller 1985). Descent and rotation of the fetus is assessed primarily by abdominal examination, with confirmation by vaginal examination. Abdominal examination is carried out every 1–2 hours and also prior to any vaginal examination (Hibbard 1988). As labour progresses and nears transition, a thick blood-stained mucus discharge referred to as 'show' is often passed through the vagina; this is usually indicative of progress. Progress in labour is confirmed by vaginal examination. Some hospitals have policies for the timing of examinations. Garforth and Garcia (1989) showed that 70% of the units surveyed had a policy on the frequency of examinations and in half of these this was fixed, although most specified 4 hours. Duignan recommends every 1–2 hours, O'Driscoll and Meagher (1980) every 2 hours and Studd *et al.* (1982) every 3 hours although there is limited rationale to support these statements. The following are indications for the performance of vaginal examinations in labour.

1. To confirm diagnosis of labour and to provide a baseline for later examinations (Crowther *et al.* 1989).
2. To assess progress. This is usually every 4–6 hours, although some units use shorter intervals.
3. Prior to giving systemic analgesia. To ensure that labour is not too far advanced for the mother to benefit from the effect before delivery or that the fetus will not be born within 2–3 hours following administration, which is the time at which the fetal respiratory system is most seriously depressed.
4. Following spontaneous rupture of membranes, especially where the presenting part is not engaged. This is to eliminate the possibility of cord prolapse (Hibbard 1988).
5. To confirm presentation or position if either of these are in doubt.
6. To confirm the onset of the second stage of labour, which might not coincide with feeling the urge to push.
7. To rupture the membranes and/or apply a fetal scalp electrode.
8. To investigate delay at any stage in labour (Hibbard 1988).

During labour, many women find vaginal examinations unpleasant. In one study, 11% of the women surveyed reported that the examination was very painful (Murphy *et al.* 1986). For this reason, the examination should be performed with the woman in her most comfortable position, following full and clear explanation of the procedure and with the assurance that she will not be examined during a contraction. It is helpful to take the mother to the toilet or to offer her a bedpan prior to the procedure. This not only increases her comfort but may also assist descent of the presenting part. The examination is most commonly performed with the mother in a semirecumbent position but if she is mobilising in labour, she may prefer to be examined whilst upright or on all fours. This may present some difficulties for the midwife in determining the fetal position as the usual landmarks are in an unusual orientation. This can be helped by making a diagram of the findings to give clarity.

To begin the procedure, the midwife washes her hands and puts on sterile gloves. The woman's vulva is usually swabbed with a warmed antiseptic solution to help prevent introducing infection, although there is limited evidence as to the effectiveness of this. It is then usual to cover the examining fingers (index and middle fingers) with (antiseptic) obstetric cream. Whilst using the other hand to separate the labia, the vulva and perineum are examined for varicose veins or scar tissue. The midwife puts one and then both examining fingers gently into the woman's vagina and assesses the tone of the pelvic floor muscles which surround the vagina.

The vagina

For the vast majority of labouring women the vagina is warm and moist. However, where labour is obstructed or in cases of maternal illness such as acute infection the vagina may feel hot and dry.

The cervix

Where the mother is lying in a semirecumbent position, the fingers are moved downwards and backwards until the cervix is identified. In early labour (especially in multiparous women), the cervix may project down into the vault of the vagina; a long uneffaced cervix feels about 2.5 cm long (Hibbard 1988). More commonly, the effaced cervix is well applied to the presenting part and can be felt as a depression which admits the width of one or two fingers or later on as a raised edge. Dilatation is assessed by measuring the diameter of the cervical os in centimetres. This requires practice. The thickness (effacement) of the rim of the cervix, whether it is firm or soft and how well it is applied to the presenting part, is also assessed. The cervix is maximally dilated 15 seconds after the peak of each contraction (Richardson *et al.* 1978).

The membranes

Before labour is established, the membranes are usually closely applied to the presenting part and difficult to identify. Later on they can project into the vaginal vault as a wedge or, if the presenting part is ill-fitting, as a loose 'sausage-shape' of membranes which can rupture easily (Hibbard 1988).

Position of the fetus

To determine fetal position, it is necessary to identify certain landmarks on the presentation. For a well-flexed fetus presenting by the head, the posterior fontanelle is usually identified lying towards the front of the pelvis. The lambda is easily recognised as a small triangular depression at the junction of three suture lines. Where the head is less well flexed, the sagittal suture can be palpated and in posterior positions the anterior fontanelle can be felt towards the front of the pelvis. When determining the fetal position, it is easier to confirm the findings of the previous abdominal examination rather than relying totally on the findings on vaginal examination. In prolonged labour and/or in posterior positions of the vertex, the presence of caput and moulding can obscure these landmarks.

Descent

The station of the presenting part is determined with respect to the level of the ischial spines. Unless these are particularly prominent or the woman is extremely relaxed, this is far from easy. With the woman in a semirecumbent position, the ischial spines can be located at an angle of 30–35° from the side walls of the vagina with the fingers pointing down into the bed. This is a skill which requires practice. Whilst withdrawing her fingers, the midwife on her first examination should assess the size of the pelvis, especially the curve of the sacrum and the angle of the pubic arch (see Chapter 24).

Following the examination, the midwife should remove any antiseptic cream from the woman's vulva with dry cotton wool balls before applying a clean vulval pad. The woman should be informed of the findings which should also be fully recorded in the notes and charted in the partogram. The following is an example of how the results are recorded:

> 03.45. Examination to assess progress. On palpation left occipito anterior position, head 1-2/5 palpable abdominally.
> On inspection, the external genitalia appear normal, there is a right medio lateral-episiotomy scar and a small left-sided vulval varicosity.
> On vaginal examination. Cervix 4–5 cm dilated, soft, 80% effaced, well applied to the present part.
> Presenting part, vertex (Vx) position LOA, descent 1 cm below ischial spines, slight moulding and caput succadeneum.
> Clear liquor draining
> Jane Grey

Maternal well-being

This section will first consider the monitoring of maternal well-being and then those aspects of midwifery care which are important for supporting mothers throughout labour.

Labour, as the name implies, is hard work (Hazle 1986). Although the woman is not consciously investing her energies in uterine activity, her body is working very hard. Observations of maternal condition in labour give an indication of how the woman is coping and of her response to stress. Recordings taken at the start of labour are regarded as a baseline for later assessment. All recordings should be charted on the partogram.

1. Temperature. This is recorded either two- or four-hourly (Hibbard 1988). There are questions regarding the usefulness of these recordings (temperature, pulse and blood pressure) in normal women (Crowther *et al.* 1989). A slight (0.5°C) rise in temperature especially during and after delivery, is quite normal (Varney 1987), but higher levels might indicate the presence of infection.

2. Pulse rate is usually recorded every half-hour. The increased metabolic activity in labour causes a small rise in the pulse rate (above the levels before labour) between contractions. During the onset of each contraction, there is a marked increase in pulse rate, due to pain and tension. Infection and ketoacidosis can result in a persistent tachycardia (Hibbard 1988).

3. Blood pressure recordings are taken two-hourly in early labour and hourly, once labour is established. This reading should be made when the uterus is fully relaxed. During contractions, the systolic blood pressure is raised by 10–20 mmHg and the diastolic by 5–10 mmHg (Varney 1987). When recording blood pressure, care should also be taken that the mother is not supine and occluding her vena cava with the weight of the uterus, giving rise to hypotension.

4. Urinalysis. To prevent overdistension of and damage to the bladder and delays in labour (especially in the third stage), it is good practice to encourage the mother to try to pass urine every 2 hours. A long labour and pressure on the bladder neck are risk factors for the occurrence of a vesico vaginal fistula (Kelly 1983). Where the mother is mobile, she can use the toilet, but for women confined to bed (such as those using epidural analgesia), a bedpan will be required.

   Each specimen should be measured and tested for protein and ketone bodies. Although the presence of a trace of protein is usually accounted for by contamination with liquor or blood, larger amounts of protein require further examination, since eclampsia can occur for the first time during labour. Specimens obtained using a catheter should contain no protein.

   The presence of ketones indicates that carbohydrates are in short supply and that fats are being metabolised (Dumoulin and Foulkes 1984). This condition can be prevented by giving a light diet in early labour (Crawford 1978). If the ketosis is severe, the contractions may be inhibited and both mother and fetus can have a tachycardia (Hibbard 1988). Treatment is with intravenous Hartmann's solution (Ringer's lactate) (Dumoulin and Foulkes 1984) but this should not be necessary if the woman is not prevented from taking sweet drinks and glucose in early labour. Glucose is usually only present where intravenous dextrose is being given which raises blood glucose, producing renal glycosuria (Rutter et al. 1980). It can also result in stimulation of fetal insulin production, causing the neonate to develop hypoglycaemia soon after birth (Singhi et al. 1982). For this reason glucose-based intravenous fluids are less frequently used in labour these days (Dumoulin and Foulkes 1984).

5. It is important to observe and record the mother's response to contractions. This gives a guide to the progress of labour and also to the mother's abilities to cope and to her level of tiredness. After giving analgesia, the effectiveness of the method should be recorded.

Maternal care in labour

Enemata and shaves

These two practices, which were an accepted part of labour management in the

1960s and 1970s, are now no longer recommended; indeed their use has been shown to be harmful (Romney 1980; Romney and Gordon 1981; Drayton and Rees 1984). One could pose the question: would the use of shaving of the pubic hair prior to childbirth have been so widespread without the introduction of the safety razor at the turn of the century? It was argued that the pubic hair could harbour bacteria and thus increase the risk of infection (Voorhees 1906). This premise was never supported by research and the practice persisted, despite evidence of the trauma caused by shaving and the lack of a reduction in infection (Johnston and Sidall 1922). Romney (1980) demonstrated in a non-randomised trial that shaving did not reduce the incidence of infection, but it did cause the mothers some discomfort. Results of this research indicate that shaving should be discontinued, except for those women requiring abdominal deliveries. Garforth and Garcia (1989) found that only 61% of women in their national survey in England and Wales had no shave at all, with 10% still having a complete shave.

Enemas were introduced with the aim of speeding up labour, reducing faecal contamination at delivery and limiting neonatal infections. Romney and Gordon (1981) and Drayton and Rees (1984) demonstrated that the use of an enema did not significantly affect the length of labour. Whilst the frequency of faecal contamination was reduced following an enema, it was more difficult to deal with, being in a liquid form. The routine use of enemas (and, indeed, any bowel preparation) has been discontinued in the United Kingdom (Garforth and Garcia 1989). Suppositories may be used where the woman is suffering from constipation or is worried about potential soiling.

Both enemas and shaves were distressing to women in labour although some women preferred them (Garforth and Garcia 1989). Their discontinuation will help to contribute to the demedicalisation of childbirth.

Activity in labour

Traditionally, women have adopted the position most comfortable for them during the first and second stages of labour (Engelmann 1882; Ploss *et al.* 1935). This is most commonly an upright posture (Engelmann 1882). Caldeyro Barcia (1979a) has demonstrated that during the first stage of labour an upright posture reduces the frequency of contractions, but that they are of a greater intensity. Read *et al.* (1981) suggest that an upright posture can be as efficient as oxytocin in stimulating effective uterine action. Other benefits of maternal activity in labour were that the length of labour was slightly reduced and that there was a reduced usage of analgesia (Flynn *et al.* 1978). Disadvantages of the recumbent position include supine hypotension with reduced cardiac output (Ueland and Hansen 1969) and diminished placental perfusion. In addition, it is more difficult for the woman to adopt a position which minimises her pain (Roberts 1989).

To aid descent of the presenting part or for the second stage of labour, Russell (1969) demonstrated that the squatting position increased diameters of the pelvic outlet by 1 cm in the transverse and 2 cm for the antero-posterior diameters. The outlet, recorded using X-rays, increased by 28% when the position altered from supine to squatting. For Western women, squatting is not an easy position to maintain (Sleep *et al*. 1989). If the woman wishes to use such a position for delivery, she must practise it during pregnancy or utilise one of the birth stools, bars, birthchairs or other aids which are now increasingly available. Low stools, such as those used by young children for reaching the wash-hand basin or lavatory, are an ideal and cheap aid for the woman adopting the supported squat position, assisted by her partner.

For the woman who wishes to remain in bed or who, due to her choice of analgesia has no chance to ambulate, wedges and pillows can provide a semirecumbent position. The lateral position is good for preventing vena-caval compression and is better for uterine action than the supine position (Turnbull 1957).

Diet in labour

Restriction of diet in labour to sips of water only is a further example of how a sensible scheme of management for one high-risk group of women (those with a high chance of general anaesthetic) becomes the rule for all (Johnson *et al*. 1989). Garforth and Garcia (1989) found that 39% of UK maternity units surveyed allowed no solid food at all during labour and half restricted it during the active phase. Few allowed women to eat and drink as they wished. Eighty-six per cent permitted women to drink water at any time.

Increasing fatigue and the use of narcotic analgesia both increase retention of gastric contents, with the higher risk of vomiting (due to analgesia) and inhalation of stomach contents (Crawford 1985). The causes of maternal mortality and morbidity from pulmonary aspiration of stomach contents are usually poor anaesthetic techniques and non-observance of protocols, rather than the taking of a light diet in early labour (Department of Health and Social Security 1985; Department of Health 1989). Labour is a time of great energy demand; Ludka (1987) estimates that the labouring woman may require 800–1100 kcals/hour. Using an intravenous infusion to meet these needs could cause more problems than it solves (Dumoulin and Foulkes 1984). These problems include fetal hyperinsulinism with neonatal hypoglycaemia, maternal and fetal hyponatraemia and maternal overhydration (Dumoulin and Foulkes 1984).

Women in labour do not require, nor do they commonly request, a full diet, although feeling hungry in the first stage of labour can be an unpleasant experience (Simkin 1986). A light diet high in carbohydrate, including sweet drinks and the use of glucose tablets is sufficient to sustain most women through labour (Crawford 1978). As a guide, once a woman reaches 5 or 6 cm of cervical dilatation, she no longer has an appetite for any solid food. Women at particular risk of ketoacidosis in labour are those who have been starved (or on a very restricted diet) for a number of days while attempts are made to initiate labour with prostaglandin pessaries. It is vital to remember their nutritional needs (Ludka 1987). For women in high-risk groups, such as those having a trial of labour, multiple birth, preterm or breech delivery, restriction of diet is a wise precaution (Crawford 1978).

Pain relief in labour

Pain is a sensation perceived by the individual, the intensity of and response to which is affected by culture, previous experience of pain, emotional state and anticipation (Melzak 1973). Pain receptors are present throughout the body; when stimulated, they relay signals to the brain, which are interpreted as pain (Brown and Deffenbacher 1979). Pain signals travelling to the brain can be altered by competing stimuli which reduce or increase the perception of pain. Pain nervous impulses travel along neurones relatively slowly and therefore 'faster' stimuli can reach the brain first and 'close the gate', reducing the perception of pain (Melzak 1973). Such competing stimuli include heat, cold and pressure.

The sensation of pain in early labour is transferred from the uterus via the sympathetic nervous system through the eleventh and twelfth thoracic dermatomes; in later labour as the pain intensity increases the tenth thoracic and first lumbar dermatomes are also involved (Bonica 1986). Pain sensations from cervix, vagina, vulva and perineum travel via the pudendal nerve, entering the spinal column between the second and fourth sacral vertebrae (Moir and Thorburn 1986).

The body produces its own natural pain killers, the endorphins, which give the effects of analgesia by attaching themselves to specific receptors in the brain and spinal cord (Mayer and Walkins 1984). Pain relief can also be obtained by blocking the nerve pathway (local anaesthesia), interfering with reception of nerve impulses (general anaesthesia, inhalational and systemic analgesia) and by inducing competing stimuli which use similar nerve pathways to the pain impulses (massage, acupuncture and the use of heat) (Bonica 1986). The perception of pain can be reduced by using distraction techniques, together with the use of relaxation, which can help relieve tension (Simkin 1989). Read (1942) postulated that fear and anxiety increase tension, leading to the release of adrenaline, which further increases pain. This cycle, unless interrupted, can become an established 'vicious circle'.

The characteristics of an ideal type of pain relief are as follows:

1. It should produce complete/acceptable analgesia (Dickersin 1989).
2. It should not interfere with the process of labour (Bonica 1986).
3. It should be free of side-effects on the mother (e.g. paralysis or sedation) (Dickersin 1989).
4. It should have no adverse effects on the fetus (Dickersin 1989).

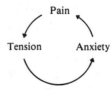

Figure 20.4 The pain, tension and anxiety circle (Read 1942).

Unfortunately, the ideal does not exist, and a woman's choice of analgesia is made after all the advantages and disadvantages of each method have been discussed. The eventual decision involves choosing which disadvantages are acceptable to that woman to achieve the benefits of that particular method.

The causation of pain in labour is still incompletely understood (Dickersin 1989). Pain in labour results from myometrial ischaemia as a consequence of stretching of the lower uterine segment and cervix, or pressure of the presenting part which restricts blood flow or from direct compression of cervical nerve ganglia (Bonica 1986). It can be perceived as backache, down the top of the thighs or as suprapubic and abdominal pain (Crawford 1982). The techniques which will be considered are psychoprophylaxis, acupuncture, transcutaneous electrical nerve stimulation (TENS), hypnosis, inhalational analgesia, systemic analgesia and local anaesthesia (including epidural).

Psychoprophylaxis is the preparation of the mind to reduce tension and therefore pain in labour (Read 1942). It seeks to break the association between labour and pain by education and information about labour (Enkin et al. 1972), the teaching of relaxation exercises and of the use of distraction and disassociation techniques (Velvovsky et al. 1960). For psychoprophylaxis to be successful, it is necessary for the woman and preferably her partner or labour companion to be taught the techniques (Lamaze 1984). Teaching about the physiology of labour is given to ensure that the woman can feel in control of her own body and fully aware of the processes which are taking place (Read 1942). Relaxation techniques are aimed at relaxing individual muscle groups and breathing exercises which can reduce intra-abdominal pressure are also advised. Different levels of breathing are employed as labour progresses, aimed at not increasing pressure and tension in the abdominal cavity. Distraction techniques involve singing, chanting nursery rhymes or counting backwards during the contraction to distract the brain from the stimuli which are bombarding it. Music has also been shown to be of help (Sammons 1984). All the above techniques are employed together with gentle abdominal massage, back rubbing (Hedstrom and Newton 1986) and the use of water in a shower or bath (Smith 1987) to produce relaxation. Psychoprophylaxis works best where the woman remains at home until labour is established, adopting the most comfortable position for her, remaining active (Carlson et al. 1986) and being accompanied by a trusted companion throughout labour. Teaching of these techniques is available in the United Kingdom through many hospital antenatal classes, the National Childbirth Trust and local Active Birth Groups.

Acupuncture is an ancient technique whose mechanism is still improperly understood, but does have a significant psychological component (Chapman 1984). It is reliant upon lines of energy, known as meridians, which pass throughout the body (Bonica 1974). Along these meridians there are acupuncture points which can be stimulated by pressure, the insertion of needles or the use of needles plus a small electrical current (Bonica 1974). For acupuncture in labour, it is necessary to utilise areas which do not restrict the mother's mobility or interfere with the conduct of labour. Skelton and Flowerdew (1988) recommend 3 points between the knee and the ankle on 1 knee only or 2 points on the ear. Individual differences require some trial and error until the trained practitioner locates the exact points. Helms (1987) in a randomised trial, showed the effectiveness of acupuncture for the relief of dysmenhorroea. Most studies of its use in labour have been either descriptive or involved non-randomised self-selected groups (Simkin 1989).

Transcutaneous Electrical Nerve Stimulation (TENS) is the passage of a small electrical current through the skin between two pairs of electrodes, attached either side of the spine in the lumbar and sacral regions. It was originally developed for the control of chronic pain. TENS acts by stimulating the release of natural endorphins (Sjolund *et al.* 1977). The woman herself controls the frequency of the current, which is kept low (below the woman's pain threshold) between contractions, but can be increased to obtain maximum pain relief by competing with the pain stimuli. Further research into the effectiveness of this technique is being carried out. The advantages of this technique are that it is self-administered and non-invasive (Simkin 1989). In a randomised controlled trial by Harrison *et al.* (1986) where, unknown to the woman or her attendant the apparatus did or did not produce an electrical current, mothers using the active machines reported that it was helpful in labour. This group used less epidural analgesia, although use of other analgesics was unaffected. Harrison *et al.* (1986) noted though, that the experimental group reported feeling more intense pain.

Hypnosis is being used antenatally and in labour to achieve relaxation and analgesia (Simkin 1989). It was first used in childbirth in the nineteenth century. Hypnosis has the following effects: an increase in physical and mental relaxation, modification (increase and decrease) of memory, focusing of concentration and control of physiological processes such as respiration and the cardiovascular system (Olson 1984). It can be achieved by a trained practitioner, but more commonly in labour it is self-induced often using an audiotape. Some general practitioners are offering hypnosis in their practice. Brann and Guzvica (1987), in their self-selected sample, reported greater satisfaction and a reduction of anxiety. Freeman *et al.* (1986), in a randomised trial of self-hypnosis amongst primiparae, demonstrated no difference in the amount of analgesia used, although the hypnosis group were more likely to be happy with their labour.

All the above have no effect on the fetus; the following methods, which involve drugs however, have constitutional effects on both mother and fetus.

Inhalational analgesia for relieving pain in childbirth was first used in 1847 by James Young Simpson in Edinburgh. From 1853, when Queen Victoria used chloroform to assist in the birth of her seventh child, it began to gain in popularity (Dickersin 1989). Its use met with opposition from medical and religious circles who deplored interventions which affected the divine order of pain in childbirth (Wakley 1858). The gas of choice now is a mixture of 50% oxygen and 50% nitrous oxide given via an apparatus known as an Entonox machine, which is approved for use by British midwives. The gas is administered via a facemask or a mouthpiece (Dolan and Rosen 1975) attached to a one-way valve on the cylinder, which delivers the gas when the woman takes a deep breath (Tunstall 1961). The two gases separate at temperatures below 6°C, the nitrous oxide liquidises and falls to the bottom of the cylinder causing the mother to breathe pure oxygen (Cole *et al.* 1970). The apparatus should therefore be kept at room temperature.

The woman should be in charge of administering the gas herself; the mask should never be held by anyone else, so she should not breathe too much nitrous oxide and become unconscious. The mother should be instructed to breathe the gas as the contraction is beginning, so she experiences maximum analgesia at the height of the contraction (Crawford 1982). She can then stop using the gas whilst having its analgesic effects for a further 20 seconds (Crawford 1982). Overbreathing should be avoided, since carbon dioxide depletion occurs and respiration may be depressed. A warning sign of this is the woman complaining of a tingling sensation in her limbs. Other disadvantages are that some women do not like the mask or the mouthpiece; it can induce feelings of nausea, can dry the mouth and the analgesic effect may be insufficient.

Systemic analgesia

The most commonly used in the United Kingdom is the narcotic pethidine (USA Demerol) which can be given both intravenously and by intramuscular injection (Crawford 1982). Given intramuscularly (IM), it reaches its maximum effect in 1 hour. The usual dose IM is 50–150 mg, depending on maternal size. If given when labour is not yet in the active phase, uterine contractions can be depressed (James 1960). Pethidine readily crosses the placenta, so it is not advisable to administer it within 2–3 hours of delivery, to avoid depression of the fetal respiratory centre (Shnider and Levinson 1987); this effect is most marked when pethidine is given intravenously (Bonica 1967). Morrison (1973) showed that neonatal respiratory depression was most common where the pethidine had been given between 3 and 6 hours prior to delivery, but did not occur at all at intervals of less than 1 hour.

When using continuous electrical fetal monitoring, a loss of beat-to-beat variation may be noted for 60–90 minutes after administration. Whether this is due to fetal vagal overactivity or direct effects upon the myocardium is unclear (Crawford 1982). The effectiveness of pethidine as an analgesic in labour is questionable (Beazley *et al.* 1967; Dickersin 1989). Women comment that it makes them drowsy and less able to cope with the pain of the contractions. Other maternal effects are a delay in gastric emptying time, and nausea (Nimmo *et al.* 1975). Because of this, pethidine is often combined with an anti-emetic to reduce the risk of vomiting.

Local/regional anaesthesia

Local anaesthesia is used by midwives when infiltrating the perineum with lignocaine prior to performance or repair of an episiotomy. Medical staff use lignocaine for this purpose and also for achieving a pudendal nerve block prior to performing a forceps delivery. Its effectiveness depends on careful accurate infiltration and allowing sufficient time for the anaesthetic to take effect before commencing the procedure. Regional anaesthesia in obstetrics is usually given via an epidural, which allows repeated doses of anaesthetic to be administered. Less commonly, a caudal block may be established, to permit the performance of a forceps delivery (Dickersin 1989).

The epidural can be inserted by an experienced anaesthetist at any stage in labour. Not all hospitals offer this facility; 24 hour anaesthetic cover is a requisite to having an epidural service (Reynolds 1986). The use of epidurals in the United Kingdom was given a boost by the 1970 decision by the Central Midwives' Board to permit midwives to 'top-up' the epidural (Doughty 1978). Analgesia from the lower abdomen downwards is achieved with an associated variable loss of mobility in the lower limbs (Crawford 1978).

Vasodilation in the lower half of the body can cause hypotension (Crawford 1982); for this reason an intravenous infusion line is established and most anaesthetists prefer to administer 500 ml of a crystalloid plasma expander prior to inserting the epidural (Crawford 1982). Epinephrine should be available to deal with a severe fall in blood pressure (Ralston *et al.* 1974). It is important that prior to giving consent to an epidural, the woman fully understands exactly how she will be affected, for example as regards loss of sensation and movement in the lower limbs.

Baseline recordings of maternal pulse and blood pressure and fetal heart rate are taken, since hypotension can reduce placental perfusion (Crawford 1982). The mother should be offered a bedpan before the epidural is inserted while she still has the ability to consciously empty her bladder.

To insert the cannula, it is necessary to emphasise the space between the vertebrae (Crawford 1978). This is achieved by the woman curling herself up either sitting or laying on the edge of the bed. Following a small injection of local anaesthetic (to numb the insertion site), a Tuohy needle is used to insert the cannula midway into the space between the spinous processes of the first and second, second and third or third and fourth thoracic vertebrae. The needle passes through the skin; supraspinous and intraspinous ligaments to meet the tough ligamentum flavum. A glass syringe containing 10 ml of normal saline is attached to the Tuohy needle; pressure is exerted on the syringe whilst pushing the needle through the ligamentum flavum. As soon as a loss of resistance is felt, the needle has passed through the ligament (Crawford 1982).

The cannula is introduced and positioned in the epidural space (which is in fact a potential rather than an actual space); a bacterial filter is fitted to the free end. A test dose of short-acting local anaesthetic (usually lignocaine) is given to confirm that the cannula is correctly positioned (that the cannula is in far enough and also that a spinal anaesthetic has not been achieved). The maternal response to the injection of lignocaine gives a rapid response and is short-acting (Crawford 1982). The cannula is then kept in position with waterproof strapping attached to the mother's back. Maternal pulse, blood pressure and fetal heart rate are checked every 5 minutes for 20 minutes to detect any hypotension (Crawford 1978). This procedure is repeated every time any anaesthetic is given. If the test dose is satisfactory, further doses of bupivacaine (Marcain) can then be given. The first full dose is always given by an anaesthetist in the United Kingdom. Since this is heavier than the fluid in the epidural space, it may be necessary to reposition the woman following a top-up dose, to obtain an even spread of analgesia.

Where a midwife takes on the topping-up of the epidural, she must observe certain precautions:

1. The top-up dose prescribed by the anaesthetist must be the same as the previous dose given.
2. The previous dose must have been effective.
3. There must be no maternal or fetal complications to blood pressure or fetal heart rate.
4. The prescribed dose must be checked by two midwives.
5. The prescription chart must be signed and maternal observations recorded.

Epidural anaesthesia is useful for women with hypertension, as it prevents further rises in blood pressure (Moir *et al.* 1972). It is also helpful in a prolonged labour to reduce maternal exhaustion or where there is a malposition or malpresentation. An epidural does have the effect of increasing the length of the first stage of labour by 1 hour on average (Studd *et al.* 1980); the second stage is also lengthened, possibly caused by relaxation of the pelvic floor, which slows down internal rotation (Crawford 1982). In cases where systemic analgesia is contra-indicated, such as preterm labour and for operative deliveries, an epidural can be appropriate. Contra-indications include coagulation disorders, spinal anomalies, hypotension, neurological disease and maternal refusal. Many women using epidural anaesthesia perceive no feelings of pressure during the second stage of labour and may either be unaware of the onset of the second stage or have difficulties in pushing (Crawford 1978). In some cases, the anaesthetic is allowed to 'wear-off' to allow active pushing, whilst in others the uterine action is sufficiently strong not to require maternal effort to expel the baby. Care should be taken before deciding not to give further doses of anaesthetic, especially when the epidural has been *in situ* since before labour (e.g. for induction of labour). It is cruel to expose a woman who has had no chance to become accustomed to the contractions to the severe pains of second stage-labour.

Complications of an epidural include having an incomplete nerve block; the mother may simply need to lay on her opposite side in order to achieve even distribution of the anaesthetic or the cannula may need to be withdrawn slightly (Crawford 1978). Very rarely the dura mater is punctured and a spinal anaesthetic is given; an early sign of this is the mother complaining that her tongue feels tingly or numb. Medical help must be sought and the woman may require ventilatory support until the effects wear off.

Fetal well-being

The primary method of assessing well-being of the fetus in labour (see also Chapter 22) is by listening to and counting the fetal heart rate. This is performed every 15 minutes when the mother is in active labour. The heart can be heard using a Pinard's stethoscope or a portable doptone machine. To use the stethoscope successfully, the mother should be recumbent (with a wedge on one side to avoid supine hypotension). Where the mother is unable to move easily, is asleep or where she is keeping mobile during the labour, the doptone is easier to use. It also has the added advantage of causing less discomfort (Garcia *et al.* 1985) and all those present can hear the heart beat clearly, which gives reassurance to the woman and her partner. Using the Pinard's stethoscope, the best time to listen is just after a contraction has finished. Recovery from any heart rate decelerations can be clearly heard. Using the doptone, it is possible to assess the fetal heart rate both during and in between contractions. It may be necessary to reposition the transducer downwards with contractions, as the fetus is being pushed further into the pelvis. All recordings of the fetal heart rate should be recorded on the partogram. The normal fetal heart baseline is between 120 and 160 beats/minute (Hon 1958). Any abnormalities, such as decelerations not associated with contractions or bradycardia or tachycardia should be recorded in the notes and reported to the relevant medical attendant (obstetrician or general practitioner).

Continuous recordings of the fetal heart can be made using cardiotocograph or via ECG readings from a scalp electrode. Ninety-six per cent of deliveries in the United Kingdom take place in units with facilities for continuous monitoring (Grant 1987a). The need for these techniques depends on whether the labour is classed as being at high or low risk and on the presence of anomalies during the current labour. For a discussion of the value of continuous monitoring see Chapter 22.

The colour of the amniotic fluid gives another indication of fetal well-being. Fresh meconium in the absence of a breech presentation is considered a sign of potential fetal distress, which requires further investigation (Miller 1985). The presence of old meconium (giving a greenish tinge to the liquor) demonstrates a previous 'insult' to the fetus; further observation is necessary to ensure normal progress through labour (Miller 1985). Both obstetricians and paediatricians need to be informed about the presence of fresh meconium staining. The former because this is now a high-risk labour and the latter because they will need to be present at delivery to ensure meconium aspiration does not occur. Passage of meconium is associated with increased rates of perinatal mortality and morbidity (Miller 1985).

Conduct of the second stage

Diagnosis and duration

The second stage of labour commences when the cervix is fully dilated and lasts until the baby has been delivered. Uterine contractions during the second stage have an intrauterine pressure of 85 mmHg, which rises to 165 mmHg with maternal effort (Caldeyro Barcia 1979b). The onset of the second stage is not always diagnosed, since a mother may feel the urge to push before or sometime after the start of the stage. Maresh (1987) divides the second stage into two phases. A latent phase, during which descent and rotation occur, and an active phase with descent and the urge to push. In the absence of complications and where the mother does not feel the urge to push, it is now acceptable to wait for the active phase when maternal effort is more appropriate (Maresh 1987). This helps to prevent maternal overexertion. In the presence of fetal or maternal complications, such as fetal distress or maternal hypertension, delivery should be expedited. The length of the second stage has been a subject of much discussion (Thomson 1988). The second stage is considered to be the time of greatest risk to the fetus and therefore there were recommendations that it should be limited (Hamilton 1861). Thomson (1988) quotes personal experience of a 30 minute time limit. Garcia *et al.* (1986) in their survey of UK maternity units, showed that many hospitals applied limits of 30 minutes for multiparae and 60 minutes for primiparae, although it is far from clear cut how the diagnosis of the second stage is made (Sleep *et al.* 1989). Pushing before the mother has the urge to push will increase the rate of forceps deliveries (Maresh 1987). Reynolds and Yudkin (1987) showed that 56.5% of primiparous women in their study had spontaneous deliveries following second stages of 90–120 minutes, 37% had 121–150 minutes and 31.8% had more than 150 minutes. Prolonged pushing has been shown to be more damaging to the fetus than a long second stage (Maresh 1987).

Position

As with the first stage of labour, the 'normal' mother has a choice of positions which she can adopt for delivery. Garcia *et al.* (1986) showed that 87% of UK maternity units surveyed respected the woman's choice of position, but only 43% of the Canadian units did so. However it must be questioned how many midwives actively encourage women to adopt alternative positions. In the West, most women prefer to remain semirecumbent upon the delivery bed supported by wedges and cushions or they are put into dorsal positions or lithotomy (this last is common in the United States). This could be due to lack of knowledge, the portrayal of birth in the media or the adoption of the 'sick role'. These positions are not physiological and they do not accord with the practices in more traditional societies (Thomson 1988). Thomson (1988) is critical of the UK practice of positioning the mother in a semirecumbent position where the midwives put her feet on their hips. This places the legs wider apart than would be achieved when squatting, is uncomfortable and puts undue strain on the perineum. Some hospitals have birthing chairs or beds which can be adapted to whatever position the woman requests. Mattresses can be placed on the floor to assist the woman who wants to deliver on 'all fours' whilst small stools can be used should she wish to adopt a supported squatting position. The midwife may find some of these positions less easy to manage than with the mother semirecumbent, especially for visibility of the perineum; this is part of the reason why delivery in bed became so popular following the intervention of doctors into childbirth in the seventeenth century (Donnison 1977). Practice in different ways of management can do much to increase a midwife's confidence and adaptability to meet the wishes of the women to whom she gives care.

Pushing

As with many practices in labour, there has been a change in the way that women are encouraged to push. The practice of organised pushing and breath-holding was first challenged by Beynon (1957) in her non-randomised study comparing 'organised' with 'voluntary' pushing. There were no differences between the groups with regard to the time taken to deliver but the voluntary group had less need for perineal repair. There has been a move to encourage spontaneous pushing which is of shorter duration (5 seconds) than organised pushing (10–15 seconds), since this causes less fetal hypoxia (Caldeyro Barcia 1979b). Organised pushing with a closed glottis (Valsalva Manoeuvre) increases maternal intrathoracic pressure, reduces venous return and cardiac output, causing a fall in blood pressure and a reduction in placental perfusion (Straddling 1984). It has also been argued that such prolonged breath-holding does not make for efficient pushing, since the abdominal muscles tighten and are displaced away from the uterus, therefore not contributing to expulsion of the fetus (Grant 1987b). In a preliminary study to compare the effect of organised maternal pushing (with the glottis closed) versus spontaneous pushing, Thomson (1990) suggests that directed efforts are disadvantageous to the baby where the second stage is long. There are no demonstrated hazards to mother or baby of spontaneous pushing techniques (Thomson 1990).

Clear, concise records of progress in the second stage must be maintained. It is required practice to record the fetal heart rate between each contraction and maternal pulse after alternate contractions, and to measure blood pressure every 15 minutes if elevated and hourly during the active phase of pushing. Stewart (1984), analysing 39 cardiotocograph traces from the second stage of labour from infants born with good Apgar scores and cord blood pHs, found that 70% had decelerations with contractions. Fifteen per cent of these were early, 50% were prolonged and 5% were late. Normal fetal heart rate response in the second stage is somewhat erratic and hard to evaluate (Stewart 1984).

The woman and her partner should be kept informed of progress; a mirror can be used so that the mother can see for herself. The decision about when to prepare for delivery depends on the mother's parity and her rate of progress. Sterile gloves are always worn for delivery, to aid grip and to prevent contamination with the mother's blood; a gown is still usual, but masks are becoming rare as their use has not shown any benefit in reducing infection.

Conduct of delivery

The vulva and perineum

The woman's vulva and perineum is swabbed with an antiseptic solution. Drapes, if used are positioned. Where the delivery is taking place with the woman in an upright position, the drapes should be placed on the floor.

Delivery of the head

The midwife's aim is to maintain the smallest diameter of the head coming through the pelvis. This is usually achieved by keeping the head well flexed, although there is limited research as to the effectiveness of this procedure. In addition, the head is delivered as slowly as possible to prevent damage to the perineum (by allowing the perineal tissues to stretch gradually) (Sleep *et al*. 1989). This may involve requesting the woman not to push during a contraction either by panting or by breathing nitrous oxide and oxygen, or with a parous woman, by giving small pushes between contractions. (There is no research to demonstrate the effect of 'guarding' the perineum on the prevention of perineal tears (Sleep *et al*. 1989).) Once the biparietal diameters are born, the grip of the delivering hand is altered to allow extension of the head.

The perineum

In circumstances where the perineum is about to tear, an episiotomy may be performed but the most usual indication is to hasten delivery in cases of fetal distress or maternal exhaustion. However there is little evidence supporting the belief that an episiotomy reduces the risks of perineal tears (Chalmers *et al*. 1976). Sleep *et al*. (1984) demonstrated that there was little difference between an episiotomy and a tear regarding pain, resumption of sexual intercourse and integrity of the pelvic floor (Sleep *et al*. 1984; Sleep and Grant 1987). Before performing an episiotomy a 'fan shaped' area of the perineum is infiltrated with lignocaine (0.5 or 1% depending on local policy). The lignocaine takes approximately 5 minutes to take effect and anaesthesia lasts up to 2 hours (Laurence 1973). Once this has taken effect an episiotomy can be performed at the height of a contraction. To expedite delivery, the head should already be well applied to the thinned perineum before the episiotomy is performed. If it is not, delivery will be delayed and all that will have been achieved is a significant blood loss from the incised unthinned perineum (Myerscough 1982).

In the United Kingdom a mediolateral episiotomy is the most common (Sleep *et al*. 1989), whereas in the United States the preference is for the midline. The latter is associated with an increased frequency of third-degree tears (Thorp *et al*. 1987). Although the frequency of performance of an episiotomy has been significantly reduced in recent years, Sleep *et al*. (1984) estimated that 69% of women will need repair of perineal trauma whether intentional or spontaneous. Logue (1990) stated that the episiotomy rate for their unit in 1987 was 12%. When she reviewed the 1985 figures in relation to the position adopted for birth, the rates for intact perineums for primiparous women were as follows (the figure for multiparous women is given in brackets): birthing chair 17% (34%), dorsal 33% (52%) and lateral 58% (67%) (Logue 1990). In addition, whilst the rate of performance of episiotomies varied with individual midwives, it was not related to the length of experience of the midwife (Logue 1990).

Restriction of the performance of an episiotomy to cases of fetal distress or imminent tearing does appear to reduce the overall rate of trauma (Sleep *et al.* 1984). The two randomly allocated groups in their study ('liberal' and 'restricted' episiotomy) showed no significant differences in subsequent dyspareunia at 3 months and 3 years after delivery, or as regards long-term urinary incontinence (Sleep and Grant 1987). Pelvic floor muscle tone is related more to overall fitness and activity level than to childbirth or a history of perineal trauma (Gordon and Logue 1985).

Checking for cord

Once the head is delivered, the chin should be freed and a careful check made to ensure that the umbilical cord is not wrapped around the baby's neck. This is done by gently pressing down on the back of the baby's head and feeling for the cord under the symphysis pubis. If a loose loop of the cord is present, it should be passed over the baby's head before checking for the presence of another loop. If the cord is tight, two artery forceps are applied to the cord and a cut made between them. The cord is then unwrapped from around the neck.

Restitution

Restitution is the undoing of the twist in the baby's neck following internal rotation of the baby's head. This occurs before a contraction, during which internal rotation of the shoulders, followed by external rotation of the head, takes place.

Delivery of the head and body

Once the shoulders are in the antero-posterior diameter of the pelvis, the mother can give a short push with the next contraction to assist in delivering the anterior shoulder. The midwife should place the palms of her hands on either side of the baby's head. When the contraction occurs, gentle downward (or backward if the mother is upright) pressure should help free the anterior shoulder from under the symphysis pubis. To aid holding the baby, the little finger of the upper hand can be gently inserted in the upper axilla. The baby is then lifted up to free the posterior shoulder and the body is delivered by lateral flexion in the direction of the Curve of Carus. The baby can be delivered onto drapes on the mother's abdomen if she wishes. The mother and/or father may also be encouraged to hold their baby as he or she is being born.

Resuscitation of the newborn

The vast majority of babies breathe spontaneously at birth and require no resuscitation at all. Rosen and Roberton (1984) estimate that 85% of babies require no resuscitation, 10% require minor attention, and only 5% will need artificial respiration. Of this final group 30–40% will have shown no previous signs of distress or compromise (Ritchie and McClure 1985; Roberton 1986). Therefore the midwife may find herself with an unexpectedly asphyxiated baby. Medical help is usually present when such a delivery is anticipated, although it is important that a midwife can assess a baby at birth or decide whether resuscitation is required and when to summon aid. She should then be able to commence the resuscitation procedure while waiting for help to arrive. Because births occur where paediatric cover is not immediately available, the midwife must be capable of initiating and continuing treatment to effect resuscitation and to maintain the baby in the best possible condition.

For the vast majority of normally delivered babies, the stimulation of birth together with being dried with a towel cause the babies to breathe spontaneously. The procedure of routinely using suction to clear the baby's airway has not been evaluated (Tyson et al. 1989). The various categories of babies for whom the midwife might need to provide resuscitation are as follows:

1. The baby who breathes normally (but not lustily) initially but then becomes cyanosed and sleepy after birth (hard to rouse and unresponsive to stimulae); these babies have often received narcotic analgesia across the placenta which depresses the neonatal respiratory centre.
2. Babies with a good heart rate but no respiratory effort.
3. The severely depressed baby who is pale and bradycardic, making no attempt at respiration.

The first baby requires respiratory support; drugs such as narcotic antagonists may be given to reverse the sedative effects. The other two categories require respiratory support. The principal method of assessing the baby's respiratory and cardiovascular status is the Apgar score, which is recorded at 1, 5 and if necessary 10 minutes after birth, although if resuscitation is needed this must begin before the 1 minute score is determined (Tyson et al. 1989). The Apgar score is a useful measure of respiratory failure and of the need for ventilatory support (Roberton 1986) but its use is more limited where the baby is preterm, especially in the presence of birth asphyxia (Catlin et al. 1986). A weakness in the Apgar score is that similar scores do not differentiate sufficiently the variations in well-being which gave rise to them (Roberton 1986) (see Table 20.1).

Scores at 1 minute of 7–10 indicate no respiratory depression, 4–6 mild/moderate depression and 3 or less denotes severe depression (Roberton 1986). For midwives, unless especially trained to intubate the baby, the management of all respiratory depressed babies is similar.

Table 20.1 The Apgar score

Clinical Score Sign	0	1	2
Heart rate	0	Less than 100	More than 100
Respiration	Absent	Gasping or irregular	Crying lustily
Muscle tone	Limp	Diminished or normal without movements	Normal with active active movements
Reponse to Stimuli	None	Slight grimace	Cough or cry
Colour of trunk	White	Blue	Pink

(Apgar 1958)

- The umbilical cord should be clamped and cut. The baby should be placed head down on a warmed resuscitaire (overhead heater switched on). The clock should be started. The baby should be dried with a warm towel and its condition assessed with respect to heart rate, colour and respiration.
- The airways should be cleared using a suction catheter. It is usual to clear the nostrils first as babies are nose breathers. These are also quicker to clear than the mouth. This suction should be performed gently; care should be taken not to advance the catheter too far, since laryngeal spasm can occur (Tyson *et al.* 1989). A suction bulb is preferred to perform the initial clearing of the airways, as this is less likely to give rise to a cardiac arythmia than a catheter performing 'blind' suctioning (Cordero and Hon 1971).
- To maintain an airway, care should be taken not to hyperextend the head, which in neonates stretches and narrows the larynx (Rosen and Roberton 1984). A neonatal airway can be inserted.
- Intermittent positive pressure ventilation (IPPV) by bag and mask is given using a well-fitting baby face mask with an oxygen supply and a paediatric ambu bag. The oxygen should be given at no more than 30 cm of water pressure; this is achieved by having a built-in pressure valve in the bag, which prevents excess pressure being applied. Alternatively, the oxygen supply can pass through a water manometer. Ritchie and McClure (1985) recommend that the lowest possible pressure is used to ensure gentle movements of the chest wall, air entry into the lungs and the achievement of an acceptable skin colour. The bag should be gently squeezed 40–60 times a minute whilst observing the chest for signs of movement. If an assistant is present, she can listen for air entry into the lungs. Once the baby is no longer cyanosed the rate can be reduced until the baby is maintaining his/her own respiration. Bag and mask ventilation is difficult to achieve where the infant has never breathed (Milner *et al.* 1984). There is controversy surrounding the use of unhumidified fast-flowing oxygen across the baby's face which can give rise to bradycardia or breath-holding in the early minutes of life (Brown *et al.* 1976).

- If the mother has received a narcotic analgesic within 2 or 3 hours of birth, the baby may require a narcotic antagonist to reverse its depressant effects on the respiratory centre (Roberton 1986). Naloxone hydrochloride (Narcan) is the narcotic antagonist for morphine and pethidine. The dosage is 0.01 mg/kg body weight or 0.03 mg for an average weight neonate. It can be given intramuscularly or intravenously and is effective intramuscularly in 2–3 minutes. If local policy permits, it can be given intravenously by the midwife but usually only intramuscular administration is permitted.
- For the more severely respiratory-depressed neonate with little or no heartbeat present, an assistant should give cardiac massage while IPPV with bag and mask is occurring (Moya *et al.* 1962). Cardiac massage is given by placing both hands around the baby's trunk with two thumbs against the lower part of the sternum (Ostheimer 1982). Care should be taken with this procedure, since excessive pressure can cause fractures of the ribs and damage to the lungs and liver (Tyson *et al.* 1989). The chest is gently compressed for 1 second every 10 seconds. In between IPPV is given. If a heartbeat is present, the lungs are ventilated 3 or 4 times before further massage until the heart rate picks up (Rosen and Roberton 1984).
- Endotracheal intubation of neonates is a difficult technique, which if incorrectly performed can cause further problems. However, all midwives need a knowledge of this technique for the occasion when, in the absence of medical assistance, the neonate fails to breathe following bag and mask treatment and there is a severe bradycardia of less than 60 beats/minute.

The technique is as follows:

1. The baby is positioned head down on the resuscitaire.
2. The neonatal laryngoscope is checked to see it is working. (The laryngoscope and resuscitation equipment should be checked frequently, preferably at each change-over of staff and always following use.)
3. Holding the laryngoscope in the left hand and opening the baby's mouth with the right, the laryngoscope is gently introduced into the mouth. The tongue is pushed to the left and the uvula can be seen between the tonsils (Figure 20.5).
4. Gently pushing the laryngoscope over the back of the tongue, suction can be used (in the right hand) to clear any secretions present. The epiglottis can then be seen (Figure 20.6).
5. By placing the laryngoscope in front of the epiglottis, the tongue can be lifted forward, revealing the larynx. Gentle pressure by an assistant on the cricoid cartilage makes this easier (Figure 20.7).
6. The neonatal endotracheal tube can then be introduced through the larynx until its broadest part is against the vocal cords. Carefully holding the ET tube, the laryngoscope is gently withdrawn.
7. Oxygen tubing connected to a blow-off valve, set at 30 cm of water to prevent excess pressure (Roberton 1986) and a Y connector is attached to the ET tube.

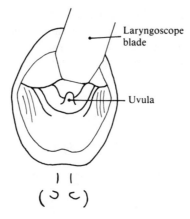

Figure 20.5 Uvula and oropharynx viewed as the laryngoscope is passed.

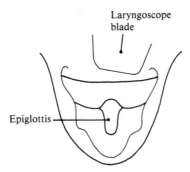

Figure 20.6 View of the epiglottis during intubation.

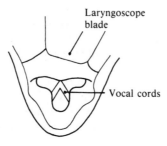

Figure 20.7 Vocal cords seen with the aid of the laryngoscope.

IPPV is given by placing the thumb over the open end of the Y in the connector, a rate of 40–60 breaths/minute is usually used (Roberton 1986). It is helpful to listen to air entry into the lungs with a stethoscope. Oxygen is given at a flow rate between 2 and 4 l/minute.

The birth of an asphyxiated baby is a great shock to the parents. It is vital to keep them informed at all stage of what is going on, since silence is even more distressing than lack of progress. When medical aid arrives, a full description of the treatment given should be made before recordings are made in the baby's records.

References

Apgar V (1958) 'Evaluation of the newborn: second repeat' *Journal of the American Medical Association* 168: 1985

Baird D (1952) 'The cause and prevention of difficult labour' *American Journal of Obstetrics and Gynecology* 63: 1200–12

Beazley J M, Leaver E P, Morewood J H M and Birkhumshaw J (1967) 'Relief of pain in labour' *Lancet* i: 1033

Beynon C (1957) 'The normal second stage of labour, a plea for reform of its conduct' *Journal of Obstetrics and Gynaecology of the British Empire* 64: 815–20

Bonica J J (1967) *Obstetric Analgesia and Anaesthesia* Davis: Philadelphia

Bonica J J (1974) 'Acupuncture anesthesia in the Peoples' Republic of China: Implications for British medicine' *Acupuncture Anesthesia* 229: 1317–25

Bonica J J (1986) 'Pain of parturition' *Clinics in Anaesthesiology* 4(1): 1–31

Brann L R and Guzvica S A (1987) 'Comparison of hypnosis with conventional relaxation for antenatal and intrapartum use' *Journal of the Royal College of General Practitioners* 37: 437–40

Brown E L and Deffenbacher K (1979) *Perception and the Senses* Oxford University Press: Oxford

Brown W, Ostheimer G, Bell G and Datta S (1976) 'Newborn response to oxygen blown over the face' *Anesthesiology* 44: 535–6

Caldeyro Barcia R (1979a) 'Physiological and psychological bases for the modern and humanised management of normal labour' *Recent Progress in Perinatal Medicine and Prevention of Congenital Anomaly* Tokyo Ministry of Health and Welfare 77–96

Caldeyro Barcia R (1979b) 'The influence of maternal bearing down efforts during the second stage of labour on foetal wellbeing' *Birth and Family Journal* 6(10): 17–21

Caldeyro Barcia R, Giussi G and Storch E (1979) 'The bearing-down efforts and their effects on fetal heart rate, oxygenation and acid base balance' *Journal of Perinatal Medicine* 9: 63–7

Cardozo L and Studd J (1985) 'Abnormal labour patterns' in J Studd (ed) *Management of Labour* Ch 12 171–87 Blackwell Scientific: Oxford

Carlson J M, Diehl J A, Sachtleben-Murray M, McRae M, Fenwick L and Friedman E A (1986) 'Maternal position during parturition in normal labor' *Obstetrics and Gynecology* 68: 443–7

Cartwright A (1979) *The Dignity of Labour* Tavistock: London

Catlin E, Carpenter M, Brann B, Mayfield S, Shaul P, Goldstein M and Oh W (1986) 'The Apgar revisited: influence of gestational age' *Journal of Pediatrics* 109: 865–8

Chalmers I, Garcia J and Post S (1989) 'Hospital policies for labour and delivery' in I Chalmers, M Enkin and M J N C Keirse (eds) *Effective Care in Pregnancy and Childbirth* Ch 50 815–9 Oxford Medical: Oxford

Chalmers I, Zlosnik J E, Johns J A and Campbell H (1976) 'Obstetric practice and outcome of pregnancy in Cardiff residents 1965–73' *British Medical Journal* 1: 735–8

Chapman C R (1984) 'New directions in the understanding and management of pain' *Social Science in Medicine* 19: 1261–77

Cole P V, Crawford J S, Doughty A G, Epstein H G, Hill I G, Rollaston W N and Tunstall M E (1970) 'Specifications and recommendations for nitrous oxide/oxygen apparatus to be used in obstetric analgesia' *Anaesthesia* 25: 317

Cordero L and Hon E H (1971) 'Neonatal bradycardia following nasopharyngeal stimulation' *Journal Pediatrics* 78: 441–7

Crawford J S (1978) *Principles and Practice of Obstetric Anaesthesia* (4th edn) Blackwell Scientific: Oxford

Crawford J S (1982) *Obstetric Analgesia and Anaesthesia* Churchill Livingstone: Edinburgh

Crawford J S (1985) 'The phases and stages of labour' *British Journal of Hospital Medicine* July 32–6

Crowther C, Enkin M, Keirse M J N C and Brown I (1989) 'Monitoring the progress of labour' in I Chalmers, M Enkin and M J N C Keirse (eds) *Effective Care in Pregnancy and Childbirth* Ch 53 833–45 Oxford University Press: Oxford

Department of Health (1989) *Confidential Enquiry into Maternal Deaths in England and Wales 1982–84* HMSO: London

Department of Health and Social Security (1969) *Confidential Enquiries into Maternal Deaths in England and Wales 1964–6* HMSO: London

Department of Health and Social Security (1985) *Confidential Enquiries into Maternal Deaths in England and Wales 1979–81* HMSO: London

Dickersin K (1989) 'Pharmacological control of pain during labour' in I Chalmers, M Enkin and M J N C Keirse (eds) *Effective Care in Pregnancy and Childbirth* Ch 57 913–50 Oxford Medical: Oxford

Dolan P F and Rosen M (1975) 'Inhalational analgesia in labour: facemask or mouthpiece' *Lancet* ii: 1030

Donnison J (1977) *Midwives and Medical Men* Heinemann: London

Doughty A (1978) 'Epidural analgesia in labour: the past, the present and the future' *Journal of the Royal Society of Medicine* 71: 879–84

Drayton S and Rees C (1984) 'They know what they're doing: The midwife and enemas' *Research and the Midwife Proceedings* 2–21

Dumoulin J G and Foulkes J E B (1984) 'Ketonuria during labour' *British Journal of Obstetrics and Gynaecology* 91: 97–8

Engelmann G J (1882) *Labor Amongst Primitive Peoples* J H Chambers: St Louis

Enkin M, Smith S L, Dermer S W and Emmett J O (1972) 'An adequately controlled study of the effectiveness of PPM training' in N Morris (ed) *Psychosomatic Medicine in Obstetrics and Gynecology* Karger: Basel

Flint C (1984) 'Cosiness in the delivery suite' *Nursing Times* June 13: 28–30

Flint C (1991) 'The Know Your Midwife Scheme' in S Robinson and A M Thomson (eds) *Midwives, Research and Childbirth* 2: 72–103 Chapman and Hall: London

Flynn A M, Kelly J, Hollins G and Lynch P F (1978) 'Ambulation in labour' *British Medical Journal* iii: 591–3

Freeman R M, Macaulay A J, Eve L, and Chamberlain G V P (1986) 'Randomised trial of self hypnosis for analgesia in labour' *British Medical Journal* 292: 657–8

Friedman E A (1955) 'Primigravid labour – a graphostatistical analysis' *Obstetrics and Gynecology* 6: 567

Garcia J, Corry M, MacDonald D, Elbourne D and Grant A (1985) 'Mothers' views on continuous electronic fetal heart rate monitoring and intermittent auscultation in a randomised controlled trial' *Birth* 12: 79–85

Garcia J, Garforth S and Ayers S (1986) 'Midwives confined? Labour ward policies and routines' *Research and the Midwife Conference Proceedings* 74–80

Garforth S and Garcia J (1989) 'Hospital admission practices' in I Chalmers, M Enkin and M J N C Keirse (eds) *Effective Care in Pregnancy and Childbirth* Ch 51 820–6 Oxford Medical: Oxford

Gordon H and Logue M (1985) 'Perineal function after childbirth' *Lancet* ii: 123–5

Grant A (1987a) 'Equipment and services' in G V P Chamberlain and P Gunn (eds) *Birthplace* 50–100 John Wiley: Chichester

Grant J (1987b) 'Reassessing second stage' *Association of Chartered Physiotherapists in Obstetrics and Gynaecology Journal* 60(1): 26–30

Grant G and Keirse M J N C (1989) 'Prelabour rupture of membranes at term' in I Chalmers, M Enkin and M J N C Keirse (eds) *Effective Care in Pregnancy and Childbirth* Ch 64 1112–7 Oxford Medical: Oxford

Hamilton G (1861) 'Clinical observations and suggestions in obstetrics' *Edinburgh Medical Journal* 7: 313–21

Harrison R F, Woods T, Shore M, Mathews G and Unwin A (1986) 'Pain relief in labour using transcutaneous electrical nerve stimulation (TENS)' *British Journal of Obstetrics and Gynaecology* 93: 739–46

Hazle N R (1986) 'Hydration in labor: Is routine intravenous hydration necessary?' *Journal of Nurse-Midwifery* 31: 171

Hedstrom L W and Newton N (1986) 'Touch in labor: A comparison of cultures and eras' *Birth* 13: 181–6

Helms J M (1987) 'Acupuncture for the management of primary dysmenhorrea' *Obstetrics and Gynecology* 69: 51–6

Hendricks C H, Brenner W E and Kraus G (1970) 'Normal cervical dilation pattern in late pregnancy and labour' *American Journal of Obstetrics and Gynecology* 106: 1065–82

Hibbard B M C (1988) *Principles of Obstetrics* Butterworths: London

Hon E H (1958) 'The electronic evaluation of fetal heart rate: preliminary report' *American Journal of Obstetrics and Gynecology* 77: 1215–30

Jackson P (1986) 'The Huddersfield Birthplan' *Maternal and Child Heath* Jan: 14–17

James L S (1960) 'The effect of pain relief for labour and delivery on the fetus and newborn' *Anesthesiology* 21: 405–30

Johnson C, Keirse M J N C, Enkin M and Chalmers I (1989) 'Nutrition and hydration in labour' in I Chalmers, M Enkin and M J N C Keirse (eds) *Effective Care in Pregnancy and Childbirth* Ch 52 827–32 Oxford Medical: Oxford

Johnston R A and Sidall R S (1922) 'Is the usual method of preparing patients for delivery necessary or beneficial?' *American Journal of Obstetrics and Gynecology* 4: 645–50

Kadar N (1985) 'The second stage' in J Studd (ed) *The Management of Labour* Ch 19 268–86 Blackwell Scientific: Oxford

Kelly J (1983) 'Vesico-vaginal fistulae' in J Studd (ed) *Progress in Obstetrics and Gynaecology* 3(25): 324–33 Churchill Livingstone: Edinburgh

Keirse M J N C, Enkin M and Lumley J (1989) 'Social and professional support during childbirth' in I Chalmers, M Enkin and M J N C Keirse (eds) *Effective Care In Pregnancy and Childbirth* Ch 49 805–14 Oxford Medical: Oxford

Kirkham M (1983) 'Admission in labour: Teaching the patient to be patient' *Midwives Chronicle* 96(2): 44–5

Kitzinger S (1987) *Freedom and Choice in Childbirth* Penguin: Harmondsworth

Lamaze F (1984) *Painless Childbirth: The Lamaze method* Contemporary Books: Chicago

Laurence D R (1973) *Clinical Pharmacology* Churchill Livingstone: Edinburgh

Logue M (1990) 'Putting research into practice: perineal management during delivery' in S
    Robinson and A M Thomson (eds) *Midwives, Research and Childbirth Vol 2* Ch 9 252–70
    Chapman and Hall: London

Ludka L (1987) 'Fasting during labour' Paper given at the 21st International Confederation
    of Midwives Conference 26/8/87

MacIntyre S (1982) 'Communications between pregnant women and their medical and
    midwifery attendants' *Midwives Chronicle* Nov: 387–94

Maresh M (1987) 'Management of the second stage of labour' *Midwife, Health Visitor and
    Community Nurse* 23(11): 498–506

Maresh M, Choong K H and Beard R W (1983) 'Delayed pushing with lumbar epidural
    analgesia in labour' *British Journal of Obstetrics and Gynaecology* 90: 623–7

Maternity Services Advisory Committee (1984) *Maternity Care In Action, II. Intrapartum
    Care* HMSO: London

Mayer D J and Watkins L R (1984) 'Multiple endogenous opiate and non-opiate analgesia
    systems' *Advances in Pain Research and Therapy* 6: 253–76

Melzak R D (1973) *The Puzzle of Pain* Basic Books: New York

Miller F C (1985) 'Significance of meconium in amniotic fluid' in J Studd (ed) *Management
    of Labour* Ch 13 188–94 Blackwell Scientific: Oxford

Milner A D, Vyas H and Hopkin I (1984) 'Effect of exogenous surfactant on total respiratory
    system compliance' *Archives of Disease in Childhood* 59: 369–71

Moir D D and Thorburn J (1986) *Obstetric Anaesthesia and Analalgesia* Balliere Tindall:
    London

Moir D D, Victor-Rodrigues L and Willcocks J (1972) 'Epidural analgesia during labour in
    patients with pre-eclampsia' *Journal of Obstetrics and Gynaecology of the British
    Commonwealth* 79: 465

Morrison J C (1973) *American Journal of Obstetrics and Gynecology* 115: 1132

Moya F, James L S, Burnard E and Hanks E (1962) 'Cardiac massage in the newborn infant
    through the intact chest' *American Journal of Obstetrics and Gynecology* 84: 798–803

Murphy K, Greig V, Garcia J and Grant A (1986) 'Maternal considerations in the use of
    pelvic examinations in labour' *Midwifery* 2: 93–7

Myerscough P R (1982) *Munro Kerr's Operative Obstetrics* (10th edn) Balliere Tindall: London

Naaktgeboren C (1989) 'The biology of childbirth' in I Chalmers, M Enkin and M J N Keirse
    (eds) *Effective Care in Pregnancy and Childbirth* Ch 48 765–804 Oxford University Press:
    Oxford

Nimmo W S, Wilson J and Prescott L F (1975) 'Narcotic analgesics and delayed gastric
    emptying in labour' *Lancet* i: 890–3

O'Driscoll K, Stronge J M and Minogue M (1973) 'Active management of labour' *British
    Medical Journal* 3: 135–7

O'Driscoll K and Meagher D C (1980) *Active Management of Labour* W B Saunders: London

O'Driscoll K, Foley M and MacDonald D C (1984) 'Active management of labour as an
    alternative to caesarean section' *Obstetrics and Gynaecology* 63: 485–90

Olson H A (1984) 'Hypnosis in the treatment of pain' *Individual Psychology* 40: 412–23

Ostheimer G W (1982) 'Resuscitation of the newborn infant' *Clinics in Perinatology* 9(1):
    177–90

Philpott R H (1972) 'Graphic records in labour' *British Medical Journal* iv: 163

Ploss H H, Bartels M and Bartels P (1935) *Woman* Heinemann: London

Ralston D H, Shnider S M and de Lorimer A A (1974) 'Effects of equipotent ephedrine
    metaraminal, mephentermine and methoxamine on uterine blood flow in the pregnant
    ewe' *Anesthesiology* 40: 354

Read G D (1942) *Revelation of Childbirth* Heinemann: London

Read J A, Miller F C and Paul R H (1981) 'Randomised trial of ambulation versus oxytocin for labour enhancement' *American Journal of Obstetrics and Gynecology* 139: 669–72

Reynolds F (1986) 'Obstetric anaesthetic services' *British Medical Journal* 293: 403–4

Reynolds Y L and Yudkin P L (1987) 'Changes in the management of labour: 1 length and management of the second stage' *Canadian Medical Association Journal* 136(10): 1041–5

Richardson J A, Sutherland I A and Allen D W (1978) 'A cervimeter for continuous measurement of cervical dilation in labour – preliminary results' *British Journal of Obstetrics and Gynaecology* 85: 178–84

Ritchie K and McClure G (1985) 'Resuscitation of the newborn' in J Studd (ed) *Management of Labour* Ch 22 312–21 Blackwell Scientific: Oxford

Roberton N R C (1986) 'Resuscitation of the newborn' in N R C Roberton (ed) *Textbook of Neonatology* Ch 15 239–56 Churchill Livingstone: Edinburgh

Roberts J (1989) 'Maternal position in the first stage of labour' in I Chalmers, M Enkin and M J N C Keirse (eds) *Effective Care in Pregnancy and Childbirth* Ch 55 882–92 Oxford Medical: Oxford

Romney M L (1980) 'Is your enema really necessary' *British Medical Journal* 282: 1269–71

Romney M L and Gordon H (1980) 'Predelivery shaving an unjustified assault' *Journal of Obstetrics and Gynaecology* 1: 33–5

Rosen M and Roberton N R C (1984) 'Resuscitation of the newborn' *Midwives Chronicle* May 142–8

Russell J G B (1969) 'Moulding of the pelvic outlet' *Journal of Obstetrics and Gynaecology of the British Commonwealth* 76: 817–20

Rutter N, Spencer A, Mann N and Smith M (1980) 'Glucose during labour' *Lancet* ii: 155

Sammons L N (1984) 'The use of music by women during childbirth' *Journal of Nurse-Midwifery* 29: 266–70

Schnider S M, Asling J H, Holl J W and Margolis A J (1970) 'Paracervial block anaesthesia in obstetrics' *American Journal of Obstetrics and Gynecology* 107: 619

Shnider S M and Levinson G C (1987) *Anesthesia for Obstetrics* Williams and Wilkins: Baltimore

Simkin P (1986) 'Stress, pain and catecholamines in labor Part 2' *Birth* 13: 324–40

Simkin P (1989) 'Non-pharmacological methods of pain relief during labour' in I Chalmers, M Enkin and M J N C Keirse (eds) *Effective Care in Pregnancy and Childbirth* Ch 56 893–912 Oxford Medical: Oxford

Simpson J Y (1847) Answer to Religious Objections Advanced Against The Employment of Anaesthetic Agents in Midwifery and Surgery. Cited by Dickersin K (1989) 'Pharmacological control of pain during labour' in I Chalmers, M Enkin and M J N C Keirse (eds) *Effective Care in Pregnancy and Childbirth* Ch 57 913–50 Oxford Medical: Oxford

Singhi S, Kang E C and Hall J, StE (1982) 'Hazards of maternal hydration with 5% dextrose' *Lancet* ii: 335–6

Sjolund B, Ternius L and Eriksson M (1977) 'Increased cerebro-spinal fluid levels of endorphins after electro-acupuncture' *Acta Physiologica Scandanavica* 100: 382–4

Skelton I F and Flowerdew M W (1988) 'Acupuncture and labour – A summary of result's *Midwives Chronicle* May 134–7

Sleep J and Grant A (1987) 'West Berkshire perineal management trial: three year follow-up' *British Medical Journal* 295: 749–51

Sleep J, Grant A, Garcia J, Elbourne D, Spencer J and Chalmers I (1984) 'West Berkshire perineal management trial' *British Medical Journal* 289: 587–90

Sleep J, Roberts J and Chalmers I (1989) 'Care during the second stage of labour' in I Chalmers, M Enkin and M J N C Keirse (eds) *Effective Care in Pregnancy and Childbirth* Ch 66 1129–44 Oxford Medical: Oxford

Smith B (1987) 'The effect of warm-tub bathing during labour' Presentation at the Third International Congress on Pre and Perinatal Psychology, San Francisco, California July 9–12

Stewart K S (1984) 'The second stage' in J Studd (ed) *Progress in Obstetrics and Gynaecology* Vol 4 Ch 14 197–216 Churchill Livingstone: Edinburgh

Straddling J (1984) 'Respiratory physiology during labour' *Midwife, Health Visitor and Community Nurse* 20(2): 38–42

Studd J (1973) 'Partograms and normograms of cervical dilatation in management of primigravid labour' *British Medical Journal* iv: 451–5

Studd J W, Crawford J S, Duignan A M, Rowbotham C J F and Hughes A O (1980) 'Effect of lumbar epidural upon cervimetric progress and the outcome of spontaneous labour' *British Journal of Obstetrics and Gynaecology* 87: 1015

Studd J W, Cardozo C D and Gibb D M F (1982) 'The management of spontaneous labour' in J Studd (ed) *Progress in Obstetrics and Gynaecology* 2: 7: 60–72 Churchill Livingstone: Edinburgh

Thomson A M (1988) 'Management of women in normal second stage of labour: a review' *Midwifery* 4(2): 77–85

Thomson A M (1990) 'Pilot study of a randomised controlled trial of pushing techniques in the second stage of labour' *Proceedings of the 22nd Congress of the International Confederation of Midwives, Kobe Japan* 225 Japanese Nursing Association: Tokyo

Thorp J M, Bowes W A and Brame R G (1987) 'Selected use of midline episiotomy: effect on perineal trauma' *Obstetrics and Gynecology* 70: 260–2

Tunstall M E (1961) 'The use of a fixed nitrous oxide and oxygen mixture from one cylinder' *Lancet* ii: 964

Turnbull A (1957) 'Uterine contractions in normal and abnormal labour' *Journal of Obstetrics and Gynaecology of the British Empire* 64: 321–3

Tyson J, Silverman W and Reisch J (1989) 'Immediate care of the infant' in I Chalmers, M Enkin and M J N C Keirse (eds) *Effective Care in Pregnancy and Childbirth* Ch 75 1293–1312 Oxford Medical: Oxford

Ueland K and Hanson J M (1969) 'Maternal cardiovascular dynamics II. Posture and uterine contractions' *American Journal of Obstetrics and Gynecology* 103: 1–8

Varney H (1987) *Nurse-Midwifery (2nd edn)* Blackwell Scientific: Oxford

Velvovsky I, Platnov K, Ploticher V and Shogum E (1960) *Painless Childbirth Through Psychoprophylaxis* Foreign language Publishing House: Moscow

Voorhees J D (1906) 'The etiology of puerperal sepsis' *American Journal of Obstetrics* 53: 762

Wakley T (1858) 'Administration of chloroform to the Queen' *Lancet* 14 May 453 Cited by Dickersin (1989)

Wood C, Ng K W, Hounslow D and Berming H (1973) 'Time – an important variable in normal delivery' *Journal of Obstetrics and Gynaecology of the British Commonwealth* 80: 295–300

21 Management of the third and fourth stages of labour

History

Following the second stage of labour, which presents the greatest potential hazard for the fetus, is the third stage, with its attendant risks for the mother. Historically in the Western world and currently in the developing world, haemorrhage has been a major cause of maternal mortality (Martin and Dumoulin 1953; World Health Organization 1989). The control of pathological blood loss was a prime aim of early obstetrics (Moir 1964). The chemical ergot, a constituent of a fungal infection occurring on rye, had been known for centuries, but was only isolated (as ergotoxine) in 1906, ergotamine was discovered in 1932 and a water-soluble form (ergometrine) in 1935 (Moir 1932; Dudley and Moir 1935). Ergometrine acts intravenously within 40 seconds and intramuscularly within 6–7 minutes, producing a non-physiological sustained contraction affecting the whole uterus (Moir 1932) including those muscle fibres in the lower uterine segment and cervix (few in number) which are unaffected by oxytocin.

The next pharmacological advance in the control of haemorrhage came with the isolation, from pituitary extract, of oxytocin (du Vigneaud *et al.* 1953). In 1954 a pure form was isolated and marketed in the United Kingdom as Syntocinon. This acts intravenously in 40 seconds and intramuscularly in 2.5 minutes, producing strong rhythmic contractions, affecting mainly the upper segment of the uterus

(Caldeyro Barcia and Heller 1961). Both ergometrine and syntocinon were originally developed for the control of haemorrhage, but were later used with various techniques in the management of the third stage of labour as prophylaxis against excess blood loss. Commenting on the widespread use of oxytocic drugs, Moore (1977), states that 'As so often with developments in obstetrics all mothers come to be treated in the same manner irrespective of the degree of risk' (p. 120).

Clinical trial of management technique

Prendiville *et al.* (1988a) in a review of trials comparing an oxytocic preparation with either a placebo or with physiological management, examined 9 trials, whose combined results implied that routine oxytocic use could reduce the risk of postpartum haemorrhage (PPH) by up to 40%. They recommended further studies to examine the effects on maternal physiology and the rate of retained placentae resulting from such a uniform use of oxytocics. Elbourne *et al.* (1988), in a similar review of trials comparing oxytocic drugs, examined 17 studies which used a randomised controlled experimental design (a further 10 studies were excluded due to methodological difficulties). These studies revealed an equivalent reduction in the risk of PPH (approximately 40%) following the routine use of oxytocics. They recommended a further trial to compare ergometrine and oxytocin (syntometrine) with oxytocin alone to assess benefits and side-effects (Elbourne *et al.* 1988).

A recent randomised trial of physiological and active management demonstrated that active management reduced the incidence of PPH from 17.9% in the physiological group to 5.9% amongst those whose third stage was actively managed (Prendiville *et al.* 1988b). Methodological problems with this trial involved inclusion of women at other than low risk into the study, including those whose labours were already being actively managed, and limited preparation of midwifery staff for the change to physiological management. Begley (1990a) compared the outcome where 1429 women at 'low' risk of postpartum haemorrhage were randomly allocated for the third stage to physiological or actively managed groups. The latter received 0.5 mg of ergometrine; this group of mothers experienced significantly more nausea, vomiting, severe after-pains, hypertension, secondary postpartum haemorrhage and they were more likely to need a manual removal of placenta (Begley 1990a). Whilst the physiological group were more likely to have a postpartum haemorrhage, there was no difference in the need amongst mothers in either group for a blood transfusion. Begley (1990a) concludes that the adverse effects of routine oxytocic group for women at low risk is not justified. In addition, further study of a subgroup of breast-feeding women from the trial showed that those who had received ergometrine were significantly less likely to continue feeding after 4 weeks (Begley 1990b).

Botha (1968) reviewing 26 000 deliveries amongst Bantu women argued that PPH is a 'man-made' condition relating to current management, which includes delivering women in bed and early clamping of the umbilical cord.

Physiological management

The role of the midwife when using physiological management of the third stage is one of watching and waiting. Once the baby is delivered it can be handed to its mother or placed between her legs if she has delivered in an upright position. The umbilical cord is neither clamped nor cut but is allowed to continue pulsating until the neonatal blood volume has equilibrated. This has the advantage of allowing the baby to receive up to 150 ml of blood which is required to provide the extra volume needed for the pulmonary circulation (Usher *et al*. 1963). This extra volume of blood is especially important for preterm infants. Leaving the cord to pulsate following the administration of an oxytocic drug can result in an overtransfused, plethoric baby. Once the cord has stopped pulsating, it is acceptable to clamp it twice and to cut between the clamps. The clamp on the maternal end of the cord can then be removed to drain the placenta of blood, facilitating its easy passage through the cervix (Clinch 1985).

Where the mother delivers in an upright position, the placenta, once separated, will fall from the upper to the lower uterine segment under the influence of gravity. This, together with maternal effort if necessary, will effect a swift delivery. For the mother lying in a semirecumbent position, gravity will have only a limited effect (Leff 1939). In this situation, the midwife must be alert for the signs of separation:

1. A lengthening of the umbilical cord at the vulva.
2. A small gush of blood at the vulva.
3. The uterine fundus rises up and becomes ballottable.

As soon as two of these signs have been seen, the mother can be encouraged to expel her placenta. To assist her efforts, the midwife can place the palm of one hand against the mother's lower abdomen to give her something to push against. Once the placenta is visible at the vulva, the midwife can assist its delivery by lifting up the cord and collecting the placenta in the lower hand. The membranes can then be gently teased out of the vagina if necessary by twisting them into a 'cord' to give strength and to prevent tearing.

Once the placenta is delivered, it, together with any blood loss, are collected in a kidney dish and put aside for later examination. The fundus of the mother's uterus is felt to ensure that it is firmly contracted. The mother's vulva is then washed with sterile water before the midwife examines the vagina and perineum for the presence of a laceration which may require suturing. Cervical tears will be suspected by the presence of a steady vaginal blood loss with a well-contracted uterus, the cervix should then be visualised to determine the extent of the damage. Grazes to the labia often cause the woman discomfort, especially when passing urine. The grazes rarely need (nor are they suitable for) suturing and normally heal quickly. A sanitary pad can then be applied and the bed linen changed before the mother is made comfortable.

Active management

Active management of the third stage of labour involves the use of an oxytocic drug as a prophylactic to prevent haemorrhage (and to a lesser extent delay), clamping and cutting of the umbilical cord and controlled cord traction (Prendiville and Elbourne 1989). Syntometrine is the most commonly used oxytocic for third stage management in the United Kingdom (Garcia *et al.* 1986). This is a combination of 0.5 mg of ergometrine and 5 units of syntocinon. It is given as an IM injection into the mother's upper thigh, usually at the time of the delivery of the anterior shoulder or, less commonly, with crowning of the fetal head (Prendiville *et al.* 1988a). The aim of active management is to deliver the placenta with the first contraction after the delivery of the baby; this usually occurs 2 or 3 minutes following administration of the oxytocic. The placenta must be delivered before ergometrine has its effect (7 minutes after administration) when the lower segment and cervix have contracted down, preventing delivery.

Following delivery of the baby, the midwife puts two clamps on the umbilical cord and cuts between them. This prevents the baby receiving an excess transfusion of blood, which can occur if the cord remains unclamped when the syntocinon-induced contractions occur (Yao and Lind 1974). These contractions are stronger than those which would occur physiologically. If desired, the maternal end of the cord can be unclamped and the blood in the placenta drained off. This creates a smaller, more compact, placenta which is easier to deliver (Botha 1968). In addition, early cord clamping followed by the drainage of blood from the maternal end of the cord reduces the occurrence of feto-maternal transfusion (Lapido 1972). This is of importance in the management of women with rhesus-negative blood.

Once the uterus has contracted, the midwife performs controlled cord traction to effect delivery of the placenta. This is achieved by the midwife (if right-handed) placing her open left hand with its radial surface downwards and the palm towards the mother's head above the mother's symphysis pubis. The umbilical cord is wrapped around the fingers of the midwife's right hand and it is then gently pulled outwards and downwards. The left hand braces the uterus and applies gentle pressure upwards, while feeling if the uterus itself is being pulled as would happen if the placenta were still adherent. Once the placenta is visible at the vulva, the midwife lifts up her right hand to bring the placenta along the direction of the Curve of Carus. The left hand, meanwhile, is brought under the placenta to hold it once it is delivered. The placenta and blood loss are put aside for later inspection and the mother is made comfortable as described for physiological management.

Cord traction to effect delivery of the placenta is an ancient technique, first described by Aristotle (Hibbard 1964). Despite being advocated by physicians such as Mauriceau (1694) and Baudelocque (1823), it did not gain great popularity, due to the risks of inverting the uterus, delivering a partly separated placenta or of breaking the umbilical cord. In 1767 Harvie, a Dublin obstetrician who was wary of the hazards of cord traction, published a pamphlet advocating abdominal pressure on the contracted uterus to expel the placenta. This was achieved by placing the flat of the hand over the uterine fundus and applying gentle pressure in the direction of the symphysis pubis. A similar procedure was recommended 100 years later by Crede, who used pressure on the fundus to create a piston with which to expel the placenta and also advocated squeezing of the fundus to assist the procedure (Crede 1854). Cord traction returned to popularity following the work of Brandt (1933) and Andrews (1940), but there were still problems of possible uterine inversion or later prolapse. In 1962, Spencer suggested the use of an oxytocic prior to cord traction and the positioning of the operator's left hand to apply upward pressure above the symphysis pubis. This is known as controlled cord traction.

Levy and Moore (1985) demonstrated that blood loss during active management of the third stage could be reduced if the midwife awaited signs of separation before performing controlled cord traction. There are, however, many unanswered questions regarding the management of the third stage. Prendiville and Elbourne (1989) suggest the following areas as requiring more examination:

a) choice of oxytocic
b) route of ocytocic
c) timing of oxytocic
d) timing of cord clamping
e) value of signs of placental separation
f) effects of controlled cord traction. (Prendiville and Elbourne 1989, p. 1165)

Examination of the placenta

Following completion of the third stage of labour, it is important to examine the placenta and membranes carefully to confirm their completeness. Retention of portions of the placenta or membranes is associated with postpartum haemorrhage, infection and subinvolution of the uterus. Examination of the placenta also yields useful information about the intrauterine environment.

A systematic approach to the examination of the placenta is helpful in preventing any aspect being overlooked. The placenta should be examined on a large flat surface in a good light. Mopping the maternal surface of the placenta can aid visualisation. The examiner should wear gloves to avoid contact with maternal blood which could be carrying hepatitis B or HIV.

The umbilical cord

The cut surface of the umbilical cord is examined and the number of fetal vessels counted. The normal cord has two umbilical arteries and one thicker-walled vein. The reasons for the presence of a single artery is unclear, although it appears that environmental factors are of greater importance than genetic ones (Altshuler *et al.* 1975). A single artery occurs in cases of renal abnormality and therefore a close watch should be kept on the baby's urinary output. However there is no other abnormality in most babies with a single uterine artery.

The average length of the umbilical cord is 50–60 cm although there is little need to measure cord length unless it is very short or unusually long. A short cord may cause traction at delivery with the risks of cord rupture, placental separation or uterine prolapse (DeSa 1984). An extremely long cord increases the risks of cord prolapse and cord entanglement. True knots are more common with long cords. False knots are extra twists of the umbilical vessels surrounded with Wharton's jelly, this is normally white in colour but which can be stained khaki or yellow by meconium or bilirubin, respectively, in the liquor.

The umbilical cord is normally inserted into either the centre or close to the centre (mediolateral) of the placenta. Less common insertions include battledore (into the edge of the placenta) and velamentous (into the membranes) (see Figure 21.1). This last is associated with an increased frequency of fetal malformations, which are thought to relate to mechanical factors such as multiple pregnancy, abnormalities of uterine blood supply and uterine anomalies including fibroids (Robinson *et al.* 1983). Velamentous insertion of the umbilical cord can give rise to vasa praevia, where the umbilical vessels lie in front of the presenting part and are at risk of rupture and subsequent fetal exsanguination during labour.

The membranes

The membranes should be carefully examined for their completeness. Lifting up the placenta by its cord, the hole through which the fetus passed can be examined. It should have smooth edges. Where these are ragged, the midwife has to decide whether the membranes are complete. Retained membranes can give rise to subinvolution of the uterus and infection. The amnion (fetal surface) is then separated from the chorion, which is easily identified by the shreds of decidua which adhere to it. The amnion can be stripped back to the base of the umbilical cord.

Battledore   Velamentous

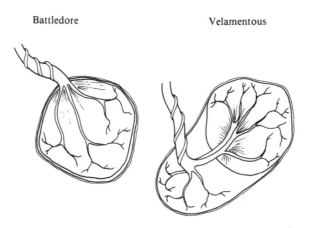

Figure 21.1 Battledore and velamentous insertions of the umbilical into the placenta.

Double folds of chorion inside the edge of the fetal surface of the placenta are known as circumvallation and are thought to be due either to lateral growth of the placenta or to too deep implantation (Fox 1978).

The chorion at the edge of the placenta on the maternal surface is then carefully examined for any vessels leading away from the main placenta. Their progress should be checked to ensure that they either return to the placenta or lead to an extra lobe (a succenturiate lobe) in the membranes. If the vessel ends at a hole in the membranes, a portion of placenta has been retained and appropriate medical staff should be informed. It is thought that succenturiate lobes result from a failure of part of the trophoblast (the chorion laeve) to atrophy during early placental development.

The maternal surface

The maternal surface of the placenta is then examined for its completeness, in particular the presence of all of its lobes. The surface is then observed for the presence of infarctions or areas of calcification (Kaplan 1987). The former are fairly common and result from disturbances in the blood supply; if extensive they can give rise to intrauterine growth retardation and fetal death in utero (Kaplan 1987). Calcification increases with ageing of the placenta.

Weight

The placenta is then usually weighed. This information is normally of only academic interest unless the fetus is growth-retarded. A healthy placenta weighs approximately one-sixth of the weight of the baby. The collected blood loss is then measured and the total loss estimated, although this is far from accurate (Levy and Moore 1985).

Record keeping

Details of the examination of the placenta together with an assessment of blood loss should be recorded in the casenotes. Any serious abnormalities, for example, an incomplete placenta, should be reported to the medical staff and all abnormalities should be brought to the attention of the midwifery staff on the postnatal ward including ragged membranes, which are usually passed in the early days after delivery.

Repair of the pelvic floor

Lacerations to the perineum, labia, vagina and cervix can occur during childbirth.

In addition, an episiotomy is still commonly performed to expedite delivery. Sleep *et al.* (1984) report an episiotomy rate of 61% (52% during spontaneous deliveries) in their hospital prior to the randomised trial of perineal management. Of mothers allocated to the group with a restricted episiotomy policy, 33.9% as against 24.3% of those in the liberal group had an intact perineum after delivery. Episiotomy rates amongst the 1000 women were 45.2% in the liberal group and 9% in the restricted group. By 1987, in the same unit the episiotomy rate was 20% (Sleep 1990) whilst Logue (1990) reported a rate of 12% during the same year in her hospital. Episiotomies and perineal tears involving skin and muscle require suturing, as do cervical and some vaginal tears. Vaginal tears are usually repaired with chromic catgut, no further treatment being necessary except to alert the mother that the fibrous tissue with which the tear heals is inelastic and may give rise to dyspareunia (pain on intercourse). Labial lacerations and grazes can usually be left to heal naturally; suturing is rarely appropriate. They can however be quite painful when healing. Discomfort on micturition is common for the first few days, sometimes giving rise to retention of urine due to fear of pain (reflex inhibition).

Trauma to the perineum is classified according to the extent of tissue damage:

First degree:	Involving the skin at the fourchette.
Second degree:	Involving the skin and superficial muscles of the perineum and perineal body; this category includes the damage resulting from an episiotomy.
Third degree:	Involving skin, muscles of the perineum and perineal body extending to and including the margins of the anal sphincter. In severe cases, the anal canal and the rectum can also be affected.

In the United States and under the ICDC-approved definitions, damage to the anal canal or to the rectum is referred to as fourth degree damage. First degree lacerations rarely require suturing, since the damaged skin edges lie naturally in apposition.

Midwives who have received a course of instruction and have been judged competent in the procedure may repair the perineum. This is helpful in providing continuity of care and in preventing long delays before the perineum is repaired. In the United Kingdom, the theory and technique of perineal repair has been a part of the midwifery syllabus since the introduction of the 18 month post-general nursing midwifery education programme. Garcia *et al.* (1986), in their survey of maternity units in England and Wales, found that midwives were repairing the perineum in over 60% of consultant units.

The repair of third and fourth degree trauma does not come under the scope of the midwife and such damage should be repaired by an experienced obstetrician. Either a general anaesthetic or regional analgesia (usually an epidural anaesthetic) are used to facilitate the repair and to prevent maternal pain. It is customary to offer such women a high fibre diet in the days following delivery, to ease the passage of the first stool and to prevent constipation. The woman's greatest difficulty is to overcome the fear following such a repair.

Perineal repair undertaken by midwives includes that of mediolateral and (more rarely) midline episiotomies and of second degree tears. The principle behind all these types of repair is the same. This is to reunite the tissues so that they lie in the same position as they were before the damage occurred. The repair is usually performed in three layers: vaginal mucosa, deeper perineal tissues and finally, the skin (Grant 1989).

The procedure is performed under aseptic conditions, with the woman usually in the lithotomy position, to ease access and visualisation. This can be uncomfortable (and undignified) for the mother and as it is known to place an extra strain on the perineum during the second stage of labour (Thomson 1988), a similar situation is likely to occur during suturing. The area must be adequately anaesthetised before the repair can begin. This can be achieved either by 'topping-up' an existing epidural or by infiltrating with a local anaesthetic agent. The area is first swabbed with an antiseptic solution and the scope of the damage assessed before a local anaesthetic agent is introduced. This is usually lignocaine 0.5% or 1%, depending on local policy. The latter has the advantage of being a smaller volume and therefore giving rise to less swelling. The lignocaine is injected along the margins of the laceration and also into the deep muscle layer. Care must be taken to allow the anaesthetic to achieve its effect, which takes 3–4 minutes (Cunningham *et al.* 1989) before beginning the repair.

The vagina is examined to find the apex of the damage. A vaginal tampon may be inserted to prevent the wound being obscured by blood trickling from the uterus. (The tape on the tampon should be attached to the drapes for safety, to prevent it being forgotten).

Beginning at the apex, the vaginal mucosa is repaired, using a continuous suture and an absorbable suture material, usually chromic catgut (Cunningham *et al.* 1989). The knot may be buried behind the fourchette, although there is no evidence that this improves healing (Grant 1989) (see Figure 21.2).

Two or three interrupted sutures are now inserted into the deep muscles of the perineum to unite the levator ani muscles. Where a mediolateral laceration is being repaired, care should be taken to maintain anatomical accuracy, since the upper edge of the wound will be longer than the lower. The sutures should not be placed too deep, to avoid impinging on the rectum. Research has shown that polyglycolic acid sutures (Dexon or Vicryl) cause less discomfort than catgut (Grant 1989) (see Figure 21.3)

The skin is now repaired, using either continuous subcuticular or interrupted polyglycolic acid sutures. This has been shown to cause less discomfort than either catgut or black silk (Grant 1989). Continuous sutures cause less pain than interrupted ones in the short term, although there is no difference in the long term (Grant 1989). Interrupted sutures are easier to use for beginners and therefore this method is usually taught until the technique becomes familiar (see Figures 21.3a and 21.3b).

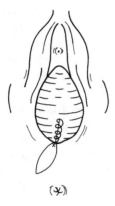

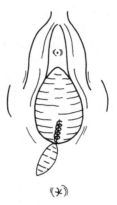

Figure 21.2 Continuous sutures from the apex of the episiotomy to the fourchette realigning the vaginal mucosa.

Deep sutures to the muscle layer. If the episiotomy is large, two or three smaller sutures may be required to align superficial muscles.

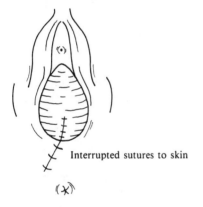

Interrupted sutures to skin

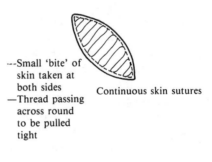

---Small 'bite' of skin taken at both sides
—Thread passing across round to be pulled tight

Continuous skin sutures

Figure 21.3 (a) Interrupted sutures to skin. (b) Continuous sutures.

The tampon is gently removed from the vagina and the vaginal wall rechecked. Finally, a rectal examination is carried out to ensure that no sutures have entered the rectum. A sanitary pad is then applied and the woman's legs carefully removed from the lithotomy stirrups. The woman should be informed how the damage has been repaired, how it will heal and whether any of the sutures will require removal. A record of the repair is then made in the casenotes and signed by the person who undertook it.

The fourth stage of labour

The fourth stage of labour refers to the early hours after delivery while the mother remains on the labour ward or, if delivered at home while the midwife remains in attendance. This is the start of the period of recovery. For the midwife, it involves close observation of the mother for the state of her uterus, vaginal blood loss and her vital signs. The placenta and membranes are examined for completeness and any perineal trauma is repaired. The parents can make acquaintance with their new baby, to continue the process of parent–infant attachment. The baby may be fed for the first time and breast feeding initiated. All mothers should be offered the opportunity to feed their baby. Newborn babies are often particularly alert in the first hour or two after birth and will feed well, although those whose mother has had narcotic analgesia during labour may be sleepy and reluctant to feed (Mathews 1989). It has been shown that early initiation of breast feeding reduces the chances of the mother stopping feeding in the first 2 weeks (Martin and White 1988) (see Chapter 34 for more information about infant feeding).

The mother should be made comfortable and left with the means of summoning help. After completion of the third stage, her temperature, pulse and blood pressure are measured and recorded. Unless abnormal, the pulse only should be rechecked every 15 minutes during the fourth stage. It is important to record the blood pressure following delivery, because eclampsia can occur for the first time in the puerperium. The pulse is recorded as an indicator of the presence of infection and for signs of shock. The fundus is palpated every 15 minutes to ensure it is well contracted and the amount of lochia observed. Relaxation of the uterus, which may occur, can give rise to a considerable blood loss. If this occurs, a contraction is obtained by firmly rubbing the uterine fundus and expelling from the uterine cavity any blood clots. Where intravenous oxytocin was used during labour, this is usually kept running slowly for 30–60 minutes following delivery to prevent uterine relaxation (Myerscough 1982). Bleeding occurring with a well-contracted uterine fundus usually indicates the existence of unrepaired lacerations, for example in the cervix.

The presence of signs of shock (pale skin, raised pulse and hypotension), with maternal perineal pain and no visible blood loss, could be the early signs of a developing vulval haematoma. This would normally appear within the first 12–24 hours following delivery. Treatment involves ligating the effected vessel under general anaesthesia and evacuation of the haematoma (Cunningham et al. 1989). A vaginal pack may be inserted to apply pressure on the damaged area. If the haematoma is large, a blood transfusion may be necessary. Whatever the blood loss, it is hard to estimate (Cunningham et al. 1989), so the mother's haemoglobin should be measured and appropriate treatment given.

After the exertions of labour, it is customary to give the couple light refreshment such as tea and toast. It is not unusual for the mother who has received narcotic analgesia or ergometrine (Begley 1990a) to feel hungry initially, but then to experience nausea and possibly to vomit after having eaten (Nimmo et al. 1975). The parents may wish to spend some time alone together with their new family member. Should they wish to examine the baby more closely, an overhead heater can be positioned over the bed to prevent the baby becoming cold. Skin-to-skin contact between mother and baby can also help prevent cooling.

Before transfer from the delivery unit or before the departure of the midwife from the home, the mother should be offered a bath, a shower or a bedbath. The choice depends upon the policy of the hospital and how the mother is feeling. Mothers who have had an epidural may not have sufficient sensation in their lower limbs to be mobile, whereas those who have had a quick labour might prefer a bath or a shower to a bedbath. The bed linen and nightclothes are changed to prepare the mother for a well-deserved rest. The mother is encouraged to pass urine (this may be easier using a toilet rather than a bedpan) and, should the post-delivery diuresis have occurred, she may pass large amounts. Before the mother leaves the care of her midwife, her vital signs must be measured and recorded together with the state of her fundus, lochia and perineum. If an epidural cannula has been *in situ*, it is carefully removed and checked for completeness, according to local policy. Where an intravenous infusion has been used, this is normally removed prior to transfer to the postnatal ward, unless there are instructions to the contrary. The midwife ideally accompanies the mother and her new baby to the postnatal ward and transfers her to the care of the midwife there.

Record keeping

Concise and accurate record keeping is a major part of the role of every midwife (United Kingdom Central Council 1986; Dimond 1990). Record keeping in labour falls into three main areas:

1. Charted recordings of observations on the partogram.
2. Contemporaneous entries into the medical and midwifery notes.
3. Summary information at the end of labour.

The partogram has already been covered in some detail in Chapter 20. All entries into the records should include the date and time of entry, together with the full signature of the individual making the entry. The midwife should record her observations of the events, an assessment of the processes behind the events and what action (if any) she has taken. It is better for the midwife to record any suspicion that things are not progressing normally as soon as she notices changes in progress, rather than waiting for the situation to worsen. The following is an example of an entry in midwifery/medical records:

11/5/90 03.30 Occasional late decelerations of the fetal heart seen on the cardiotocograph. Mrs Brown turned from her right to her left side. Dr White informed.   Jane Grey
04.00 Trace now satisfactory, will continue to observe.   Jane Grey
04.45 Thick meconium stained liquor seen. Two late decelerations seen, with slow recovery. Dr White called. Mrs Brown experiencing an urge to push.
                                                                 Jane Grey

> 05.00 Dr White has not arrived; called again. Fetal heart decelerations continue. Contractions becoming expulsive. Vaginal examination performed; cervix 8–9 cm dilated, station-vertex at the level of the ischial spines, position left occipito transverse.   Jane Grey
> 05.05 Dr White has still not arrived, Mrs Green called and informed of events. She says she will come straight away.   Jane Grey
> 05.12 Mrs Green has arrived.   Jane Grey

It is just as important to record events which do not happen as those which do. It is also advisable to document the mother's wishes regarding the conduct of her labour and delivery, particularly where there is no birthplan in the notes.

> 8/11/90 20.10 Advantages and disadvantages of artificial rupture of the membranes discussed with Donna Brown and her partner. They decide that they would rather wait with the membranes intact to see how things develop. If progress is slow at the next vaginal examination, they will reconsider their decision.   Jane Grey

In the very rare situation of a mother or her partner refusing to accept the midwife's advice regarding management, it may be advisable to request that the mother co-signs the entry in the notes. It is unusual for the mother to resist the midwife's advice where a relationship of mutual trust has been established. The midwife should act with great care when a disagreement occurs, since an action contrary to the mother's wishes could be construed as an assault or a trespass against the person (Dimond 1990).

Summary entries in the notes are made at the end of labour and as their name implies, they summarise the whole proceedings. In addition to calculations of the lengths of the stages of labour, the completeness of the placenta and the condition of the newborn, there are explanations about certain procedures. This may include the rationale for the performance of an episiotomy and a description of the method used for its repair. When transferring the mother to the postnatal ward, the records of analgesia received (whether the mother has passed urine and how she wishes to feed her baby) for example, will form the basis for planning the care of mother and baby in the puerperium. Although a verbal report is given on transfer, written records can be more accurate.

The labour ward record book (or computerised entry) must be completed, together with the local format for the notification of birth. Under the 1936 United Kingdom Public Health Act, it is a legal requirement for the father, or any other person present within 6 hours following the birth, to notify the event to the appropriate local medical officer (District Medical Officer in England or Chief Administrative Medical Officer in Wales) within 36 hours of the birth. This duty is commonly undertaken by the midwife. This procedure applies to all live births and any stillbirths occurring after 24 weeks of gestation. This notification initiates the provision of primary health services such as health visiting and invitations for the mother to bring the baby for immunisations or developmental tests. It also alerts the local Registrar to expect registration of birth by the parents within 42 days of the event. Copies of the notification are also dispatched to The Office of Population Censuses and Surveys which compiles national statistics.

Initial examination of the newborn

Within the first hour following birth, the midwife examines the baby to look for any obvious signs of abnormality. This examination is usually performed in the delivery room; parents often like to watch, giving the midwife an opportunity to teach them about their new baby. The examination should be performed in a systematic fashion, to avoid overlooking any aspect. If the first examination is delayed for any reason, it is important to ensure that the baby does not leave the delivery room until two name-bands, which have been checked with the parents, have been applied. In some hospitals, the umbilical cord is not cut until the name-bands have been attached. The initial examination should take place in a light, draught-free environment; an overhead heater may be used.

Before starting to examine the baby, it is important to observe his/her skin colour, movements and respiratory rate.

The head

The baby's head is examined to check its shape and the presence of moulding and caput succadeneum. The examiner's fingers are gently run over the suture lines and fontanelles to feel for overriding of the bones. The ears are observed for their position (the top of the ear should be level with the eyes), presence of accessory auricles or skin tags. The baby's eyes are examined to make sure they are normal (the baby will open his/her eyes if given something to suck, for example, whilst being held away from any bright lights). The mouth is carefully examined in a good light for the presence of teeth and abnormalities of the hard and soft palate.

The neck and trunk

The neck is carefully examined for signs of any webbing. This is achieved by extending the head allowing the neck to be visualised. The trunk is observed for its uniformity of shape and to check the presence of two nipples which should be located midway between the sternum and the side wall of the chest. The umbilical cord is examined to confirm that it is securely clamped.

The arms

Free movement of both arms is demonstrated and the axilla are examined for the presence of any lumps or skin tags. The hands are carefully observed for the presence of the correct number of digits. It is important to open the palm (helped by gently tapping the back of the hand), to observe the existence of palmar creases (usually two or three) and to eliminate the existence of extra digits.

The legs

As with the arms, the legs are gently put through the full range of movements. The feet are examined for the presence of skin creases and the number of toes. The feet and ankles are observed for their normal positioning to detect the existence of talipes. The hips are not normally examined until 24 hours after birth to allow them to stabilise. Local policy will determine the timing of this test as well as who should undertake it.

The genitalia

The genitalia are carefully examined to confirm the baby's sex. With boys it is customary to check that both testes are descended. The external urinary meatus on the end of the penis should be examined to determine that its position is not on the underside. The anal sphincter is checked for patency. This is normally done by using a rectal thermometer.

The back

The baby is placed chest down over the hand of the midwife while the back is examined for the presence of obvious defects, dimples or hairy patches, especially in the lumbar region, which could indicate the existence of spina bifida occulta.

Weight

The baby is weighed shortly after birth. This is the important piece of information for the parents and the family; it is also required for the notification of birth and for the records.

Records

The weight and the results of the first examination are recorded in the notes and signed. If the parents did not watch the examination they should be informed of the results.

Should any anomaly be found, it should first be shown to the parents before informing a paediatrician, who will come and examine the baby. For a home birth, the GP should be notified. Where a major anomaly exists, the baby should not be removed from the room until the parents have seen the anomaly, since this can increase the risks of rejection. With minor anomalies, such as the presence of extra digits, it is not uncommon to find that one of the parents also shares this.

References

Altshuler G, Tsang R C and Ermocilla R (1975) 'Significance of single umbilical artery: Correlation of clinical status and umbilical cord histology' *American Journal of Disease in Childhood* 129: 697–700

Andrews C J (1940) 'The third stage of labor with an evaluation of the Brandt method of expression of the placenta' *Southern Medicine and Surgery* 102: 605–8

Baudelocque J L (1823) *Midwifery (3rd edn)* Thomas Desilver: Philadelphia

Begley C M (1990a) 'A comparison of "active" and "physiological" management of the third stage of labour' *Midwifery* 6(1): 3–17

Begley C M (1990b) 'The effect of ergometrine on breastfeeding' *Midwifery* 6(2): 60–72

Botha M C (1968) 'The management of the umbilical cord in labour' *South African Journal of Obstetrics and Gynaecology* 16(2): 30–3

Brandt M L (1933) 'The mechanism and management of the third stage of labor' *American Journal of Obstetrics and Gynecology* 25: 662–6

Caldeyro Barcia R and Heller H (1961) *Oxytocin* Pergamon Press: New York

Clinch J (1985) 'The third stage' in J Studd (ed) *Management of Labour* Ch 20 287–300 Blackwell Scientific: Oxford

Crede C S (1854) *Klinische Vortrage uber Geburtshuelfe* Verlag August Hirschwald: Berlin

Cunningham F G, MacDonald P C and Gant N F (1989) *William's Obstetrics (11th edn)* Prentice Hall: London

DeSa D J (1984) 'Diseases of the umbilical cord' In E V D K Perrin (ed) *Pathology of the Placenta* 121–40 Churchill Livingstone: New York

Dimond B (1990) *Legal Aspects of Nursing* Prentice Hall: Hemel Hempstead

Dudley H W and Moir J C (1935) 'The substance responsible for the traditional clinical effect of ergot' *British Medical Journal* i: 520–3

du Vigneaud V, Ressler C and Tippett S (1953) 'The sequence of amino acids in oxytocin with a proposal for the structure of oxytocin' *Journal of Biological Chemistry* 205: 949

Elbourne D, Prendiville W and Chalmers I (1988) 'Choice of oxytocic preparation for routine use in the management of the third stage of labour: an overview of the evidence from controlled trials' *British Journal of Obstetrics and Gynaecology* 95(1): 17–30

Fox H S (1978) *Pathology of the Placenta* Saunders: Philadelphia

Garcia J, Garforth S and Ayers S (1986) 'Midwives confined? Labour ward policies and routines' *Research and the Midwife Proceedings* 1986: 2–30

Grant A (1989) 'Repair of perineal trauma after childbirth' in C Chalmers, M Enkin and M J N C Keirse (eds) *Effective Care in Pregnancy and Childbirth* Ch 68 1170–81 Oxford Medical: Oxford

Harvie J (1769) *Practical Directions Showing a Method of Preserving the Perineum in Childbirth and Delivering the Placenta Without Violence* London

Hibbard B M (1964) 'The third stage of labour' *British Medical Journal* 2: 1485–8

Kaplan C (1987) 'Gross and microscopic abnormalities of the placenta' in J P Lavery (ed) *The Human Placenta: Clinical Perspectives* Ch 4 47–66 Aspen: Rockville, Maryland

Lapido O A (1972) 'Management of the third stage of labour' *British Medical Journal* i: 721–3

Leff M (1939) 'Management of the third and fourth stages of labor' *Surgical Gynecology and Obstetrics* 68: 224–9

Levy V and Moore J (1985) 'The midwife's management of the third stage of labour' *Nursing Times* 25 Sept: 47–50

Logue M (1990) 'Putting research into practice: Perineal management during delivery' in S Robinson and A M Thomson (eds) *Midwives Research and Childbirth* Vol 2 Ch 9 252–70 Chapman and Hall: London

Martin J and White A (1988) *Infant Feeding 1985* HMSO: London

Martin J D and Dumoulin J G (1953) 'Use of intravenous ergometrine to prevent post partum haemorrhage' *British Medical Journal* i: 643–6

Mauriceau F (1694) *Traite des Maladies des Femmes Grosse Vol 1 (4th edn)* Paris

Mathews M K (1989) 'The relationship between maternal labour analgesia and delay in the initiation of breastfeeding in healthy neonates in the early neonatal period' *Midwifery* 5(1): 3–10

Moir J C (1932) 'The action of ergot preparation on the puerperal uterus' *British Medical Journal* i: 1119–22

Moir J C (1964) 'The obstetrician bids and the uterus contracts' *British Medical Journal* ii: 1025–9

Moore W M O (1977) 'The conduct of the second stage' in T Chard and M Richards (eds) *Benefits and Hazards of the New Obstetrics* Ch 8 116–25 Spastics International: London

Myerscough P R (1982) *Munro Kerr's Operative Obstetrics (10th edn)* Balliere Tindall: London

Nimmo W S, Wilson J and Prescott L F (1975) 'Narcotic analgesia and delayed gastric emptying in labour' *Lancet* i: 890–3

Prendiville W J and Elbourne D R (1989) 'Care during the third stage of labour' in I Chalmers, M Enkin and M J N C Keirse (eds) *Effective Care in Pregnancy and Childbirth* Ch 67 1145–69 Oxford Medical: Oxford

Prendiville W, Elbourne D and Chalmers I (1988a) 'The effects of routine oxytocic administration in the management of the third stage of labour: an overview of the evidence from controlled trials' *British Journal of Obstetrics and Gynaecology* 95(1): 3–16

Prendiville W J, Harding J E, Elbourne D R and Stirrat G M (1988b) 'The Bristol third stage trial: active versus physiological management of the third stage of labour' *British Medical Journal* 297: 1295–1300

Robinson L K, Jones K L and Benirschke K (1983) 'The nature of structural defects associated with velamentous and marginal insertion of the umbilical cord' *American Journal of Obstetrics and Gynecology* 146: 91–3

Sleep J M, Grant A, Garcia J, Elbourne D, Spencer J and Chalmers I (1984) 'West Berkshire perineal management trial' *British Medical Journal* 289: 587–90

Sleep J M (1990) 'Spontaneous delivery' in J Alexander, V Levy and S Roch (eds) *Midwifery Practice, Intrapartum Care – A Research Based Approach* Ch 6: 122–36 Macmillan: Basingstoke

Spencer P M (1962) 'Controlled cord traction in the management of the third stage of labour' *British Medical Journal* 1: 1728–32

Thomson A M (1988) 'Management of women in normal second stage labour: a review' *Midwifery* 4(2): 77–85

Usher R, Shepherd M and Lind J (1963) 'The blood volume of the newborn infant and placental transfusion' *Acta Paediatrica Scandanavica* 52: 497–512

United Kingdom Central Council (1986) *Handbook of Midwives Rules* UKCC: London

World Health Organization (1989) *Maternal Mortality* World Health Organization: Geneva

Yao A C and Lind J (1974) 'Placental transfusion' *American Journal of Diseases in Childhood* 127: 128–41

22 Active management of labour

Acceleration of labour

Any discussion concerning the augmentation of labour needs to be accompanied by an awareness of what constitutes normal progress. In the past, labour could be prolonged and women became exhausted, with poor outcomes for both mother and baby (Butler and Bonham 1963). Barlow (1822) reports that in the case of the first mother to survive a caesarean section, the mother had been in labour for several days with little progress. In today's highly technological delivery units, women and their labour can be controlled; in some cases this can imply linear progression of labour along a set time-scale (O'Driscoll and Meagher 1980). For today's obstetrician, physiology is not so regimented: some women will labour well and swiftly; others may take some time for labour to be established, whilst a few require medical intervention to achieve the desired outcome. Ploss *et al.* (1935), in their historical and anthropological review of women, describe in detail the processes of labour and birth in other societies and their understanding of physiology. It appears that much of this knowledge has been discarded and not passed on to the current generation.

Assessing progress in labour is a complex skill (Crowther *et al.* 1989). Many midwives are taught to rely on clinical judgement, gaining information from the contractions (length, strength and frequency), the maternal response to pain, the colour and quantity of per vaginum loss and the descent of the presenting part on abdominal examination over a period of time (Bennett and Brown 1989). These recordings give an overall picture of the state reached in the labour, which can be confirmed (if necessary) by vaginal examination. The assessment of progress by the medical staff is more likely to be based upon the periodic visits to see the mother, with only a small proportion of the labour being observed. This may result in reliance on measurement of cervical dilatation to assess progress, which can give a misleading picture (Crowther *et al.* 1989). The midwife's assessment of progress can be confirmed on vaginal examination by the position, consistency and application of the cervix to the presenting part in addition to dilatation itself. Progress may be 'slow' but fetal descent and a strengthening of contractions can augur well for improved and sustained progress.

It is known that both fetal and maternal risks increase where the labour lasts longer than 24 hours (Butler and Bonham 1963), but modern definitions of normal labour may include the time limit of 12 hours for their completion (O'Driscoll and Meagher 1980). The partogram, as instituted by Philpott and Castle (1972a,b), was devised for rural doctors and midwives in developing countries to detect a tardy labour and effect transfer to the urban hospital while the mother and fetus were still in good condition. This was based on work by Friedman (1954, 1955) and later by Hendricks *et al.* (1970) who analysed the rates of progress in normal labour.

The Friedman (1955) curve (see Figure 20.1a, p. 291) showed that the first stage of labour was divided into four phases: a latent phase, an acceleration phase, a phase of maximal slope (fastest rate of cervical dilatation and descent of the presenting part) and, prior to full dilatation, a deceleration phase. O'Driscoll *et al.* (1969) however, concluded that normal progress in labour was only confirmed by cervical dilatation of at least 1 cm/hour; women failing to conform to these limits should, they suggest, have their labour augmented.

Such an arbitrary time-scale has been subject to criticism; Friedman (1981) argued that labour is more accurately divided into latent and active phases. The maximum duration of labour for any individual should be decided with reference to the effects of that labour on mother and fetus (Crowther *et al.* 1989).

With good support for the mother from family and midwife, adequate pain relief and a light diet (Crawford 1978), the deleterious results of a long labour can be prevented. Stress and a strange or changed environment have been shown in animal studies to interfere with the normal progress of labour (Bontekoe *et al.* 1977). Whereas Klaus *et al.* (1986) have demonstrated that the presence of a supportive companion in labour (in their study a female doula, or birth companion), significantly reduces the length of the labour. Flynn *et al.* (1978) reported that ambulation in labour leads to reduced use of oxytocic drugs to enhance labour.

Donald (1979) was of the opinion that the causes of slow labour include a faulty definition of true labour, together with maternal fear and anxiety, all of which can be helped by a sympathetic and knowledgeable midwife. Other causes are:

> *Hypotonic uterine action* (worsened by a poorly fitting presenting part and maternal exhaustion). This can include a prolonged latent phase; Cardozo and

Studd (1985) define this as the time taken (from admission in labour) to reach a cervical dilatation of 3 cm; they set an upper time limit of 6 hours for primiparae and 4 hours for multiparae. They state that women who take longer than this need careful observation. Friedman and Sachtleben (1961) state that the normal rate of progress for 95% of women in established labour is 1.2 cm/hour for primiparae and 1.5 cm/hour for multiparae.

Incoordinate uterine action.

Malposition and malpresentation (especially occipito-posterior position (Cardozo and Studd 1985).

Cephalo-pelvic disproportion (Cardozo and Studd 1985).

Primiparity. Uterine action in primiparous women is less likely to be efficient than in multiparae. Miller *et al.* (1976) demonstrated that the primiparous woman requires a much greater degree of uterine activity for each centimetre of cervical dilatation than does the multipara.

Postmaturity. The fetal head may be less able to mould to the pelvis.

Misuse of narcotics especially in the latent phase of labour. The use of epidural analgesia is also known to increase the length of labour (Studd *et al.* 1980).

Stress. Evidence from animal studies has shown that invasions of privacy, bright lighting and moving the labouring female can inhibit labour (Naaktgeboren 1989). Such results cannot, however, be extrapolated directly from animals to humans.

Augmentation of labour is usually by encouraging maternal mobility (Flynn *et al.* 1978), artificial rupture of the membranes (Friedman and Sachtleben 1963), breast stimulation (Curtis *et al.* 1986) and the use of intravenous oxytocin (the latter is discussed later in the chapter).

Caldeyro Barcia (1980) has demonstrated that intrauterine pressure increases during contractions to a greater degree when the woman is upright than when she is horizontal. Material mobility during labour reduces the duration of the first stage (Flynn *et al.* 1978). There are other advantages to such management, including the elimination of aorto-caval compression and the relief of pain, especially in the lumbosacral area, by adopting the position most comfortable for that individual (Odent 1983; Balaskas and Balaskas 1979).

Artificial rupture of the membranes was first recommended by Denman (1785) to induce preterm labour. Due to its irreversibility, it fell out of fashion during the nineteenth century. It was reintroduced in the 1930s, but was a controversial procedure due to disagreement about its effectiveness and concern about a 'dry' labour (Eastman 1938). O'Driscoll *et al.* (1969) stated that this procedure alone was sufficient to hasten delivery in 70% of the women in their study. Whilst the labour is shortened, it has been shown that cord blood gas and pH levels are improved where the membranes have been left intact or rupture late in labour (Martell *et al.* 1976). This is possibly due to the even pressure within the uterus, exerted upon the placenta and cord. The formation of caput succedaneum is increased following early rupture of the membranes, as is the amount of moulding produced (Lindgren

1959; Schwartz *et al.* 1969), with its attendant risks of cerebral damage, if severe. Schwarz (1973) has demonstrated that rupture of the membranes increases head compression and therefore the risk of changes in fetal heart rate (type 1 dips), although Keirse (1989) is critical of the methodology employed in this study. If left to their own devices, many women would labour with intact membranes until delivery. Schwartz (1974) found that 66% of women in their study had intact membranes at full cervical dilatation and 12% were still intact at delivery.

The rupturing of a woman's membranes is a procedure for which the midwife must obtain permission, after a full discussion of its advantages and disadvantages. Henderson (1984) discovered that the giving of information and the obtaining of consent were rare. In a number of cases, the lack of any specific objection was taken by the midwife as consent, although the grounds for the procedure were more influenced by local hospital policy than by personal decision-making. Medical staff, however, felt that the woman's presence in hospital implied consent and that the existence of any degree of cervical dilatation was sufficient grounds for the membranes to be ruptured (Henderson 1984). Since many mothers have little or no choice over their place of delivery, it must be questioned whether their presence in hospital can be taken to imply consent.

Breast stimulation, that is gentle massage of the breasts, is a method of encouraging labour and preventing postpartum haemorrhage with a well-founded historical basis (Curtis *et al.* 1986). Massage of the breasts at or after term encourages the release of oxytocin and can promote uterine contractions in cases of spontaneous rupture of the membranes, hypotonic uterine action and uterine inertia in the second stage of labour. It has also been shown to be of use as a simple, cheap, non-invasive method to achieve cervical ripening prior to induction of labour (Salmon *et al.* 1986).

The psychological effects of augmentation for a woman previously feeling in control of her labour can be severe (Cartwright 1977). The contractions are more painful, in addition to which the woman may feel that she has relinquished control over her body (Cartwright 1979). The midwife must keep the woman fully informed about the management and try to involve her as much as possible. Fear and anxiety can depress uterine activity, worsening the situation (Klaus *et al.* 1986; Naaktgeboren 1989).

Disordered uterine action

Prior to the introduction of synthetic oxytocics, disordered uterine action was a major cause of prolonged labour and of fetal and maternal distress (O'Driscoll *et al.* 1969).

Hypotonic uterine action (primary inertia)

This can also be referred to as primary dysfunctional labour (Cardozo and Studd 1985). It is said to occur when the active phase of labour progresses at less than

1 cm/hour of cervical dilatation (Cardozo and Studd 1985) and the normal slope of progress in labour is not achieved (Friedman 1954). In this state, the resting tone in the uterus is reduced, the contractions are weaker and less frequent than is necessary for progress, and maternal perception of pain is slight. While the triple descent gradient is present (see Chapter 19) there is limited progress, and labour may be prolonged without the use of oxytocic therapy.

This is the commonest abnormal labour pattern reported in 26.3% of primiparous women (Cardozo et al. 1982) and in 8.1% of multiparae (Gibb et al. 1982). Some women, diagnosed as having primary hypotonic uterine action, may be experiencing a prolonged latent phase and are best managed conservatively (Friedman 1973). In the absence of any complications, women with hypotonic uterine action are usually allowed to rest, preferably overnight, awaiting an improvement. If the woman is experiencing pain necessitating the use of analgesia, Friedman (1973) recommends that this should be given as it can help to differentiate between true and false labour. However, Cardozo et al. (1982) recommend that women with a prolonged latent phase respond well to being actively managed using intravenous oxytocin. The authors report that 80% of women in primary dysfunctional labour in their study responded well to augmentation with oxytocin, having a caesarean section rate of 6.2%, whereas those who had little response had a caesarean rate of 80% (Cardozo et al. 1982).

Primary inertia should not be confused with secondary uterine inertia, which follows a period of normotonic uterine activity and may indicate the presence of cephalopelvic disproportion. The woman with primary inertia has never had satisfactory uterine activity.

Inefficient uterine action

In this situation, the resting tone and frequency of contractions may be normal, although the triple descent gradient can be reversed or absent. All contractions begin in the fundus; they last longer and are stronger in the fundus and the peak of the contraction occurs simultaneously in all areas of the uterus. The intensity and duration of contractions may be increased (Donald 1979). The woman will experience prolonged pain and backache; this is caused by the contractions starting in the lower portion of the uterus or, in the case of a 'colicky' uterus, the lack of a period of total uterine relaxation. In some cases, the urge to push is present before full dilatation of the cervix. Whatever the precipitating factor, these conditions are usually managed using small doses of intravenous syntocinon (with maternal analgesia) to increase flexion of the presenting part, thus encouraging descent and rotation (Studd et al. 1982).

Reversed polarity (where the contraction begins in the lower uterine segment) is associated with malpositions, malpresentations and minor degrees of cephalopelvic disproportion, where the cervix is poorly applied to the presenting part (Hibbard 1988). These conditions are associated with slow progress, as the triple descent gradient is necessary to coordinate contraction and retraction of the upper uterine segment, together with thinning and stretching of the lower segment and cervical dilatation.

Secondary arrest of cervical dilatation

This is said to occur when, following good uterine action, the cervix ceases to dilate and the contractions diminish (Cardozo and Studd 1985). The cause of this condition is usually cephalopelvic disproportion or a malposition. Friedman *et al.* (1977) noted that amongst primigravid women with this condition, 29% had a caesarean section and 40% an instrumental delivery. When treated with intravenous syntocinon, 70% of the mothers were helped and the caesarean delivery rate was reduced to 5.6% (Friedman *et al.* 1977).

Hypertonic uterine action

Hypertonic activity can occur spontaneously or following overstimulation with oxytocic drugs (Donald 1979). The result of this type of labour is dependent upon whether or not cephalopelvic disproportion is present. In the absence of disproportion, precipitate delivery will occur, with all its attendant risks (Myerscough 1982). Hibbard (1988) defines a precipitate labour as one with a duration of under 2 hours. Maternal dangers include perineal lacerations and postpartum haemorrhage, apart from any shock or psychological consequences of such a precipitate delivery (Hibbard 1988). The fetus may suffer intrauterine hypoxia, especially where there is little interval between contractions, resulting in a severe reduction in placental perfusion (Hibbard 1988). Due to a speedy passage through the birth canal, moulding may be rapid and the fetal head may be damaged should delivery occur while the mother is standing (Donald 1979).

Where there is a degree of cephalopelvic disproportion, this excess uterine activity may be a diagnostic sign of the uterus (especially for a multiparous woman) attempting to overcome an obstruction (Hibbard 1988). In such cases, there is a risk of uterine rupture, which is preceded by the palpation abdominally of Bandl's ring (Donald 1979; Hibbard 1988). This is an exaggeration of the normal retraction ring formed at the junction of the retracted upper uterine segment and the thinned lower segment. The lower segment is so stretched that this ridge rises above the symphysis pubis; it can be palpated abdominally and may, if the mother is slim, be visible. The woman may also complain of suprapubic pain. This is an obstetric emergency which requires reporting to the medical staff and immediate treatment (usually delivery by caesarean section) to prevent uterine rupture (Hibbard 1988).

Cervical dystocia is a rare occurrence, where the cervical os fails to dilate (Donald 1979). This can be caused by an anatomical abnormality or as a result of scarring following treatment such as cone biopsy, cautery or amputation of the cervix (Hibbard 1988). At the start of labour, the cervix is rigid, effaced but only partly dilated (Donald 1979); later it can be felt so thinly stretched over the presenting part that sutures and fontanelles are recognisable. This may be mistaken for a fully dilated cervix. The treatment is for the obstetrician to make two small incisions in the cervix (cervicotomy) to permit delivery to occur (Hibbard 1988). If treatment is delayed, pressure ischaemia can occur, causing oedema and leading to necrosis and detachment of the affected part. This is known as annular detachment of cervix (Jeffcoate and Lister 1952).

Management of incoordinate labour

1. This type of uterine activity is abnormal and therefore the midwife is obliged to inform the obstetrician or general practitioner who will decide what principle of management needs adopting.
2. It is important for the obstetrician to exclude cephalopelvic disproportion as the cause. This may be done by using X-ray pelvimetry or ultrasound scanning if available, but if there is any doubt the obstetrician may decide to perform a caesarean section while mother and fetus are still in good condition.
3. If labour has been prolonged and the mother has been denied a light diet during labour, it may be necessary to correct ketoacidosis, but such an approach is becoming controversial (Dumoulin and Foulkes 1984).
4. It is necessary to ascertain that the bladder is empty; a full bladder is more susceptible to damage.
5. The woman will require artificial rupture of the membranes, and continuous fetal monitoring and either:
   (a) stimulation with oxytocic drugs. These should be used with caution especially for multiparous women (Keirse 1989); or
   (b) analgesia and rest for the mother, followed by gentle stimulation of the uterus with oxytocics, if the rest and relaxation are not sufficient to stimulate labour (Keirse 1989).
6. Women experiencing incoordinate uterine action require much moral support especially if experiencing pain without appreciable progress. The woman and her partner or labour companion need to be kept fully informed of what is happening so that they can understand the situation.

Induction of labour

Donald (1979) states that 'An induced labour is one in which pregnancy is terminated artificially any time after the 28th week of gestation by a method that aims to secure delivery per vias naturales' (p. 480), by a way as natural as possible.

In his review of induction of labour, Calder (1983) states that the continuation of pregnancy is a balancing act. In normal pregnancy, the dangers of intervening far outweigh those of allowing events to take their natural course. In complicated pregnancies, the reverse is true; the obstetrician has to decide at what point the risks of continuing are greater than the problems of prematurity and of establishing labour before term (Calder 1983). In the mid-1970s, once the techniques for inducing labour had been developed, the frequency of induction rose. In some UK hospitals, the rates were over 40% (Howie 1977). The indications for induction at that time had more to do with the staffing level, both medical and midwifery of labour wards (Cartwright 1979) than with proven benefits for the mother and child. Public criticism of massive obstetric intervention without an adequate research base made the rate of induction of labour a subject for debate (Calder 1983). Over recent years, the grounds for inducing labour have changed; improved fetal monitoring has allowed pregnancies previously considered at risk to continue on a day-to-day basis while observing for deleterious changes (Calder 1983).

The following obstetric indications for induction of labour have been advanced:

Gestational proteinuric hypertension (especially where fetal growth is compromised). If the maternal condition is worsening, delivery may be expedited to prevent eclampsia and other complications. Even where fetal and maternal condition are stable, labour may be induced at or around term, due to premature ageing of the placenta which can produce a falling off in fetal growth (Turner 1985).

Post-maturity. With improved fetal monitoring, many obstetricians will allow the pregnancy to continue beyond 42 weeks in the absence of any complications (Cardozo *et al*. 1986). Term is defined as the period between the thirty-seventh and forty-second completed weeks of pregnancy.

Intrauterine growth retardation. Where there are maternal complications, fetal growth may slow or cease, due to placental insufficiency. The fetus is often better delivered than remaining in a hazardous environment (Beischer *et al*. 1984).

Intrauterine death. Induction of labour can prevent increasing the psychological distress the mother is already experiencing, being worsened by the knowledge that she is carrying a dead baby. Bourne (1983) found that some women wanted to have the pregnancy ended as soon as possible, whereas Jolly (1987) discovered that some preferred to have time to come to terms with their loss. Kellner *et al*. (1984) found that 53% of the 69 women they studied preferred to wait for labour to start spontaneously.

Antepartum haemorrhage (Myerscough 1982).

Rhesus isoimmunisation. In the management of rhesus disease, the obstetrician has to balance the maintenance of fetal well-being in utero against the risks of prematurity, if a decision is made to induce labour (Whitfield 1982).

Multiple pregnancy (especially if polyhydramnios is present). Due to the increased risk of maternal complications, there may be reduction in placental function after term (see Chapter 16). Multiple pregnancies may be delivered at or before term (MacGillivray 1984).

Maternal diabetes. There is still a risk of fetal death in utero after 38 weeks gestation, especially where diabetic control has been poor (West 1983).

Cephalopelvic disproportion. In the presence of mild degrees of cephalopelvic disproportion, it is occasionally decided to attempt an early vaginal delivery before the fetus grows too large. In such cases, there are usually contra-indications to the performance of a caesarean section, such as intolerance of general anaesthesia or the presence of a pre-existing medical condition (Myerscough 1982).
Chronic renal disease (Davison 1984).

Prerequisites for successful induction

Hendricks (1983) has shown that there is a period of prelabour lasting up to 4 weeks before delivery, during which the uterus changes from the state of pregnancy to one of readiness for labour. The uterus becomes more contractile and sensitive to oxytocin and there are alterations in the structure of the cervix and pelvic joints and ligaments are relaxed (for more information see Chapter 19). Cervical effacement and dilatation occur progressively, so that the cervix is on average 2 cm dilated during the last half week prior to spontaneous labour (Hendricks *et al.* 1970). For induction of labour to succeed, it is necessary for the technique(s) chosen to produce sufficient uterine contractions and other changes to bring the uterus from the state it has reached in 'prelabour' to the active phase of labour and to maintain progress thereafter (Hendricks 1983). Bishop (1964) devised a system to assess the readiness of the uterus for labour regardless of gestation or maturity of the fetus (see Table 22.1). By assessing the state of the cervix and the descent of the presenting part it can be predicted if labour is imminent. The score is added up; a total of 8 and over is associated with a failure of induction for less than 3% of women, whereas a score of 4 or less indicates that it will take at least 4 hours before the active phase of labour is reached (Friedman *et al.* 1966).

Methods of induction

Prostaglandins PGE_2 and PGF_2 have been used in clinical practice for over 20 years (Pickles *et al.* 1965). Biologically, prostaglandins are produced in all areas of the body, having a local action depending on the particular site and being rapidly metabolised (Calder 1983). Prostaglandins are produced in the myometrium and cervix (Schwartz 1982). Their release can be encouraged by mechanical effects, such as vaginal examination, a 'stretch and sweep' or sexual intercourse (Mitchell *et al.* 1977). Due to their local action and speed of metabolism, prostaglandins are rarely given systemically since, to be effective, large doses are required, which produce severe side-effects such as nausea, vomiting and pyrexia (Calder 1983). Recent use of prostaglandins has involved the use of pessaries, gels or tablets, which are placed in the posterior fornix of the vagina or cervix. Intra- and extra-amniotic solutions may be used, the latter being administered via a Foley catheter, which is inserted through the cervix. The prostaglandin solution is then given via an infusion pump.

Table 22.1 The Bishop score

Score Points	0	1	2	3
Dilatation (cm)	0	1–2	3–4	5–6
Effacement (%)	0–40	40–60	60–80	80 +
Station of presenting part in relation to ischial spines (cm)	− 3	− 2	− 1, 0	+ 1, + 2
Consistency	Firm	Medium	Soft	−
Position of cervical os	Posterior	Central/ anterior	−	−

(Bishop 1964, p. 267)

Prostaglandins are the treatment of choice where the cervix is unfavourable, but they can also be used where intravenous therapy is to be avoided, allowing labour to progress 'naturally' and artificial rupture of the membranes be delayed. Use of prostaglandins in these ways can greatly reduce the rate of failed induction (Shepherd *et al.* 1981).

If prostaglandins are to be used, the woman should remain at rest while the gel or pessary dissolves (usually 30–60 minutes). It is necessary that a cardiotocograph of fetal response to the treatment is obtained for at least the first hour after its administration, to detect intrauterine and therefore fetal hypoxia should the resulting contractions be more than the fetus can cope with. Adverse responses are not uncommon (Keirse and Chalmers 1989). The individual response to prostaglandins varies, some primiparous women requiring repeated doses. In such cases, morale must be maintained and the woman encouraged to eat so she is not in a starved condition when labour does commence, increasing her risks of maternal distress. The maximum dose of PGE_2 recommended by the manufacturer is 3 mg of gel or 6 mg in vaginal tablet form (Upjohn 1989).

Oxytocin

Pituitary extracts were first noted to cause uterine contractions by Dale in 1905 when assessing their effect on a laboratory cat. The first therapeutic use was by Bell in 1909 in the treatment of postpartum haemorrhage. At that stage, the oxytocin was heavily contaminated with other pituitary hormones. Pure oxytocin was available in the early 1930s and was usually administered subcutaneously, intramuscularly or nasally (Thiery *et al.* 1989). In the 1940s intravenous usage was introduced (Page 1943). Du Vigneaud *et al.* (1953) described the chemical structure of oxytocin prior to its synthetic synthesis.

Originally devised to be given sublingually or in the buccal cavity, oxytocin in its synthetic form, syntocinon, is now given intravenously for the induction and augmentation of labour. Syntocinon is of limited effectiveness prior to 34 weeks gestation (Hendricks and Brenner 1964). It is also less potent prior to artificial rupture of the membranes (ARM) (Keirse and Chalmers 1989). In certain cases, such as polyhydramnios or with a high head, contractions may be induced prior to ARM, but great care should be taken as the contractions may become hypertonic when the membranes rupture. As with prostaglandins, individual sensitivity varies and it is necessary to increase the dose given until a satisfactory response is obtained (Turnbull and Anderson 1968). In many cases, the woman's endogenous oxytocin will then take over, especially if the presenting part is well applied to the cervix, and the syntocinon dosage can be reduced without reduction in uterine activity (Calder 1983). To regulate the dose carefully, the infusion should be given via a syringe pump or using a drip counter. The contractions produced using syntocinon tend to be more painful and severe than those occurring naturally (Cartwright 1977, 1979). Unlike physiological contractions, they do not build-up gradually, nor is a strong contraction followed by a couple of weaker ones while the uterus recovers. Some women find the infusion site painful and that the apparatus restricts their movements.

Side-effects of syntocinon are few, but include allergy, overstimulation of the uterus with resulting fetal distress and overhydration of the mother if large quantities of fluid are given (Hatch 1969; Dumoulin and Foulkes 1984). It is thought that fluid retention may result due to the slight antidiuretic effect of oxytocin. Neonatal jaundice is more common in an infant whose mother has received syntocinon in labour (Keirse and Chalmers 1989). It is as yet unclear whether the cause is due to a direct toxic effect, increased neonatal red blood cell haemolysis or simply to the relatively immature bilirubin conjugation mechanism in the liver (Keirse and Chalmers 1989). Fetal condition requires close observation especially if intrauterine hypoxia or placental insufficiency is present.

Amniotomy

Amniotomy was first advocated by Denman in 1785, who supported the technique of forewater rupture to induce preterm labour in women thought to be at risk of cephalopelvic disproportion. The procedure went out of favour, due to the risk of infection if labour was not quickly established. Amniotomy is effective in inducing labour only if the cervix and uterus are on the verge of labour (Keirse and Chalmers 1989). Its effectiveness is increased if used in conjunction with intravenous oxytocin (O'Driscoll *et al.* 1969).

Failure and hazards of induction

Induction of labour may fail because the uterus and cervix are not prepared for labour or because the wrong method is used (Hendricks 1983). It may also fail because the mother or fetus are unable to withstand the treatment chosen. Artificial rupture of the membranes (ARM) may damage the fetus, especially hindwater rupture (Russell *et al.* 1956), introduce infection (Muldoon 1968), provoke a cord prolapse, or even vasa praevia (MacDonald 1970). The mother may suffer a uterine rupture if the uterus has been overstimulated (Keirse and Chalmers 1989). Discontinuing oxytocin therapy at delivery has been associated with an increased risk of postpartum haemorrhage (Donald 1979).

The maternal response to induced labour has been negative in many cases. Work by Kitzinger (1978) and Cartwright (1977, 1979) has shown that induction is less well accepted than spontaneous labour and that it can lead to increased medical interference and worsened outcomes for psychological acceptance, maternal–infant bonding and breast feeding. Kitzinger's (1978) survey results should be treated with a little caution, since her sample was a self-selected group of mothers who were members of an organisation advocating natural childbirth. Cartwright (1979) found that women's greatest dislike was the loss of control over their labour.

Maternal distress in labour

Maternal distress is a term used to describe a mother who is ketotic, pyrexial, with a tachycardia and possibly poor uterine action (Munro Kerr *et al.* 1944). The woman may also be exhausted from the effect of prolonged labour or severe pain. This can be the result of a mismanaged labour. Argument surrounds whether the presence of maternal ketosis alone is a pathological condition or a physiological state normal in pregnancy and labour (Sabata *et al.* 1968; Dumoulin and Foulkes 1984). Ludka (1987) equates uterine activity in labour as being similar to the energy expenditure of a woman walking uphill with a heavy load. She argues that it is no wonder women who are starved in labour experience problems. A hospital is described where women who were previously allowed to eat lightly and drink as desired were then only allowed sips of water during labour. Over a 6 month period following the change in practice there was a fivefold increase in the augmentation of labour, a 35% and 38% rise in forceps and caesarean section deliveries, respectively, and a 69% increase in use of intensive care of the newborn. The figures returned to their previous levels once women were again permitted to eat in labour (Ludka 1987).

The risk of aspiration of stomach contents is advanced as a reason for denying food during labour; it is however noticeable that, once in established labour, women usually only desire fluids. The antacids routinely prescribed present danger if aspirated (Scott 1978). Specific antacid preparations can be given prior to anaesthesia; these include sodium citrate and aluminium hydroxide (Taylor and Pryse-Davies 1966), hydrogen ion antagonists (such as cimetidine) (McCaughey *et al.* 1981), and metoclopramide, which increases the speed of gastric emptying (Howard and Sharp 1973). The anaesthetic should be given by a well-qualified anaesthetist with an assistant to perform cricoid pressure until intubation is complete (Sellick 1961; Crawford 1986). Only in this way will aspiration be prevented. Denying fluid to the woman only serves to increase the acidity of gastric contents and hence the risk should aspiration occur (Roberts and Shirley 1976).

Hydration with parenteral glucose and electrolyte solutions to correct ketosis is going out of favour, due to the associated problems of fetal hypernutraemia with iatrogenic hyperinsulinsim and neonatal hypoglycaemia (Lucas *et al.* 1980).

Maternal overhydration is also dangerous, since the labouring woman has an impaired ability to excrete water. Tarno-Mordi *et al*. (1981) state that an intravenous intake of 1200 ml/day is adequate in labour. Feeney (1982) demonstrated that intravenous intakes of more than 3500 ml can give rise to postpartum cerebral oedema, fits and coma.

Fetal distress and monitoring

Fetal distress in labour arises due to disruption in the flow of oxygen and nutrients to the fetus, and of waste products from the fetus (Whittle 1985). Most normal fetuses at term can withstand the temporary hypoxia which occurs during contractions. Amongst the causes of distress in labour are:

1. Pre-existing placental insufficiency, which is worsened by uterine contractions (Ramsey *et al*. 1963).
2. Cord compression, due to position, true knots, the cord being around the neck or cord prolapse (James *et al*. 1976).
3. Obstructed labour.
4. Head compression (Whittle 1985).

The aim of monitoring is to differentiate those babies who are able to cope with the stresses of labour from those who cannot.

Meconium

In utero passage of meconium is most common amongst term and post-term fetuses (Knox *et al*. 1979). It can occur spontaneously, but anoxia (for example, as a result of cord compression) produces stimulation of the vagus nerve which increases gastric mobility resulting in passage of meconium (Walker 1959). The presence of meconium staining (especially if slight), in the absence of other signs of fetal distress, is not itself a dangerous sign (Miller *et al*. 1984); however meconium, with or without fetal heart rate anomalies, should not be ignored (Miller 1985).

In cases of meconium staining, expert resuscitation by a paediatrician is required, involving clearing the airways as soon as the head is delivered, careful suctioning and examination of the vocal cords for meconium staining (Carson *et al*. 1976). Aspiration is most likely to occur where there is thick meconium and the fetus/neonate is acidotic (Carson *et al*. 1976). In these circumstances, gasping (and therefore inhalation of liquor) can occur, both in utero and during delivery (Miller 1985). If aspiration has occurred, bronchial lavage is required to prevent inhalational pneumonia (Miller 1985). The stomach contents should also be checked as meconium is a gastric irritant which can provoke vomiting; if necessary, a gastric washout should be performed. This is important because Carson *et al.* (1976) report that neonatal mortality rates can be increased twentyfold following aspiration.

Assessing fetal well-being

Monitoring fetal condition in labour involves observation of the fetal heart rate, either intermittently with a Pinard's stethoscope or continuously with a cardiotocograph (external) or electrocardiograph (ECG – internal) machines. Midwives develop the necessary skills to assess fetal heart patterns by listening before, during and just after contractions. To minimise disturbance to the mother, a portable Doptone machine may be used, which is more convenient, especially where the mother wishes to be upright.

Fetal cardiac muscle has an intrinsic rhythm, with a rate between 120 and 160 beats/minute. This is as a consequence of the balance achieved and stimulation of the autonomic nervous system, in which parasympathetic input comes to predominate with maturity (Wladimiroff and Seelan 1972). Changes in the heart rate can be brought about through stimulation of the fetal autonomic nervous system; sympathetic nervous system stimulation causes acceleration of the heart, whereas the parasympathetic nervous system causes deceleration via the vagus nerve (Rudolph and Heymann 1973). Depending on which system is receiving most stimulation, the fetal heart rate changes accordingly (Wladimiroff and Seelan 1972). The speed of response to a stimulus will be apparent in the heart rate pattern, for example, head compression is quickly mediated via the vagus nerve, producing a rapid change in heart rate. Placental hypoxia is much slower to produce a response and therefore the alterations in fetal heart rate occur later. Fetal activity stimulates the sympathetic nervous system, giving rise to an acceleration in the fetal heart rate (Dalton *et al.* 1977).

- Baseline variability is when the fetal heart has a beat-to-beat variation of 10–15 beats/minute; reduced or increased variability requires reporting to medical staff. Following maternal narcotic analgesia, the pattern may be 'flat' for a while before recovering (Yeh *et al.* 1974). The variability of the fetal heart rate (that is, the beat-to-beat variation), indicates fetal well-being and its absence may signal the presence of fetal compromise (Kubli *et al.* 1969). Hammacher *et al.* (1968) define a beat-to-beat variation of less than 5 beats/minute as being an abnormal/silent pattern; 5–10 beats/minute as at the lower limit of normal; 10–25 beats/minute as normal and over 25 beats/minute as abnormal/excess variability. Increased variability may be associated with the early onset of acute hypoxia (Martin 1978).
- Baseline fetal heart rates above 160 and below 120 beats/minute are regarded as tachycardia and bradycardia, respectively. Tachycardia can be caused by maternal ketosis or pyrexia and early fetal hypoxia and acidosis. Bradycardias are usually associated with hypoxia, especially if combined with a loss of beat-to-beat variation (Hon 1968).
- Fetal heart rate decelerations.

Early decelerations

The lowest point in the deceleration coincides with the peak of the contraction; recovery is swift (Hon 1968). These are usually caused by head compression, in which the fetal parasympathetic nervous system is quickly stimulated, giving an instantaneous response although the exact mechanism is unclear (Whittle 1985). This type of deceleration requires noting, but is not thought to be ominous; it is very common in the second stage of labour (Whittle 1985).

Late decelerations

These occur when there is a time delay (lag time) between the height of the contraction and the lowest point in the deceleration; the recovery may also be slow (Hon 1968). Cord or placental compression take longer than head compression to affect the fetal nervous system, hence the delay in the heart rate response. Prolonged hypoxia causes direct depression of the myocardium and brain, producing deceleration in the heart rate (Whittle 1985). These are associated with fetal acidosis and must be reported to the medical staff, who will decide what action is to be taken. To confirm acidosis, fetal blood sampling may be performed (Zanini et al. 1979), or if the obstetrician is sufficiently concerned, delivery will be effected by forceps or caesarean section. The use of fetal blood sampling has been shown to reduce the caesarean section rate for fetal distress (Zalar and Quiligan 1978).

Effectiveness of continuous fetal monitoring

Midwives have argued that by listening intermittently they can detect heart rate anomalies and then if necessary institute continuous monitoring (Flint 1986). Medical staff, fearful of litigation (Prentice and Lind 1987) and unsure of the midwives' skills, may have more faith in machinery, especially since intermittent monitoring only samples 7% of the total heart beat (MacDonald et al. 1985), is subject to wide margins of error (Hon 1958) and gives poor assessment of beat-to-beat variation (Miller et al. 1984). It has been documented by MacDonald et al. (1985) that the introduction of continuous monitoring, especially if unsupported by corroborative evidence of acidosis from fetal blood sampling, is associated with a rise in the caesarean section rate. Fetal blood sampling is the only definitive method of differentiating the baby who is coping, although showing decelerations from the one with deceleration who is hypoxic (Grant 1989). Tejani et al. (1976) showed that only 50% of newborns who had had an ominous fetal heart rate pattern were depressed at birth when the Apgar was measured. In another 73% of newborns with a cord arterial blood pH of more than 7.10 had an Apgar score less then 7 and 86% had a five minutes score of over 7 (Sykes et al. 1982).

In addition to their doubtful effectiveness, the use of scalp electrodes is a further hindrance to maternal mobility (the availability of telemetry is not uniform) and of necessity, the membranes need to be ruptured. However, when considering the already 'at risk' fetus the use of continuous electronic fetal monitoring supported by fetal blood sampling is all that can be advised to ensure fetal well-being with the proviso that there are still arguments as to the interpretation of the data (Prentice and Lind 1987). Prentice and Lind (1987) state that there is no evidence to support the routine use of continuous fetal monitoring in labour.

In the largest study to date involving 12 964 women, MacDonald *et al.* (1985) found little difference in outcomes where fetuses were randomly assigned to being monitored continuously or intermittently; all diagnoses of fetal distress were subject to confirmation by fetal blood sampling. The rates of delivery by caesarean section were similar, although there were slightly more instrumental deliveries amongst mothers in the continuously monitored group. The authors could find no benefit in a particular method of monitoring to mother or fetus where the labour lasted for less than 5 hours, although there was an excess of neonatal convulsions amongst the intermittently monitored group when the labour lasted longer than this. At a follow-up at 1 year of age, there was no significant difference in the neurological wellbeing of babies in either group (MacDonald *et al.* 1985). Few midwives or obstetricians would argue against the monitoring of the fetal condition in women at high obstetric risk, but the argument is about extending yet another procedure to normal women, further increasing the medicalisation of childbirth (Grant 1989).

References

Balaskas A and Balaskas J (1979) *New Life* Sidgwick and Jackson: London

Barlow J (1822) *Essays on Surgery and Midwifery* Baldwin, Cradock and Joy: London

Beischer N A, Abell D A and Drew J H (1984) 'Intra-uterine growth retardation' in J Studd (ed) *Progress in Obstetrics and Gynaecology* Vol 4 Ch 6 82–91 Churchill Livingstone: Edinburgh

Bell W B (1909) 'The pituitary body' *British Medical Journal* 2: 1609–13

Bennett V R and Brown L K (1989) *Myles Textbook for Midwives (11th edn)* Churchill Livingstone: Edinburgh

Bishop E H (1964) 'Pelvic scoring for elective induction' *Obstetrics and Gynecology* 24: 266–8.

Bontekoe E H M, Blacquiere J F, Naaktgeboren C, Dieleman S J and Willems P P M (1977) 'Influences of environmental disturbances on uterine motility during pregnancy and parturition in rabbit and sheep' *Behavioural Processes* 2: 41–73

Bourne S (1983) 'Psychological impact of stillbirth' *The Practitioner* 227(1): 53–60

Butler N R and Bonham D G (1963) *Perinatal Mortality* E and S Livingstone Ltd: Edinburgh

Calder A (1983) 'Methods of induction of labour' in J Studd (ed) *Progress in Obstetrics and Gynaecology Vol III* 86–100 Churchill Livingstone: Edinburgh

Caldeyro Barcia R (1980) 'Physiological and psychological bases for the modern and humanised management of labour' in Tokyo Ministry of Health and Welfare *Recent Progress in Perinatal Medicine.* Government of Japan: 77–96.

Cardozo L, Fysh J and Pearce J M (1986) 'Prolonged pregnancy: the management debate' *British Medical Journal* 293: 1059–63

Cardozo L D, Gibb D M F, Studd J W W, Vasant R V and Cooper D J (1982) 'Predictive value of cervimetric labour patterns in primigravidae' *British Journal of Obstetrics and Gynaecology* 80: 33

Cardozo L and Studd J (1985) 'Abnormal labour patterns' in J Studd (ed) *Management of Labour* Ch 12 171–87 Blackwell Scientific: London

Carson B S, Losey R W, Bowes W H and Simmons M A (1976) 'Combined obstetric and pediatric approach to prevent meconium aspiration syndrome' *American Journal of Obstetrics and Gynecology* 126: 712

Cartwright A (1977) 'Mothers' experiences of induction' *British Medical Journal* 2: 745–9

Cartwright A (1979) *The Dignity of Labour?* Tavistock: London

Chalmers I (1976) 'British debate on obstetric practice' *Pediatrics* 58: 308–12

Crawford J S (1978) *Principles and Practice of Obstetric Anaesthesia* (4th edn) Blackwell Scientific: Oxford

Crawford J S (1986) 'Maternal mortality from Mendelson's syndrome' *Lancet* i: 920–1

Crowther C, Enkin M, Keirse M J N C and Brown I (1989) 'Monitoring the progress of labour' in I Chalmers, M Enkin and M J N C Keirse (eds) *Effective Care in Pregnancy and Childbirth* Ch 53 833–45 Oxford University Press: Oxford

Curtis P, Evans S, Resnick J, Rimer R, Lynch K and Carlton J (1986) 'Uterine responses to three techniques of breast stimulation' *Obstetrics and Gynecology* 67(1): 22–8

Dale H H (1905) 'On physiological actions of ergot' *Journal of Physiology* 34: 163–205

Dalton K J, Dawes G S and Patrick J E (1977) 'Diurnal, respiratory and other rhythms of foetal heart rate in lambs' *American Journal of Obstetrics and Gynecology* 127: 414–24

Davison J (1984) 'Renal disease' in M de Swiet (ed) *Medical Disorders in Obstetric Practice* Ch 7 192–259 Blackwell Scientific: Oxford

Denman T (1785) *Principles of Midwifery on Puerperal Medicine* E. Cox: London

Donald I (1979) *Practical Obstetric Problems* (5th edn) Lloyd-Luke: London

Dumoulin J G and Foulkes J E B (1984) 'Ketonuria during labour' *British Journal of Obstetrics and Gynaecology* 91(2): 97–8

du Vigneaud V, Ressler C and Trippett S (1953) 'The sequence of amino acids in oxytocin with a proposal for the structure of oxytocin *Journal of Biological Chemistry* 205: 949–57

Eastman N J (1938) 'The induction of labor' *American Journal of Obstetrics and Gynecology* 35: 721–30

Feeney J G (1982) 'Water intoxication and oxytocin' *British Medical Journal* 284: 243

Flint C (1986) *Sensitive Midwifery* Heinemann: London

Flynn A M, Kelly J, Hollins G and Lynch P F (1978) 'Ambulation in labour' *British Medical Journal* 2: 591–3

Friedman E A (1954) 'The graphic analysis of labor' *American Journal of Obstetrics and Gynecology* 68: 1568–75

Friedman E A (1955) Primigravid labor – a graphostatistical analysis' *Obstetrics and Gynecology* 6: 567–89

Friedman E A (1973) 'Patterns of labor – as indication of risk' *Clinical Obstetrics and Gynecology* 6: 567

Friedman E A (1981) 'The labor curve' *Clinics in Perinatology* 7: 15–25

Friedman E A, Niswander K R, Bayonet-Rivera N P and Sachtleben M R (1966) 'Relation of prelabour evaluation in inducibility and the course of labour' *Obstetrics and Gynecology* 29: 495–501.

Friedman E A and Sachtleben M R (1961) 'Dysfunctional labor' *Obstetrics and Gynecology* 17: 135

Friedman E A and Sachtleben M R (1963) 'Amniotomy and the course of labour' *Obstetrics and Gynecology* 22: 755–70

Friedman E A, Sachtleben M R and Bresky P A (1977) 'Dysfunctional labor: XII Long-term effects on infants' *American Journal of Obstetrics and Gynecology* 127: 779

Gibb D M F, Cardozo L D, Studd J W W, Magos A L and Cooper D J (1982) 'Outcome of spontaneous labour in multigravidae' *British Journal of Obstetrics and Gynaecology* 89(9): 708

Grant A (1989) 'Monitoring the foetus in labour' in I Chalmers, M Enkin and M J N C Keirse (eds) *Effective Care in Pregnancy and Childbirth* Ch 54 846–82 Oxford Medical: Oxford

Hammacher K, Huter K A, Bokelmann J and Werners P H (1968) 'Foetal heart frequency and perinatal condition of the foetus and newborn' *Gynaecologia* 166: 349–60

Hatch M C (1969) 'Maternal death associated with induction of labour' *New York State Journal of Medicine* 69: 599–602

Henderson C (1984) 'Influences and interactions surrounding the midwife's decision to rupture membranes' *Research and the Midwife Proceedings* 68–85

Hendricks C H (1983) 'Second thoughts on induction of labour' in J Studd (ed) *Progress in Obstetrics and Gynaecology Vol 3* Ch 8 101–12 Churchill Livingstone: Edinburgh

Hendricks C H and Brenner W E (1964) 'Patterns of increasing uterine activity in late pregnancy and the development of uterine responsiveness to oxytocin' *American Journal of Obstetrics and Gynecology* 90: 485–92

Hendricks C H, Brenner W E and Kraus G (1970) 'Normal cervical dilatation pattern in late pregnancy and labour' *American Journal of Obstetrics and Gynecology* 106: 1065–82

Hibbard B M (1988) *Principles of Obstetrics* Butterworth: London

Hon E H (1958) 'The electronic evaluation of the fetal heart rate: a preliminary report' *American Journal of Obstetrics and Gynecology* 75: 1215–30

Hon E H (1968) *An Atlas of Fetal Heart Rate Patterns* Harty Press: New Haven

Howard F A and Sharp D S (1973) 'Effect of Metoclopramide on gastric emptying during labour' *British Medical Journal* 1: 446–8

Howie P W (1977) 'Induction of labour' in T Chard and M Richards (eds) *Benefits and Hazards of New Obstetrics* 83–99 Spastics International Medical Publications: London

James L S, Yeh M, Marishma H O, Daniel S S, Cartis S M, Niemannn D V M and Indyk L (1976) 'Umbilical vein occlusion and transient acceleration of FHR ' *American Journal of Obstetrics and Gynecology* 126: 276

Jeffcoate T N A and Lister U (1952) 'Annular detachment of the cervix' *Journal of Obstetrics and Gynaecology of the British Empire* 54: 327–35

Jolly J (1987) *Missed Beginnings. Death Before Life has been Established.* Austen Cornish Publishers: Reading

Keirse M J N C (1989) 'Augmentation of labour' in I Chalmers, M Enkin and M J N C Keirse (eds) *Effective Care in Pregnancy and Childbirth* Ch 58: 951–66 Oxford Medical: Oxford

Keirse M J N C and Chalmers I (1989) 'Methods for inducing labour' in I Chalmers, M Enkin and M J N C Keirse (eds) *Effective Care in Pregnancy and Childbirth* Ch 62 1057–79 Oxford Medical: Oxford

Kellner K R, Donnelly W H and Gould S D (1984) 'Parental behaviour after perinatal death' *Obstetrics and Gynecology* 63: 809–14

Kitzinger S (1978) *Some Mothers' Experiences of Induced Labour* National Childbirth Trust: London

Klaus M H, Kennell J H, Robertson S S and Sosa R (1986) 'Effects of social support during parturition on maternal infant morbidity' *British Medical Journal* 293: 585–7

Knox G E, Huddleston J F and Flowers C E (1979) 'Management of prolonged pregnancy: Results of a prospective randomised controlled trial' *American Journal of Obstetrics and Gynecology* 134: 376

Kubli F W, Hon E H, Khazin A F and Takemura H (1969) 'Observations on heart rate and pH in the human fetus at term' *American Journal of Obstetrics and Gynecology* 104: 1190

Lindgren L (1959) 'The courses of foetal head moulding in labour' *Acta Obstetric and Gynaecologica Scandanavica* 38: 211

Lucas A, Adrian T E, Aynsley-Green A and Bloom S R (1980) 'Iatrogenic hyperinsulimism at birth' *Lancet* i: 144–5

Ludka L (1987) *Fasting During Labour* Paper given at the 21st International Confederation of Midwives Congress The Hague 26.8.87

MacDonald D (1970) 'Surgical induction of labour' *Americal Journal of Obstetrics and Gynecology* 107: 908–11

MacDonald D, Grant A, Sheridan-Pereira M, Boylan P and Chalmers I (1985) 'The Dublin randomised controlled trail of intrapartum fetal heart rate monitoring' *American Journal of Obstetrics and Gynecology* 152(5): 524–39.

MacGillivray I (1984) 'The maternal response to twin pregnancy' in J Studd (ed) *Progress in Obstetrics and Gynaecology Vol 4* Ch 10 139–50 Churchill Livingstone: Edinburgh

McCaughey W, Howe J P, Moore J and Dundee J W (1981) 'Cimetidine in elective caesarean section. Effect on gastric acidity' *Anaesthesia* 36: 167–72

Martell M, Belizan J M, Nieto F and Schwarz R (1976) 'Blood acid base balance at birth in neonates from labours with early and late rupture of membranes' *Journal of Pediatrics* 89: 963–7

Martin C B (1978) 'Regulation of fetal heart rate and genesis of fetal heart rate patterns' *Seminars in Perinatology* 2: 13

Miller F C (1985) 'Significance of meconium in amniotic fluid' in J Studd (ed) *Management of Labour* Ch 13 188–94 Blackwell Scientific: Oxford

Miller F C, Pearce K E and Paul R H (1984) 'Fetal heart rate pattern recognition by the method of auscultation' *Obstetrics and Gynecology* 64: 332–6

Miller F C, Yeh S-J and Schifrin B S (1976) 'Quantification of uterine activity in 100 primiparous patients' *American Journal of Obstetrics and Gynecology* 124: 398–405

Mitchell M D, Flint A P F, Bibby J, Brunt J, Anderson A B M and Turnbull A C (1977) 'Rapid increases in plasma prostaglandin concentrations after vaginal examination and amniotomy' *British Medical Journal* 2: 1183–5

Muldoon M J (1968) 'A prospective study of intrauterine infection following surgical induction of labour' *Journal of Obstetrics and Gynaecology of the British Commonwealth* 75: 1144–50

Munro Kerr J M, Johnstone R W, Young J, Hendry J, McIntyre D, Baird D and Fahmy E C (1944) *Combined Textbook of Obstetrics and Gynaecology (4th edn)* Livingstone: Edinburgh

Myerscough P R M (1982) *Munro Kerr's Operational Obstetrics (10th edn)* Balliere Tindall: London

Naaktgeboren C (1989) 'The biology of childbirth' in I Chalmers, M Enkin and M J N C Keirse (eds) *Effective Care in Pregnancy and Childbirth* Ch 48 795–804 Oxford Medical: Oxford

Odent M (1983) 'Birth under water' *Lancet* ii: 1476

O'Driscoll K, Jackson R J A and Gallagher J T (1969) 'Prevention of prolonged labour' *British Medical Journal* 2: 477–80

O'Driscoll K and Meagher D (1980) *Active Management of Labour* W B Saunders: London

Page E W (1943) 'Response of human pregnant uterus to Pitocin tannate in oil' *Proceedings of the Society of Experimental Biological Medicine* 52: 195–7

Philpott R H and Castle W M (1972a) 'Cervicographs in the management of labour in primigravidae: 1. The alert line for detecting abnormal labour' *Journal of Obstetrics and Gynaecology of the British Commonwealth* 79: 592–8

Philpott R H and Castle W M (1972b) 'Cervicographs in the management of labour in primigravidae: 2. Action line and treatment of abnormal labour' *Journal of Obstetrics and Gynaecology of the British Commonwealth* 79: 599–602

Pickles V R, Hall W J, Best F A and Smith G N (1965) 'Prostaglandins in endometrium and menstrual fluid from normal and dysmenorrheic subjects' *Journal of Obstetrics and Gynaecology of the British Commonwealth* 72: 185–92

Ploss H H P, Bartels M and Bartels P (1935) *Woman Vol II* Heinemann Medical: London

Prentice A and Lind T (1987) 'Fetal heart rate monitoring during labour – too frequent intervention, too little benefit?' *Lancet* ii: 1375–7

Ramsey E M, Corner G W and Donner M W (1963) 'Serial and cineradioangiographic visualization of maternal circulation in the primate placenta' *American Journal of Obstetrics and Gynecology* 86: 213

Roberts R B and Shirley M A (1976) 'The obstetricians role in reducing the risk of aspiration pneumonitis' *American Journal of Obstetrics and Gynecology* 124: 611–7

Rudolph A M and Heymann M A (1973) 'Control of foetal circulation' *Proceedings of the Sir Joseph Barcroft Symposium* 89 Cambridge University Press: Cambridge

Russell J K, Smith D F and Yule R (1956) 'Foetal exsanguination associated with surgical induction of labour' *British Medical Journal* 2: 1414–5

Sabata V, Wolf H and Lansmann S (1968) 'The role of free fatty acids, glycerol, ketone bodies and glucose in the energy metabolism of the mother and fetus during laour' *Biology of the Neonate* 13: 7–17

Salmon Y M, Kee W H, Tans L and Jen S W (1986) 'Cervical ripening by breast stimulation' *Obstetrics and Gynecology* 67(1): 21–4

Schwarz R (1973) 'Fetal heart rate patterns in labour with intact and ruptured membranes' *Journal of Perinatal Medicine* 1: 152

Schwarz R (1974) 'Effect of late rupture of membranes on labour and the neonate' in L Gluck (ed) *Modern Perinatal Medicine* 432 Yearbook Medical Publishers: Chicago

Schwartz R (1982) 'The onset of labour' in J Studd (ed) *Progress in Obstetrics and Gynaecology Vol 2* Ch 1 3–9 Churchill Livingstone: Edinburgh

Schwartz R, Strada-Saenz G, Althabe O, Fernandez-Funes J and Caldeyro-Barcia R (1969) 'Pressure exerted by uterine contractions on the head of the human fetus during labor' in R Caldeyro-Barcia (ed) *Perinatal Factors Affecting Human Development* 115–26 Pan American Health Organisation: Washington

Scott D B (1978) 'History of Mendelson's syndrome' *Journal of International Medical Research* 6: 47–51

Sellick B A (1961) 'Cricoid pressure to control regurgitation of stomach contents during induction of anaesthesia' *Lancet* ii: 404–6

Shepherd J H, Bennett M J, Lawrence D, Moore F and Sims C D (1981) 'Prostaglandin vaginal suppositories: a simple and safe approach to the induction of labour' *Obstetrics and Gynecology* 58: 596

Studd J W W, Cardozo L D and Gibb D M F (1982) 'The management of spontaneous labour' in J Studd (ed) *Progress in Obstetrics and Gynaecology Vol 2* Ch 7 60–72 Churchill Livingstone: Edinburgh

Studd J W W, Crawford S J, Duignan N M, Rowbotham C J R and Hughes A O (1980) 'The effect of lumbar epidural analgesia in the rate of cervical dilatation and the outcome of labour of spontaneous onset' *British Journal of Obstetrics and Gynaecology* 87: 1015

Sykes G S, Johnson P S and Ashworth F (1982) 'Do apgar scores indicate asphyxia?' *Lancet* i: 494–6

Tarno-Mordi W O, Shaw J C L, Liv D, Gardner D A and Flynn F V (1981) 'Lactrogenic lyponatraemia of the newborn due to maternal fluid overload' *British Medical Journal* 283: 639–42

Taylor G and Pryse-Davies J (1966) 'The prophylactic use of antacids in the prevention of acid-pulmonary-aspiration syndrome (Mendelson's syndrome)' *Lancet* i: 288–91

Tejani N, Mann L I, Bhakthavathsalan A (1978) 'Correlations of fetal heart rate patterns and fetal pH with neonate outcome' *Obstetrics and Gynecology* 48: 460–3

Thiery M, Baines C J and Keirse M J N C (1989) 'The development of methods for inducing labour' in I Chalmers, M Enkin and M J N C Keirse (eds) *Effective Care in Pregnancy and Childbirth* Ch 59 969–80 Oxford Medical: Oxford

Turnbull A C and Anderson A B M (1968) 'Induction of labour III: Results with amniotomy and oxytocin titration' *Journal of Obstetrics and Gynaecology of the British Commonwealth* 75: 32–41

Turner G M (1985) 'Management of pre-eclampsia and eclampsia' in G Chamberlain (ed) *Contemporary Obstetrics* Butterworth: London

Upjohn (1989) *Prescribing Information for Prostin E2 Vaginal Gel and Vaginal Tablets* Upjohn: Crawley

Walker J (1959) 'Fetal distress' *American Journal of Obstetrics and Gynecology* 79: 94–107

West T E T (1983) 'Diabetic pregnancy' *Update* 26(4): 633–42

Whitfield C R (1982) 'Future challenges in the management of rhesus disease' in J Studd (ed) *Progress in Obstetrics and Gynaecology Vol 2* Ch 6 48–59 Churchill Livingstone: Edinburgh

Whittle M J (1985) 'Fetal physiology in labour' in J Studd (ed) *Management of Labour* Ch 18 252–67 Blackwell Scientific: Oxford

Wladimiroff J W and Seelen J C (1972) 'Fetal heart action in early pregnancy' *European Journal of Obstetrics and Gynaecology* 2: 55

Yeh S-Y, Paul R H, Cordero L and Hon E H (1974) 'A study of diazepam during labour' *Obstetrics and Gynecology* 43: 363–73

Zalar R W and Quiligan E J (1978) 'The influence of scalp sampling on the cesarean section rate for fetal distress' *American Journal of Obstetrics and Gynecology* 135: 239

Zanini B, Paul R H and Huey J R (1979) 'Intrapartum fetal heart rate: correlation with scalp pH in the preterm fetus' *American Journal of Obstetrics and Gynecology* 136: 43

23   Preterm labour and delivery

The World Health Organization (1977) defines preterm labour as one occurring before the completion of 37 weeks of gestation. No lower limit is established and therefore countries rely on their own definitions for differentiating preterm labour from late abortion (Lumley 1987b). In the United Kingdom a baby born alive before 28 weeks gestation would be classified as a live birth, whereas one born dead would be a late abortion rather than a stillbirth. Mugford (1983) noted that whilst most European countries used a 28 week (of gestation) dividing line, Norway registered stillbirths after 16 weeks, Australia from 20 weeks and Japan from as early as 12 weeks.

Approximately 5% of births occur before 37 completed weeks of gesation, but these deliveries account for two-thirds of perinatal deaths (stillbirths and deaths in the first week of life) (McCormick 1985; Hibbard 1987). In addition to the risks of mortality for the fetus/baby, there is a considerable risk of morbidity for the mother (especially psychological (Astbury and Bajuk 1987)) and for the baby (Kumar *et al.* 1980).

Causes

The causes of preterm birth are complex and poorly understood. Certain conditions, such as multiple pregnancy, are associated with spontaneous preterm delivery (McKeown and Record 1952), whereas maternal complications, such as severe hypertensive disease of pregnancy, may result in a planned preterm birth (Kaltreider and Kohl 1980). Rush *et al*. (1976) studied 400 preterm deliveries and concluded that in 12% of cases there was no scope for the improvement of outcome, since the fetus either had a lethal malformation or was dead prior to admission to hospital. Twenty-eight per cent of the deliveries resulted from elective preterm induction of labour for maternal or fetal complications, the most common being hypertensive disease, antepartum haemorrhage and intrauterine growth retardation (Rush *et al*. 1976). Multiple pregnancy accounted for 10% of the deliveries, and in a further 24% there was a recognised precipitating cause. There still remained a significant proportion of preterm deliveries with no obvious cause, except for the multifactorial influences of stress (Newton *et al*. 1979), poverty, cigarette smoking and socio-economic status (Garn *et al*. 1977), which provide a confusing picture (Lumley 1987a). Fredrick and Anderson (1976) have shown that having had one or more previous spontaneous preterm deliveries significantly increases a woman's risk of having another.

Creasy *et al*. (1980) developed a scoring system which could be used antenatally to determine a woman's risk of having a preterm delivery (see Table 23.1). Women

Table 23.1 Risk scoring for preterm delivery

Points	Socio-economic	Past history	Daily habits	Current pregnancy
1	Two children at home Low SES	One abortion < 1 year since birth	Work outside home	Unusual fatigue
2	< 20 years > 40 years	Two abortions	> 10 cigarettes/days	< 13 kg weight gain by 32 weeks Albuminuria Hypertension Bacteruria
3	Very low socio-economic status	Three abortions	Heavy work long tiring trip to work	Breech at 32 weeks, weight loss of 2 kg, head engaged, febrile illness.
4	< 18 years	Pyelonephritis		Bleeding after 12 weeks, effacement, diliatation, uterine irritation
5		Uterine anomaly second trimester abortion		Placenta praevia polyhydramnios
6		Premature delivery Repeated second trimester abortion		Twins Abdominal surgery

(Creasy *et al*. 1980)

have their risk assessed at the start of antenatal care and they are reassessed at 26–28 weeks gestation. In Creasy *et al.* (1980), the initial assessment detected 44% of the preterm deliveries, with the number successfully anticipated rising to 66% following the second assessment. Using this system, women scoring less than 5 are said to be at low risk with those over 10 being at high risk.

Diagnosis of preterm labour

The term labour implies progressive uterine activity, producing cervical dilatation and resulting in expulsion of the fetus.

However, over 50% of women in apparently established preterm labour will stop contracting spontaneously and continue with their pregnancy (Anderson 1981). These figures refer to the proportion of women who cease their preterm labour when treated with bed rest or a placebo. The onset of preterm labour may be insidious, so making a diagnosis is difficult. King (1987) supports the recommendation that apparent preterm labour should not be treated medically unless the diagnosis is supported by progress in labour, such as dilatation of the cervix. Castle and Turnbull (1983) have used the absence of fetal breathing movements as an indicator that preterm labour will continue. Those women whose fetuses showed no breathing movements (FBM) in a 45 minute period all delivered within 48 hours, whereas those with intact membranes where FBM were present continued their pregnancy for at least a week in 25 out of 27 cases. Where the membranes rupture spontaneously before 37 weeks gestation and there are no contractions, the pregnancy may be allowed to continue, as long as infection or fetal complications do not develop (Keirse *et al.* 1989a).

The obstetrician's dilemma is to detect the woman who is on the threshold of preterm labour, without allowing her to progress 'too far' so that she has passed beyond the period where treatment could be effective, whilst avoiding giving potentially harmful therapy to those women who do not need it. Anderson (1981) states that with the current state of development of neonatal intensive care, little is to be gained by trying to stop labour in women over 34 weeks gestation.

Management of preterm labour

Psychological care

The onset of preterm labour is a very worrying time for the parents and their close relatives. Preparations so carefully made can fall apart; other children will need to be cared for and given explanations, the father may need to negotiate time away from work and plans for early transfer home from hospital will be disrupted. The parents will experience great uncertainty whether the labour will continue and, if it does, what will be the condition of the baby when it is born. Following delivery, the parents may grieve for the child they were expecting (Kaplan and Mason 1960), one born at term looking like the typical pink, round-cheeked ideal (Astbury and Bajuck 1987).

During the labour the parents must be fully involved (should they so wish) when decisions are being made concerning care and everything that is happening must be explained to them. This should help to reduce anxiety resulting from non-verbal communication by carers, which is at variance with the information given. If at all possible, it is helpful for parents to visit the neonatal intensive care unit before the delivery to prepare them for the care their baby will receive. Equipment can appear frightening to those unfamiliar with it and a visit to inspect the unit before their baby is admitted may help reduce later anxiety. The midwife should use her judgement before arranging such a visit, since it may not be appropriate for all couples. If the labour is too far advanced, a member of staff from the unit should visit the labour ward to explain what will occur.

Bedrest

Saunders *et al.* (1985) in a randomised trial of women at risk of preterm delivery showed that women allocated to the bedrest group had more preterm deliveries than the 'active' group. Admission to hospital for rest gives rise to considerable psychological stress (Jonas 1963) and much disruption (Rosen 1975). Rest at home does have the advantage that the woman feels that she is doing something, although as Lumley (1987b) comments, it is questionable how much rest women get without adequate support at home.

Drug therapy

The two main groups of drugs employed to stop labour are the betamimetics and the prostaglandin synthetase inhibitors (Keirse *et al.* 1989b). Drugs used to inhibit labour are referred to as tocolytics. Anderson (1981) argues that the use of tocolytics is justified in only 10% of women in preterm labour, although it is difficult before the event to identify those who will benefit. Factors to be taken into account include the estimated size of the fetus, its normality, its gestational age, the condition of the membranes, cervical dilatation and maternal well-being (Anderson 1981).

Betamimetics act by stimulating the beta receptors in smooth muscle resulting in a decrease in free calcium ions and therefore muscle relaxation (Pearce 1985). The most commonly used betamimetics in Europe are ritodrine and salbutamol (Keirse *et al.* 1989b). These drugs are both non-specific to the uterus (although better than others in this group) and their use gives rise to various side-effects including hypotension, tachycardia, palpitations and nausea. These effects may sometimes be so severe as to necessitate discontinuing the treatment. Betamimetic drugs are contra-indicated in women with cardiac disease, diabetes mellitus and hypothyroidism (Keirse *et al.* 1989b). Their use is questionable in cases of spontaneous rupture of the membranes and antepartum haemorrhage. If the fetus is already compromised, environmental changes resulting from betamimetic therapy together with placental transfer may give rise to fetal tachycardia and loss of beat-to-beat variation (Ingermarsson 1976).

Treatment begins with an intravenous infusion of the drug, with the dosage being increased until uterine contractions cease. The dosage is maintained at that level for a period of time before oral therapy begins and the intravenous dose is slowly reduced while observing for signs of renewed uterine activity. During administration of betamimetics, regular recordings of maternal pulse rate must be made. Depending upon local protocols and the pulse before therapy, the maximum permitted pulse rate is usually between 130 and 140 beats/minute (Keirse et al. 1989b). Should the tachycardia be greater than this level or in the presence of an adverse maternal response, medical assistance should be sought and the dosage reduced or discontinued. During treatment, close observation of the fetal condition is necessary and this is usually achieved using a cardiotocograph.

Betamimetic drugs are quickly metabolised so that, should labour continue, there is no risk of uterine atony in the third stage of labour. Where the woman is receiving oral therapy, the doses need to be taken regularly and frequently to prevent a drop in the circulating amounts of the drug and the return of contractions. Although these drugs have been shown in randomised trials to postpone delivery, the picture is far from clear regarding their effect on neonatal mortality and morbidity, which appear unchanged following treatment (Anderson 1981; Keirse et al. 1989b).

Prostaglandin synthetase inhibitors directly inhibit prostaglandin release by suppressing its formation from locally occurring precursors (see Chapter 19). They appear to be more effective than betamimetics, in inhibiting uterine contractions (Keirse et al. 1989b). Drugs in this category which can be used include aspirin (salicylic acid) and indomethacin. Unlike the betamimetics the actions of the individual drugs in this group tend to differ, making generalised statements about their use and side-effects difficult (Keirse et al. 1989b). Identified potential side-effects include peptic ulceration, masking of infection, gastrointestinal bleeding and allergic reactions (Keirse et al. 1989b). Fetal/neonatal effects include a risk of premature closure of the ductus arteriosus (Andersson et al. 1983).

Corticosteroids

Corticosteroids are sometimes used before 34 weeks gestation to help prevent respiratory disease of the newborn. Liggins and Howie (1972) demonstrated a reduction in respiratory disease in infants whose mother had received steroids prior to preterm delivery. They are of limited effect after 34 weeks gestation, since at this time there is a surge in fetal glucocorticoid production, stimulating fetal pneumocytes to produce phospholipids necessary for surfactant production. Surfactant is required to lower the surface tension within the lung alveoli, preventing their collapse on expiration. The lack of surfactant predisposes to respiratory disease of the newborn. Giving corticosteroids to the mother mimics the response of the fetus to stress; that is, it accelerates surfactant production. Liggins and

Howie (1974) demonstrated that the greatest effect of glucocorticoids occurred amongst infants born 1–7 days following their administration.

Antenatal administration of corticosteroids has been superseded to some extent by the neonatal administration of artificial surfactant via an endotracheal tube (see Chapter 36).

Cervical cerclage

Cervical cerclage involves placing a non-absorbable suture in the cervix at 16–20 weeks gestation in women with a history of late abortion or preterm delivery. The diagnosis of cervical incompetence is not clear, although most obstetricians rely on history (MRC/RCOG 1988). Harger (1983) is sceptical that the condition actually exists, arguing that, at term, women can spend some time with a partly dilated cervix without going into labour. The suture is inserted under general or regional anaesthesia, with the mother resting in bed for 12–24 hours afterwards. The suture is removed at 36–37 weeks gestation or when the woman goes into labour, whichever is earlier. The MRC/RCOG (1988) multicentre randomised trial of cervical cerclage failed to demonstrate significant advantages for the technique.

Preterm rupture of the membranes

Preterm rupture of the membranes is a subject of controversy regarding its management. Where preterm labour follows the rupture, as occurs in the majority of cases, usually within 1 week (Taylor and Garite 1984), labour is usually allowed to proceed, especially where infection is present (Keirse et al. 1989a). In cases where labour does not occur or until it does, the situation is commonly managed 'conservatively'. Keirse et al. (1989a) highlight the wide range of care that this term can encompass, from doing nothing to routine speculum examination, prophylactic antibiotics or tocolytics and the administration of corticosteroids.

Preterm delivery

Once it is apparent that labour will continue (or a decision has been made to initiate labour), the obstetrician must choose the most appropriate place for and mode of delivery. Transferring mother and fetus to a regional centre prior to delivery ensures that the neonate has expert care in the moments surrounding birth. Lobb et al. (1983) however, failed to demonstrate significant differences in outcome between infants who were transferred in utero and those moved after birth in one English region. In New York, Paneth et al. (1987) showed significantly reduced mortality rates amongst preterm infants delivered in tertiary care centres. Keirse (1989) comments that the very worst place for a preterm baby to be born is one in which the care givers hold the mistaken belief that they have the skills and equipment needed to give care.

The next decision to be made concerns the mode of delivery. Factors to be taken into account include the mother's previous obstetric history, the gestation and normality of the fetus, its presentation and the presence of any maternal complications. The data comparing the outcomes of preterm infants delivered vaginally or by caesarean section are confusing (Healy 1987). However, Lamont (1985) showed that for a preterm baby presenting by the breech or the vertex before 30 weeks gestation, an operative delivery may be of advantage. A multicentre trial has been established to evaluate this. Data regarding the ideal management for the preterm breech are confusing, since those delivered vaginally may be less likely to have received corticosteriods or to have benefited from a planned delivery (Keirse 1989). It does appear, however, that caesarean section is of benefit before 33 weeks gestation amongst infants presenting by the breech and weighing between 1000 and 1500 g (Yu et al. 1984).

The aims of the management of labour are to minimise intrapartum asphyxia and birth trauma (Healy 1987). These aims are in addition to the care and support that the mother and her partner require during any labour, remembering that the couple may be more anxious than for a labour at term. During labour it is best to avoid any narcotic analgesia, although the need for adequate pain relief is as important as in any labour. Crawford (1975) suggested that epidural anaesthesia in preterm labour improves outcome, especially for breech presentations. Unfortunately this subject has not been researched further.

Fetal well-being requires careful observation using continuous fetal heart rate monitoring; this has been shown to improve the outcome for the infant (Paul 1977). Where the trace obtained using a cardiotocograph is of insufficient quality, a scalp electrode may be applied, but care should be taken to avoid any trauma when applying it.

The next controversy surrounds whether or not prophylactic episiotomy or forceps should be employed to minimise pressure on the fetal head. Bishop et al. (1965) reported that elective use of forceps and an episiotomy to aid delivery produced lower neurological morbidity at 1 year of age than spontaneous delivery. There is no conclusive evidence as to the effectiveness of forceps in reducing trauma, especially when O'Driscoll et al. (1981) suggest that the forceps themselves may give rise to trauma. Laufe (1968) has designed a pair of forceps, designed to minimise head compression, which are used in preterm deliveries in preference to the standard forceps, which can put pressure on the head (Healy and Laufe 1985). Beazley and Lobb (1983) are of the opinion that a vaginal delivery of a preterm infant by an experienced midwife is as good as, if not better than, a forceps delivery by an obstetrician. Keirse (1989) states that, until there is evidence to demonstrate that an elective episiotomy has greater neonatal benefits than maternal disadvantages, its use must continue to be questioned.

The parents should be prepared for the presence of a paediatrician at delivery and for the fact that, depending on the baby's condition, it may be taken for resuscitation before they have a chance to hold him. The parents must be kept informed of their baby's progress during stabilisation of its condition. Once the baby is breathing well, either spontaneously or with the assistance of a ventilator, the parents will be able to see and possibly hold their baby before his/her transfer to the neonatal intensive/special care baby unit. Where the baby is in a transport incubator, it may not be possible for the parents to hold or touch their baby. In some units, a photograph of the baby is taken and given to the parents at this early stage before monitors and equipment are attached.

References

Anderson A B M (1981) 'Second thoughts on stopping labour' in J Studd (ed) *Progress in Obstetrics and Gynaecology Vol 1* Ch 10 125–38 Churchill Livingstone: Edinburgh

Andersson K E, Forman A and Ulmsten U (1983) 'Pharmacology of labour' *Clinics in Obstetrics and Gynaecology* 26: 56–81

Astbury J and Bajuck B (1987) 'Psychological aspects of preterm birth' in V Y H Yu and E C Wood (eds) *Prematurity* Ch 12 246–56 Churchill Livingstone: Edinburgh

Beazley J M and Lobb M O (1983) *Aspects of Care in Labour* 125 Churchill Livingstone: Edinburgh

Bishop E H, Israel S L and Briscoe C C (1965) 'Obstetric influences on the premature infant's first year of development' *Obstetrics and Gynecology* 26: 628–35

Castle B M and Turnbull A (1983) 'The presence or absence of fetal breathing movements predicts the outcome of preterm labour' *Lancet* ii: 471–7

Crawford J S (1975) 'Lumbar epidural analgesia for the singleton breech presentation' *Anaesthesia* 30: 119–20

Creasy R K, Gummer B A and Liggins G C (1980) 'System for predicting spontaneous preterm birth' *Obstetrics and Gynecology* 55: 692–5

Fredrick J and Anderson A B M (1976) 'Factors associated with spontaneous preterm birth' *British Journal of Obstetrics and Gynaecology* 83: 342–50

Garn S M, Shaw H A and McCabe K D (1977) 'Effects of socio-economic status and race on weight defined and gestational prematurity in the United States' in D M Reed and F J Stanley (eds) *The Epidemiology of Prematurity* 127 Urban and Schwarzenberg: Baltimore

Harger J H C (1983) 'Cervical cerclage: patient selection, morbidity and success rates' *Clinics in Perinatology* 10(2): 321–41

Healy D L (1987) 'Obstetric management of preterm birth' in V Y H Yu and E C Wood (eds) *Prematurity* Ch 5 76–96 Churchill Livingstone: Edinburgh

Healy D L and Laufe L E (1985) 'A survey of obstetric forceps residency training in North America' *American Journal of Obstetrics and Gynecology* 151: 54–8

Hibbard B (1987) 'The aetiology of preterm labour' *British Medical Journal* 294: 594–5

Ingermarsson I (1976) 'Effect of terbutaline on premature labour: a double-blind placebo controlled study' *American Journal of Obstetrics and Gynecology* 125: 520–4

Jonas E G (1963) 'The value of prenatal bed rest in multiple pregnancy' *Journal of Obstetrics and Gynaecology of the British Commonwealth* 70: 461–4

Kaltreider D F and Kohl S (1980) 'Epidemiology of preterm delivery' *Clinical Obstetrics and Gynecology* 23: 17–31

Kaplan D M and Mason E A (1960) 'Maternal reactions to premature birth viewed as an acute emotional disorder' *American Journal of Orthopsychiatry* 30: 539–52

Keirse M J N C (1989) 'Preterm delivery' in I Chalmers, M Enkin and M J N C Keirse (eds) *Effective Care in Pregnancy and Childbirth* Ch 74 1270–92 Oxford Medical: Oxford

Keirse M J N C, Ohlsson A, Treffers P E and Kanhai H H H (1989a) 'Prelabour rupture of membranes preterm' in I Chalmers, M Enkin and M J N C Keirse (eds) *Effective Care in Pregnancy and Childbirth* Ch 43 666–93 Oxford Medical: Oxford

Keirse M J N C, Grant A and King J F (1989b) 'Preterm labour' in I Chalmers, M Enkin and M J N C Keirse (eds) *Effective Care in Pregnancy and Childbirth* Ch 44 694–745 Oxford Medical: Oxford

King J F (1987) 'Dilemmas in the treatment of preterm labour and delivery' in J Bonnar (ed) *Recent Advances in Obstetrics and Gynaecology Vol XV* Ch 3 65–82 Churchill Livingstone: Edinburgh

Kumar S P, Anday E K and Sacks L M (1980) 'Follow-up studies of very low birthweight infants born and treated within a perinatal centre' *Pediatrics* 66: 348

Lamont R F (1985) 'Factors influencing the route of delivery of the preterm infant' *Proceedings of the 13th Study Group of the Royal College of Obstetricians and Gynaecologists* 1985: 263–71

Laufe L E (1968) 'A new divergent outlet forcep' *American Journal of Obstetrics and Gynecology* 101: 509–14

Liggins G C and Howie R N (1972) 'A controlled trial of antepartum glucocorticoid treatment for the prevention of respiratory distress syndrome in premature infants' *Paediatrics* 50: 515

Liggins G C and Howie R N (1974) 'The prevention of RDS by maternal steroid therapy' in L Gluck (ed) *Modern Perinatal Medicine* Year Book Publishers: Chicago

Lobb M O, Morgan M E I, Bond A P and Cooke R W I (1983) 'Transfer before delivery on Merseyside: an analysis of the first 140 patients' *British Journal of Obstetrics and Gynaecology* 90: 338–41

Lumley J (1987a) 'Epidemiology of prematurity' in V Y H Yu and E C Wood (eds) *Prematurity* Ch 1 1–24 Churchill Livingstone: Edinburgh

Lumley J (1987b) 'Prevention of preterm birth' in V Y H Yu and E C Wood (eds) *Prematurity* Ch 4 54–75 Churchill Livingstone: Edinburgh

McCormick M C (1985) 'The contribution of low birthweight to infant mortality and morbidity' *New England Journal of Medicine* 312: 82–90

McKeown T and Record R (1952) 'Observations of growth in multiple pregnancies in man' *Journal of Endocrinology* 8: 386–94

MRC/RCOG Working Party on Cervical Cerclage (1988) 'Interim report on the Medical Research Council/Royal College Of Obstetricians and Gynaecologists multicentre randomized trial of cervical cerclage' *British Journal of Obstetrics and Gynaecology* 95(5): 437–45

Mugford M (1983) 'A comparison of reported differences in definitions of vital events and statistics' *World Health Organization Statistics Quarterly* 36: 201–12

Newton R W, Webster P A C, Binu P S, Maskrey N and Phillips A B (1979) 'Psychosocial stress in pregnancy and its relation to the onset of premature labour' *British Medical Journal* ii: 411–3

O'Driscoll K, Meagher D, MacDonald D and Geoghegan F (1981) 'Traumatic intracranial haemorrhage in firstborn infants and delivery with obstetric forceps' *British Journal of Obstetrics and Gynaecology* 88: 577–81

Paneth N, Kiely J L, Wallenstein S and Susser M (1987) 'The choice of place of delivery. Effect of hospital level on mortality in all singleton births in New York City' *American Journal of Disease in Childhood* 141: 60–4

Paul R H (1977) 'Fetal heart rate monitoring and low birthweight' in A B M Anderson, R W Beard, J M Brudenell and P M Dunn (eds) *Preterm Labour* Ch 6 308 Royal College of Obstetricians and Gynaecologists: London

Pearce J M (1985) 'The management of preterm labour' in J Studd (ed) *Management of Labour* Blackwell Scientific: Oxford

Rosen E L (1975) 'Concerns of an obstetric patient experiencing long-term hospitalisation' *Journal of Obstetrical, Gynecological and Neonatal Nursing* 4: 15–19

Rush R W, Keirse M J N C, Howat B, Baum J D, Anderson A B M and Turnbull A C (1976) 'Contribution of preterm delivery to perinatal mortality' *British Medical Journal* ii: 965–8

Saunders M C, Dick J S, Brown I, McPherson, K. and Chalmers I (1985) 'The effects of hospital admission for bed rest on the duration of twin pregnancy: A randomised trial' *Lancet* ii: 793–5

Taylor J and Garite T J (1984) 'Premature rupture of membranes before fetal viability' *Obstetrics and Gynecology* 64: 615–20

World Health Organization (1977) 'Recommended definitions, terminology and format for statistical tables related to the perinatal period and use of a new certificate for cause of perinatal deaths' *Acta Obstetrica and Gynaecologica Scandanavia* 56: 247–53

Yu V Y H, Bajuk B and Cutting D (1984) 'Effect of mode of delivery on outcome of very low birthweight infants' *British Journal of Obstetrics and Gynaecology* 91: 633–9

24 Malpositions and malpresentations

Please Note. Due to a lack of primary sources for some of the information contained in this chapter, the author has drawn upon recently published obstetric texts (Hibbard 1988; Cunningham *et al.* 1989). Because this knowledge has no identifiable origin but rather been quoted by many authors over the years, there is always the possibility of perpetuating myths unsubstantiated by research.

Malpresentation

The definition of a malpresentation refers to a fetus presenting other than by the vertex, which includes breech, face, brow and shoulder presentations. The term malposition refers to a fetus presenting by the vertex in which the occiput (the denominator) is facing the posterior of the pelvis.

At the beginning of labour, most fetuses are of cephalic presentation with the occiput, laying either anteriorly or laterally (Hibbard 1988). The most common malposition of the vertex, approximately 10% of cases (Myerscough 1982), is that of occipito-posterior position. Breech is the most frequently encountered malpresentation, its frequency decreasing with increasing gestational age (Sheer and Nubar 1976). At 32 weeks gestation, approximately 20% of fetuses present by the breech (Myerscough 1982). Other rarer malpresentations include face, brow, shoulder and compound malpresentations. The midwife will frequently manage the care of mothers with malpositions and give care to those with malpresentations under medical supervision. However, such conditions are often diagnosed by the midwife and in an emergency she must be able to take action as required and to conduct the delivery. Before considering the malpositions and malpresentations themselves, this chapter will describe the pelvic variations which may give rise to them. Techniques for pelvic assessment are also discussed.

Abnormal pelves

As with all other human characteristics, there are variations in the size and shape of the female pelvis. Their origin may be genetic, hormonal, nutritional or related to previous injury (Myerscough 1982). Minor variations of the pelvis may or may not cause difficulties in labour, depending on the size and type of the pelvis and the size of the fetus (Moir 1947). In addition to variants of the normal pelvis there are also pelvic deformities; both of these can give rise to pelvic contraction. The term cephalopelvic disproportion refers to a misfit between a given pelvis and a particular fetal head. It is rarely an absolute diagnosis for all time (Hibbard 1988). The next pregnancy could result in a preterm or growth-retarded fetus which might be small enough to pass through the pelvis.

Caldwell and Molloy (1940) classified four genetic types of the pelvis which were appropriate for the vast majority of women. Most are normal variants which cause no difficulties, unless their dimensions are significantly reduced. These pelvises can exist both in a 'pure' form and also as a mixed type (Hibbard 1988). The cause of these types of pelvis is related to nutrition in childhood, to genetic and endocrine factors (Hibbard 1988).

1. The most frequently seen form of female pelvis is the gynaecoid. The gynaecoid pelvis is present in approximately 33% of women who have a 'pure' pelvis (Bernard 1952) and 50% of those with a pelvic variant (Caldwell *et al.* 1939). Its characteristics are as follows (see Figure 24.1):

   Brim   – Round, with its largest transverse diameter almost central.
   Cavity – With straight side walls and a well-curved sacrum, the cavity is round.
   Outlet – The ischial spines are not prominent, which together with a wide subpubic angle give a roomy outlet.

   In labour, the fetus presents with the bulky occiput anteriorly where there is most room. This escapes easily under the wide subpubic arch.

2. The android or male type of pelvis is present in about 33% of women with a

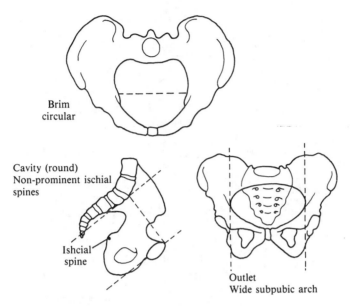

Brim
circular

Cavity (round)
Non-prominent ischial
spines

Ishcial
spine

Outlet
Wide subpubic arch

Figure 24.1 Gynaecoid pelvis.

'pure' type of pelvis (Caldwell *et al*. 1939). Its characteristics are as follows (see Figure 24.2):

Brim   – Heart-shaped with a prominent sacrum and an acute angle of the pubic bones. The largest transverse diameter is close to the sacrum, reducing the area in the posterior part of the brim.

Cavity – The side walls are convergent giving a funnel shape in the cavity. The heavy sacrum, with a poor sacral curve, further reduces the area.

Outlet – Sharp, prominent and inward-facing ischial spines, together with an acute subpubic angle (as small as 65°) create a small outlet.

In labour the fetus is most likely to present with the occiput posterior, where there is more room. However, the flat sacrum might prevent further descent through the cavity. If rotation does occur, progress may be prevented by the prominent ischial spines, which can result in deep transverse arrest (Cunningham *et al*. 1989).

3. Approximately 26% of women have an anthropoid pelvic variant (Donald 1979); for non-white women this proportion rises to almost 50% (Cunningham *et al*. 1989). Its characteristics are as follows (see Figure 24.3):

Brim   – Oval with short transverse and long antero-posterior diameters.

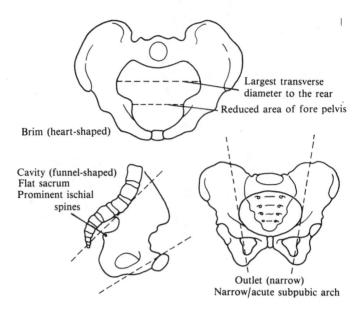

Largest transverse
diameter to the rear

Reduced area of fore pelvis

Brim (heart-shaped)

Cavity (funnel-shaped)
Flat sacrum
Prominent ischial
spines

Outlet (narrow)
Narrow/acute subpubic arch

Figure 24.2 Android pelvis.

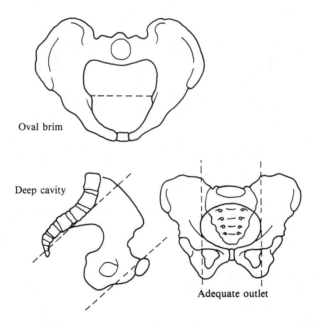

Oval brim

Deep cavity

Adequate outlet

Figure 24.3 Anthropoid pelvis.

Cavity – Rather deep, but adequate.
Outlet – Wide subpubic arch.

The fetus presents with its occiput directly anterior or posterior. Rotation is not required. Posterior positions are more common, due to available space in the hollow of the sacrum. Delivery is in an occipito-anterior position or a spontaneous face-to-pubes (Hibbard 1988).

4. The final pelvic type described by Caldwell *et al.* (1940) is the platypelloid or flat pelvis. This is present in its 'pure' form amongst less than 3% of white women (Caldwell *et al.* 1939). Whilst this type of pelvis can occur due to genetic variation, it can also arise due to childhood (or less commonly adult) dietary deficiencies, for example rickets (Myerscough 1989). The effect of weight bearing on a 'fragile' pelvis results in antero-posterior flattening. Its main features are as follows (see Figure 24.4):

Brim   – Bean-shaped with long transverse and short antero-posterior diameters.
Cavity – The cavity is rather shallow, but more roomy than the gynaecoid.
Outlet – The subpubic angle is wide and the outlet spacious.

In labour, difficulties may be encountered at the pelvic brim. The head, which presents in the transverse, nods from side-to-side (asynclitism) to facilitate engagement. If the head can negotiate the brim, the rest of the

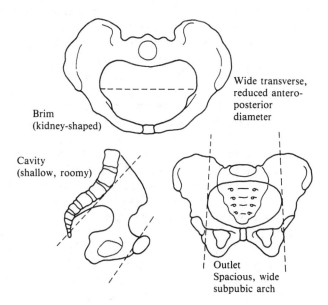

Brim
(kidney-shaped)

Wide transverse,
reduced antero-
posterior
diameter

Cavity
(shallow, roomy)

Outlet
Spacious, wide
subpubic arch

Figure 24.4 Platypelloid pelvis.

mechanism is relatively straightforward. In some cases of delay at the brim, extension of the fetal head may occur, to produce a face presentation (Myerscough 1982).

The pelvic variations described above are not absolute. They can occur as combinations or in lesser or greater degrees (Hibbard 1988). It is the overall diameters of the pelvis rather than its type which govern progress in labour. The miniature gynaecoid pelvis (justo-minor) found in petite women can accommodate a small fetus, but may be inadequate for one of average or above average size (Myerscough 1982).

Pelvic deformities are now very rare in the Western world (Hibbard 1988). They are usually related to the presence of some disease or abnormality. Thoms (1940) demonstrated that the size of the antero-posterior diameter of the pelvic brim is related to socio-economic status. Rickets in children and osteomalacia (adult rickets) produce a pelvis similar to the platypelloid type with a 'squashed' brim (which in severe cases is almost obliterated) and a wide outlet with splayed-out ischial tuberosities (Myerscough 1982). Abnormalities or injuries to the knee, hip or spine which alter walking patterns can cause deformities of the developing pelvis, producing assymetry (Hibbard 1988).

Pelvic assessment

In the later stages of pregnancy and during labour, much effort is expended in assessing whether the pelvis is large enough to permit passage of the fetal head. When taking an antenatal booking history, the midwife seeks information about the woman's previous births, which include the weight of the baby and the type of delivery. Such knowledge can help assess pelvic adequacy. For the primiparous woman, however, there are no such data. Careful questioning about previous illnesses or road traffic accidents can help elicit possible deformities. Observing the way the woman stands and walks is of great assistance. Abnormalities of posture and/or gait will only be present with the grosser types of abnormality. Detection of minor degrees of pelvic contraction must wait until late pregnancy or labour.

Frame et al. (1985) demonstrated a correlation between shoe size and labour outcome in an ethnically mixed inner city population. They found that shoe size was related to ethnic group with 50% of mothers of Asian origin having shoe size less than 5 and 33% of those of African origin with shoes over size 7. Women with a shoe size of under 5 had an increased incidence of rotational forceps deliveries and caesarean sections. Those with feet larger than size 7 had on average shorter first and second stages of labour. A further study by Mahmood et al. (1988) on a homogenous group of white women found no such correlation.

Antenatal assessment of the adequacy of the pelvic brim is by the non-invasive technique of 'head fitting'. This is usually performed on primiparous women whose fetal head has not already engaged by 38 weeks of gestation (Hibbard 1988). However, Bader (1936), reporting a study of 499 primiparae with a non-engaged fetal head at the onset of labour, showed that 87% had a normal labour. Engagement of the head in multiparous women usually occurs during labour. One technique of many to assess 'head fitting' is to have the woman (having previously emptied her bladder) lie on an examination couch. The midwife, standing on the mother's right-hand side, gently places her fingers on either side of the fetal head. The mother is then given assistance to sit up. As she does so the midwife should feel the head move through her fingers and down into the pelvis. This test, however, gives no indication as to the size of the pelvic outlet.

The most common method of assessing the adequacy of the pelvis is by vaginal examination. This used to be a routine examination by obstetricians from 38 weeks gestation, but it is more commonly performed at the time of the first vaginal examination in labour. It is not advisable to perform this examination earlier in pregnancy since, without the relaxation in joints and ligaments which occurs prior to labour, the procedure can be painful and the results inaccurate (Cunningham *et al.* 1989). After a full explanation to the mother of the procedure to be followed, the midwife should request that the mother informs her at the start of any contractions (if in labour), so that the examination can cease. If the mother is severely distressed by her contractions this examination should be delayed until adequate analgesia has been ensured.

Smout *et al.* (1969) developed a guide to pelvic assessment by vaginal examination, commonly known as the 'rule of threes'. This concerns the three areas of the pelvis and the three aspects within each:

1. The brim – diagonal conjugate, iliopectineal line and posterior surface of the symphysis pubis.
2. The cavity – the sacrum (curve, shape, length), ischial spines and sacrospinous ligament.
3. The outlet – subpubic arch and angle, intertuberous diameter and sacrococcygeal joint.

Not all of these measurements are used by midwives.

The procedure where the woman is in labour is as follows: as for any vaginal examination (VE), the woman is first encouraged to empty her bladder. She is then positioned on her back with a wedge under one side to prevent supine hypotension. The midwife washes her hands, dons sterile gloves and swabs the mother's vulva. Using antiseptic cream, two fingers are gently inserted into the vagina.

> *Assessment of the brim* – This is better assessed by determining the engagement or otherwise of the presenting part on abdominal examination. On VE, the midwife should assess the diagonal conjugate by trying to reach the sacral promontory (see Chapter 19). It should not be felt by a woman's hands of average size; this indicates that the antero-posterior diameter is at least 11 cm (Cunningham *et al.* 1989).
> *Cavity* – The curve of the sacrum should be roomy and the ischial spines should not be felt, unless the mother is very relaxed or has an epidural *in situ*,

in which case the spines should not be prominent. It should be possible to fit at least two fingers along the sacrospinous ligament to assess the side wall of the pelvis (Caldwell *et al.* 1939).

Outlet – Again the ischial spines should not be prominent. The subpubic arch should be more than 90°; this is usually assessed by seeing if two fingers together can be placed under the arch. On removing the fingers from the vagina, the intertuberous diameter can be assessed. It should be possible to fit four knuckles of one hand between the tuberosities; this is on average 8 cm (Cunningham *et al.* 1989).

The findings of the examination should be recorded in the notes and then signed. Where cephalopelvic disproportion or pelvic contraction are suspected, pelvic size is assessed by X-ray pelvimetry in which accurate measurements of diameters and planes of the pelvis are obtained (Cunningham *et al.* 1989). When using this technique, care should be taken to avoid exposing the mother or fetus to excess radiation. Cohen and Friedman (1983) reported a very slight increase in the incidence of childhood leukaemia following X-rays in late pregnancy. X-ray pelvimetry is usually only performed in the last weeks of pregnancy.

Occipito-posterior position

This occurs where the fetal head is in a deflexed vertex presentation. The occiput lies towards one of the sacroiliac joints. It occurs in approximately 10% of labours and is the most common malposition of the vertex (Myerscough 1982). Right occipito-posterior occurs more than left, since the uterus is usually dextrorotated and the descending colon (on the left) may be bulky (Myerscough 1982). Posterior positions of the occiput are less advantageous to the fetus than anterior positions. There is less room at the back of the pelvis (in the sacrocotyloid diameter (8.8 cm)) for the broad biparietal diameter than there is at the front. Where the fetal back aligns itself to the maternal spine, it is difficult for the fetus to increase flexion (Rydberg 1954). The flat surface of the maternal spine encourages the fetus to straighten its spine and to adopt a 'military' attitude (see Figure 24.5).

Causation

In most cases there is no obvious cause for the posterior position. Certain types of pelvis predispose to this position, including the anthropoid (or high assimilation) pelvis, which predisposes to direct anterior or posterior positions which cause few problems in labour (Myerscough 1982) and the android pelvis, where there is limited space in the front of the pelvic brim for the occiput (Rydberg 1954). Where the sacrum is flattened and the head poorly flexed, further deflexion can occur, causing the sinciput to become the leading part. The significance of posterior position in labour has reduced over the past 20 years, due to the availability of oxytocic drugs

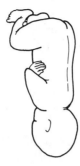

Figure 24.5 Fetus in a 'military' attitude.

to augment inefficient labour. Phillips and Freeman (1974) found that a persistent occipitoposterior position increased the average length of labour by 1 hour for multiparae and 2 hours for primiparae.

Diagnosis

Antenatally posterior positions are diagnosed on abdominal examination. On inspection, a dip or depression may be seen around the umbilicus. Fetal limb movements may also be visible. On palpation, the back may be felt far out to one flank or not be palpable at all. Limbs may be easily felt. The head may feel rather large and high, due to the ease of feeling an anterior sinciput which is higher than the occiput. However, Snow (1952) showed that the incidence of non-engaged heads at the start of labour was the same for anterior and posterior positions of the vertex. On auscultation, the fetal heart may be difficult to hear. It may be found far out on the right flank in the right occipito-posterior position and in the midline for those on the left.

Diagnosis in labour includes abdominal examination and an assessment of the rate of progress of labour and findings on vaginal examination. Posterior positions prolong labour because there are larger presenting diameters and the presenting parts fit badly over the cervix, poorly stimulating contractions and dilatation. Due to the badly fitting presenting part, the membranes may rupture early. Where early spontaneous rupture of the membranes occurs, in only a quarter of these labours does the occiput rotate spontaneously to an anterior position (Miller 1930). Pressure of the occiput on the sacral nerves causes severe backache and later, when pressing on the rectum, the mother feels a premature urge to push. There is also an associated difficulty in passing urine.

On vaginal examination, the head may be high and hard to reach. It will be poorly applied to the cervix. If the membranes are intact, they may be protruding through the cervix in a 'sausage' shape rather than the more common wedge. The sagittal suture will be palpated in the oblique. Where the head is poorly flexed, it may be possible to feel both fontanelles, with the anterior to the front of the pelvis. The anterior fontanelle may feel more obvious than the posterior (Hibbard 1988). There may be a large amount of caput present (Myerscough 1982).

Outcomes of labour

Long rotation to an anterior position occurs in 70% of cases. Uterine action is sufficient to increase flexion, so that the occiput becomes the leading part and rotates to the front (Myerscough 1982). This can take a considerable time. The engaging diameter is the suboccipito-frontal (10 cm) which is slightly larger than the more usual suboccipito-bregmatic (9.5 cm) in the well-flexed vertex. A normal delivery results. Where the occiput is at or behind the sacroiliac joint, the occiput rarely rotates to the front (Beard 1937).

Short rotation to a direct occipito-posterior position (face-to-pubes) occurs in 20% of cases, especially with an anthropoid pelvis (Hibbard 1988). Where flexion is deficient, the sinciput becomes the leading part and rotates to the front. Seven to 13% of persistent occipito-posterior positions deliver as spontaneous face-to-pubes (Myerscough 1982). As delivery approaches, the large biparietal diameter distends the perineum. Delivery is effected by flexing the sinciput under the symphysis pubis before the occiput sweeps the perineum. The sinciput is then delivered by extension. The remainder of the delivery continues as normal. Because of the larger diameters distending the perineum (occipito-frontal 11.5 cm) there is an increased risk of trauma to the perineum (Hibbard 1988).

Extension to a brow or face presentation can occur in rare circumstances where, due to contraction of the pelvis, the head extends in an attempt to overcome the obstruction.

Deep transverse arrest occurs in 10% of cases, where the fetus is attempting long rotation to an anterior position (Hibbard 1988). It never occurs with short rotation. There are two main causes. In the first, the prominent ischial spines (as in an android or funnel-shaped pelvis) prevent further descent (Myerscough 1982). The fetal head is forced by the contractions to nod (asynclitism) to try to overcome the obstruction. The second cause is where uterine action is insufficient to flex the fetal head. The occiput and sinciput both reach the pelvic floor together and there is no leading part and no rotation. This situation is predisposed by the existence of epidural anaesthesia in labour (Crawford 1982).

Deep transverse arrest is usually diagnosed where there is delay in the second stage of labour. Diagnosis is by vaginal examination, when the sagittal suture can be felt in the transverse of the pelvis. Excess caput formation can confuse the examiner into thinking that the head is further descended than it actually is (Cunningham *et al.* 1989). Deep transverse arrest is an abnormal situation requiring medical aid. Where the size of the pelvis permits, and using good anaesthesia, preferably an epidural or caudal block (Hibbard 1988), a forceps delivery using Kjelland's forceps to correct any asynclitism and to rotate the occiput to the front will effect delivery

(Myerscough 1982). Where the pelvis is severely contacted, a caesarean section will be required (Hibbard 1988).

Care of women with posterior positions in labour

It is in the care of such mothers that the midwife requires all her skill and sensitivity. Posterior positions are the commonest cause of delay in labour (Myerscough 1982). The mother will require support and encouragement, together with explanations as to why the labour is taking so long. Due to the extreme backache, the mother may require analgesia. Lying in a warm bath, adopting an upright posture or kneeling forward have been found to be of help in easing the discomfort. Where the pain is severe, an epidural (if available and acceptable to the mother) has been shown to be of help, especially where it is necessary for the labour to be augmented (Hibbard 1988). Because the labour is prolonged, it is vital to prevent dehydration and ketosis. This is ideally achieved by initially giving a light diet and, when labour is established, giving clear fluids and glucose.

It may be necessary to catheterise the bladder if the mother is unable to pass urine (Hibbard 1988). The deflexed sinciput presses the urethra and bladder neck against the pubic symphysis. Because the presenting part may not be a good fit over the cervix, there is a risk of cord prolapse when the membranes rupture. A vaginal examination should be performed immediately to exclude this possibility. Fetal condition in prolonged labour requires careful monitoring. If there is any sign of abnormality, such as meconium staining of the liquor or alterations in the fetal heart rate using the Pinnard's stethoscope, continuous electric fetal monitoring may be required.

Dangers to the mother include the results of a prolonged labour, such as exhaustion, dehydration and risks of postpartum haemorrhage. Due to the number of vaginal examinations, there is a risk of infection, and trauma may result from spontaneous or instrumental delivery (Hibbard 1988). There is also the attendant danger of obstructed labour. This causes excessive moulding of the fetal head ('sugar-loaf' moulding) and possible cerebral injury. The baby is also at risk of hypoxia (due to cord prolapse), jaundice (from excessive bruising at delivery) and infection (from prolonged rupture of the membranes).

Breech presentation

This is a malpresentation where the fetal buttocks lie in the lower pole of the uterus. The frequency of breech presentation at term is about 3% (Duignan 1982). At 32 weeks gestation it is 20% (Myerscough 1982), due to the greater amount of liquor present in the uterus allowing freer fetal movement. Breech delivery is dangerous for the fetus, carrying a mortality rate nearly four times that for cephalic presentations, even when prematurity and abnormality rates have been excluded (Coltart 1984). Rovinsky *et al.* (1973) recorded a perinatal mortality rate for babies delivered by the breech of 32/1000 total births compared with 8.4/1000 for babies with a cephalic presentation.

There are three types of breech presentation (see Figure 24.6). The complete breech occurs where the fetal legs and hips are fully flexed. This is most common in multiparous women (Coltart 1984). The complete breech is a poorly fitting presenting part, with the risks of early rupture of the membranes and cord prolapse. The frank or extended breech occurs most frequently in primiparous women who have firm abdominal muscles. Over 70% of frank breeches occur in primiparous women (Stabler 1945). The legs are fully extended at the knee, with the feet lying near the fetal head. The legs splint the fetal back preventing easy version. The frank breech is a well-fitting presenting part which encourages cervical dilatation and stimulates contractions. The final and rarer type of breech is the footling or knee presentation, where one or both feet or knees are below the level of the breech. This is an especially ill-fitting presenting part, with a high risk of cord prolapse (Cunningham *et al.* 1989).

Causation

In many cases there is no obvious cause, but the following are contributory factors:

1. Prematurity (Hay 1959).
2. Multiple pregnancy (Hibbard 1988).
3. Polyhydramnios (Tomkins 1946).
4. Major fetal abnormality, e.g. hydrocephalus. Some anomalies also cause polyhydramnios (Brenner *et al.* 1974).
5. Firm abdominal muscles in a primipara with extended fetal legs (Stabler 1945).
6. Grand multiparity – giving lax abdominal muscles (Tomkins 1946).
7. Uterine abnormality, such as bicornuate uterus (Tomkins 1946).

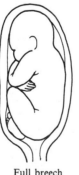

Full breech

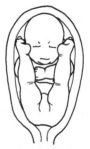

Frank breech

Figure 24.6 Types of breech presentation.

8. Lack of space in the lower segment – placenta praevia, contracted pelvis, fibroids or pelvic tumours (Tomkins 1946).
9. Cornual or fundal implantation of the placenta (Fianu and Vaclavinkova 1978).

Prematurity and fetal anomaly are the most common factors.

Diagnosis

Breech presentation is commonly diagnosed by abdominal examination. On inspection, there may be little to see, except in the case of a frank breech, where the uterus can appear long and thin. If the mother has a history of previous breech presentations this is helpful to alert one's suspicions. On palpation, the breech may feel somewhat soft and bulky. However, a frank breech may be well into the pelvis giving the examiner the impression of a deeply engaged head (Hibbard 1988). In the fundus, there should be a hard ballottable mass. The head, if posterior and well under the ribs, may be difficult to reach. The mother may complain of discomfort and pressure under her ribs. If the legs are extended and the fetal feet hooked over the shoulders, it may be difficult to ballote the head (Myerscough 1982). The fetal heart is usually heard higher up than for cephalic presentations. However, if the placenta is anterior and/or the legs extended auscultation may be difficult. Diagnosis of a breech presentation is far from easy and confirmation is often sought using an X-ray or an ultrasound scan (Cunningham *et al.* 1989). This has the added advantage of screening for fetal structural abnormality and assessing fetal size.

In labour, the findings on vaginal examination can also be confusing. The presenting part may feel soft, with few identifying features (Cunningham *et al.* 1989). It can easily be confused with a face presentation; the triangular sacrum and the anal cleft can be felt. Meconium may be seen on the examining finger. The genitalia are soft and difficult to distinguish. In a footling presentation, the foot can be distinguished from a hand by the fact that it is at right angles to the leg and unlike a hand, a foot does not grip the examining finger.

Management of breech presentation

Any midwife suspecting the presence of a breech presentation from 32 weeks gestation should inform the mother's obstetrician. The woman should be booked for delivery in a consultant unit if this is not already the case. Between 34 and 36 weeks gestation external cephalic version (ECV) may be attempted (Cunningham *et al.* 1989). Before this time the fetus is too mobile and later there is insufficient liquor to permit easy movement. Obstetricians are divided as to the usefulness of ECV (Duignan 1982). They are usually either totally in favour of or against it. One argument is that if the version is easy the fetus would have turned itself and if it is hard, it should not be attempted (Hay 1959). Duignan (1982) reports a series of cases in which 194 fetuses were successfully turned (9 were not), in which 185 fetuses remained cephalic. The procedure is performed with the woman (having previously emptied her bladder) lying supine (Hibbard 1988). The whole procedure should be gentle and unrushed. The fetal heart should be checked frequently (Hibbard 1988). The obstetrician using gentle pressure behind the head and the breech moves the fetus so that it 'follows its nose' (Myerscough 1982). The heart rate is rechecked and the woman examined to ensure that there is no vaginal bleeding and that the membranes have not ruptured. Because there is a slight risk of placental separation, premature rupture of the membranes and cord entanglement, ECV is not attempted in women with hypertension, multiple pregnancies, rhesus isoimmunisation, antepartum haemorrhage, fetal abnormality or uterine scar (Hibbard 1988). For rhesus-negative women, anti-D will need to be given to prevent rhesus isoimmunisation (Gjode et al. 1980) although some obstetricians will not perform ECV on rhesus-negative women. ECV is rarely performed under general anaesthesia, since excessive force may be employed (Myerscough 1982). In some cases, tocolytics are used prior to the procedure to help relax the uterus (Cox 1986).

If ECV is unsuccessful or contra-indicated, the woman needs assessment to decide the mode of delivery. X-ray pelvimetry is usually performed together with ultrasound determination of the size of the baby (Rovinsky et al. 1973). The choice of mode of delivery is dependent on maternal parity, pelvic and fetal size, gestational age and upon the normality of the fetus. The greatest benefit for preterm infants has been found by delivering those weighing under 1500 g by caesarean section (Ingermarsson et al. 1978). Coltart (1984) cautions against delivering all breech presentations by caesarean section, due to the effects that this will have on maternal mortality and morbidity (Collea et al. 1980). This is further compounded when one considers the effect of an operative delivery on a woman's childbearing future (Myerscough 1982).

Care in labour

Management of the first stage proceeds as for any woman with a high-risk labour. A vaginal examination should be performed when the membranes rupture to exclude the possibility of cord prolapse (Brenner et al. 1974). A mother with a well-fitting frank breech can be mobile during labour but, due to the risk of cord prolapse with other types of breech, it is safer if the mother stays in bed. Due to the risk of fetal hypoxia from cord compression, continuous electrical fetal monitoring is advisable (Hill et al. 1976). If available, telemetry can be used. Progress in labour should be closely monitored, since slow progress may indicate a degree of disproportion (Rovinsky et al. 1973). It is impossible to rule out cephalopelvic disproportion until delivery is almost complete, so a cautious approach is adopted (Cunningham et al. 1989). In addition, the smaller breech and trunk can slip through a partially dilated cervix (especially if the infant is preterm), leaving the head trapped. To avoid this, the second stage is always confirmed by vaginal examination before the mother is allowed to push (Hibbard 1988). To prevent premature pushing, an epidural analgesic may be advised (Crawford 1974). If not available or not acceptable to the mother, she should be encouraged to lie on her side and to use inhalational analgesia to prevent pushing during the transition stage.

Mechanism

Descent occurs with increasing compaction. This results in the passage of meconium.

The anterior buttock reaches the gutter shape of the pelvic floor and rotates to the front. This brings the engaging diameter, the bitrochanteric (10 cm), into the antero-posterior diameter of the pelvis.

By lateral flexion, the anterior buttock escapes under the symphysis pubis and the posterior sweeps the perineum and is born.

After delivery of the buttocks, the shoulders descend into the pelvis. The anterior shoulder hits the pelvic floor and rotates to the front.

The anterior shoulder (and arm) escape under the symphysis pubis and the posterior sweeps the perineum.

The head enters the brim in the transverse. The occiput rotates internally to the front. The face now lies in the hollow of the sacrum.

With further descent, the occiput escapes under the symphysis pubis. The chin, face and sinciput and vertex sweep the perineum and the head is born by a process of flexion.

Conduct of delivery

The mother should be prepared prior to the delivery for the presence of an obstetrician, a paediatrician (for resuscitation) and an anaesthetist (in case of emergency). The delivery is the time of greatest risk to the fetus. The woman is usually delivered in the lithotomy position. Although the delivery in the United Kingdom is usually conducted by an obstetrician, the midwife must know how to carry out the procedures in an emergency situation. It is now normal to perform an assisted breech delivery. Spontaneous delivery and breech extraction are both considered too dangerous (Hibbard 1988).

The buttocks. The mother is encouraged to push with contractions. Adequate anaesthesia is required, so in the absence of an epidural or caudal block a pudendal nerve block is established. The perineum is infiltrated and when the buttocks distend the perineum, an episiotomy is performed (Hibbard 1988). Myerscough (1982) cautions against doing this too early, due to the blood loss which results from continued trickling. The buttocks are allowed to deliver themselves with no help from the doctor (Myerscough 1982).
The legs. If the legs are extended it will be necessary to ease their delivery. This is achieved by placing a finger in the popliteal fossa and gently flexing the knee.

If the umbilical cord appears taut, a loop can be pulled down. Otherwise the cord should be left alone, since handling can cause the vessels to go into spasm (Hibbard 1988).

The shoulders. The weight of the buttocks will bring the shoulders into the pelvis. If necessary, slight downward traction during a contraction can be used. Care should be taken to grasp the baby around the pelvis with the thumbs on the sacrum to avoid damage to internal tissues (Hibbard 1988). When the anterior shoulder has escaped under the symphysis pubis, the trunk is elevated to permit the posterior to sweep the perineum. If the arms are extended, it may be necessary to perform the Lovset manoeuvre to effect their delivery (Myerscough 1982). Since the head and the arms cannot both pass through the pelvis the arms must be delivered first. The principle of the Lovset manoeuvre is that, due to the inclination of the pelvic brim, the posterior arm enters the pelvis before the anterior. By gently turning the fetus so that the back comes uppermost, the posterior arm is drawn down across the chest and can be easily delivered (Myerscough 1982). Repeating the manoeuvre frees the other arm.

The head. There are three main methods of delivering the head:

1. Most obstetricians will use forceps to cradle the head from excessive moulding and effect a slow controlled delivery (Cox 1986). Once the mouth is free, it can be cleared of mucus and the baby encouraged to breathe while the remainder of the head is delivered slowly.
2. Burns-Marshall method, where the head is flexed: the fetal head descends into the pelvis by the weight of the body, which is allowed to hang. When the hair line is seen, the feet are grasped and swung through 180° and held on the stretch until the chin, mouth and nose are seen. These can then be cleared (Hibbard 1988). The mother is then encouraged to breathe out the remainder of the head (see Figure 24.7).
3. Mauriceau-Smellie-Veit manoeuvre for a non-flexed head: for a person delivering by themselves, this technique gives good control of the fetus whether the head is flexed or not (Myerscough 1982). The fetal body is laid along one arm (usually the left), with the palm supporting the chest. The index and ring fingers of that hand are placed on the malar bones of the baby's face and the middle finger in its mouth. The first and third fingers of the right hand are hooked over the baby's shoulders, with the middle finger on the occiput. The baby's head is then flexed (see Figure 24.8). This can be aided by gentle suprapubic pressure from an assistant (the bladder must be empty). As the head descends, gentle traction is exerted in an outward direction. When the face is born, the baby's body is lifted upwards to permit breathing and slow delivery of the head.

Syntometrine can now be given to assist delivery of the third stage (Myerscough 1982).

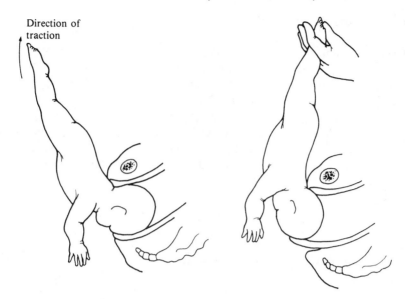

Direction of traction

Figure 24.7 Burn's Marshall method of delivering the head.

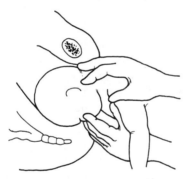

Figure 24.8 Mauriceau–Smellie–Veit manoeuvre.

Dangers of breech presentation

The risks to the mother are those of prolonged labour and obstetric interference, with increased chances of trauma and infection. She is also more likely to require an operative delivery at short notice (Collea *et al.* 1980).

Breech delivery is risky to the fetus. In addition to any problems of prematurity, the short time available for moulding of the head (unlike the hours taken in a cephalic presentation), the risk of cord compression or premature separation of the placenta and the manoeuvres at delivery all place the baby in danger (Brenner *et al.* 1974).

The major dangers are as follows:

1. Cerebral haemorrhage due to either too rapid delivery (tentorial tears) or, more commonly, hypoxia, giving intraventricular haemorrhage (Cox 1986).
2. Hypoxia and anoxia from cord compression, premature placental separation and premature inspiration (Cox 1986).
3. Trauma – soft tissue damage, especially to liver and spleen from an incorrect hold on the body. Fractures of the humerus, clavicle or cervical vertabrae (Tank *et al.* 1971). Nerve damage, especially to the brachial plexus and facial nerve (Tank *et al.* 1971). Trauma and bruising to genitalia (especially in boys), excess caput formation (on the breech) and sternomastoid haematoma are examples of possible soft tissue damage (Tank *et al.* 1971).
4. Hypothermia, due to the time taken delivering the head.

All babies presenting as a frank breech should be carefully screened for the presence of congenital dislocation of the hip as there is an increased occurrence.

Face presentation

This occurs where the area from the glabella to the under surface of the chin lies over the cervical os. The head is fully extended (see Figure 24.9). The incidence is 1 : 5–600 births (Cruikshank and White 1973). A face presentation can arise, before the start of labour, when it is known as a primary face (Hibbard 1988). The cause is usually some form of abnormality such as anencephaly, spasm of the neck muscles or fetal goitre (Cunningham *et al.* 1989). A secondary face presentation arises during labour when a deflexed-posterior position is held up at the pelvic brim, causing extension. This can occur where there is anterior uterine obliquity, which causes the body to flop forward and the head to extend (Cunningham *et al.* 1989). It can also occur where the pelvic brim is contracted, for example with a platypelloid pelvis or with polyhydramnios, where the head extends when the membranes rupture (Hellman *et al.* 1950).

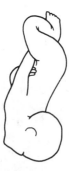

Figure 24.9 Fetus presenting with the head fully extended.

Antenatal diagnosis of a face presentation is difficult. The fetal head and back may be palpated on the same side with a deep groove between. Diagnosis is more usually made on vaginal examination in labour. The presenting part is high, with a soft irregular appearance. Caput makes landmarks hard to identify, as they may be confused with those of a breech (Cunningham *et al.* 1989). The malar bones and chin can usually be felt. Diagnosis is confirmed by X-ray, which will also demonstrate skeletal abnormalities (Hibbard 1988). Where a face presentation is suspected, medical assistance should be called to manage this abnormal situation.

Labour

The denominator in a face presentation is the chin (mentum) for which there are 8 possible positions. Mento-anterior positions will deliver spontaneously, although the first stage is slower, due to the poorly fitting presenting part and the lack of moulding of the face (although the skull does mould). The engaging diameter is the submento-bregmatic (9.5 cm). In 75% of cases, the chin rotates to the front (Myerscough 1982). It escapes under the pubic arch, aided by pressure on the sinciput to maintain extension. The sinciput, vertex and occiput then sweep the perineum. The mother should be prepared for her baby's appearance (Cunningham *et al.* 1989). The face will appear bruised and congested; this will disappear in the first 48 hours, although establishment of feeding may be delayed (Hibbard 1988). In 25% of cases, the chin is posterior (Myerscough 1982). Unless rotation to the front occurs there is no mechanism. Management is by rotating to the front with Kjellands forceps and delivering anteriorly or by operative delivery by caesarean section (Myerscough 1982).

The baby may have head retraction for a day or so after delivery. There is a risk of jaundice due to the extensive bruising. The baby should be assessed for any nerve or cerebral damage. Mortality and morbidity are higher than for babies presenting by the vertex (Hibbard 1988).

Brow presentation

This is an intermediate presentation between a 'military' attitude (see Figure 24.5) and a face presentation. The head is partly extended, with the brow presenting. This is the area between the anterior fontanelle and the supraorbital ridges. The frequency of this presentation is 1 : 5000 (Cunningham *et al.* 1989). Cunningham *et al.* (1989) reported an incidence of 11 cases amongst 50 000 singleton fetuses over a 4 year period. The causes are the same as those for face presentation, with the exception of anencephaly (Cunningham *et al.* 1989).

The fetus presents with the mentovertical as the potential engaging diameter (13 cm). Unless the fetus is small and the pelvis large, there is no mechanism. In most cases, the head remains above the pelvic brim (Cunningham *et al.* 1989). Diagnosis is difficult, with a large head palpable abdominally. On vaginal examination the pelvis may feel empty although it may be possible to reach a high presenting part. The landmarks of the anterior fontanelle, supraorbital ridges and frontal suture may be obscured by caput formation. The membranes may rupture early, due to the poorly fitting presenting part. Diagnosis is confirmed by X-ray. Medical assistance should be sought to cope with this abnormal situation. Delivery is usually by caesarean section, although it is possible for the obstetrician to use forceps to convert it to a vertex presentation. In 40% of cases, the brow extends to a face presentation or flexes to a vertex (Cruikshank and White 1973).

Shoulder presentation

Shoulder presentation occurs when the lie is transverse or oblique and the shoulder lies in the lower uterine segment (see Figure 24.10). The incidence of this presentation is 1 : 322 deliveries (Cruikshank and White 1973). If labour ensues, it will be obstructed and therefore labour with a shoulder presentation should be prevented if possible. The causes are related to laxity of the abdominal muscles (linked to high parity), multiple pregnancy and polyhydramnios (Cunningham *et al.* 1989). Shoulder presentation is 10 times more common at parities over 4 than in primiparous women (Hall and O'Brien 1961). It can also occur in cases of pelvic contraction or placenta praevia. Hall and O'Brien (1961) recorded that placenta praevia was present in 10% of the cases of shoulder presentation in their study.

Diagnosis is usually made antenatally. On inspection, the uterus appears wide. The fundus is empty and a fetal pole can be grasped at each side of the uterus. Nothing is done before 34 weeks gestation. After this time, the mother is admitted to hospital because there is a risk of cord prolapse should the membranes rupture (Hibbard 1988). An ultrasound scan is performed to exclude the presence of placenta praevia, and X-ray pelvimetry to assess the adequacy of the pelvis (Hibbard 1988).

An attempt may be made to use version to convert the fetus to a longitudinal lie, preferably with a cephalic presentation. In cases of polyhydramnios, a stabilising induction may be performed (Edwards and Nicholson 1969). The fetus is maintained as a cephalic presentation while liquor is allowed to drain slowly. The head should

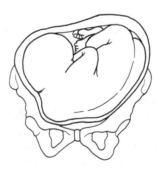

Figure 24.10 Shoulder presentation.

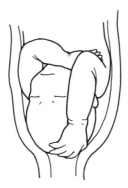

Figure 24.11 Compound presentation.

then descend into the pelvis (Edwards and Nicholson 1969). Checks must be made that the umbilical cord does not precede the head. In cases of difficulty, the mother will be delivered by elective or emergency caesarean section.

Compound presentation

This occurs when a hand or foot lie alongside the head (see Figure 24.11). Gopelrud and Eastman (1953) estimate that this occurs in 1 : 700 deliveries. Unless the fetus is very small they cannot both enter the pelvis together. In most cases, the limb concerned recedes as the presenting part advances (Gopelrud and Eastman 1953). If this does not occur and the pelvis is adequate, it may be possible to push the limb back behind the head. If the pelvis is contracted or the limb cannot be moved, it may be necessary to deliver by caesarean section.

References

Bader A (1936) 'The significance of the unengaged head in primiparous labor' *Ber. ges. Gynaekologika und Geburtshuelfe* 31: 395 (Abstract)

Beard R J (1937) *The Occipito-posterior Position (2nd edn)* Adelaide

Bernard R M (1952) 'The shape and size of the female pelvis' *Edinburgh Medical Journal* 1951/2: 1–1610

Brenner W E, Bruce R D and Hendricks C H (1974) 'The characteristics and perils of breech presentation' *American Journal of Obstetrics and Gynecology* 118: 700

Caldwell W E, Moloy H C and D'Esposo D A (1940) 'More recent conceptions of pelvic architecture' *American Journal of Obstetrics and Gynecology* 40: 558–65

Caldwell W E, Moloy H C and Swenson P C (1939) 'The use of the roentgen ray in obstetrics' *American Journal of Roentgenology* 41: 305

Cohen D and Friedman E A (1983) *Management of Labour* 33 University Press: Baltimore

Collea J V, Chein C and Quilligan E J (1980) 'The randomised management of term frank breech presentation' *American Journal of Obstetrics and Gynecology* 137: 235

Coltart T M (1984) 'Management of breech presentation' in G Chamberlain (ed) *Contemporary Obstetrics* Ch 16 126–34 Butterworth: London

Cox L W (1986) 'Breech presentation – A review' *Midwifery* 2(2): 71–80

Crawford J S (1974) 'An appraisal of lumbar epidural blockade in patients with a singleton fetus presenting by the breech' *Journal of Obstetrics and Gynaecology of the British Commonwealth* 81: 867–72

Crawford J S (1982) 'The effect of epidural block on the progress of labour' in J Studd (ed) *Progress in Obstetrics and Gynaecology Vol 2* Ch 9 85–93 Churchill Livingstone: Edinburgh

Cruikshank D P and White C A (1973) 'Obstetric malpresentations: 20 years experience' *American Journal of Obstetrics and Gynecology* 116: 1097

Cunningham F G, MacDonald P C and Gant N F (1989) *Williams Obstetrics (18th edn)* Prentice Hall: London

Donald I (1979) *Practical Obstetric Problems (5th edn)* Lloyd-Luke: London

Duignan N M (1982) 'The management of breech presentation' in J Studd (ed) *Progress in Obstetrics and Gynaecology Vol 2* Ch 8 73–84 Churchill Livingstone: Edinburgh

Edwards R L and Nicholson H O (1969) 'The management of unstable lie in late pregnancy' *Journal of Obstetrics and Gynaecology of the British Commonwealth* 76: 713–8

Fianu S and Vaclavinkova V (1978) 'The site of placental attachment as a factor in the aetiology of breech presentation' *Acta Obstetrica and Gynaecologica Scandanavica* 57: 371

Frame S, Moore J, Peters A and Hall D (1985) 'Maternal height and shoe size as predictor of pelvic disproportion: an assessment' *British Journal of Obstetrics and Gynaecology* 92: 1239–45

Gjode P, Rasmussen K and Jorgensen J (1980) 'Fetomaternal bleeding during attempts at external bleeding' *British Journal of Obstetrics and Gynaecology* 87: 571

Gopelrud J and Eastman N J (1953) 'Compound presentation: Survey of of 65 cases' *Obstetrics and Gynecology* 1: 59

Hall S C and O'Brien F B (1961) 'Review of transverse lie at the Methodist Hospital Brooklyn 1924–58' *American Journal of Obstetrics and Gynecology* 82: 1180–5

Hay D (1959) 'Observations on breech presentation and delivery' *Journal of Obstetrics and Gynaecology of the British Empire* 66: 529–47

Hellman L M, Epperson J W W and Connally F (1950) 'The experience of the Johns Hopkins Hospital, 1896–1948' *American Journal of Obstetrics and Gynecology* 59: 831

Hibbard B M (1988) *Principles of Obstetrics* Butterworths: London

Hill J G, Elliot B W, Campbell A J and Pickett-Heaps A A (1976) 'Intensive care of the foetus in breech labour' *British Journal of Obstetrics and Gynaecology* 83: 271–5

Ingermarsson J, Westgren M and Svenningsen N W (1978) 'Long term follow-up of pre-term infants and breech presentation delivered by Caesarean section' *Lancet* ii: 172–5

Mahmood T A, Campbell D M and Wilson A W (1988) 'Maternal height, shoe size and outcome of labour in white primigravidas: a prospective anthropometric study' *British Medical Journal* 297: 515–7

Miller D (1930) *British Medical Journal* i: 1036

Moir J C (1947) 'The use of radiology in predicting difficult labour' *Journal of Obstetrics and Gynaecology of the British Empire* 54: 20–33

Myerscough P R (1982) *Munro Kerr's Operative Obstetrics (10th edn)* Balliere Tindall: London

Myerscough P R (1989) 'Cephalopelvic disproportion' in A Turnbull and G Chamberlain (eds) *Obstetrics* 813–22 Churchill Livingstone: Edinburgh

Phillips R D and Freeman M (1974) 'The management of persistent occipito posterior position: A review of 552 consecutive cases' *Obstetrics and Gynecology* 43: 171

Rovinsky J J, Miller J A and Kaplan S (1973) 'Management of breech presentations at term' *American Journal of Obstetrics and Gynecology* 115: 497

Rydberg E (1954) *The Mechanism of Labour* Charles C Thomas: Springfield, Illinois

Sheer K and Nubar J (1976) 'Variation of fetal presentation with age' *American Journal of Obstetrics and Gynecology* 125: 269–70

Smout C F V, Jacoby F and Lillie E W (1969) *Gynaecological and Obstetrical Anatomy (4th edn)* H K Lewis: London

Snow W (1952) *Roentgenology in Obstetrics and Gynecology* 95 Charles C Thomas: Sringfield, Illinois

Stabler F (1945) 'The cause of polar lie' *Journal of Obstetrics and Gynaecology of the British Empire* 54: 345

Tank E S, Davis R, Holt J F and Morley G W (1971) 'Mechanism of trauma during breech delivery' *Obstetrics and Gynecology* 38: 761

Thoms H (1940) 'Clinical application of roentgen pelvimatry and study of results in 1100 white women' *American Journal of Obstetrics and Gynecology* 42: 957–75

Tomkins P (1946) 'An enquiry into the causes of breech presentation' *American Journal of Obstetrics and Gynecology* 51: 595

25   Instrumental and operative delivery

This chapter will consider the measures available to obstetricians to effect delivery when the maternal or fetal condition warrant intervention. The indications for instrumental delivery will be considered, together with the conduct of the delivery. Both obstetric forceps and ventouse deliveries will be described. The grounds for elective and emergency caesarean section will then be discussed. The care of the mother prior to, during and after the operation will be described. Some thought will be given to the causes of the recent rise in the caesarean section rate. Finally, the conduct and management of labour for a mother having a trial of labour or trial of scar will be described. Although the management of these deliveries is not normally within the remit of the midwife, she will provide support and assistance to both parents and medical staff.

Instrumental delivery

Instrumental delivery is most commonly employed either to speedily effect the delivery of the fetal head or to protect the fetus and/or mother from trauma and exhaustion (Cunningham *et al.* 1989).

Indications

- Delay in the second stage, where the woman is tiring and progress is absent or slow. The cause could be a malposition of the vertex, poor uterine action, rigidity of the pelvic floor or a lack of understanding of the physiology of the second stage's latent and active phases.
- To prevent maternal exhaustion or trauma. In women for whom pushing is contra-indicated, such as those with cardiac or respiratory disease (Cunningham *et al*. 1989). Where the woman is already exhausted or she is experiencing distress.
- To prevent fetal morbidity (Myerscough 1982). In cases of fetal distress. To protect the fetal head from trauma as when premature or with the aftercoming head of a breech presentation (Chamberlain 1980).

In the United Kingdom, most instrumental deliveries involve the use of obstetric forceps (Chalmers and Chalmers 1989). In other places such as Scandanavia, vacuum extraction (also known as ventouse deliveries after the apparatus) is more common (Chalmers and Chalmers 1989). The ventouse is suitable for use on term babies with a cephalic presentation. It should not be used when the fetal head is above the level of the ischial spines (Ryden 1986). The ventouse can be particularly effective in cases of transverse or occipito-posterior positions. Since the suction cap is applied over the presenting part, traction and maternal effort increase flexion and spontaneous internal rotation to anterior positions can occur (Barclay and Fraser 1988). Vacuum extraction causes less maternal trauma, such as injury to the birth canal, than does obstetric forceps (Vacca *et al*. 1983) although Grant (1986) argues that fetal trauma to the scalp is similar in occurrence to facial trauma following delivery by forceps. When the vacuum is formed between the suction cup and the scalp (over the occiput), oedema forms within the cap (Hibbard 1988). This is known as a 'chignon' (French for 'bun'). This swelling subsides in the hours following delivery. There is, however, an increase in the occurrence of cephalhaematoma and mild jaundice (not requiring phototherapy or exchange transfusion) (Ryden 1986; Herabutya *et al*. 1988). Unlike forceps, vacuum extraction can be used when the cervix is not fully dilated, but only in multiparae with a soft cervix of at least 7 cm dilation (Ryden 1986). These conditions reduce the time taken for delivery to an acceptable maximum of 30 minutes. Ventouse delivery is less forceful than that by forceps and is reliant on maternal effort. In situations where speed is not of the essence, this maternal involvement can do much to improve the mother's perception of the events (Ryden 1986).

There are three main types of obstetric forceps used in the United Kingdom. These were developed to aid the mother, especially in cases of obstructed labour. They were not designed to maximise the health of the baby and consequently some can exert considerable trauma to the foetal head (Hibbard 1988). The various types available include the following:

1. Short forceps with a cephalic and a pelvic curve and short handles, used when

the head is on the perineum, often employed to assist delivery at caesarean section. Type: Wrigley's, a small and light pair of forceps (Myerscough 1982).

2. Midcavity forceps. Larger than Simpson's, but still having a cephalic and pelvic curve. The handle is more substantial and there is the ability to attach an axis traction handle, which enables the obstetrician to exert traction at right angles to the Curve of Carus. Axis traction is rarely used nowadays (Myerscough 1982). Types: Neville Barnes, Haig Ferguson and Simpson (the latter type is sometimes also used as short forceps (Hibbard 1988)).

3. Rotational forceps. Long, straight forceps having a cephalic but no pelvic curve. Unlike short and midcavity forceps, they have a sliding rather than fixed lock. This permits the obstetrician to use the forceps to correct asynclitism (nodding of the head) (Vacca and Keirse 1989). The absence of a pelvic curve makes these forceps suitable for use in rotating the fetal head from a posterior or transverse position. In some cases rotation is effected using long, straight forceps; these are then replaced with mid- or low-cavity forceps for the delivery. Type: Kjelland (Myerscough 1982).

Conditions for a forceps delivery:

1. There must be a legitimate reason for using forceps (Vacca and Keirse 1989).
2. The head must be engaged and there should be no obvious disproportion (forceps deliveries are rarely performed where the fetal head is not at or below the ischial spines) (Crichton 1974; Cunningham *et al.* 1989).
3. The position of the occiput should be known (Cunningham *et al.* 1989).
4. The cervix should be fully dilated (Moolgaoker 1970).
5. There must be adequate anaesthesia, either regional (epidural or caudal block) or local (pudendal nerve block) (Vacca and Keirse 1989).
6. Unless the fetal head is on the perineum, the bladder should be empty (Hibbard 1988).
7. Uterine action must be satisfactory. This reduces the effort required to effect delivery and lowers the risk of an atonic postpartum haemorrhage (Vacca and Keirse 1989).
8. The membranes should be ruptured. Intact membranes may be the cause of the delay (Cunningham *et al.* 1989).
9. An episiotomy is usually performed to reduce the risk of perineal trauma (Hibbard 1988).
10. Informed consent must be obtained from the mother (Beazley and Lobb 1983).

The mother and her partner must be fully prepared for the procedures which are about to take place, including the indications for their use. It is unusual for the woman's companion to be requested to leave. The woman is placed in the lithotomy position, with a wedge under one side to move the weight of the uterus off the inferior vena cava. It is important to place the legs simultaneously and symmetrically in the stirrups to prevent strain on the sacroiliac joints (Hibbard

1988). Some birthing chairs can be tilted to permit their use for forceps deliveries. The pudendal nerve block (if required) is established. It is necessary to allow sufficient time to elapse so that the local anaesthetic can take effect before commencing the delivery. The midwife should encourage the woman to push with the contractions (Hibbard 1988). The baby is often delivered on the mother's abdomen. In cases of fetal distress or rotational forceps delivery, it is usual to have a paediatrician in attendance to ensure the onset of respiration and to check for any signs of cerebral irritation. In accordance with local policy, syntometrine is given to assist in completion of the third stage. The episiotomy is then repaired and the woman's legs removed from the stirrups. She can now rest and get to know her baby. Davidson *et al.* (1976) demonstrated that the ease of performance of a forceps delivery was directly related to the time taken for the cervical os to dilate from 7 to 10 cm. An 'easy' delivery could be anticipated where the interval was less than 2 hours. The greater the time period, the greater the chance of a difficult forceps delivery.

Complications of forceps delivery

Maternal

Lacerations can occur, especially if the cervical os is not completely dilated (Hibbard 1988). Tears to the vaginal wall or lower uterine segment and cervix can occur during rotational forceps deliveries. Where the pelvis is small and the fetal head a tight fit, the vaginal wall can be damaged by being compressed between the fetal head and the forceps (Hibbard 1988). Unless an episiotomy is performed at the right time, perineal damage will occur. Myerscough (1982) cautions against doing an episiotomy too early, in view of the blood loss which can result.

Pressure on the woman's bladder neck or bladder by the fetal head can lead her to retain urine postnatally. Catheterisation prior to delivery can help prevent some problems (Hibbard 1988).

Neonatal

Pressure of the forceps blades on the fetal head can produce depression fractures of the skull or intracranial haemorrhage (Chiswick and James 1979). This should not occur if the blades are applied correctly and the force used is not excessive. The blades can also cause bruising and temporary paralysis to the facial nerve (Eastman *et al.* 1962). Friction of the fetal scalp on the cranium caused by a tight fit in the pelvis or traction of the forceps blades may result in a cephalhaematoma (Dierker *et al.* 1985).

Caesarean section

Caesarean section is the delivery of the fetus through the uterine and abdominal walls after the twenty-eighth week of gestation. It can be performed as an elective technique (usually prior to the onset of labour) or as an emergency procedure at any time during labour (including during the second stage). Caesarean sections are increasingly being performed with the mother having an epidural anaesthetic, which allows her to hold her baby straight after birth (Pearson and Rees 1989). This also reduces the risks of mortality and morbidity resulting from general anaesthesia (Pearson and Rees 1989). The maternal death rate amongst women delivered by caesarean section is 37:100 000 as opposed to an overall maternal mortality rate of 8.6:100 000 total births (DOH 1989). The caesarean section rate in England and Wales is 10.6% (Currie 1987). This rate (it was 10.1% in 1982) compares with an increasing rate in other developed countries (Macfarlane 1988). Figures from Canada give a rate approaching 20% and from the United States, one in excess of 25% (Lomas 1988). Even wider variations exist within countries (Thiery and Derom 1986). Some countries with a low caesarean section rate (such as The Netherlands) also have amongst the lowest perinatal mortality rates (Macfarlane and Mugford 1986).

Indications for operative delivery

The decision to deliver by caesarean section is based on an analysis of various factors, which include fetal gestation, well-being and presentation and maternal health (Lomas and Enkin 1989). Whilst in many cases operative delivery improves the baby's chances of survival, this is at the increased cost of maternal mortality and morbidity (Cunningham *et al.* 1989). When confronted with a case of preterm labour, the obstetrician must balance the chances of a good neonatal outcome against maternal risks, including the effect of the presence of a scar on the uterus on future pregnancies (Hibbard 1988). Major indications (Hibbard 1988), none of which are absolute, are as follows:

1. Maternal disease, such as hypertensive disease of pregnancy.
2. Fetal jeopardy, including acute or chronic asphyxia due to antepartum haemorrhage, cord prolapse and placental insufficiency.
3. Difficult labour, such as cervical dystocia or fetal malpresentation. Taffel *et al.* (1987) showed that 79% of babies in their study presenting by the breech were delivered by caesarean section.
4. In some countries, most notably the United States, having had one baby delivered by caesarean section almost guarantees a repeat (Grandjean 1986).

The 1982–1984 report of the Confidential Enquiry into Maternal Deaths (Department of Health 1989) gives the indications for the performance of operative deliveries as follows: hypertensive disease (33%), delay in labour (19%), fetal distress (14%) and antepartum haemorrhage (14%).

The operation most commonly performed today is a lower uterine segment caesarean section with a Pfannenstiel (bikini line) incision (Pearson and Rees 1989) or more rarely a longitudinal skin incision. The latter is more commonly used to aid delivery in pregnancies with triplets or more (Pearson and Rees 1989). The classical caesarean section with a longitudinal incision in the upper uterine segment does not heal well due to uterine contractibility in the puerperium and has a risk of rupture during the next pregnancy (Myerscough 1982). The lower segment incision, being in a less muscular and active part of the uterus, heals better and, should rupture occur in subsequent labour (a risk of 0.09% (Lomas 1988)), it is usually a simple dehiscence of the scar without severe haemorrhage (Myerscough 1982).

Given the increasing frequency of operative deliveries, it is common to find caesarean section being covered in antenatal education. This helps prepare both the mothers who know they will be having an elective operative delivery and also those for whom it will become necessary during labour. Hayward (1975) demonstrated that giving detailed information before surgery speeds recovery time and reduces the need for analgesia. Although plans can be made for caesarean section, where an emergency procedure is instituted in labour the outcome may produce disruption of all the family's personal arrangements. Not only does the woman have to accept having a surgical rather than a vaginal delivery with all the attendant feelings of loss of control, but she will have a prolonged stay in hospital. If she has a general anaesthetic, she will miss the moment of her baby's birth and her period of recuperation will be lengthened (Hibbard 1988). Her partner or other family members may need to take time off work to care for her and any other children. In order to assist the woman in coming to terms with the change in delivery route, it is vital to keep her informed of everything which is happening in labour. Except in the cases of sudden acute fetal distress or haemorrhage, the decision is rarely made quickly. The couple can be prepared for the possibility of a caesarean section before the final decision is made. Should things progress normally, no harm has been done by giving the earlier warnings.

It is necessary to prepare the mother, as for any other surgical operation. Where the procedure is elective, these preparations will be more extensive. Blood should be taken for haemoglobin estimation and for cross-matching (Hibbard 1988). The doctor, after explaining the procedure, should obtain written consent. The abdomen and pubic hair are shaved to reduce the risk of infection (Cunningham et al. 1989). If an elective procedure, suppositories are usually given the night before to empty the bowel. Because of the risk of inhalation of stomach contents, it is helpful if the stomach is empty and an antacid such as sodium citrate has been given (Gibbs et al. 1981). Occasionally, it is necessary to empty the stomach using a Ryles tube, especially where the mother has eaten shortly before being admitted. To avoid damaging the bladder, a catheter is inserted and left on free drainage (Hibbard 1988). This can be inserted prior to the mother going to theatre and a spigot used until the operation starts. The operation is performed using either epidural or general anaesthesia. If an epidural is used, it is possible for the woman's partner to accompany her into theatre and to give her support (Pearson and Rees 1989). Because of the risk of deep venous thrombosis, antiembolism boots may be used during the operation and for 12–24 hours afterwards until the woman is starting to mobilise.

After the operation, the mother (and usually her baby) remain under close observation in the recovery room. Once she has regained full consciousness and her vital signs are stable, she can be transferred to the postnatal ward. It is important to check pulse and blood pressure every 15 minutes and also to observe the wound and vulval pad for signs of haemorrhage. The uterine fundus can be gently palpated to ensure it is well contracted. It is possible to initiate breast feeding in the recovery area. This both increases the chances of successfully establishing breast feeding (Martin and White 1988) and promotes maternal–infant bonding.

The woman should be allowed to rest, with analgesia given as necessary. She should be bed-bathed initially and later assisted to use the bidet and shower. Because the mother has had a major abdominal operation, she will need more help with caring for her baby and the midwife should use her judgement when to offer help and when to leave the mother to get on with things herself. The midwife should beware of taking over the care of the baby.

Observations for any developing infection should be made. These include four-hourly recordings of temperature and pulse, observations of the wound and lochia and a routine midstream specimen of urine on the third or fourth day. Early ambulation is encouraged, to aid healing and reduce the risk of deep venous thrombosis (Hibbard 1988); any leg pain or dyspnoea should be reported to the obstetrician at once. A high fibre diet should be taken to encourage normal bowel action, but delays in eating (following non-return of bowel sounds) and limited activity may necessitate the use of a mild laxative or suppositories. Wound dressings are rarely used and the closure is often with a subcuticular stitch or clips. These are removed as directed. When fit (usually from 6 days onwards), the woman and her baby are transferred home. The family must be aware that being fit to go home does not mean that the woman can resume her normal roles and responsibilities.

Psychological aspects of caesarean section

More attention is being paid to the woman's perceptions of her birth experience. An operative delivery, especially one performed as an emergency procedure, may be at variance with the woman's expectations. She may feel somehow that she has either failed or has done something wrong (Marut and Mercer 1979).

Cranley et al. (1983) and Kirchmeier (1984) have both shown that women who had an emergency caesarean section had fewer positive feelings about their birth than did those who had either vaginal or elective caesarean deliveries. The type of anaesthesia used is also important, with regional (epidural) anaesthesia giving more positive attitudes than a general anaesthetic (Marut and Mercer 1979; Cranley et al. (1983). The presence of the woman's partner during the caesarean section also improved the woman's perceptions.

Garel and Kaminski (1986) comment that an operative delivery places considerable physiological, psychological and economic burdens on the woman and her family. Studies of the father's reactions to caesarean section have reported anger that labour was allowed to continue for far too long and guilt due to the pain that their partner had experienced (Erb *et al.* 1983). Many also mentioned the lack of information for fathers to prepare them for the experience.

The rise in the caesarean section rate

Causes

Both technological and social changes have contributed to the increase in the caesarean section rate (Lomas and Enkin 1989). With a reduction in family size and the expectation that every pregnancy ends in a healthy outcome, pressure has been placed on obstetricians to adopt a proactive approach (Cunningham *et al.* 1989). In countries where maternity care is paid for personally or by health insurance, caesarean rates are higher (McPherson *et al.* 1981). Even in the United Kingdom, Macfarlane and Mugford (1986) report a 1980 caesarean section rate of 19.6% amongst women in private care against 9.0% for other NHS cases. The fear of litigation especially in North America, has led some obstetricians to avoid potentially difficult procedures such as breech delivery (Haynes de Regt *et al.* 1986; Lomas 1988). In the Maternity Alliance (1983) survey of trends in operative delivery 'defensive' obstetrics was given as the second commonest reason for the increase in caesarean births.

Technological changes include the increasing safety of operative delivery, but, despite this, a caesarean birth is still more than four times more likely than a vaginal one to result in a maternal death (Department of Health 1989). Resulting morbidity, including pain, infection and difficulties with breast feeding are hard to quantify. The introduction of continuous fetal monitoring in labour has resulted in an increase in emergency caesarean sections for 'fetal distress'. MacDonald *et al.* (1985) argue that if fetal blood sampling is used to assess fetal acidosis before embarking on surgery, the caesarean rate is not increased. 'Failure to progress' is a common reason for caesarean section. Derom *et al.* (1987) blame misdiagnosis of the onset of labour and a lack of understanding of progress in the latent stage. O'Driscoll and Meagher (1980) found no increase in the rate of operative delivery where women with 'tardy' labour were actively managed with artificial rupture of the membranes and an oxytocin infusion.

The improved safety of operative delivery has led some obstetricians to balance this against the fetal risks of some obstetric procedures, such as breech and high forceps deliveries. Only 4% of fetuses in labour present by the breech so even if all breech babies were to be delivered operatively, this could not account for all the increase in operative deliveries. With improvements in neonatal intensive care and better survival chances, there is pressure from neonatologists to deliver the baby in the best possible condition. In the United States repeated caesarean sections are an ever-increasing proportion of operative deliveries (Derom *et al.* 1987). In many places, the dictum 'once a caesarean section always a caesarean section' seems to be adhered to. Molloy *et al.* (1987) have reviewed 2176 consecutive women who had undergone one previous caesarean section. There was a repeat elective caesarean rate of 18.2%, with 81.8% of the remaining women achieving a vaginal delivery. Women most likely to need a repeat caesarean section were those whose earlier labour did not progress beyond 4 cm, those who had elective sections and those who needed augmentation in the later labour. They also give a rate of 0.45% for rupture of the uterine scar amongst those women who went into labour (Molloy *et al.* 1987).

Implications

Increased delivery rates by caesarean section could result in loss of skills by both midwives and obstetricians. The midwives will lack practice in managing a woman with a high-risk labour and the doctors may lose (or never learn) the techniques of complicated delivery. Economically, use of the operating theatre, longer stays in hospital and the need for family members to be absent from work can place heavy burdens. Fear of litigation and defensive practice could result in legal action where the parents object to what they perceive as unnecessary intervention. Increased use of technology in obstetrics has been accompanied by a fall in the perinatal mortality rate. Cause and effect have not been demonstrated. Antenatal screening, developments in neonatal intensive care and improvements in general health could also be responsible for improving outcomes. Lomas (1988) has called for increased use of auditing procedures, forcing doctors to question their actions and to measure outcomes before the high rate of operative deliveries becomes established.

Trial of labour/trial of scar

A trial of labour occurs where the outcome of the labour is in doubt (Myerscough 1982). Extra supervision is given to the woman and her fetus while it is ascertained whether the presenting part is capable of flexing sufficiently to pass through the birth canal. A trial of scar is a similar exercise performed when the previous delivery has been by caesarean section. Ideally the labour should be spontaneous. It is conducted in a unit with all the facilities available for operative delivery if required. The two main criteria of progress are progressive dilatation of the cervix and progressive descent of the presenting part (Donald 1979). In the case of a trial of scar, it is also necessary to observe for any pain or discomfort over the area of the scar (Ruddick *et al.* 1984). Time limits should be set for the labour by which time a minimum amount of progress should have been achieved (American College of Obstetricians and Gynaecologists 1988). If progress does not occur, if the contractions are ineffective, if fetal distress occurs or in the case of a previous operative delivery, there is pain over the scar, a caesarean section is usually performed.

References

American College of Obstetricians and Gynaecologists, Committee on Maternal and Fetal Medicine (1988) *Guidelines For Vaginal Delivery After a Previous Cesarean Section* ACOG: Washington

Barclay C and Fraser R C (1988) 'The history of the use of vacuum extraction' *Midwife, Health Visitor and Community Nurse* 24(8): 328–31

Beazley J M and Lobb M O (1983) *Aspects of Care in Labour* Churchill Livingstone: Edinburgh

Chalmers J A and Chalmers I (1989) 'The obstetric vacuum extractor is the instrument of first choice for operative vaginal delivery' *British Journal of Obstetrics and Gynaecology* 96(5): 505–6

Chamberlain G V P (1980) 'Forceps and vacuum extraction' in I MacGillivray (ed) *Operative Obstetrics* Ch 7 511–28 W B Saunders: Philadelphia

Chiswick M L and James D K (1979) 'Kjelland's forceps: Association with neonatal morbidity and mortality' *British Medical Journal* 1: 7

Cranley M S, Hedahl K J and Pegg S (1983) 'Women's perceptions of vaginal and caesarean deliveries' *Nursing Research* 32: 10–14

Crichton D (1974) 'A reliable method of establishing the level of the fetal head in obstetrics' *South African Medical Journal* 48: 784–7

Cunningham F J, MacDonald P C and Gant N F (1989) *William's Obstetrics (18th edn)* Prentice Hall: London

Currie E (1987) 'Parliamentary written answer' *House of Commons Report (Hansard)* 24 July 120: Col 713 (No 26 part II)

Davidson A C, Weaver J B, Davies P and Pearson J F (1976) 'The relation between ease of forceps delivery and speed of cervical dilatation' *British Journal of Obstetrics and Gynaecology* 83(4): 279–83

Department of Health (1989) *Report on Confidential Enquiries into Maternal Deaths in England and Wales 1982–4* HMSO: London

Derom R, Patel N B and Thierry C (1987) 'Implications of increasing rates of caesarean section' in J Studd (ed) *Progress in Obstetrics and Gynaecology Vol 6* Ch 9 175–94 Churchill Livingstone: Edinburgh

Dierker L J, Rosen M G, Thompson K, Debanne S and Linn P (1985) 'The midforceps: maternal and neonatal outcomes' *American Journal of Obstetrics and Gynecology* 152: 176

Donald I (1979) *Practical Obstetric Problems (5th edn)* Lloyd Luke: London

Eastman N J, Kohl S G, Maisel J E and Kaveler F (1962) 'The obstetrical background of 753 cases of cerebral palsy' *Obstetrical and Gynaecological Survey* 17: 459

Erb L, Hill G and Houston D (1983) 'A survey of parents' attitudes towards their caesarean birth in Manitoba Hospitals' *Birth* 10: 85–91

Garel M and Kaminski M (1986) 'Psychosocial outcomes of caesarean births' in M Kaminski (ed) *Perinatal Care Delivery Systems* Ch 10 156–66 Oxford University Press: Oxford

Gibbs C P, Sophr L and Schmidt D (1981) 'In vitro and in vivo evaluation of sodium citrate as an antacid' *Anesthesiology* 55: A31

Grandjean H (1986) 'Determinents of caesarean section' in M Kaminski (ed) *Perinatal Care Delivery Systems* Ch 8 114–28 Oxford University Press: Oxford

Grant A (1986) 'Vacuum extraction or forceps?' *British Medical Journal* 292: 343–4

Haynes de Regt F H, Minkoff H L, Feldman J and Schwarz R H (1986) 'Relation of private or clinic care to the cesarean birth rate' *New England Journal of Medicine* 315: 619

Hayward J (1975) *Information – a Prescription Against Pain* Royal College of Nursing: London

Herabutya Y, Prasertsawat P and Boonrangsimant P (1988) 'Kjelland's forceps or ventouse – a comparison' *British Journal of Obstetrics and Gynaecology* 95(5): 483–7

Hibbard B M (1988) *Principles of Obstetrics* Butterworths: London

Kirchmeier R (1984) 'Influences on mothers' reactions to caesarean birth' *Research and the Midwife Proceedings* 86–101

Lomas J (1988) 'Holding back the tide of caesareans' *British Medical Journal* 297: 569–70

Lomas J and Enkin M (1989) 'Variations in operative delivery rates' in I Chalmers, M Enkin and M J N C Keirse (eds) *Effective Care in Pregnancy and Childbirth* Ch 69 1182–95 Oxford Medical: Oxford

MacDonald A, Grant A and Pereira M (1985) 'The Dublin randomised controlled trial of intrapartum electronic fetal heart rate monitoring' *American Journal of Obstetrics and Gynecology* 154: 524–39

Macfarlane A (1988) 'Holding back the tide of caesareans' *British Medical Journal* 297: 852

Macfarlane A and Mugford M (1986) 'An epidemic of caesareans?' *Maternal and Child Health* 11(2): 38–42

McPherson K, Strong P M, Epstein A and Jones L (1981) 'Regional variations in the use of common surgical procedures: within and between England and Wales, Canada and the United States of America' *Social Science and Medicine* 15A: 273–88

Martin J and White A (1988) *Infant Feeding 1985* HMSO: London

Marut J S and Mercer R T (1979) 'Comparison of primipara's perceptions of vaginal and caesarean births' *Nursing Research* 28: 260–6

Maternity Alliance (1983) *One Birth in Nine* Maternity Alliance: London

Molloy B G, Sheil O and Duignan N M (1987) 'Delivery after caesarean section: a review of 2176 consecutive cases' *British Medical Journal* 294: 1645–8

Moolgaoker A (1970) 'A safe alternative to caesarean section?' *Journal of Obstetrics and Gynaecology of the British Commonwealth* 77: 1077–87

Myerscough P R (1982) *Munro Kerr's Operative Obstetrics (10th edn)* Bailliere Tindall: London

O'Driscoll K and Meagher D (1980) *Active Management of Labour* Saunders: London

Pearson J and Rees G (1989) 'Technique of caesarean section' in I Chalmers, M Enkin and M J N C Keirse (eds) *Effective Care in Pregnancy and Childbirth* Ch 72 1234–45 Oxford Medical: Oxford

Ruddick V, Niv D, Hetman-Peri C, Geller C, Avni A and Golan A (1984) 'Epidural analgesia for planned vaginal delivery following previous cesarean section' *Obstetrics and Gynaecology* 64: 621

Ryden G (1986) 'Vacuum extraction or forceps' *British Medical Journal* 292: 76–7

Taffel S M, Placek P J and Liss T (1987) 'Trends in the United States cesarean section rate for the 1980–85 rise' *American Journal of Public Health* 77: 955

Thiery M and Derom R (1986) 'Review of evaluation studies of caesarean section Part I: Trends in caesarean section and perinatal mortality' in M Kaminski (ed) *Perinatal Care Delivery Systems* Ch 7 93–113 Oxford University Press: Oxford

Vacca A, Grant A, Wyatt G and Chalmers I (1983) 'A comparison of vacuum extraction and forceps delivery' *British Journal of Obstetrics and Gynaecology* 90: 1107–12

Vacca A and Keirse M J N C (1989) 'Instrumental vaginal delivery' in I Chalmers, M Enkin and M J N C Keirse (eds) *Effective Care in Pregnancy and Childbirth* Ch 71 1217–33 Oxford Medical: Oxford

26 Postpartum haemorrhage and complications of the third stage of labour

This chapter considers the causes and management of third stage abnormalities. After the birth of the baby, the midwife must not relax her concentration on the mother's well-being, since this is the time when rapid deterioration in condition can occur. Donald (1979) states that since such events escalate very quickly, it is preferable to intervene early rather than to wait for the situation to get out of hand. Postpartum haemorrhage caused nine maternal deaths in the 1979–1981 triennium and three deaths in 1982–1984 in England and Wales (Department of Health and Social Security 1985; Department of Health 1989). This chapter will first define the types and causes of postpartum haemorrhage before discussing their management. The causes of retained placenta and the process of manual removal will be described.

Postpartum haemorrhage

This is a serious emergency occurring after the birth of the baby. The maternal condition can deteriorate alarmingly in a matter of seconds (Clinch 1985). Because haemorrhage can follow the most normal of deliveries, every midwife must be able to both diagnose and commence treatment while awaiting aid. Prompt treatment is a lifesaving measure. Postpartum haemorrhage refers to excessive bleeding from the genital tract occurring within 6 weeks of the birth of the baby. It is subdivided into three main time periods:

- Third stage haemorrhage – Before delivery of the placenta.
- Primary postpartum haemorrhage – Within the first 24 hours after delivery of the baby (including the third stage).
- Secondary postpartum haemorrhage – After the first 24 hours and up to 6 weeks after delivery. This is sometimes also called puerperal haemorrhage.

Primary postpartum haemorrhage

The amount of blood loss which constitutes a postpartum haemorrhage (PPH) depends on the time of occurrence and its effect on the maternal condition. The accepted definition is an estimated blood loss of more than 500 ml. Begley (1990) is critical of this definition. In her comparative study of physiological and active management (using ergometrine) of the third stage of labour, although there was a higher incidence of PPHs using the above definition, this increased blood loss had no significant effect on maternal well-being and there was no need for any blood transfusions (Begley 1990). An estimated loss of more than 500 ml occurs in between 1.1% (Clinch 1985) and 5% (Cunningham *et al.* 1989) of deliveries. Estimates of blood loss are notoriously inaccurate (Pritchard *et al.* 1962). A blood clot if measured does not always include the plasma, which can be absorbed by drapes. Levy and Moore (1985) showed that blood loss estimation following delivery may be only 50% of the true amount. It is thought that blood losses of 500 ml are normal. Newton (1966) estimated average blood loss at delivery and in the first 24 hours after birth as 650 ml by measuring the fall in haemoglobin. DeLeeuw *et al.* (1968), measuring the fall in erythrocytes, estimated average blood loss as 600 ml. When considering primary postpartum haemorrhage, it is usual to classify as haemorrhage any blood loss, however small, which adversely affects the mother's condition, as well as losses over 500 ml. Pritchard *et al.* (1962) estimate that in 5% of vaginal deliveries the actual blood loss exceeds 1000 ml.

There are three main types of primary postpartum haemorrhage: those where bleeding comes from the placental site, (the majority), those due to trauma and finally haemorrhage due to coagulation defects.

Bleeding from the placental site

This is usually caused by a failure of the myometrium to contract and thus seal off the blood sinuses to the placental site (Hibbard 1988). There are a number of factors which contribute to poor muscle tone, but which themselves do not directly give rise to haemorrhage:

1. High degrees of parity (Fuchs *et al.* 1985). With each successive pregnancy,

more uterine muscle fibres are replaced by fibrous tissue which does not contract and retract. Donald (1979) postulates that, whilst contractions in the first and second stages are vigorous, the uterus may have lost its ability to retract. This only becomes apparent in the third stage of labour. In addition, if the intervals between births are short, the mother may be anaemic and malnourished (Fuchs *et al.* 1985).

2. Anaemia. Any woman embarking upon labour with a haemoglobin level below 10 g/100 ml is at an increased risk of the effects of haemorrhage, since even a normal blood loss could worsen her condition (Cunningham *et al.* 1989).

3. Fibroids. These can predispose to haemorrhage, since they both impede uterine action and, if the placenta has implanted into them, may produce adhesions of the placenta and delay its expulsion (Donald 1979).

4. Women with a previous history of haemorrhage or retained placenta are at risk of repeating the event (Myerscough 1982). For this reason, such women should give birth in a consultant unit. Blood for transfusion if necessary should be on hand and an intravenous line should be *in situ* for the third stage of labour. In some cases, prophylactic intravenous ergometrine is given by a member of the medical staff with delivery of the shoulders (Myerscough 1982). The placenta must be delivered rapidly before constriction occurs between the upper and lower uterine segments. If this is not achieved, the woman must remain under observation for at least 45 minutes until the effects of the ergometrine reduce and the placenta can be delivered (Myerscough 1982).

Causes of atonic uterus

1. Incomplete separation of the placenta. If the placenta is fully adherent, there is usually no bleeding. However, if separation is incomplete, torrential haemorrhage can occur from torn maternal sinuses (Cunningham *et al.* 1989). Until the placenta is delivered, control of bleeding cannot occur. Similarly, retained portions of the placenta (such as a succenturiate lobe) or fragments of membranes may prevent efficient control of bleeding by contractions (Hibbard 1988).

2. Overstretching of the uterus. The overstretched myometrium is less efficient at contracting in the third stage and after delivery. This can occur in cases of polyhydramnios or multiple pregnancy (Cunningham *et al.* 1989). Pritchard (1965) calculated that average blood loss during a vaginal twin delivery was almost 1000 ml. In addition, in multiple pregnancies there is a larger placental site and an increased risk of low implantation.

3. Antepartum haemorrhage. If the placenta is low lying (placenta praevia), the retractile power of the muscles in the lower segment is poor, giving an increased risk of haemorrhage. In cases of abruptio placentae (especially if resulting in a couvelaire uterus), blood seeping into the myometrium can interfere with contraction and retraction (Donald 1979).

4. Precipitate labour. Over vigorous uterine activity in the first and second stages may not have permitted the myometrium sufficient time to retract (Cunningham *et al.* 1989).

5. Mismanagement of the third stage. This includes having a full bladder and squeezing or mishandling the uterus. Inefficient contractions may be produced which cause partial separation of the placenta and haemorrhage (Cunningham *et al.* 1989).

6. Prolonged labour. There is disagreement as to whether it is the length of labour which results in uterine exhaustion or the resulting maternal dehydration, ketosis, augmentation of labour or the use of narcotic analgesics (Donald 1979).

7. General anaesthetic agents, especially halothane, relax the myometrium and therefore can give rise to haemorrhage. They are also sometimes used to overcome spasms of the myometrium, such as hourglass constriction (Gilstrap *et al.* 1987).

8. No known cause. A large number of haemorrhages occur in the absence of any defined cause or predisposing factor (Hibbard 1988).

Diagnosis can be easy when there is profuse bleeding and a worsening in maternal condition. However, in many cases the onset is an insidious, slow trickling of blood over a few hours which can give rise to significant blood loss (Cunningham *et al.* 1989). The uterus may feel enlarged and soft, and there may be little external blood loss, or else a slight trickle. The uterus fills up with blood clots. The mother may become restless and tachycardic, although maternal pulse is a poor guide to the extent of the blood loss. It may rise with quite small losses, yet remain normal in conditions of hypovolaemia (Jansen 1978). Her blood pressure may fall and she could look pale. The existence of a normal blood pressure cannot be used as indication that the circulating blood volume is satisfactory (Cunningham *et al.* 1989). Because of the insidious nature of some cases of haemorrhage, the mother's condition is observed frequently in the hours immediately after delivery (Cunningham *et al.* 1989).

The condition must be managed aggressively before it worsens. The midwife (without leaving the mother) must summon medical assistance, try to stop the bleeding and then, when aid has arrived, the mother's condition can be improved.

Medical aid

A midwife should always call for medical assistance as early as possible. Should the mother be at home or in peripheral unit without medical staff, the general practitioner and the local obstetric flying squad should be alerted. If the delivery is taking place at home, it is important that the midwife calls for medical assistance as soon as she suspects that the situation is not progressing normally. She must allow sufficient time for help to arrive before the mother becomes shocked (Hibbard 1988). If the situation is under control by the time aid arrives, nothing has been lost (Myerscough 1982). Women in a collapsed condition or those who are actively haemorrhaging should not be transferred to hospital in the absence of medical assistance and equipment for resuscitation.

Treatment

Controlling the bleeding

Whether the placenta is *in situ* or not, the action of the midwife is the same. She should assess the state of contraction of the uterus. If it is soft, she should gently massage the fundus with a circular motion until a contraction is produced. When this occurs, the hand remains in contact with the fundus to check for any relaxation. An oxytocic drug such as syntometrine (0.5 mg ergometrine and 5 units syntocin) can be given intramuscularly to help sustain the contractions. If experienced in intravenous administration, or if an intravenous line is *in situ*, 0.25 mg of ergomentine can be given (Hibbard 1988), which produces a sustained uterine contraction in 45 seconds. Further doses should be used with caution because of the risk of hypertension and vomiting (Myerscough 1982). Physiological oxytocin production can be increased by putting the baby to the breast. Once the uterus is well contracted, the midwife should ensure that it is empty. If the placenta is still *in situ*, it should be delivered (check first that the bladder is empty). Where the placenta has been delivered, it should be examined for its completeness. Any clots or shreds of membrane present in the uterus should be expelled by gentle pressure on the uterus. Under no circumstances should the mother be positioned head down, as this will cause blood to collect in the uterine cavity, which is capable of containing up to 1 l of blood (Cunningham *et al.* 1989).

To improve maternal condition, an intravenous line should be established. This is better done earlier while peripheral veins are still visible. This permits the giving of fluids, plasma and blood to restore circulating blood volumes and intravenous syntocinon (10 units/500 ml) to maintain uterine contractions (Cunningham *et al.* 1989). Before establishing the infusion, blood should be taken for cross-matching and haemoglobin estimation. The intravenous infusion is usually allowed to run slowly over a number of hours to maintain contractions. In certain circumstances of severe haemorrhage, it may be necessary to establish full intensive care procedures, including central venous pressure lines, electrocardiograph readings and hourly measurement of urinary output (Cunningham *et al.* 1989).

If the placenta is still *in situ*, the medical staff will prepare for a manual removal of placenta (see later). In emergencies a midwife must be capable of carrying out this procedure. If bleeding is continuing, manual removal of the placenta will need to be carried out as soon as possible. The woman who has a placenta *in situ* after the birth of the baby must never be left alone (Clinch 1985). If the placenta has been removed and bleeding continues, bimanual compression may be performed (Hibbard 1988). This is an emergency procedure performed in the absence of oxytocic drugs or where they have failed to be effective (Hibbard 1988). A hand is introduced into the vagina and the uterus is squeezed between this internal fist and the external hand which surrounds the uterine fundus (Cunningham *et al.* 1989). This is a tiring procedure which is difficult to maintain for long. When aid arrives or when facilities are prepared, the woman is transferred to a setting where exploration of the uterus and vagina can be carried out under general or epidural anaesthesia. The presence of a coagulation disorder should be excluded before embarking on this procedure. On rare occasions, a hysterectomy may be the only method of controlling the bleeding (Fox 1972).

Prophylaxis

The best treatment is prevention. For this reason, it is important to ensure that every woman begins labour in the best possible physical condition. During the antenatal period it is important to detect and treat any anaemia as early as possible (Myerscough 1982). With good history taking, risk factors such as previous precipitate deliveries, retained placentae and postpartum haemorrhage can be highlighted and the woman delivered in an appropriate setting. During labour, it is important to ensure that the woman does not become dehydrated or ketotic and that the labour progresses at an appropriate pace. The bladder should be empty in the second and third stages of labour. In the woman at risk of a postpartum haemorrhage it is important that oxytocic drugs are employed in the management of the third stage.

Manual removal of the placenta

Separation of the placenta is usually complete within 15 minutes using active management and 30 minutes with physiological management of the third stage of labour (Clinch 1985). If a haemorrhage occurs, action is taken more swiftly than in its absence. The causes of retained placenta include inefficient uterine action to produce separation, partial separation (often resulting from mismanagement), the formation of a constriction ring between the upper and lower uterine segments (due to internal manipulations or ergometrine use) and a morbidly adherent placenta (Hibbard 1988). This last problem occurs during implantation of the placenta, where decidual reaction (a laying down of fibrous tissue in the lower layer of the decidua to resist implantation) has not occurred. The placenta has implanted through the spongy layer of the decidua and into the myometrium (Cunningham *et al.* 1989). There is no proper line of cleavage, so separation cannot occur (Cunningham *et al.* 1989). Breen *et al.* (1977) estimate the occurrence rate for morbid adherence of the placenta as 1 : 7000 deliveries.

It is not usually possible to determine the cause of the delay in delivery of the placenta until examination under general anaesthesia. Preparations are made to take the mother to theatre. Blood is taken for cross-matching and an intravenous infusion is established. The mother must remain under close observation during this time, because there is a risk of partial separation of the placenta and haemorrhage

(Clinch 1985). Before inducing anaesthesia, a last attempt is made to deliver the placenta (Cunningham *et al.* 1989). General anaesthesia is preferred to an epidural, although it carries a slightly higher risk for the mother, because the anaesthetic agents will relax the uterus, especially in the presence of a constriction ring (Myerscough 1982).

Although manual removal of the placenta is not a normal part of the work of the midwife, she should be aware of the techniques involved should the need arise in an emergency. Manual removal of the placenta is carried out as an aseptic procedure. The anaesthetised woman is placed in the lithotomy position, her vulva swabbed with an antiseptic solution and she is draped. Her bladder is emptied with a catheter. Wearing extra-long gloves, the obstetrician covers his/her hand and forearm with antiseptic cream before introducing it into the vagina and following the umbilical cord up to the placenta. Using his/her external hand to steady (and guard) the uterus (felt through sterile drapes), the obstetrician searches around the edge of the placenta for an area which has started to separate. The ulnar border of this hand is then moved in a sweeping motion to separate the placenta from the uterine wall (Cunningham *et al.* 1989). When it is separated, the hand is slowly withdrawn holding the placenta while the external hand rubs up a contraction (Hibbard 1988). The anaesthetist then either gives syntometrine or intravenous syntocinon to maintain the uterine contraction (Hibbard 1988).

If a constriction ring is encountered, a deeper anaesthetic may be needed to achieve relaxation. If the placenta is morbidly adherent (placenta accreta), it is usually removed piecemeal. Occasionally it will be necessary to perform a hysterectomy to control bleeding and prevent infection (Fox 1972).

Following manual removal, a close watch is maintained on the mother's condition. An intravenous infusion, often with syntocinon, is maintained for 8–12 hours after delivery of the placenta. Prophylactic antibiotic cover may be given (Clinch 1985).

Should the placenta be retained following a home delivery, medical assistance is sought. The mother is not moved in the absence of skilled assistants with the placenta *in situ*, as there is the possibility of separation at any time. If it is not possible to effect delivery at home and the obstetric flying squad will be called to transfer the woman to hospital (Myerscough 1982).

Trauma

In the case of trauma, bleeding continues, despite a well-contracted uterus. An episiotomy itself gives rise to an average blood loss of 200 ml (Odell and Seski 1947). Lacerations can occur in the uterus itself (rare), the cervix, vagina, vulva, perineum and labia (Cunningham *et al.* 1989). Internal trauma is most common following an instrumental delivery (Gilstrap *et al.* 1984). In order to isolate the source of the bleeding, it may be necessary to put the woman into the lithotomy position and to use a speculum with a good light source to examine the upper vagina and cervix (Hibbard 1988). Should a bleeding point be seen, this can be stopped by applying a pair of artery forceps until a repair can be carried out. General anaesthesia may be required, depending on the type and scope of the damage (Hibbard 1988). If no bleeding point is visible, but blood is still oozing from the uterus, a laparotomy may be needed to identify the source (Hibbard 1988). External sources of bleeding are easily identified and bleeding controlled with mosquito forceps until a repair is performed.

Within 12–48 hours of delivery, a vulval haematoma may develop from ruptured vulval varicosities or an inadequately repaired episiotomy or perineal tear. This is a rare but serious complication. A large swelling can develop which extends up the vaginal wall. The area is at best tender and at worst excruciatingly painful. The mother may be shocked from both the pain and the blood loss (Hibbard 1988). If left, the haematoma could re-absorb, but abscess formation is a risk, so the clot is usually evacuated under general anaesthesia. Before embarking upon this, it will be necessary to reverse the maternal state of shock and collapse (Cunningham *et al.* 1989). During evacuation of the clot, the bleeding point is isolated and if visible, sutured. A vaginal pack can also be used to control bleeding. A urinary catheter should be inserted and left *in situ* for the first 12 hours after the repair. Antibiotic cover is usually required in the early postnatal period (Cunningham *et al.* 1989). Early haemaglobin estimation will determine the extent of the blood loss and any need for transfusion (Hibbard 1988).

Coagulation disorders

These are rare conditions where the serum fibrinogen level is low. They arise as a result of some antepartum haemorrhages (abruptio placentae), intrauterine deaths, missed abortions, fulminating pre-eclampsia, sepsis and amniotic fluid embolism (Myerscough 1982). The uterus is usually well contracted, but blood loss (which does not clot) continues. There may also be bleeding from other areas such as the site of an intravenous infusion. Expert medical assistance, including haematology support, is required (Hibbard 1988). Treatment involves a combination of intravenous fresh whole blood, extra clotting factors and fibrinogen (see Chapter 27).

Secondary postpartum haemorrhage

Although this can occur any time from 24 hours to 6 weeks after delivery, it is most common between 7–12 days by which time the mother is normally at home (Cunningham *et al.* 1989). Fresh blood loss should have ceased and the mother is alarmed to discover that she is bleeding again and/or passing clots. Bleeding is usually due to a retained portion of the placenta and/or membranes. If infection is present, the lochia will be offensive and there may also be maternal pyrexia, tachycardia and subinvolution of the uterus (Hibbard 1988). Lee *et al.* (1981) from a study of 3822 women, estimate that secondary postpartum haemorrhage occurs in 0.7% of women.

The midwife may be summoned to the woman's home as an emergency or the bleeding may be noticed at a postnatal visit. If the former, the mother should be advised to rest in bed until the midwife arrives and to keep any blood loss to allow estimation of the size of the haemorrhage. On arrival, the midwife must assess the mother's condition and vital signs. Her uterus should be felt to see if it is palpable and, if possible, any clots expelled. If the mother is in a poor condition, arrangements will need to be made to transfer her to the nearest maternity unit. An obstetric flying squad may need to be called. An oxytocic drug should be given to try to control the bleeding (Goldstein *et al.* 1983). When medical help arrives, an intravenous infusion will be established. When the mother's condition permits, a manual exploration of her uterus will be performed under general anaesthesia. Lee *et al.* (1981) have had some success using ultrasound scanning to detect retained portions of the placenta.

For less severe conditions, the general practitioner is summoned. If the lochia is offensive, a high vaginal swab will be taken and sent to bacteriology for culture and sensitivity. Oral ergometrine tablets and antibiotics may be adequate to resolve this condition. If blood loss persists, the woman may be transferred to hospital for evacuation of the uterus of intramuscular antibiotic therapy. Measurement should be made of the woman's haemoglobin level to assess the need for iron therapy.

References

Begley C M (1990) 'A comparison of "active" and "physiological" management of the third stage of labour' *Midwifery* 6(1): 3–17

Breen J L, Neubecker R, Gregori C A and Franklin J E (1977) 'Placenta accreta, increta and percreta: A survey of 40 cases' *Obstetrics and Gynecology* 49: 43

Clinch J (1985) 'The third stage' in J Studd (ed) *Management of Labour* Ch 20 287–300 Blackwell Scientific: Oxford

Cunningham F G, MacDonald P C and Gant N F (1989) *William's Obstetrics (18th edn)* Prentice Hall: London

DeLeeuw N K M, Lowenstein L, Tucker E C and Dayal S (1968) 'Correlation of red cell loss at delivery with red cell mass' *American Journal of Obstetrics and Gynecology* 84: 1271

Department of Health (1989) *Confidential Enquiry into Maternal Deaths in England and Wales 1982–4* HMSO: London

Department of Health and Social Security (1985) *Confidential Enquiry into Maternal Deaths in England and Wales 1979–81* HMSO: London

Donald I (1979) *Practical Obstetric Problems* Lloyd Luke: London

Fox H (1972) 'Placenta accreta: a review' *Obstetrical and Gynaecological Survey* 27: 475–90

Fuchs K, Peretz B A, Marcovici R, Paldi E and Timor-Tritsh I (1985) 'The "grand multipara" – Is it a problem? A review of 5785 cases' *International Journal of Gynaecology and Obstetrics* 23: 321

Gilstrap L C, Hauth J C, Hankins G D V and Patterson A R (1987) 'Effect of type of analgesia on blood loss at cesarean section' *Obstetrics and Gynecology* 69: 328

Gilstrap L C, Hauth J C, Schiano S and Connor K D (1984) 'Neonatal acidosis and method of delivery' *Obstetrics and Gynecology* 63: 681

Goldstein A I, Kent D R and David A (1983) 'Prostaglandin E2 vaginal suppositories in the treatment of intractable late onset postpartum hemmorrhage' *Journal of Reproductive Medicine* 28: 425

Hibbard B M (1988) *Principles of Obstetrics* Butterworth: London

Jansen R P S (1978) 'Relative bradycardia: A sign of acute intraperitoneal bleeding' *New Zealand Journal of Obstetrics and Gynecology* 18: 206

Lee C Y, Madrazo B and Drukker B H (1981) 'Ultrasonic evaluation of the postpartum uterus in the management of postpartum bleeding' *Obstetrics and Gynecology* 58: 227

Levy V and Moore J (1985) 'Midwife's management of the third stage of labour' *Nursing Times* 81(39): 47–50

Myerscough P R (1982) *Munro Kerr's Operative Obstetrics (10th edn)* Balliere Tindall: London

Newton M (1966) 'Postpartum hemmorrhage' *American Journal of Obstetrics and Gynecology* 94: 711

Odell L D and Seski A (1947) 'Episiotomy blood loss' *American Journal of Obstetrics and Gynecology* 54: 51

Pritchard J A (1965) 'Changes in blood volume during pregnancy and delivery' *Anesthesiology* 26: 393

Pritchard J A, Baldwin R M, Dickey J C and Wiggins K M (1962) 'Blood volume changes in pregnancy and the puerperium II' *American Journal of Obstetrics and Gynecology* 84: 1271

27 Shock and Obstetric Emergencies

This chapter will first consider the phenomenon of shock: the circumstances which prevail when the woman's circulatory system is unable to fulfil the demands of the body for oxygenation, nutrition and excretion. It will then describe the causes, diagnosis and management of disseminated intravascular coagulation. The obstetric emergencies whose detection and management are included are rupture of and inverted uterus, amniotic fluid embolism and hazards of obstetric general anaesthesia. Finally, the fetal emergencies of prolapsed umbilical cord and shoulder dystocia will be discussed.

Emergencies

This chapter contains purely abnormal obstetrics. Although this is the realm of the obstetrician rather than the midwife, it is vital for midwives to be able to detect these conditions and, while awaiting medical assistance, to initiate treatment. The very rarity of these conditions requires theoretical instruction in advance of any practical experience. Emergencies need a rapid response and there is limited time to refer either to more experienced colleagues or to textbooks. Swift, accurate management is a life-saving measure.

417

Midwives caring for women in both low- and high-risk labours should be aware of how quickly an emergency can occur and the woman's condition deteriorate. An obstetric emergency can result in maternal morbidity and mortality. In the 1982–84 report of the Confidential Enquiries into Maternal Deaths in England and Wales (Department of Health 1989), there were 2 deaths due to confirmed amniotic fluid embolism (6 in 1979–1981 (Department of Health and Social Security 1985)), 3 from rupture of the uterus, 69 following delivery by caesarean section, of which 44 were directly related to the operation, and 18 deaths directly related to obstetric anaesthesia.

Shock

The mechanisms which cause shock in obstetric situations are no different from those in other circumstances, although the initiating factors may be. The three main types of shock will be considered followed by the physiological response to shock, its severity then its management.

Hypovolaemic shock

This is shock due to a reduction in circulating blood volume. It is characterised by the individual showing signs of relative hypotension, a rapid but thready pulse, fast but shallow respirations, a pale clammy skin and either restlessness or torpor. This can occur in cases of internal and external haemorrhage. Hypovolaemic shock can also be accompanied by pain, for example in abruptio placentae, where blood has seeped into the uterine muscle (Pritchard and Brekken 1967), or in surgical shock where dehydration and bleeding both internal and external contribute with wound shock (from the pain of the incision) to the total picture. In the case of burns, the reduction in plasma volume and the raised haematocrit cause problems.

In pregnancy, vital signs such as pulse and blood pressure can be misleading. Relative hypertension is not uncommon in later pregnancy, resulting in normotension being taken, in some cases mistakenly, as a sign of adequate circulating blood volume (Cunningham et al. 1989). In addition, maternal pulse is a poor guide to the extent of the blood loss. It may rise with quite small losses and yet remain normal in conditions of hypovolaemia (Jansen 1978)

Cardiogenic shock

This is rarely seen in obstetrics. Heart failure produces a fall in cardiac output. Venous return is reduced and the lungs and other internal organs become congested with blood. This situation is most commonly seen following a myocardial infarction, which is rare, occurring in fewer than 1 in 10 000 pregnancies (de Swiet 1989).

Low resistance shock

In these cases, whilst the volume of blood circulating is normal, the capacity of the circulatory system is increased by vasodilation. Into this category fall bacteraemic shock, due to the presence of endotoxins (most commonly from gram-negative bacteria) (Myerscough 1982), and anaphylactic shock which occurs when the woman comes into contact with an antigen against which she has previously been sensitised (Myerscough 1982). In obstetrics this is a rare condition, which occurs most commonly following the administration of certain drugs such as anaesthetic agents and antibiotics. When challenged with the antigen again, there is a rapid release of histamine, which increases capillary permeability while dilating arteries and capillaries. Anaphylactic shock is treated by administering adrenaline, ephidrene and more rarely intravenous hydrocortisone (Myerscough 1982).

Physiological effects of shock

The sympathetic nervous system regulates blood flow by releasing adrenaline to cause peripheral vasoconstriction (Hibbard 1988). This occurs when pressure falls in the large arteries and veins whose walls contain pressure receptors (Herbert and Alison 1988). This measure reserves scarce blood supplies for vital body organs including the brain, heart and kidneys. Due to lack of blood flow in the periphery, the woman appears pale and feels cold and clammy. She may complain of a dry mouth. On no account should she be warmed up as this will divert blood from vital areas. Due to limited peripheral blood flow, heat is not adequately dispersed and burns can result from heat sources such as hot water bottles.

When circulating blood volume, cardiac output and venous return fall, certain mechanisms come onto action to preserve blood pressure (Herbert and Alison 1988). Constriction of the arterial system can initially maintain blood pressure but its capacity to do so is limited, resulting in an eventual fall in pressure (Cunningham et al. 1989). Because this fall is not immediate, blood pressure is an unreliable sign for detecting blood loss or reductions in circulating blood volume. In women with hypertensive disease of pregnancy, the situation is even more confused (Cunningham et al. 1989).

In order to maintain oxygenation, there is an increase in the pulse rate; this may become thready and weak. A reduction in blood flow through the carotid and aortic sinuses, together with a build-up of carbon dioxide (due to reduced cardiac output) stimulate an increase in the respiratory rate (Stocks 1988). Diminution of blood flow through the kidneys results in the release of aldosterone and antidiuretic hormone to conserve sodium and water (Goodinson 1988). In severe cases where systolic blood pressure falls below 80 mmHg, renal filtration ceases, resulting in anuria (Donald 1979). The longer this reduced blood flow continues, the less the ability of the kidneys to recover their functional capacities.

Severity of shock

Hardaway (1968) developed the following classification of the severity of shock:

1. Early reversible shock. Caused by small amounts of blood loss or minor injuries. Peripheral vasoconstriction occurs; the situation is easily reversed by blood transfusion.
2. Late reversible shock. This occurs after a more serious blood loss or injury and also where there has been a delay in treating more serious conditions. The person will experience marked hypotension. The situation can be reversed by infusion of blood volumes greater than the perceived blood loss. This should be of the correct ABO and rhesus group and it should be warmed. A central venous pressure line may be necessary to avoid overtransfusion.
3. Refractory shock. Hardaway (1968) defined this as shock complicated by infection, severe trauma, cardiac failure or delay in treatment. It may be associated with disseminated intravascular coagulation producing a clotting defect. Because tissue perfusion is poor, the replacement of circulating blood volume (with blood, plasma and plasma expanders) may be accompanied by the administration of vasodilators or beta adrenergic drugs (Hibbard 1988).
4. Irreversible shock occurs when all treatment has failed and death results. It is a rare event.

Management of shock

The principles of management are similar, whatever the cause of the shock. Medical assistance must be sought if not already present. A full assessment of the woman's condition is vital and then resuscitative measures should be taken. If the collapse occurs at home, the obstetric flying squad should be called.

If the mother is semiconscious or unconscious she should be placed in the recovery position and, if available, an airway inserted. Fluids should be replaced intravenously. If peripheral veins have collapsed, a 'cut down' may be required in order to insert an intravenous cannula. Cross-matched blood is an ideal replacement but plasma or plasma expanders can be used as an interim measure (Hibbard 1988). To avoid undertransfusion or overtransfusion, a central venous pressure line is advisable. By measuring pressure in the superior or inferior vena cava close to their entry into the heart, an indication of venous return can be obtained. Normal pressure is between 5 and 10 cms of water (Herbert and Alison 1988). Below this, there is a risk of hypovolaemia (Brantigen 1982). Care must be taken when obtaining readings to ensure that the mother is laying in a position where the zero point of the manometer is level with the right atrium. Movements of the water in the manometer occur with respirations.

In addition to restoring circulating blood volume, it is necessary to measure urinary output. The most accurate method is to insert a urinary catheter, which is left on free drainage connected to a urometer, allowing hourly measurement and testing of output. Anuria or oliguria with blood-stained urine indicate poor or absent renal blood flow. If shock is prolonged, blood flow is reduced in the anterior pituitary gland causing necrosis. This condition is called Sheehan's syndrome and is characterised by pituitary failure resulting in failure of lactation, amenorrhoea, premature ageing and an early death (Sheehan and Murdoch 1938).

Because emergencies occur swiftly and rapid deterioration can occur, the onset of shock is very distressing to relatives. Uncertainty over the outcome should not prevent the giving of information as and when it is available. The mother may remember little about the events, and needs to have them explained to her. Once she has recovered, the couple should be seen together to discuss any long-term effects and the prospects for future pregnancies.

Disseminated intravascular coagulation (DIC)

This is a disorder of coagulation in which the blood is slow to clot or fails to clot (Letsky 1985). It can be caused by a number of conditions in pregnancy, including abruptio placentae, retention of a dead fetus, amniotic fluid embolism and eclampsia (Hibbard 1988). Before describing the events which result in DIC, it is useful to consider the normal processes of coagulation (Macfarlane 1964):

1. Damage to the tissues or breakup of platelets releases thromboplastins.
2. In the presence of circulating calcium ions prothrombin is converted to thrombin.
3. Thrombin has the ability to convert fibrinogen into fibrin.
4. Fibrin forms itself into a scaffold of protein strands which entrap platelets and blood cells to form a clot.
5. When the clot is fully formed it exudes serum. This is plasma minus the clotting factors necessary to complete the clotting process.
6. When the tissue damage has been repaired or when clots occur in the absence of damage, the enzyme plasmin, formed from its precursor plasminogen, breaks down the clot. This produces fibrin degradation products (FDPs) which can be detected in the blood. FDPs themselves inhibit the clotting process (Letsky 1985).

The whole system is maintained in a state of dynamic equilibrium by clotting inhibitors and potentiators (antithrombin and antiplasmin) which are present in the general circulation (Bonnar 1975).

In disseminated intravascular coagulation, two events can occur; most commonly the available fibrinogen and clotting factors are exhausted due to the presence of one very large clot or numerous micro-clots in the general circulation (Letsky 1985). If tissue thromboplastins (which are present in high concentrations at the placental site and in amniotic fluid) enter the circulation, microthrombi will be formed using much of the available fibrinogen (Bonnar 1981).

In the second phase, which is not always present, activators of plasminogen (which are present in certain areas sensitive to clotting such as the lungs, placenta and uterus) may be produced to excess, resulting in the breakdown of any clot which is formed (Bonnar 1981). Plasminogen activator production is increased in times of stress or in the presence of shock.

Events relating to childbirth which can give rise to DIC are as follows:

1. Placental abruption. Thromboplastins from the placental site are released into the general circulation (Bonnar 1981). In addition, the clot behind the placenta will use up clotting factors (Redman 1979).
2. Intrauterine death. Dead fetal tissues can release thromboplastins which are absorbed into the maternal circulation. This happens 3 weeks or more after the fetal death (Pritchard 1959).
3. Eclampsia. Due to disruptions in the cascade system which maintains homeostasis of physiological functions, DIC can occur. Its exact aetiology is unclear (Letsky 1985).
4. Septicaemia. Endotoxins in the general circulation release thromboplastins when they damage blood vessels (Boulton and Letsky 1985).
5. Amniotic fluid embolism. Thromboplastins are present in large amounts in liquor (Bonnar 1981).

It is necessary for the midwife to be aware of conditions which can give rise to DIC. One of the principles of management in such cases is to exclude DIC before embarking upon procedures which could provoke bleeding (such as caesarean section). A screening test for coagulation must be performed. This includes measurement of:

Blood count and platelets.
Whole blood clotting time.
Plasma fibrinogen estimation.
Prothrombin time.
Thrombin time.
Estimation of fibrin degradation products (Letsky 1985).

Treatment is aimed at replacing fibrinogen and clotting factors. This can be achieved by using fresh (less than 24 hours old) whole blood, but more commonly involves platelets, plasma, plasma substitutes, such as haemaccel, but not dextran which interferes with platelet function (Letsky 1985) and clotting factors. The most recent report of Confidential Enquiries into Maternal Deaths (Department of Health 1989) recommended that each obstetric unit should have an agreed policy for managing cases of catastrophic haemorrhage.

Obstetric emergencies

This section considers maternal emergencies including hazards of obstetric anaesthesia, before considering prolapsed cord and shoulder dystocia, both of which can have adverse fetal outcomes.

Ruptured uterus

This is a rare but very serious complication which accounted for 3 deaths in England and Wales in 1982–1984 (Department of Health 1989). In addition, it gives rise to considerable maternal morbidity (Cunningham *et al.* 1989). Schrinsky and Benson (1978) found that the incidence of rupture amongst a number of hospitals in the United States varied from 1:100 to 1:11 000 deliveries. It rarely occurs in primiparous women, increasing in frequency with parity (Fuchs *et al.* 1985). This is possibly due to replacement of uterine muscle fibres with fibrous tissue each successive pregnancy. Rupture can occur before the onset of labour but it is more common as labour progresses. Cunningham *et al.* (1989) state that it is important to differentiate between rupture of a caesarean section scar (which occurs most commonly following a classical incision) and scar dehiscence, where the membranes are intact and the fetus remains within the uterine cavity.

Cause

1. Rupture of a uterine scar. This is most commonly a caesarean section scar with the classical (longitudinal) incision being most rupture-prone. In some cases rupture occurs in late pregnancy (especially with a classical scar), when Braxton Hick's contractions aid formation of the lower uterine segment (Myerscough 1982). Case *et al.* (1971) reported that over half the cases of scar dehiscence in their study were discovered during an elective repeat caesarean section, prior to or during very early labour.

    Other uterine scars which predispose to rupture include previous hysterotomy, excision of a uterine septum and previous uterine rupture (Pearce and Steel 1987). A woman with a scarred uterus should always be cared for in a consultant unit during future pregnancies.

2. Obstructed labour. Most commonly occurring in multiparous women where overthinning of the lower uterine segment occurs in order to overcome the obstruction. In primiparous women, uterine inertia is usually the result of obstruction (Myerscough 1982).

3. Hypertonic uterine action without or more commonly with the use of oxytocic drugs. The latter is more common when syntocinon is given to women of high parity who fail to progress (Awais and Lebherz 1970) or when it is administered with intact membranes.

4. Traumatic rupture. Following intrauterine manipulations including internal

podalic version, external cephalic version, breech extraction, difficult forceps delivery (high or rotational), destructive procedures and the after-coming head of a hydrocephalic breech presentation (Eden *et al.* 1986).

In the Developing World, most cases of uterine rupture occur as a result of neglected labour or poor obstetric practice (Skelly *et al.* 1976).

Diagnosis is far from simple although it is made easier by including maternal history. In some cases, a 'silent rupture' occurs, the only sign of which is fetal distress with variable decelerations of the fetal heart (Cunningham *et al.* 1989). At caesarean section, the baby may be found laying in the abdominal cavity. In other cases the rupture is not complete, with a bag of amniotic fluid protruding from the uterine rupture (Myerscough 1982). Usual signs of rupture include:

1. Maternal tachycardia usually over 100 bpm.
2. Sudden and severe abdominal pain with a sensation of 'giving way'.
3. Low abdominal pain with vomiting.
4. Sudden stopping of contractions.
5. Severe fetal distress of rapid onset. This includes variable decelerations or profound bradycardia.
6. Vaginal bleeding of variable quantity.
7. Maternal shock.
8. Fetal parts may be easily palpable abdominally. (Cunningham *et al.* 1989)

As midwives give most of the care to women in labour, they are the most likely people to detect these signs. Prompt recognition of an abnormal situation and the summoning of appropriate medical assistance is vital to the outcome for mother and baby. While the anaesthetist begins resuscitative procedures, preparations will be made to transfer the mother to theatre. Once there, a caesarean section or laparotomy will be performed. Where possible following delivery of the baby (which may be asphyxiated or stillborn), a uterine repair is effected. If the damage is too severe, it may be necessary to undertake a hysterectomy (Hibbard 1988). The woman will require diligent nursing in the immediate post-operative period, since there is a risk of further haemorrhage as the uterus contracts, with possible disruption of sutures. Both parents need clear explanations of what has happened and of the prospects for future pregnancies. These include hospitalisation in late pregnancy and delivery by early elective caesarean section (Hibbard 1988).

Inversion of the uterus

This is a rare emergency occurring in 1 : 20 000–25 000 deliveries (Myerscough 1982). However some American studies have given a much greater frequency of 1 : 2148 (Platt and Druzin 1981) to 1 : 2284 deliveries (Kitchin *et al.* 1975). It is a serious complication of the third stage of labour, in which part or all of the uterus is turned inside out and prolapsed down into the vagina. In cases of complete inversion, the whole uterus can lie outside the vulva (Myerscough 1982). The causes are usually related to mismanagement of the third stage of labour, although spontaneous inversion can occur in multiparous women with fundal insertion of the placenta (Watson *et al.* 1980) or with suddenly increased intraabdominal pressure from coughing or sneezing (Myerscough 1982). The most common causes are:

1. Using cord traction when the uterus is not contracted.
2. Using cord traction without guarding the uterus above the symphysis pubis.
3. Using fundal pressure to deliver the placenta when the uterus is relaxed.
4. Where the placenta is morbidly adherent (placenta accreta).

Where the inversion is severe, the mother quickly becomes profoundly shocked (Greenhill and Friedman 1974). This is accompanied by great lower abdominal pain caused by traction on the peritoneum and the ovaries (Hibbard 1988). If the placenta has been delivered there may be severe bleeding (Cunningham *et al.* 1989). The best opportunity for replacing the uterus is to do so as soon as the inversion occurs (Myerscough 1982). After summoning medical assistance, the midwife should use manual pressure on the part of the uterus nearest the cervix. It may be possible to reduce the inversion (Cunningham *et al.* 1989). The placenta should not be removed, since the uterus will not contract and severe bleeding may occur (Cunningham *et al.* 1989). To relieve shock, the foot of the bed may be raised (to reduce traction on the ovaries), an intravenous infusion commenced and an analgesic such as morphine administered (Myerscough 1982). Once the maternal condition has been stabilised, attempts will be made to replace the uterus using hydrostatic pressure (O'Sullivan's method) or if there is a constriction ring present, under general anaesthesia (Myerscough 1982).

For the hydrostatic method, a sterile douche can is positioned at the top of a drip stand. An intravenous giving set is connected. Several litres of warmed normotonic solution (usually saline) are emptied into the douche can. The end of the tubing is placed into the vagina and the vulva is sealed off with the operator's hands. The fluid is turned on and, as fluid pressure increases in the vagina, the uterus is pushed back to its normal situation (O'Sullivan 1945). The placenta (if *in situ*) can now be removed manually before an oxytocic drug is given to ensure contraction of the uterus (Cunningham *et al.* 1989). The mother should remain on bedrest for the first 24 hours. An indwelling catheter is helpful to avoid distension of the bladder. It is usual for the obstetrician to prescribe prophylactic antibiotics to prevent puerperal infection (Hibbard 1988).

Amniotic fluid embolism

This is a condition with a reported incidence between 1:3360 to 1:80 000 pregnancies (Duff and Kopelman 1987) in which amniotic fluid is forced into the maternal circulation, forming an embolism which blocks small blood vessels in the heart or lungs. In addition, particulate matter (such as skin squams) and prostaglandin produce pulmonary vasoconstriction and complement activation (Duff and Kopelman 1987). Thromboplastins in the fluid result in DIC (Bonnar 1981).

Diagnosis of amniotic fluid embolism is confirmed by detecting elements of the fluid in the maternal circulation, either via a CVP line or at post-mortem (Peterson and Taylor 1970). Confirmed cases of amniotic fluid embolism accounted for 14 deaths in England and Wales in the 1982–1984 report into maternal deaths (Department of Health 1989).

The exact mechanism of entry of the fluid into the maternal circulation is not always clear, but it has been linked to the following events:

1. Hypertonic uterine action which forces liquor through a weak point in the placenta or membranes.
2. Artificial or spontaneous rupture of membranes at the height of an enormous contraction.
3. The risks increase with parity.
4. Lacerations to the uterus, for example during manipulations.
5. At caesarean section. (Myerscough 1982; Cunningham *et al.* 1989)

The woman shows acute signs of collapse, including respiratory distress with cyanosis, dyspnoea and circulatory collapse, followed by cardiac arrest (Hibbard 1988). In these cases, the prognosis is poor, with 85% of women dying (25% of the deaths occur in the first hour) (Duff and Kopelman 1987) whilst fetal mortality approaches 40% (Duff 1984). In less acute cases the following signs may occur:

- Shock.
- Tachypnoea, dyspnoea and cyanosis.
- Maternal anxiety.
- Haemorrhage (due to DIC).
- Convulsions. (Pearce and Steel 1987)

Emergency action is vital if the mother is to stand any chance of survival. Medical assistance should be called immediately. Since the management is similar to that for other forms of collapse, treatment is commenced before the diagnosis is confirmed.

1. Ensure adequate respiration, if necessary using a ventilator. Initial support includes giving 100% oxygen via a face mask (Price *et al.* 1985).
2. Maintain the circulation. Suitable intravenous fluids, with necessary drugs to correct cardiac function, are given to correct shock. A CVP line may be used (Boulton and Letsky 1985).
3. A clotting screen will be performed. Fresh-frozen plasma may be required to correct defects (Hibbard 1988).
4. As soon as the mother's condition permits, the baby should be delivered. If the collapse occurs in the second stage of labour, an immediate forceps delivery may be attempted.

Clear explanations should be given to the woman's partner who will be shocked at the rapid progress of events. Although no information on prognosis can be given, the events which have occurred and procedures being implemented can be explained.

If the mother survives the hour following the collapse, her chances improve slightly. It is advisable that when her condition permits she is transferred to an Intensive Care Unit for expert assessment and observation.

Hazards of general anasthesia

The hazards we will consider are Mendelson's syndrome and failed intubation.

Pulmonary aspiration syndrome, also known as Mendelson's syndrome (Mendelson 1946) occurs due to the aspiration of acid stomach contents into the bronchial tree (Crawford 1972). The resulting chemical pneumonitis and oedema lead to destruction of the endotracheal lining and capillaries. The final stage is necrosis of pulmonary tissue. In severe cases, death can occur as it did to seven mothers in England and Wales reported in the 1982–1984 Confidential Enquiry (Department of Health 1989). Mendelson's syndrome is preventable by good midwifery, obstetric and anaesthetic practice (Crawford 1986). The woman in labour is prone to acid inhalation, due to the slowed gastric emptying time in women at term. This is further worsened by the giving of narcotic analgesia which severely delays gastric emptying (Nimmo *et al.* 1975).

Women at risk of requiring a general anaesthetic should receive only clear fluids during labour. Prior to anaesthesia, non-particulate antacids should be administered by the anaesthetist (Johnson *et al.* 1989). During induction of anaesthesia, a trained assistant should apply cricoid pressure to occlude the oesophagus and maintain this until the endotracheal tube is in place and the cuff inflated (Crawford 1978). The cuff prevents 'silent regurgitation' of stomach contents. After the anaesthetic, the woman should be turned on her side and not extubated until the cough reflex has returned (Cunningham *et al.* 1989). Suction should be on hand to remove any secretions.

If inhalation does occur, the woman must be intubated and ventilated with high doses of oxygen. Anti-inflammatory and steroidal drugs may be given where the pH of bronchial fluids is less than 3.5, although this has not always been shown to be beneficial (Bynum and Pierce 1976). Bronchial lavage is not advised, as this can worsen the situation (Pearce and Steel 1987). The woman should then be transferred to the Intensive Care Unit for respiratory support.

Failed intubation, a minor degree of laryngeal oedema, is common in the pregnant woman at term. This may impede the anaesthetist's vision of the vocal cords and prevent introduction of the endotracheal tube. If a systemic muscle relaxant has been given, the woman cannot be oxygenated without intubation. Pre-oxygenation for 5 minutes before inducing anaesthesia increases the time available to the anaesthetist for achieving intubation. It is vital that the anaesthetist maintains a clear airway and oxygenation during the anaesthetic. All operating theatres should have a clearly understood procedure which is followed in cases of failed intubation (Department of Health 1989). The Confidential Enquiry into Maternal Deaths 1982–1984 in England and Wales (Department of Health 1989) reported 10 deaths directly related to problems with endotracheal intubation.

Fetal emergencies

Presentation and prolapse of the umbilical cord

Cord presentation occurs when the umbilical cord lies in front of the presenting part while the membranes are intact. Once the membranes have ruptured, it is known as cord prolapse (Hibbard 1988). The cord can be palpated in the vagina and occasionally it may be visible at the vulva. The predisposing factors for both conditions are those in which the presenting part is poorly fitting in the pelvis. These include non-engagement of the head, prematurity and malpresentations. In both a footling and a complete breech presentation, the umbilical cord can easily slip down between the baby's legs (Cunningham et al. 1989). This can also occur in cases of an oblique or transverse lie, shoulder presentation or polyhydramnios (Hibbard 1988).

Cord presentation is diagnosed on vaginal examination. The membranes must be left intact and medical assistance summoned. As labour cannot progress without cord compression, an operative delivery is often performed (Hibbard 1988). To exclude the diagnosis of cord prolapse, it is routine to perform a vaginal examination when the membranes rupture spontaneously. This is especially important in the presence of any of the predisposing factors (Hibbard 1988).

When the cord is felt, the midwife must send someone for medical assistance. She should asertain whether or not the cord is still pulsating (and therefore whether the fetus is alive) (Hibbard 1988). The situation should be explained to the parents. The midwife should keep her examining hand in the vagina to prevent the presenting part from pressing on the cord. She should also assess the degree of cervical dilatation since, if in the second stage of labour, a multiparous woman could push the baby out quickly and a primipara could be delivered with forceps. Care should be taken to avoid excess handling of the cord, which could cause the vessels to go into spasm (Rhodes 1956). If the cord is outside the vagina, it should be gently replaced in order to keep it warm (Rhodes 1956). To assist in removing pressure from the cord, the woman may be placed in an exaggerated left lateral or knee-chest position (Hibbard 1988). The latter helps to move the presenting part out of the pelvis under the influence of gravity. When this condition occurs at home, the management is similar, with the midwife reducing pressure on the cord while an assistant summons the obstetric flying squad and the mother is transferred to hospital.

The aims of management are to deliver the fetus as quickly as possible before hypoxia and death result from cord compression. Relieving pressure on the cord is a temporary measure which provides extra time before delivery. Unless the cervix is fully dilated and the presenting part well descended in the pelvis, it is usual to perform a caesarean section. If the cord is not pulsating and the lie is longitudinal, preparations are made for the vaginal delivery of a stillbirth (see Chapter 31).

Shoulder dystocia

Shoulder dystocia is a serious emergency which occurs when, following the birth of the baby's head, there is difficulty delivering the shoulders. It occurs in 0.15–0.38% of deliveries (Kahn 1986; Gross *et al.* 1987). This complication carries with it a high risk of perinatal morbidity and mortality. The two major causes are an overlarge baby (usually weighing over 4.5 kg) (Swartz 1960) and failure of the shoulders to rotate into the antero-posterior of the outlet. The latter is sometimes caused by over eagerness by the midwife who attempts to deliver the shoulders before they have had time to rotate. The next contraction may occur more than 2 minutes after the one with which the baby's head was delivered.

The presence of a large baby should be recognised antenatally. In addition, the midwife during the delivery should be alerted to the possibility of shoulder dystocia where the head seems large and is difficult to deliver.

Shoulder dystocia is diagnosed when gentle pressure on the foetal head fails to reveal the anterior shoulder under the symphysis pubis. Rapid management is vital to safeguard the baby's well-being at this same time, without using excess force which can cause damage to the brachial plexus and skeletal injuries, including fractures of the humerus and clavicle (Benedetti and Gabbe 1978). Delay results in fetal/neonatal hypoxia or asphyxia (McCall 1962).

Principles of management

1. Summon medical assistance.
2. Check that the shoulders are in the antero-posterior diameter of the pelvis. If not, the midwife should aid rotation by placing two fingers into the anterior axilla and rotating the shoulder until it comes under the pubic arch (Hibbard 1988). When this is done, the shoulders can be delivered in the usual way. Gentle pressure on the anterior shoulder above the symphysis pubis applied by an assistant may be needed if the anterior shoulder is high (Resnik 1980).
3. Where the shoulders are correctly positioned in the pelvis, a change of maternal position to widen the pelvic outlet may aid delivery. This can be achieved by placing the mother in the left lateral position or preferably in lithotomy with her buttocks overhanging the end of the bed and the woman's thighs flexed upon her abdomen (McRobert's manoeuvre (Gonik *et al.* 1983)). Delivery can be attempted with an assistant applying suprapubic pressure. Fundal pressure should not be used, since this can cause uterine rupture (Gross *et al.* 1987).
4. If an episiotomy has not been performed, one can be made to further extend the outlet (Cunningham *et al.* 1989).

5. If it is not yet possible to deliver the anterior shoulder, it may be possible by gentle upward traction of the head aided by a finger in the posterior axilla to deliver the posterior shoulder (Cunningham *et al.* 1989).

6. If this fails, rotating the whole fetus through 180° will bring the posterior shoulder, anterior. The angle of inclination of the pelvis will bring it under the pubic symphysis by the same method used in the Lovset manoeuvre (Woods 1943).

7. Very rarely, the obstetrician has to break the clavicle to effect delivery. Symphysiotomy is rarely used in Western countries, but may be employed if all else has failed and the baby is still alive (Pearce and Steel 1987).

Once delivered, the baby should be carefully examined by the paediatrician for signs of skeletal or neuromuscular damage. Jaundice may result from severe bruising. The baby's neurological state should be observed for signs of hypoxic brain damage. The mother should be examined for the presence of lacerations to the cervix, vagina and perineum (Benedetti and Gabbe 1978). In addition to advice and support regarding this delivery, she will need information about subsequent pregnancies. It is possible that an elective caesarean section would be performed should the couple choose to have a further pregnancy for a fetus assessed as being of similar size.

References

Awais G M and Lebherz T B (1970) 'Ruptured uterus, a complication of oxytocic usage and high parity' *Obstetrics and Gynecology* 36: 465

Benedetti T J and Gabbe S G (1978) 'Shoulder dystocia. A complication of fetal macrosomia and prolonged second stage of labor with mid-pelvic delivery' *Obstetrics and Gynecology* 52: 526

Bonnar J (1975) 'The blood coagulation and fibrinolytic systems during pregnancy' *Clinics in Obstetrics and Gynaecology* 2: 321–44

Bonnar J (1981) 'Haemostasis and coagulation disorders in pregnancy' in A L Bloom and D P Thomas (eds) *Haemostasis and Thrombosis* 454–71 Churchill Livingstone: Edinburgh

Boulton F E and Letsky E (1985) 'Obstetric haemorrhage: Causes and management' *Clinics in Haematology* 14(3): 683–728

Brantigen C O (1982) 'Hemodynamic monitoring: Interpreting values' *American Journal of Nursing* 82: 86–9

Bynum L J and Pierce A K (1976) 'Pulmonary aspiration of gastric contents' *American Review of Respiratory Diseases* 114: 1129

Case D B, Corcoran R and Jeffcoate N (1971) 'Caesarean section and its place in modern obstetric practice' *Journal of Obstetrics and Gynaecology of the British Empire* 78: 203–14

Crawford J S (1972) 'Maternal mortality associated with anaesthesia' *Lancet* i: 72

Crawford J S (1978) *Principles and Practice of Obstetric Anaesthesia (4th edn)* Blackwell Scientific: Oxford

Crawford J S (1986) 'Maternal mortality from Mendelson's syndrome' *Lancet* i: 920–1

Cunningham F G, MacDonald P C and Gant N F (1989) *William's Obstetrics (18th edn)* Prentice Hall: London

Department of Health (1989) *Report on Confidential Enquiries into Maternal Deaths in England and Wales* 1982–4 HMSO: London

Department of Health and Social Security (1985) *Report on Confidential Enquiries into Maternal Deaths in England and Wales* 1979–81 HMSO: London

de Swiet M (1989) 'Cardiovascular problems in pregnancy' in A Turnbull and G Chamberlain (eds) *Obstetrics* Ch 37 543–56 Churchill Livingstone: Edinburgh

Donald I (1979) *Practical Obstetric Problems (5th edn)* Lloyd Luke: London

Duff P (1984) 'Defusing the dangers of amniotic fluid embolism' *Contemporary Obstetrics and Gynaecology* Aug: 127–49

Duff P and Kopelman J N (1987) 'Sudden post partum collapse' in J Studd (ed) *Progress in Obstetrics and Gynaecology Vol 6* 223–40 Churchill Livingstone: Edinburgh

Eden R D, Parker R T and Gall S A (1986) 'Rupture of the pregnant uterus: a 53 year review' *Obstetrics and Gynecology* 68: 671

Fuchs K, Peretz B-A, Marcovici R, Paldi E and Timor-Tritsh I (1985) 'The "grand multipara" – Is it a problem?' *International Journal of Obstetrics and Gynecology* 23: 321

Gonik B, Stringer C A and Held B (1983) 'An alternative maneuvre for management of shoulder dystocia' *American Journal of Obstetrics and Gynecology* 145: 882

Goodinson S M (1988) 'Renal function' in S M Hinchliff and S E Montague (eds) *Physiology for Nursing Practice* Ch 5.4 512–45 Balliere Tindall: London

Greenhill J P and Friedman E A (1974) *Biological Principles and Modern Management of Obstetrics* 687 Saunders: Philadelphia

Gross S J, Shime J and Farine D (1987) 'Shoulder dystocia: Predictors and outcome' *American Journal of Obstetrics and Gynecology* 156: 334–6

Hardaway J (1968) *Clinical Management of Shock* C C Thomas: Springfield, Illinois

Herbert R A and Alison J A (1988) 'Cardiovascular function' in S M Hinchliff and S E Montague (eds) *Physiology for Nursing Practice* Ch 4.2 315–91 Balliere Tindall: London

Hibbard B M (1988) *Principles of Obstetrics* Butterworth: London

Jansen R P S (1978) 'Relative bradycardia: A sign of acute intraperitoneal bleeding' *New Zealand Journal of Obstetrics and Gynaecology* 18: 206

Johnson C, Keirse M J N C, Enkin M and Chalmers I (1989) 'Nutrition and hydration in labour' in I Chalmers, M Enkin and M J N C Keirse (eds) *Effective Care in Pregnancy and Childbirth* Ch 52 827–32 Oxford Medical: Oxford

Kahn G Q (1986) 'Shoulder dystocia – an unexpected emergency' *Maternal and Child Health* 11(3): 79–83

Kitchin J D, Thiagarajah S, May H V and Thornton W N (1975) 'Puerperal inversion of the uterus' *American Journal of Obstetrics and Gynecology* 123: 51

Letsky E A (1985) *Coagulation Problems During Pregnancy* Churchill Livingstone: Edinburgh

Macfarlane R G (1964) 'An enzyme cascade in the blood clotting mechanism and its function as a biochemical amplifier' *Nature* 202: 494–9

McCall J O (1962) 'Shoulder dystocia. A study of after effects' *American Journal of Obstetrics and Gynecology* 83: 1486

Mendelson C L (1946) 'The aspiration of stomach contents into the lungs during obstetric anesthesia' *American Journal of Obstetrics and Gynecology* 52: 191–205

Myerscough P R (1982) *Munro Kerr's Operative Obstetrics (10th edn)* Balliere Tindall: London

Nimmo W S, Wilson J and Prescott L F (1975) 'Narcotic analgesics and delayed gastric emptying time during labour' *Lancet* i: 890–3

O'Sullivan J V (1945) 'Acute inversion of the uterus' *British Medical Journal* 2: 282–3

Pearce J M and Steel S A (1987) *A Manual of Labour Ward Practice* Wiley: Chichester

Peterson E P and Taylor H B (1970) 'Amniotic fluid embolism. An analysis of 40 cases' *Obstetrics and Gynecology* 35: 787–93

Platt L D and Druzin M L (1981) 'Acute puerperal inversion of the uterus' *American Journal of Obstetrics and Gynecology* 141: 187

Price T M, Baker V V and Cefalo R C (1985) 'Amniotic fluid embolism: Three case reports with a review of the literature' *Obstetrical and Gynecological Survey* 40: 462

Pritchard J A (1959) 'Fetal death in utero' *Obstetrics and Gynecology* 14: 573–80

Pritchard J A and Brekken A L (1967) 'Clinical and laboratory studies on severe abruptio placentae' *American Journal of Obstetrics and Gynecology* 97: 681

Redman C W G (1979) 'Coagulation problems in human pregnancy' *Postgraduate Medical Journal* 55: 367–71

Resnik R (1980) 'Management of shoulder girdle dystocia' *Clinics in Obstetrics and Gynaecology* 23: 559

Rhodes P (1956) 'Prolapse of the umbilical cord' *Proceedings of the Royal Society of Medicine* 39: 937–40

Schrinsky D C and Benson R C (1978) 'Rupture of the pregnant uterus: A review' *Obstetrical and Gynecological Survey* 33: 217

Sheehan H L and Murdoch R (1938) 'Postpartum necrosis of the anterior pituitary: pathological and clinical aspects' *Journal of Obstetrics and Gynaecology of the British Empire* 45: 456

Skelly H R, Duthie A M and Philpott R H (1976) 'Rupture of the uterus' *South African Medical Journal* 50: 505

Stocks J (1988) 'Respiration' in S M Hinchliff and S E Montague (eds) *Physiology for Nursing Practice* Ch 5.3 465–511 Balliere Tindall: London

Swartz D P (1960) 'Shoulder girdle dystocia in vertex delivery: clinical study and review' *Obstetrics and Gynecology* 15: 194

Watson B, Besch N and Bowes W E (1980) 'Management of acute and subacute puerperal invasion of the uterus' *Obstetrics and Gynecology* 55: 12–16

Woods C E (1943) 'A principle of physics is applicable to shoulder delivery' *American Journal of Obstetrics and Gynecology* 45: 796

28   Postnatal care

The puerperium

The puerperium is the period after childbirth, during which the mother recovers from labour, adapts to her new role and reverts physically to the non-pregnant state (Cunningham *et al.* 1989). The time of anticipation and waiting are over; the baby has arrived and the life of the mother, her partner and other family members has been changed by the presence of the new person (Murphy-Black 1989). Whilst the puerperium is considered to last 6–8 weeks, the midwives' rules (United Kingdom Central Council 1986) define the postnatal period as

> '...a period of not less than 10 and not more than twenty-eight days after the end of labour, during which the continued attendance of the midwife on a mother and baby is requisite.' (United Kingdom Central Council 1986, p. 6)

The midwife must be able to use her knowledge and discretion in deciding just how long (after the 10 day minimum) the mother and baby require her care (Murphy-Black 1989). The current flexibility, which allows the midwife to use her discretion in deciding when to visit the puerperal woman, is a significant change from the previous prescriptive ruling that the mother must be visited at least twice daily for the first 3 days and at least daily up until 10 days after birth (Central Midwives' Board for Scotland 1968).

The aims of a midwife's care during this time include the following:

1. Encouragement and development of the woman's new or changed role as mother.
2. Education and support for the mother in the care of her baby.
3. Guidance and support for the mother in the feeding of her baby.
4. Observation of the physiological and psychological changes which occur during the puerperium for deviations from normal.

Although the above aims refer almost totally to the mother and baby, the midwife should use her judgement in deciding the appropriateness (or otherwise) of including the father and other family members (Hanson and Bozett 1986). The role of the midwife should be one of support, education and the encouragement of self-care and independence by the mother (Rider 1985; Laryea 1989). Unfortunately, many midwives appear to be concentrating upon the physical aspects of care at the expense of the social and emotional support required by the mother (Ball 1987; Laryea 1989; Robinson 1989).

Postnatal care has been described as the Cinderella of the maternity services (Ball 1987; Royal College of Midwives 1987). The reason for this could be that Cinderella was the poor member of the family (little money), she had very little in the way of clothing (poor equipment), no-one wanted to know her (medical staff, central government) and so no one bothered with her (limited research), although this last area is now receiving attention. For many medical staff, the completion of the third stage of labour signals the end of their involvement (and possible interest). (It is right that the responsibility for supervising the normal mother and her baby should lie with the midwife. Medical staff have left this care to the midwife, unlike their inappropriate involvement in the care of women experiencing normal pregnancy and labour.) For the mother and her family, the hard work is only just beginning. Adjustments will need to be made and, especially for first-time parents, their lives will never be the same. Midwives have long recognised the disparity in the allocation of resources expended on the areas of maternity care. The Maternity Services Advisory Committee (1985) recommends that postnatal care be given equal status with the other parts of the maternity services. Fortunately, the postnatal period is becoming an area for midwifery research, with the findings being employed to improve the service provided for women (Murphy-Black 1989). A change has occurred in hospital care, from task allocation (Laryea 1984) to one where the mother and baby are viewed as a discrete unit, although this approach is not universal. This change has highlighted the social and psychological aspects of the puerperium, while reducing the emphasis on physical care (and associated pathology) which used to be apparent (Ball 1987). As Murphy-Black (1989) has reported, some midwives in the community still give more emphasis to the physical than to the educational or psycho-social needs of the mother.

As family size has reduced in the developed world, childbirth has become an increasingly rarer event. The informal networks of support for the new mother are less developed than in the past. In addition the mother is less likely to possess knowledge about childcare. The woman, due to the reduction in family size, may not have witnessed or assisted in the rearing of younger siblings (Simkin and Enkin 1989). For this reason, the midwife must assess those in her care and devise an individual plan for the education and support she will offer (Ball 1987). One cannot assume that all primiparous women know little of childcare, in the same way that some women with children may request teaching or prefer to be allowed to get on with things alone (Laryea 1984).

Reception on the postnatal ward

For the mother who gives birth in a maternity hospital (as opposed to at home, a GP unit or under team midwifery care), the greeting of the mother and her new baby by the midwife on the postnatal ward is a vital link in the personalisation and continuity of care. The midwife who has cared for the women during the birth passes the care of the mother and baby to the midwife on the postnatal ward. A full account of her labour, birth and the immediate postnatal period should be given. If a plan for midwifery care is already in place, this is useful in acting upon the mother's wishes, for example in the conduct of feeding, the need for instruction in childcare or the desired length of stay after birth (Murphy-Black 1989). The Maternity Services Advisory Committee (1985) advises that each mother should have a plan for the care of herself and her baby which has been drawn up in consultation with the woman, her GP and the community midwife.

The mother should be encouraged to talk about her labour if she so wishes. The first step in the forming of the relationship between mother and baby is, according to Mercer (1981), for the mother to review the events surrounding birth. She needs to reconcile the actual events with those which were expected (Konrad 1987). An example of a possible area of conflict for the mother is where she wished for no intervention during labour but, due to changed circumstances beyond her control, required an epidural anaesthetic and a forceps delivery. By listening to and counselling the mother, the midwife can help her to accept that she did her best and that she is not a failure. Reassurance alone is not enough.

A major part of the admission procedure will involve an examination of the mother's physical state. Due to the risk of postpartum haemorrhage, close observation is maintained on all mothers for the first 24 hours after birth (Cunningham et al. 1989). For this reason, the uterine fundus should be palpated to ensure that it remains well contracted and that there is not an excess of lochia. Where labour has been either very rapid or unduly prolonged, the uterus is more likely to become hypotonic after delivery of the placenta. Rubbing the uterine fundus firmly will expel clots and stimulate a contraction. The mother's pulse and blood pressure are assessed as a baseline for the postpartum period and to use as an indicator of the presence of haemorrhage. Temperature will be measured as a baseline in case infection occurs. Where a perineal repair has been performed, this should be observed for any swelling, as vulval haemotoma can occur after delivery (Hibbard 1988). The mother should also be asked whether or not she suffers from haemorrhoids, as these can be extremely painful and debilitating in the puerperium. Retention of urine can occur, especially if labour was prolonged or if forceps were employed (Kerr-Wilson *et al.* 1984); it is important to record when the mother passed urine after birth (Cunningham *et al.* 1989). Concern will be expressed if the woman has not passed urine within the first 12 hours after delivery (Hibbard 1988) (see later for an explanation of postpartum haemodilution).

Most maternity units prefer mothers to rest in bed after birth with the baby in a cot beside them, although there is no rationale for this period of rest, except in the case of the the woman with reduced sensations following epidural analgesia. If the mother has not had an opportunity to feed her baby and wishes to do so, this should be arranged. However long the mother remains in bed (commonly 6–8 hours although there is no rationale for this (Thomson 1990)), it is advisable that when she first gets up she is accompanied, in case she should feel faint. Some women are able to walk from the delivery bed, others are able to get up after 2–3 hours, but a few need a longer rest (more than 8 hours). Before the woman goes to sleep (if she wishes to do so), the midwife should make sure that the mother knows how to summon aid should she require it and that she has a jug of water and a glass in case of thirst. Where the birth occurred after a mealtime (especially if in the late evening or during the night), the woman should be offered something to eat; she may be unable to rest if hungry. It may be many hours (if not more than a day) since the woman last ate, especially if her labour was induced, with a long time period before labour became established. Other women may still feel nauseous as a result of narcotic analgesia.

Physiological changes in the puerperium

The uterus

After birth, the uterus weighs approximately 900–1000 g; by the end of the puerperium (6 weeks) it weighs 100 g, although it never returns to its size prior to the first pregnancy ($7.5 \times 5 \times 2.5$ cm) measuring on average $8 \times 6 \times 4$ cm (Cunningham *et al.* 1989). Immediately after delivery of the placenta, the fundus is firmly contracted and about 2 finger breadths (5 cm) below the level of the umbilicus. By 24 hours after birth when the uterus relaxes and the pelvic floor regains some of its tone, the fundus can usually be felt at the level of the umbilicus. The fundal height reduces by 1–2 cm/day until it is no longer palpable abdominally by 8–10 days after birth. By 1 week after birth, the uterus weighs approximately 500 g and by the end of the second week 375 g (Marshall and Moir 1952). This process is known as involution. Following completion of the third stage of labour, the uterine muscle is well contracted and there is a resulting degree of ischaemia (Hibbard 1988). The mechanism of reduction in uterine size is unclear, but it appears that a proteolytic enzyme is produced which results in autolysis (self-digestion) of the uterine muscle (Cunningham *et al.* 1989). The broken-down products may be reused (such as amino acids), excreted (as urea via the kidneys) or discharged from the uterus, together with the remains of the decidua, blood and serum from the uterine site and lanugo as lochia (Marshall and Moir 1952). If the process of involution is delayed (usually due to retained products of conception or infection), it is called subinvolution.

Lower abdominal pain from uterine contractions is common in the immediate postnatal period, being experienced twice as frequently by multiparous women than by the primiparous (Murray and Holdcroft 1989). Breast feeding exacerbated the pain in most of the sample of 100 women of Murray and Holdcroft (1989). Marshall and Moir (1952) explained the occurrence of more severe pain in multiparous women as an effect of their intermittent uterine contractions, as opposed to the almost continual contraction which occurs in the primiparae.

Lochia

Uterine vaginal loss after birth is called lochia. It is described according to its colour, which changes with the length of time since birth (Marshall and Moir 1952; Oppenheimer *et al.* 1986). Blood loss in the 12 hours immediately after birth accords in quantity with a heavy menstrual loss; the amount reduces thereafter. Lochia rubra is lost for the first 2–6 days (Oppenheimer *et al.* 1986). It is red from to the presence of a large number of red blood cells (Marshall and Moir 1952). Fresh blood loss is commonly seen after a breast feed, although the total quantity of lochia is less amongst breast-feeding mothers (Adams and Flowers 1960). The release of oxytocin on suckling causes uterine contractions and a temporary increase in the amount of lochia (Marshall and Moir 1952).

Lochia serosa is pale pink or brown; it contains some cells and serum (Marshall and Moir 1952). It persists after lochia rubra, on average until 28 days after birth (Oppenheimer *et al.* 1986). Lochia alba, which is white or cream in colour, may persist until 4–8 weeks after birth before it is replaced by normal non-pregnant vaginal and cervical secretions (Marshall and Moir 1952).

The cervix

The cervix is open after a vaginal birth but within 1–3 days the internal os is closed (Marshall and Moir 1952; Cunningham *et al.* 1989). The shape of the cervical os is changed after a first and subsequent birth to become a slit rather than a round hole; this change is caused by small lacerations which occur in the external os during birth (Marshall and Moir 1952).

The vagina

The vagina, having been stretched during delivery does not completely regain its nulliparous tone. If tears have occurred to the vaginal walls, these heal with the creation of non-elastic fibrous tissue. There is a tendency amongst some parous women for their introitus to gape slightly (Marshall and Moir 1952).

The pelvic floor

The pelvic floor regains its strength, especially if the woman has exercised prior to pregnancy (Gordon and Logue 1985). Each successive delivery leaves the pelvic floor progressively weakened, resulting in a shortening of the second stage of labour. Pelvic floor muscle tone is related to the level of general exercise undertaken by the woman (Gordon and Logue 1985) rather than to the type of delivery, damage to the pelvic floor or pelvic floor exercises after birth (Sleep and Grant 1987). Swimming, walking and other exercise are the best method of avoiding prolapse of the uterus in later life.

The pelvis

With the reduction in oestrogen level after delivery, the ligaments and joints in the pelvis become fixed. This is a gradual process which can take up to 3 months; backache may persist until the pelvis is fully stable (Hibbard 1988).

The bladder

During labour, the bladder becomes an abdominal organ, producing stretching of the urethra and possible bruising to the bladder neck as it is compressed between the rear of the symphysis pubis and the presenting part of the fetus (usually the head). If this pressure is severe, as in obstructed labour, necrosis can occur and fistulae may result (Swash 1988) although this is rare in the developed world. Retention of urine during labour can cause overdistension and atony of the detrusor muscle of the trigone, causing postnatal urinary retention with overflow (Hibbard 1988). Due to fear (of pain or of damaging the sutures), many women experience some difficulty passing urine after delivery. This is known as reflex inhibition and can be helped by taking the mother to the toilet (rather than giving her a bedpan), running taps or using the spray from the bidet on the vulva to encourage micturition (Hibbard 1988).

The bowels

With the discontinuation of the routine use of bowel preparations in early labour and the policy of early ambulation, postnatal constipation is less of a problem than previously. Fear of damaging perineal sutures or of painful haemorrhoids can exacerbate the situation (Cunningham *et al.* 1989). Where narcotic analgesia has been administered, dehydration has occurred or there is insufficient fibre in the diet, problems can occur (Hibbard 1988). Increasing fibre intake is difficult in hospital, but much easier at home. If she has not managed to open her bowels within 3 days of the birth, and depending on her usual non-pregnant bowel action, an oral vegetable laxative may be given. In certain circumstances glycerine suppositories may be advised (Hibbard 1988).

The breasts

Following birth, there is an increase in blood supply to the breasts which peaks on day 3 or 4 (Waller 1946). Unfortunately this coincides with the onset of milk production causing both venous and milk engorgement (Applebaum 1970) (see Chapter 34).

The extra blood volume

The extra blood volume and to a lesser extent intracellular fluid volume which were required to supply the uterus, placenta and increased demands upon the kidneys are no longer needed. Marked diuresis usually occurs within 24–48 hours of birth (Marshall and Moir 1952), resulting in an increase in blood constituents such as red and white cells, platelets and clotting factors (Letsky 1985). This helps to prevent haemorrhage from the placental site, but also unfortunately increases the risk of occurrence of thromboembolic conditions (Letsky 1985).

Psychological changes in the puerperium

Psychological changes after birth are many and varied (Sneddon 1987). It can be difficult for a midwife who has not known the woman prior to the pregnancy or birth to assess the psychological state accurately (Cox 1986). Ball (1987) showed that a woman was more likely to have problems with her emotional well-being if she had recently experienced major life events (in addition to childbirth) such as the death of a close relative or moving house. Additional factors increasing the risk were where there was marital conflict, where the mother suffered from lack of sleep, where she perceived that the advice she received was conflicting and amongst those mothers with little support at home (Ball 1987).

Amongst the factors which contribute to psychological change are the following:

1. Responsibility for caring totally for another human being (Laryea 1989). The baby may not conform to the common picture of happiness and contentment but will cry, may be difficult to feed and does not respond to his/her mother (Raphael-Leff 1989).

2. Following completion of the third stage of labour there is a rapid alteration in maternal hormone levels (especially of progesterone) (Cunningham *et al*. 1989).
3. In hospital, the woman is in an alien environment without the constant presence of family or friends (Ball 1987).
4. Labour may not have been in accordance with the mother's labour plans or expectations; the experience may have been frightening or disappointing (Konrad 1987).
5. The woman may well be experiencing physical discomfort from a sore perineum, enlarged haemorrhoids, abdominal wound or engorged breasts.
6. Especially with the first baby, many mothers suffer from a lack of confidence in their abilities for baby care or feeding (Ball 1987). This may be the first time that she has handled a newborn baby (Murphy-Black 1989). Midwives care for babies with such ease and assurance (from years of practice) that mother may feel dispirited or inadequate.
7. The woman may have other worries, such as concerns about housing, money or having to stop work which are realised now that the baby has arrived (Martin *et al*. 1989).

Midwifery care of the postnatal woman

Continuity of postnatal care from one or two midwives at home or in hospital is the ideal to make repetitive or conflicting advice less likely (Ball 1987; Murphy-Black 1989). The mother and midwife can come to know and trust each other, this is easier if they have met antenatally (Murphy-Black 1989; Flint 1990).

Physical and psychological problems are easier to detect where the same midwife gives care. The postnatal woman will normally be seen at home twice daily for the first 3 days and then daily for 10 days or more in accordance with the previous midwive's rules (Central Midwives' Board for Scotland 1968) which were superseded in 1983 permitting more scope to visit according to need (United Kingdom Central Council 1986). Where the mother and baby are managing well some later visits can be omitted, but the midwife should visit at least on alternate days. Ideally, both mother and baby should be cared for together, which allows the midwife to discuss the baby's progress with the mother and to gain an insight into the mother's adaptation to her new role, her level of confidence and her ability to cope (Laryea 1984). Whilst it is easier to assess the woman's physical than her psychological status, by talking to the mother before and during her examination, clues to any problems in adaptation to her new role can be identified. In one study, it was found that mothers rated the need for assessment of their adjustment to their new role much more highly than did the nurses caring for them (Morales-Mann 1989).

Examination of the postnatal woman

During the examination, it is easier for the midwife to use a systematic approach so nothing is forgotten:

1. Generalised information about the woman's state of health, well-being of the baby and any specific problems can be obtained in an informal manner before beginning the examination. Tiredness or signs of crying are easily seen while enquiries about the previous day's progress can elicit useful clues to the type of advice, teaching or support required. It is also helpful to enquire as to the woman's quality of sleep, since this is more important than the quantity (Bourne 1982).

2. The main method of assessing maternal well-being is still by undertaking a physical examination. This traditionally includes assessment and recording of the maternal pulse and temperature. Murphy-Black (1989) considers the rationale for this as a routine procedure for women who have experienced a normal labour and birth as unclear, although if the temperature and pulse are elevated, this can be an early indication of puerperal infection. If the mother is ill, there are other signs which should alert the midwife who can carry out a full examination. Where the woman is unwell or has an obvious sign of infection appropriate medical staff should be informed as soon as possible. The midwife is able to facilitate proceedings by, for example, obtaining from the mother a midstream sample of urine or taking a high vaginal swab where appropriate.

3. The breasts are examined to assess the onset of lactation or engorgement and to detect the presence of infection. Depending on the method of feeding chosen, the examination of the breasts will differ slightly. For the mother who is not breast feeding, it is important that the breasts are adequately and comfortably supported. Where venous engorgement occurs, oral analgesia such as paracetamol can be taken (Hibbard 1988). Engorgement resolves itself within 48–72 hours without treatment. Hormones and diuretics are no longer recommended for the suppression of lactation, as they are of limited effectiveness and can in some cases have serious side effects (Parazzini et al. 1989).

   The breast-feeding mother should be taught to examine her own breasts for blocked ducts which, if untreated, can lead to mastitis or abscess formation (Devereux 1970). Care should be taken that the nursing bra supporting the breasts does not cause undue pressure. The mother should be asked whether her nipples are sore; they should be examined for bruising, cracks or blisters. If any of these are present, the midwife must observe the mother's feeding method, especially her technique of fixing the baby to the breast (Woolridge 1986). Tactful advice should be given if there are faults in the technique. Cracks in the nipples are best treated by being kept dry and the mother continuing to feed with help being given in fixing the baby to the breast (Inch and Renfrew 1989) (see Chapter 34).

4. To assess involution, the woman's uterine fundus should be palpated. If the fundus is high or deviated to one side, the midwife must ascertain that the bladder is empty and whether the woman had her bowels open, before investigating further (Cunningham et al. 1989).

5. To assess healing of the placental site and to detect any infection which may be present, the colour and quantity of the lochia should be observed and the mother asked about the passing of any clots. Where the lochia remains red after 6 days or is offensive, medical staff should be informed (Cunningham *et al.* 1989). It is important to instruct mothers in the necessity of good perineal and vulval hygiene. Sanitary pads should be changed frequently. Where the woman does not have access to a bidet or hand-held shower, twice daily washing is advised. If available, the bidet or shower attachment should be used after each visit to the toilet.

6. To confirm healing of the perineum where the mother has perineal sutures, the perineum should be examined for signs of healing, haematoma formation, bruising or wound breakdown. Whilst good hygiene is needed for healing, it has been shown that the the addition of salt or an antiseptic to the bath water does not speed healing or reduce discomfort (Sleep and Grant 1988a). Oral analgesia such as paracetamol may be taken and some women find relief from the use of ice packs, although this has not been evaluated (Sleep and Grant 1988b). Other non-evaluated techniques for the relief of perineal pain include ultrasound and topical use of steroids (Sleep and Grant 1988b).

7. Because of the concentration of clotting factors in the blood following birth the postnatal woman is at risk of developing a deep vein thrombosis (Letsky 1985). She should be asked whether she has any pain in her legs, which are then examined for the presence of swelling (Hibbard 1988). Any deviation from normal should be reported to the woman's doctor (see Chapter 29).

8. Since excretion and micturition may take a little time to return to normal after the birth, the midwife should enquire whether the woman has had her bowels open. If not, advice about diet and fluid intake should be given before a laxative or suppositories are suggested. Any pain on micturition, loin pain or unusual odour of the urine should be investigated, as urinary tract infections can occur, especially where the woman has required catherisation during labour (Harris *et al.* 1977).

9. Where the mother was delivered by caesarean section, the state of wound healing must be assessed. Sutures should be removed on the specified day and with earlier transfer from hospital this may be when she is in the care of the community midwife.

10. The care of the baby is described in Chapter 33.

Following examination of the mother, a record of the findings, any problems, their suggested improvements and any deviations from normal be made. In this way, where there is a change in care giver, the new midwife is aware of existing problems, advice and support (Ball 1987). The decision as to how much baby care a woman needs to be taught and when is the best time to teach it is an individual one (Laryea 1984). Inquiring how much the mother already knows will prevent repetition, although it is a good idea to give non-breast-feeding mothers a refresher course in the preparation of feeds, as errors are more common with increasing parity (Jones and Belsey 1978).

The mother should be encouraged to stay in hospital for as long as she feels is necessary (Ball 1987). This may be from 2–4 hours after birth until 10 days. The average length of stay after birth in England in 1985 was 4.1 days (Her Majesty's Stationery Office 1988). Where the maternal or neonatal condition makes a stay longer than she would wish advisable, this should be discussed with her. Ball (1987) deprecates the fact that many mothers go home on the third day, just when they are at their lowest physical and mental state. If those mothers who so wished were encouraged to return home before this time, some potential problems could be lessened (Ball 1987). Discussing the desired length of stay prior to delivery is helpful, especially if done with the community midwife in the woman's own home, where support networks can be assessed (Sadler 1989). The woman should be informed that this is not a binding decision and it will depend on her health and that of her baby. She may need to stay longer or feel confident and wish to go home earlier than planned. It is necessary to point out that being 'fit to go home' does not mean that the woman is fit to resume all her duties and responsibilities, especially where there are other young children (Ball 1987). The lack of social support for many (often poorer) women in the early days after birth, especially where early transfer home becomes the norm on grounds of health economics, has been highlighted as an increasing problem (Thomson 1990).

In many areas, where the woman has had a normal birth and an uneventful early postpartum period, transfer home is arranged by the midwives without the need to call a doctor (Lewis 1987). The responsibility for care is transferred from the hospital midwife to the community midwife. Clear records and detailed plans of care can aid a smooth hand over. Close liaison between hospital and community allows for a less stereotyped form of care (Lewis 1987). The involvement of medical staff in the decision that a normal woman can go home is seen by Robinson (1989) as another example of duplication of care. This would be even greater waste of resources, since it is usually the midwife who guides the junior doctor in the decision-making (Rider 1985).

Early transfer home from hospital after the birth is not associated with poor outcomes for mother or baby (Norr and Nacion 1987). In a study of 9 schemes of early transfer home, Norr and Nacion (1987) noted an increase in re-admission of the baby, most frequently for the treatment of jaundice. Despite generally favourable outcomes, they believe care should be taken before routinely extending this policy to women from socially disadvantaged groups.

Ball (1987) remarks that it is unfortunate that many postnatal wards seem to run for the benefit of the midwifery, medical or ancillary staff rather than for the mothers and babies. There has been some relaxation in ward routine to encourage mothers who have had a disturbed night to get some sleep during the day and to make meal times more flexible. There is no need for all examinations of mothers and babies to be performed in the morning; indeed, with some current staffing levels, if this is attempted, the overall standard of care may suffer. Mothers should be encouraged to draw the curtains around their bed if they wish for more privacy. Where there are open hours for visiting, it is important to restrict the numbers present at any one time to avoid disturbing the other women (Fardell 1982). This is not usually possible where visiting times are limited, although the woman can have some quiet between times.

Fourth day blues

This is a very common type of emotional upset on the third or fourth day following birth and passes after a day or two (Sneddon 1987). The mother may have sudden unprovoked episodes of crying and find it hard coping with the baby (Levy 1986). Laryea (1984) suggests that the woman may be grieving over her lost freedom. Possible causes for this transient depression and sadness are changes in hormonal status, loss of euphoria after birth and physical discomfort from engorged breasts or a tender perineum. The midwife can give support by listening to the mother and trying to minimise physical symptoms. Increasing maternal confidence is helpful, as the blues are more common amongst first-time mothers (Priest 1979). Early transfer home after birth can help prevent feelings of isolation and loneliness, helping the woman relax in her home environment (Ball 1987). McIntosh (1986) postulates that, with a more sympathetic environment for birth and the early postpartum period and good antenatal preparation for baby care, the severity of this condition can be reduced. As this condition is self-limiting, relatives who are often distressed by it can be assured of a quick resolution. (For a more detailed description of psychological disturbances in the puerperium see Chapter 29.)

Bonding

The subject of maternal–infant attachment (known as bonding) has attracted much interest in recent years. Initial work was by Bowlby (1969), who highlighted the importance of a loving relationship between mother and child. Whilst the importance of affection and trust between children and adults has not been denied, what has been questioned is the speed with which this relationship is formed. Macfarlane (1977) comments that the process of childbirth in the past was far from risk-free, resulting on occasion in the death of the mother and/or the baby. Of necessity the mother must be able to grieve and recover from her loss before having further children whilst the orphaned baby needed to form relationships with other care givers (Macfarlane 1977). On this last point Prince and Adams (1987) emphasise that infants and children can become attached to more than one person, for example a sibling and a grandparent. Within extended families, there is much greater opportunity for such relationships to develop than there is in some of today's more isolated nuclear families.

Before discussing attachment-formation after birth, it is important to consider bonding which occurs in utero. Reading and Cox (1982) have demonstrated that a mother shown her fetus during diagnostic ultrasound had less anxiety and a more positive attitude to the pregnancy. They postulate that such effects might be utilised to increase acceptance of advice on diet or smoking, for example (Reading and Cox

1982). One must consider that if a spontaneous abortion should occur, would having seen the baby aid the grieving process?

The importance of the first hour after birth, when the newborn baby is awake and alert, has been examined extensively by Klaus and Kennell (1976) in their work with South American mothers. They have concluded that skin-to-skin contact between mother and baby at this time produces long-term differences in maternal-infant behaviour. Such conclusions have been criticised by Barrie (1986), who wonders how long it takes the 'glue' (the bond between mother and baby) to set. In addition he says that it is amazing that

> '... no practising obstetrician or midwife has become accidentally bonded to a baby whose naked skin he or she has held or into whose limpid eyes he or she has gazed at the crucial time.' (Barrie 1986, p. 335)

One could point out that since midwives and obstetricians are not caring for their own eagerly and long-anticipated baby, they are hardly likely to develop an attachment.

A useful effect of the debate about delivery room, postnatal ward and special care unit procedures has been a relaxation in routines and regimes. de Chateau (1986) cautions that care must be taken not to replace one inflexible dogma with another, that individual needs should be met within a flexible framework. Rooming in of infants with their mother is commonplace, visiting by parents to the special care baby unit is unrestricted, and where the mother is unable to visit, photographs and even videolinks have been provided to help her to keep in touch.

Admission of the newborn baby to a special care baby unit has been cited as a possible factor in the cause of child abuse. Such babies may, however, be more difficult to raise due to feeding problems and other health disorders. Cause and effect is not so easily demonstrated (Slukin et al. 1983). The fact that adoptive parents become properly attached to their baby suggests that the early hours and sustained contact may not always be necessary (Barrie 1986). There is certainly a place for further research in the area, although anything which increases parental comfort and confidence is to be welcomed.

The 6 week postnatal examination

Following the discharge of the woman from midwifery supervision, the next time she encounters a health professional on her own account will be at the time of the 6 week postnatal examination. For many women this signals that she should be physically recovered and is ready to resume her full role in society (Bowers 1984). Unfortunately this is not always the case. Tulman and Fawcett (1988) surveyed 70 women on their return to normal after birth. By the end of the sixth week after birth, 72% of women following normal births but only 34% after caesarean births had regained their physical energy (Tulman and Fawcett 1988). Field et al. (1983)

showed that 50% of women in their survey took more than 3 months to regain their physical health after birth.

The postnatal examination is usually carried out by the general practitioner or at the local hospital. The latter is helpful for women who have had complications in their pregnancy, labour or birth to be advised of future risks and to assess any residual deficits. Although Bowers (1984) showed that the majority of women visited their GP for the examination, they were not always convinced of its worth. Traditionally the visit concentrated on physical recovery and involved the following:

1. Maternal weight.
2. Urinalysis.
3. Blood pressure.
4. Bimanual examination to confirm size and position of the uterus.
5. Cervical smear.
6. Contraceptive advice (Morrell 1985).

The women in Bowers' (1984) study were more likely to wish to discuss infant feeding, tiredness or sexual difficulties than to be concerned with physical symptoms. A number were still experiencing vaginal discharge, backache and painful haemorrhoids. Bowers (1984) suggests that seeing mother and baby together, having more woman doctors or midwives carrying out the examination and giving mothers more opportunity to discuss their concerns may improve efficiency, uptake and satisfaction with this consultation.

References

Adams H and Flowers C E (1960) 'Oral oxytocic drugs in the puerperium' *Obstetrics and Gynecology* 15: 280

Applebaum R M (1970) 'The modern management of successful breast feeding' *Paediatric Clinics of North America* 17(1): 203–25

Ball J A (1987) *Reactions to Motherhood* Cambridge University Press: Cambridge

Barrie C (1986) 'The epoxy plague' *Maternal and Child Health* 11(10): 334–6

Bourne M A (1982) 'Sleep in the puerperium' *Midwives Chronicle* Mar: 91

Bowers J (1984) 'The six week postnatal examination' *Research and the Midwife Proceedings* 28–50 University of Manchester: London

Bowlby J (1969) *Attachment and Loss Vol 1* Hogarth Press: London

Central Midwives' Board for Scotland (1968) *Rules* Scottish Academic Press: Edinburgh

Cox J L (1986) *Postnatal Depression* Churchill Livingstone: Edinburgh

Cunningham F G, MacDonald P C and Gant N F (1989) *William's Obstetrics (18th edn)* Prentice Hall: London

de Chateau P (1986) 'Bonding: What is new?' *Maternal and Child Health* 11(10): 331–2

Devereux D P (1970) 'Acute puerperal mastitis' *American Journal of Obstetrics and Gynecology* 108: 78

Fardell J (1982) 'Longer visiting hours' *Midwives Chronicle* Nov: 399–401

Field S, Draper J, Kerr M and Hare M J (1983) 'Women's illness in the postnatal period' *Maternal and Child Health* 8(7): 302–4

Flint C (1990) 'The know your midwife scheme' in S Robinson and A M Thomson (eds) *Midwives, Research and Childbirth Vol 2* Chapman and Hall: London

Gordon H and Logue M (1985) 'Perineal muscle function after childbirth' *Lancet* ii: 12–5

Hanson S M H and Bozett F W (1986) 'The changing nature of fatherhood: the nurse and social policy' *Journal of Advanced Nursing* 11: 719–27

Harris R E, Thomas V L and Hui G W (1977) 'Postpartum surveillance for urinary tract infections: Patients at risk of developing pyelonephritis after catheterisation' *Southern Medical Journal* 70: 1273

Her Majesty's Stationery Office (1988) *Hospital In-patient Enquiry: Maternity Tables 1982–5* HMSO: London

Hibbard B M (1988) *Principles of Obstetrics* Butterworth: London

Inch S and Renfrew M J (1989) 'Common breastfeeding problems' in I Chalmers, M Enkin and M J N C Keirse (eds) *Effective Care in Pregnancy and Childbirth* 1375–89 Oxford Medical: Oxford

Jones R A K and Belsey E M (1978) 'Common mistakes in infant feeding: a survey from a London borough' *British Medical Journal* 2: 112–5

Kerr-Wilson R J H, Thompson S W, Orr J W, Davis R O and Cloud G A (1984) 'Effect of labour on the postpartum bladder' *Obstetrics and Gynecology* 64: 115

Klaus M H and Kennell (1976) *Maternal Infant Bonding* Mosby: St Louis

Konrad C J (1987) 'Helping mothers to integrate the birth experience' *Maternal Child Nursing* 12: 268–9

Laryea M G G (1984) *Postnatal care. The Midwives' Role* Churchill Livingstone: Edinburgh

Laryea M G G (1989) 'Midwives' and mothers' perceptions of motherhood' in S Robinson and A Thomson (eds) *Midwives, Research and Childbirth Vol 1* 176–88 Chapman and Hall: London

Letsky E A (1985) *Coagulation Problems During Pregnancy* Churchill Livingstone: Edinburgh

Levy V (1986) 'Third day blues' *Research and The Midwife 1985, Proceedings* 31–45 University of Manchester

Lewis P (1987) 'The discharge of mothers by midwives' *Midwives Chronicle* Jan: 16–8

Macfarlane A (1977) *Psychology of Childbirth* Fontana: London

Marshall F H A and Moir J C (1952) 'Parturition' in A S Parkes (ed) *Marshall's Physiology of Reproduction* 496–524 Longmans, Green and Co: London

Martin C J, Brown G W, Goldberg D P and Brockington I F (1989) 'Psycho-social stress and puerperal depression' *Journal of Effective Disorders* 16: 283–93

Maternity Services Advisory Committee (1985) *Maternity Care in Action. Part III: Care of the mother and baby* HMSO: London

McIntosh J (1986) 'Postnatal blues: a bio-social phenomenon?' *Midwifery* 2(4): 187–92

Mercer R T (1981) 'The nurse and maternal tasks of the early postpartum' *Maternal Child Nursing* 6: 341–5

Morales-Mann E T (1989) 'Activities in a postpartum unit' *Nursing Times* 85(40): 50

Morrell D C (1985) 'The final postnatal examination' in G N Marsh (ed) *Modern Obstetrics in General Practice* 364–70 Oxford Medical: Oxford

Murphy-Black T (1989) *Postnatal Care at Home: A descriptive study of mothers' needs and the maternity services* Department of Nursing Studies: University of Edinburgh

Murray A and Holdcroft A (1989) 'Incidence and intensity of postpartum lower abdominal pain' *British Medical Journal* 298: 1619

Norr K F and Nacion K (1987) 'Outcomes of postpartum early discharge 1960–86' *Birth* 14(3): 135–41

Oppenheimer L W, Sherriff E A, Goodman J D S, Shah D and James C E (1986) 'The duration of lochia' *British Journal of Obstetrics and Gynaecology* 93: 754–7

Parazzini F, Zanaboni F, Liberati A and Tognoni G (1989) 'Relief of breast symptoms in women who are not breastfeeding' in I Chalmers, M Enkin and M J N C Keirse (eds) *Effective Care in Pregnancy and Childbirth* 1390–1402 Oxford Medical: Oxford

Priest R (1979) 'Puerperal depression and its treatment' *Maternal and Child Health* 4(8): 312–7

Prince J and Adams M E (1987) *The Psychology of Childbirth (2nd edn)* Churchill Livingstone: Edinburgh

Raphael-Leff J (1989) 'Your mother should know' *Midwife, Health Visitor and Community Nurse* 25(9): 372–6

Reading A E and Cox D N (1982) 'The effect of ultrasound examination on maternal anxiety levels' *Journal of Behavioral Medicine* 5: 237–47

Rider A C E (1985) 'Midwifery after birth' *Nursing Times* 81(7 Aug): 27–8

Robinson S (1989) 'The role of the midwife: opportunities and constraints' in I Chalmers, M Enkin and M J N C Keirse (eds) *Effective Care in Pregnancy and Childbirth* 162–80 Oxford Medical: Oxford

Royal College of Midwives (1987) *Towards a Healthy Nation* R C M: London

Sadler C (1989) 'Unconditional discharge' *Nursing Times* 85(7): 18

Simkin P and Enkin M (1989) 'Antenatal classes' in I Chalmers, M Enkin and M J N C Keirse (eds) *Effective Care in Pregnancy and Childbirth* 318–34 Oxford Medical: Oxford

Sleep J and Grant A (1987) 'Pelvic floor exercises in postnatal care' *Midwifery* 3(4): 158–64

Sleep J and Grant A (1988a) 'Routine addition of salt or savlon bath concentrate during bathing in the immediate post partum period – A randomised controlled trial' *Nursing Times* 84 (21): 55–7

Sleep J and Grant A (1988b) 'Relief of perineal pain following childbirth: A survey of midwifery practice' *Midwifery* 4(3): 118–22

Slukin W, Herbert M and Slukin A (1983) *Maternal Bonding* Blackwell: Oxford

Sneddon J (1987) 'Postnatal illness' *Midwives Chronicle* Nov: 342–7

Swash M (1988) *Midwifery* 4(1): 13–8

Thomson A M (1990) 'Choices in childbirth' *Midwifery* 6: 1–2

Tulman L and Fawcett J (1988) 'Recovery from childbirth' *Nursing Times* 84(39): 62

United Kingdom Central Council (1986) *Midwives Rules* UKCC: London

Waller H (1946) 'Early failure of breastfeeding' *Archives of Disease in Childhood* 21: 1–12

Woolridge M W (1986) 'Aetiology of sore nipples' *Midwifery* 2: 172–6

29 Complications of the puerperium

This chapter will consider some of the more serious complications which can occur in the puerperium. Psychological disorders will be discussed, then physical problems, including infection, urinary disturbances and thromboembolic conditions.

Psychological disturbances in the puerperium

More than 60% of women will experience some alteration of mood following delivery (Kumar 1985). Over 50% of all women will have the transient emotional disorder known as 'the blues' occurring in the first week after birth (Kumar 1984). A further 10% of all women will suffer from a true depressive illness which has a later onset, or at least a later referral for professional help (even up until 1 year after delivery), and a prolonged period of recovery (Cox 1986). A very few women (1 in 500) will have a severe postnatal psychotic illness usually occurring within the first 2 weeks after birth (Sneddon 1987). The midwife has a role in the detection of psychological disturbances and in assisting the woman in her adaptation to motherhood. These psychological disturbances are discussed in greater detail later in this chapter.

Adaptation to motherhood

No adult is in a psychological vacuum and any one person's reaction to a particular event is heavily influenced by their previous experiences. Amongst the important factors governing adaptation to motherhood are the mother's personality, her attitudes towards childbirth, her marriage and her cultural group (Price 1988). Personality is influenced by upbringing, previous experience and past successes or failures. Parenting skills can be learned subconsciously by a young child who sees examples in his/her immediate environment (Price 1988; Bergum 1989). There are, however, many other influences exerted, or every daughter would simply repeat her mother's mistakes. Attitudes to childbirth and motherhood result from a complex interplay of social and psychological events, including education, social ambition, religious conviction, family and personal relationships, culture and emotional stability (Bergum 1989). All these, together with the stability of the marital/ interpersonal relationship, will influence the woman's ability to cope with the transition from woman to mother (Oakley 1980). Although this change is greatest with the birth of a first child, subsequent children alter the existing relationships as the family grows to include a new member (Raphael-Leff 1991). For further information concerning adaptation to motherhood see Nuckolls *et al.* 1972, Pines 1972, Chalmers 1982, Arizmendi and Affonso 1986, Nicolson 1986, Oakley 1986, Rich 1986.

Coping

As adults we constantly use strategies to help us cope with the demands and stresses of everyday life (Price 1988). When extraordinary events occur, such as bereavement, job loss, childbirth or marriage, such coping mechanisms may be overstretched and a psychological change (such as anxiety) can result (Bond 1986). Coping mechanisms are learnt; they depend on personality and upon having previously met a similar situation (Bond 1986). Factors which can ease and improve coping include having sympathetic support systems (Oakley 1980), anticipating the event (such as by attending antenatal classes) (Gordon and Gordon 1960), attacking the event (such as by imposing rigid regimes), avoidance (running away from the event, e.g. denying a pregnancy) and apathy (as occurs in depression) (Lazarus 1966). Maternal self-image is very important in determining whether a woman can cope with the new demands being put upon her (Bergum 1989). As Bergum (1989) comments, women have little or no preparation for the changing role and the demands placed upon them by motherhood. An interesting discussion of some of the issues involved can be found in work by Rich (1986), Ball (1987) and Bergum (1989).

Ball's (1987) research into women's adaptation to motherhood highlighted some characteristics of the mothers and the care they received. Women who were classed as 'emotionally distressed' 6 weeks after delivery were more likely to perceive that they had a lack of support and had received conflicting advice regarding infant feeding (Ball 1987). Midwives' conflicting advice was also reported by some of the mothers who were satisfied with their care and managed to cope, but were simply irritated rather than upset by it (Ball 1987). Social class influenced a woman's feeling of ease. The most vulnerable were women in social class 4, who on further study were seen to have some socio-economic problems (such as partners having more than one job in order to pay for housing) and were rather quiet and reluctant to bother people for advice, especially while still in hospital (Ball 1987). Ball (1987) suspects that on a busy postnatal ward, these women are simply overlooked by the midwives because they are undemanding.

A strong correlation between feelings after delivery (within 24–36 hours of birth) and satisfaction with motherhood was discovered (Ball 1987). Mothers who described themselves as 'disappointed' or 'too tired to care' were less likely to feel happy with motherhood at 6 weeks postpartum. Ball (1987) has some guidelines for good midwifery care, including using more flexible regimes in hospital, allowing a mother to discuss with the midwife the length of stay she requires, trying to avoid conflicting advice and that midwives must be always aware of a woman's emotional needs.

Social support given in pregnancy (Oakley et al. 1990) and increased contact with professionals in the puerperium (as occurred with Sleep and Grant's (1987) reinforcement of a postnatal pelvic floor exercise programme) have been shown to improve psychosocial well-being. Such findings support work by Martin et al. (1989) and Stein et al. (1989) into the importance of psychosocial stress and social adversity rather than the occurrence of perinatal complications as causes of puerperal depression.

The 'blues'

This is a term used to describe a transient mood disruption which most commonly occurs on the third or fourth day after delivery (Kumar 1985). This is a self-limiting condition, affecting more than 50% of mothers, regardless of class, ethnic group or cultural factors (Kumar 1984). If severe, it can be the forerunner of more serious disturbances, but in most cases it is benign (Kendell et al. 1981). The major characteristic of this condition is lability of the emotions, with episodes of weeping or laughing at nothing (Pitt 1973). These often coincide with an increase in physical symptoms such as perineal pain, breast engorgement or wound discomfort. There is no treatment for this condition, which is possibly due to changes in hormone levels after delivery (Dalton 1971). Listening and support from the midwife can assist the mother to understand what is happening and help her to cope until the situation resolves itself (Cox 1986).

Postnatal depression

Postnatal depression affects approximately 10% of women to some degree following childbirth (Kumar 1985). Because its existence is now being recognised and publicised, there is an impression that it is on the increase, although this is not proven. The cause is far from clear, with popular theories using a medical model relating to biochemical and physical changes, a psychoanalytical perspective involving role conflict and regression, or a social approach involving lack of home support and incorrect expectations (Romito 1989). Romito (1989) is especially critical of the medical/illness model, with its unrealistic expectations of the new mother.

The diagnosis of postnatal depression is problematic, since it may well be concealed by the mother (Cox 1986). Also, the onset of this disorder is at a time when she has less contact with health professionals. It is also important to differentiate postnatal depression from previously existing depression which has worsened since childbirth (Sneddon 1987). The two manifestations require different treatments (Sneddon 1987).

Cox (1986) highlights seven factors which would lead a doctor to make a diagnosis of postnatal depression:

1. Depressed mood. Most mothers are aware that their mood changed and that they do not feel normal. The mother may complain of feeling weepy; this situation may have existed since the tearfulness of 'the blues'.
2. Sleep disturbance is a characteristic symptom. It is important that the insomnia is not related to physical discomfort or a crying baby. The mother may complain of waking early (although still tired) or of being unable to fall asleep.
3. A feeling of being unable to cope when all the images provided by the media are of capable, organised mothers. The mother feels guilty at this but may hide it by being outwardly organised.
4. Thoughts of self-harm or of harming the baby. These are very serious symptoms to which great importance should be given especially if the mother reports making plans. In the United Kingdom, infanticide by a mother within one year of the birth is not seen as a criminal offence, since the 1938 Infanticide Act recognises the effects of severe postnatal psychological disturbance.
5. Rejection of the baby. The mother may report wanting the baby to be adopted or of having no feelings towards her child. This can be particularly painful for the mother, especially where she has previously felt a loving relationship. Mothers are aware that these feelings are abnormal and they may feel frightened by them.
6. Altered libido. A reduction in sexual activity following childbirth is fairly common, although it can be due to factors such as tiredness or dyspareunia rather than depression.
7. Anxiety may accompany depression. (Cox 1986)

Treatment can be through counselling or the establishment of postnatal support groups, if the depression is not severe (Cox 1986). There are voluntary groups such as the Marce Society and the Association for Post-natal Illness, which give support to women suffering from postnatal depression. If medication is required, tricyclic antidepressants are effective, although their effects take some time to achieve (Sneddon 1987). Treatment should be continued until it is certain that the condition is cured, since relapse is common, especially premenstrually (Sneddon 1987). Where there is a risk of suicide or infanticide or where the depression is severe, the general practitioner should arrange for a psychiatric referral (Cox 1986). Admission to a Specialist Mother and Baby Unit (if available) may be arranged as an alternative to separating the two. Long-term follow-up is necessary, usually on an out-patient basis (Sneddon 1987). Support for the family is vital, as society still has taboos regarding any form of psychiatric illness. The woman will need much assistance from her family if recovery is to be complete (Cox 1986).

Puerperal psychosis

This is a rare condition, occurring in 1:500–1000 births early in the postnatal period, often before the mother has been discharged from the care of the midwife (Kumar 1985). The mother shows abnormal behaviour, which is unlikely to be missed (Kumar 1985). In addition, 50% of women who have had this condition will experience another but in the future, not necessarily at the time of childbirth (Sneddon 1987).

The mother is usually normal for a few days after delivery, before having an acute attack of abnormal behaviour (Kumar 1985). This may include emotional lability, anxiety, lack of concentration, insomnia, agitation, auditory and visual hallucinations, memory loss, delusions and an inability to speak (Sneddon 1987). The mother may also express suicidal thoughts. A psychiatric referral is vital, usually followed by admission to hospital (Kumar 1985).

If the mother is at home at this time, the community midwife may be summoned to visit, as the family report that the woman is behaving strangely. The general practitioner should be summoned and he/she can arrange referral and admission.

The preferred type of unit is a Mother and Baby Unit which allows the mother to form relationships with her child while recovering (Margison and Brockington 1982). The units also have the advantage of being staffed by people who have developed an expertise in this specialist area of work (Margison and Brockington 1982). If such a unit is not available, it may be necessary to admit the woman alone, especially where there is a risk of her harming herself or the baby. Antidepressant and other drugs will be used, though these can take up to 3 weeks to become effective (Sneddon 1987). A rapid improvement in the mother's condition can occur in 6 weeks (Cox 1986). Breast feeding is usually contra-indicated, both because of excretion of the drugs in breast milk and because the mother may be unsafe or unable to care for her baby (Sneddon 1987).

Recurrence rates in later pregnancies are fairly high (10–20%) (Kumar 1985), although Sneddon (1987) argues that, since the condition is usually identical to the first, its recognition and treatment can begin earlier. She recommends the psychiatrist liaising with the obstetrician throughout any subsequent pregnancy. Also, since this condition has an early onset, discharge from the maternity unit should be delayed until after the time equivalent to when the previous episode occurred (Sneddon 1987). Should admission to a psychiatric unit be necessary, it is far easier to do this from a maternity hospital than from home.

Infection in the puerperium

Before considering infection in the postnatal period, it is necessary to review the body's defence mechanism which prevents infection and to discuss why the postnatal woman is susceptible to infection. The subject of infection with HIV is covered in Chapter 17.

> *First line of defence.* This is formed by the skin and mucus membranes. In addition to their normal flora which serve to maintain the balance of microbes, there are secretions and cellular adaptations which prevent infection. These include the production of perspiration, saliva and tears, which contain lysozymes, to attack cell walls of bacteria, digestive juices, acid mucus (as found in the vagina) which creates a hostile environment and the action of ciliated cells lining the respiratory tract which can move bacteria away from susceptible areas.
>
> *Second line of defence.* At the cellular level, phagocytes in the blood ingest and destroy invading pathogens (Simpson *et al.* 1988). Bacteria are immobilised and inactivated by the plasma protein complement and interferon, produced by infected cells, can be absorbed by the non-infected ones increasing their resistance to infection (Simpson *et al.* 1988).
>
> *Third line of defence.* The final obstacle for an invading pathogen to overcome is the immune response. This is an altered reaction to any antigen, produced by a process of sensitisation. When the antigen is present, antibodies which neutralise its effects are formed (Simpson *et al.* 1988). Immunity can be passive, as with the immunoglobulins passed from mother to fetus in utero, or active where individuals produce their own antibodies. Vaccination challenges an individual with the whole or a part of the microorganism to stimulate antibody production. The pathogen used is either dead or has had its toxic effects diminished (attenuated).

Women are susceptible to infection after childbirth because of the changes which have occurred during and after delivery. These include the presence of the raw placental site, lacerations and incisions (such as an episiotomy or caesarean section wound), the production of lochia (an ideal growth medium for microorganisms), and the changes in the urinary tract during pregnancy and labour (Cunningham *et al.* 1989). There are also certain predisposing factors which can increase the risk or severity of infections. These include anaemia (Cook and Lynch 1986) or obesity (especially following caesarean section) (Rehu and Nilsson 1986), whether the woman has had an instrumental or operative delivery (Farrell *et al.* 1980) and the presence of any retained dead tissue, such as a lobe of the placenta.

The organisms involved fall into two groups; first endogenous bacteria, which exist normally in the body but are only pathogenic when there is tissue damage or when they are moved from their normal position (cross-contamination) (Cunningham *et al.* 1989). Into this group come the organisms usually found in the lower genital tract or in the bowel. They include coliforms such as *Escherichia coli, Clostridium perfringens, Streptococcus faecalis* and *Pseudomonas aeroginosa* (Simpson *et al.* 1988). The second group of microorganisms are exogenous, that is, they arise from outside the individual, from attendants, the environment or from contamination from another infected person (Cunningham *et al.* 1989). They include the virulent Group A beta-haemolytic Streptococci and endemic hospital contaminations such as *Staphylococcus aureus* (Simpson *et al.* 1988). Group B streptoccoci are becoming increasingly important in the occurrence of postpartum urinary tract infections (Wood and Dillon 1981) and of neonatal sepsis (Parker 1977).

Sites of infection in the postnatal period include:

The genital tract (puerperal infection).
The urinary tract.
The breast (see Chapter 34).
Thrombophlebitis (see later in this chapter).

Puerperal infection

Up until 50 years ago, puerperal sepsis or 'childbed fever', as it was known, claimed many lives (Charles and Larson 1986). The necessity for handwashing and hygiene was demonstrated by Semmelweis (1981) who connected a high maternal mortality rate with the attendance of doctors at both delivery and post-mortem examinations.

Midwives must inform the relevant doctor when a postnatal woman has pyrexia, tachycardia or other signs of infection. For this reason, close observation is kept on women in the postnatal period for at least the first 10−14 days, until the risk of infection has passed (Cunningham *et al.* 1989).

The symptoms of a woman with puerperal sepsis depend on the location and severity of the infection. The severity can range from localised infection in vulval lacerations or in an abdominal wound, to a more generalised spread of infection from the uterus and vagina into the pelvic cellular tissue, the fallopian tubes or the pelvic peritoneum (Cunningham *et al.* 1989). If especially virulent, generalised peritonitis or septicaemia can result, with all the attendant risks of mortality (Hibbard 1988).

Signs of infection depending on the severity include:

Pyrexia (can be as high as 40° C).
Tachycardia (if severe up to 140 bpm).
Rigors (with spiking of temperature).

Subinvolution of the uterus (not present in cases of vaginal, perineal, vulval or cervical infected trauma).

Constitutional symptoms (headache, malaise, lower abdominal pain).

Offensive heavy lochia (Simpson *et al.* 1988; Cunningham *et al.* 1989).

Management

The mother and baby should be isolated (Hibbard 1988) while the doctor is summoned to assess the situation. Even for an apparently localised infection such as vulval lacerations, the pathogen involved might be very virulent, so extra effort must be taken to prevent its spread (Simpson *et al.* 1988). On arrival the doctor will review the labour history for predisposing factors such as retained membranes (any portions of placenta which were missing after completion of the third stage are usually removed shortly afterwards under general anaesthetic). A detailed physical examination will be performed and specimens sent to the laboratory. These can include any exudate from wounds, cervical secretions obtained on a high vaginal swab, and a midstream specimen of urine.

A full blood count (for signs of the body's reaction to the infection) and a blood culture may also be performed.

A broad spectrum antibiotic (or a combination of therapies) is usually commenced (Ledger 1988). These can be changed if the bacteria isolated are resistant to that treatment. If the infection is severe, the mother will require intensive nursing care. Tepid sponging and antipyretics may be used to control the temperature. The taking of oral fluids should be encouraged and, if not tolerated, an intravenous infusion may be commenced. While recovering the woman must be kept warm, clean and comfortable. Meticulous records of maternal well-being including temperature, pulse and urinary output should be maintained. The woman should also be confident that her baby is being well-looked after. It is usual to nurse mother and baby together, in case the infant is a symptomless carrier of the infection (Simpson *et al.* 1988). Even if the mother wishes to breast feed, her milk supply may diminish during the acute phase of the infection. Antibiotics approved for use by breastfeeding mothers could be used. If the mother is unable to continue feeding, the milk supply should be maintained, using a breast pump, until her condition is sufficiently improved to feed her baby. The infant meanwhile should preferably be fed expressed breast milk from the milk bank if available. Many of these have been closed due to the risk of transmission of HIV in breast milk, but the World Health Organization (1989) has suggested that pasteurisation at 56°C for 30 minutes should inactivate any virus present.

Subinvolution of the uterus occurs when the uterine fundus does not reduce in size at the expected rate (Cunningham *et al.* 1989). It is important to ensure that a full bladder or rectum are not causing the uterus to rise in the pelvis, relax and appear larger on palpation, which would confuse the assessment. Involution takes longer in women following a multiple pregnancy and in the grand multipara. Amongst the causes of subinvolution are uterine infection and retained products of conception (Cunningham *et al.* 1989). In the case of retained products of conception, the uterus may initially involute normally and the lochia progress through their usual colour changes. The uterus then fails to involute or becomes larger than it was on the previous day's examination and the lochia may become red again or even be offensive. This happens most commonly between 7 and 10 days after birth. Treatment involves emptying the uterus, combating any infection and preventing any haemorrhage. Depending on the severity of the bleeding and infection, the haemorrhage may be managed at home with antibiotics and oral ergometrine (Cunningham *et al*. 1989). Admission to hospital may be required, with evacuation of the uterus under general anaesthesia and intensive antibiotic therapy. If the bleeding is severe, the midwife should massage the uterus to expel clots and cause it to contract; it may be necessary to transfer the woman to hospital by obstetric flying squad. It is also important to ensure that the bladder is empty.

Urinary tract infection

Changes in the urinary tract during pregnancy and labour predispose to infection (Davison 1984). These include the dilatation of the uteters, which produces stasis (Davison 1984), and the overdistension of the bladder, which can occur if it is not emptied frequently during labour (Cunningham *et al* 1989) (see Chapter 28 for changes in the urinary tract in the puerperium). In the case of a forceps delivery, the bladder may have been catheterised, with the risk of an introduced infection (Hibbard 1988). Some authorities recommend the routine screening of all mothers who have had instrumental or operative delivery for the presence of a urinary tract infection (Cunningham *et al*. 1989). *Escherichia coli*. is the organism usually involved.

The diagnosis depends on the site of the infection. Cystitis is manifested by suprapubic pain, frequency of micturition and a slight pyrexia. For pyelonephritis, the woman experiences severe loin pain, which may radiate to the groin. There is a marked pyrexia of up to 40°C, with attendant rigors. The woman may vomit and complain of feeling very unwell. The urine may be cloudy or offensive. The diagnosis is confirmed by bacteriological and microscopic examination of a midstream specimen of urine. Treatment involves making the urinary tract alkaline by using potassium citrate mixture, thus reducing the growth of *Escherichia coli*. The use of antibiotics specifically designed for use in urinary tract infections will be prescribed, with care in the choice being taken if the mother is breast-feeding. Treatment may need to be prolonged, since the infection can recur if not completely treated.

Urinary tract disturbances in the puerperium

In addition to urinary tract infections, many women experience problems in the short and long term following delivery. Problems in the short term are related to trauma (including bruising) occurring to the urethra and bladder neck at delivery, overdistention of the bladder or fear that micturition will be painful (due to lacerations or stitches) (Hibbard 1988). Any bruising to the urethra or bladder neck can cause retention of urine after delivery (Kerr-Wilson *et al.* 1984). This can predispose to urinary tract infections.

Where the bladder has been overdistended, retention of urine with overflow may occur (Kerr-Wilson *et al.* 1984). The woman appears to be passing urine normally, but the bladder is either palpable abdominally or is displacing the uterus to the side (Cunningham *et al.* 1989).

Longer-term effects of childbirth include stress incontinence, the involuntary passage of urine following sudden movement, laughter, physical exercise or coughing (Cardozo 1984). Treatment can involve weight loss for overweight women and physiotherapy to strengthen the sphincter control (Heap 1987), although these can be of limited use where the cause is nerve dehiscence. Cardozo (1984) estimates that approximately 10% of the adult female population in the United Kingdom experience stress incontinence so it is vital to differentiate them from those women whose incontinence is a result of childbirth. Heap (1987) argues that better preparation for childbirth and increased knowledge of their own body can help women to avoid stress incontinence.

Thromboembolic disorders

Thromboembolic disorders are more common in pregnancy and the puerperium, because of changes in blood composition, producing an increase in clotting factors (de Swiet 1985). Risks are increased by dehydration following delivery, stasis of blood either during labour, especially following operative deliveries, or due to raised progesterone levels causing impeded venous return and the possible presence of varicosities (de Swiet 1985). Although primarily considered a disorder of the puerperium, thromboembolic disorders with their attendant risk of fatal pulmonary emboli were responsible for 29 maternal deaths in the United Kingdom between 1985–1987 of which 9 occurred during pregnancy (Department of Health 1991). The Royal College of General Practitioners (1967) calculated that a pregnant or delivered woman was 6 times more likely to experience a thromboembolic condition than if she was not pregnant.

Thrombophlebitis is the commonest and most minor form of thromboembolism occurring in 2:1000 pregnancies and after 11:1000 births (Aaro *et al.* 1967; Aaro and Juergens 1971). It is caused by a clot formed most commonly in a superficial varicosed vein (Leclerc and Hirsh 1988). These cases are unlikely to progress to pulmonary embolism, although they can be distressing to the mother. There will be a tender area over the thrombosed vein, which may be reddened (Cunningham *et al.* 1989). This may be accompanied by a small increase in pulse and temperature (Hibbard 1988). Treatment is to use correctly-fitted antithromboembolic stockings or tights, which are put on before rising. Mobility is encouraged and when sitting, the legs should be elevated with the ankle only or the whole calf supported. Anti-inflammatory drugs may be required (Cunningham *et al.* 1989). The woman should be closely observed for the signs of any deep venous thrombosis (DVT).

DVT is a less common but more serious condition which carries the risk of a part of the clot becoming dislodged, causing a pulmonary embolism (de Swiet 1985). The risk factors for this condition include women who have experienced a DVT while taking oral contraceptives, those of high parity or over 35 years of age, the overweight and in any women following operative deliveries (Department of Health 1991).

The diagnosis of this disorder is complex, since physical signs can be confusing (Simpson *et al.* 1980). Some women may have no symptoms at all. The woman may complain of pain and or swelling in the calf and there might be a slight rise in temperature (Leclerc and Hirsh 1988). Where the vessel is a major one, venous return from the leg may be stopped, the lower limb may feel cold and be white and oedematous (phlegmasia alba dolens). If prolonged, gangrene of the toes can occur (Cunningham *et al.* 1989). Resolution depends on the amount of time necessary to form a collateral circulation. Where a DVT is suspected, measurements of the calves should be taken. A difference of more than 1 cm in the diameter of the calves is considered significant (Kakkar 1984). Because of the non-specific nature of clinical signs, diagnosis should be confirmed before treatment is commenced (de Swiet 1985; Leclerc and Hirsh 1988). The diagnosis is usually confirmed by either Doppler ultrasound or impedence plethysmography, both of which rely on detecting alterations in blood flow (Leclerc and Hirsh 1988). In the puerperium, venography may also be employed (Leclerc and Hirsh 1988). Venography is not commonly used during pregnancy or lactation, because the radioactive iodine used as a contrast medium crosses the placenta and is passed in breast milk before being concentrated by the fetal and neonatal thyroid glands (Letsky 1985).

Treatment involves using anticoagulants to prevent further clots, and careful observation for signs of emboli (Leclerc and Hirsh 1988). Fibrinolytic agents cannot be given in pregnancy, since they can cause placental and fetal haemorrhage and preterm labour (Amias 1977). They may be utilised after the first postnatal week (Letsky 1985). The anticoagulant of choice in pregnancy is calcium heparin, since it does not cross the placenta (due to its high molecular weight) and its effects are easy to reverse (using protamine sulphate) should its action be too extreme (Leclerc and Hirsh 1988). Its main disadvantage is that it must be given parenterally (Letsky 1985). For initial therapeutic use, a slow intravenous injection of 40 000 units of heparin over 24 hours is used (de Swiet 1985). This will be maintained for 5–7 days before changing to subcutaneous self-administered heparin until 6 weeks after birth (de Swiet 1985). Bonnar (1989) suggests that intravenous Dextran 70, given in labour, is helpful in reducing the occurrence of pulmonary embolism following DVT. For prophylactic purposes in women with a previous history of DVT, twice daily subcutaneous doses of heparin can be given until 6 weeks postnatally (Letsky 1985).

Warfarin is not often used, since it is teratogenic in early pregnancy (its low molecular weight allows it to cross the placenta) and there is a risk of haemorrhage in later pregnancy (Letsky 1985). The control of dose is more complicated than with heparin and frequent visits (usually twice weekly) to hospital for assessment of blood coagulation profiles are necessary (Leclerc and Hirsh 1988). In addition, its action is not easily reversed, requiring 24 hours of vitamin K administration or the use of an infusion of fresh frozen plasma (Letsky 1985). Women who are unable to self-administer subcutaneous heparin may be prescribed Warfarin from 16 to 36 weeks of pregnancy and from 10 to 14 days onwards postnatally (Letsky 1985). Breast feeding is no longer contra-indicated.

For women at risk of developing a DVT and who require an operative delivery, prophylactic electric leg compression boots may be used in theatre and during the early puerperium (Hibbard 1988). The care of a woman with or at high risk of a DVT is very similar, since observations of bleeding (such as the colour and amount of lochia), encouragement of gentle mobility and avoidance of any pressure on the legs are common to both (Cunningham *et al.* 1989). There is argument as to the necessity for prophylaxis in later pregnancies, although there is agreement that oestrogen containing oral contraceptives are contra-indicated (Letsky 1985).

Pulmonary embolism is an obstetric emergency, with a high risk of maternal death (responsible for 29:209 deaths in the 1982–1984 report (Department of Health 1989). The condition may follow a known case of DVT but in most situations, it occurs without warning (Leclerc and Hirsh 1988). Pulmonary embolus presents with sudden collapse, acute chest pain, cyanosis, dyspnoea, haemoptysis, pyrexia and shock (Leclerc and Hirsh 1988). The clinical picture, however, may be somewhat unspecific, requiring a differential diagnosis to be made from Mendelson's syndrome, acute anaphylaxis, acute myocardial failure, and amniotic fluid embolism (Leclerc and Hirsh 1988). Further investigations include chest X-ray and ultrasound scan of the lungs (Leclerc and Hirsh 1988).

This is an obstetric emergency and medical aid should be sought immediately. Any case of chest pain should be reported to the medical staff to exclude pulmonary embolism as the cause. The woman should be sat up to aid breathing and given oxygen. Her vital signs should be measured and recorded. These should be repeated every 15 minutes. Medical management includes the use of heparin as an anticoagulant and a powerful analgesic such as morphine to control the pain (Hibbard 1988). In severe cases, resuscitation measures with artificial ventilation may be necessary. Enzymes to dissolve the clot (such as streptokinase) may be used in the puerperium, but if the embolism is large (and the woman survives) or during pregnancy, embolectomy may be required (Kakker 1984). If the embolus is small, the situation can be treated conservatively with anticoagulants and gentle mobility (Cunningham *et al.* 1989).

References

Aaro L A, Johnson T R and Juergens J L (1967) 'Acute superficial venous thrombophlebitis associated with pregnancy' *American Journal of Obstetrics and Gynecology* 97: 514

Aaro L A and Juergens J L (1971) 'Thrombophlebitis associated with pregnancy' *American Journal of Obstetrics and Gynecology* 109: 1128

Amias A G (1977) 'Streptokinase, cerebral vascular accident – and triplets' *British Medical Journal* 1: 1414–5

Arizmendi T C and Affonso D D (1986) 'Stressful events related to pregnancy and the post partum' *Journal of Psychosomatic Research* 31(6): 743–56

Ball J A (1987) *Reactions to Motherhood* Cambridge University Press: Cambridge

Bergum V (1989) *Woman to Mother: A transformation* Bergin and Garvey: Massachusetts

Bond M (1986) *Stress and Self Awareness* Heinemann: London

Bonnar J (1989) 'Venous thrombosis and pulmonary embolism in pregnancy and the puerperium' in A Turnbull and G Chamberlain (eds) *Obstetrics* 933–46 Churchill Livingstone: Edinburgh

Cardozo L D (1984) 'Surgery for stress incontinence' *Journal of Obstetrics and Gynaecology* 5(Suppl) 55–9

Chalmers B (1982) 'Psychological aspects of pregnancy: some thoughts for the eighties' *Social Science in Medicine* 16: 323–31

Charles D and Larson B (1986) 'Streptoccocal puerperal sepsis and obstetric infections: a historical perspective.' *Review of Infectious Disease* 8(3): 411–22

Cook J D and Lynch SR (1986) 'The liabilities of iron deficiency' *Blood* 68: 803

Cox J L (1986) *Postnatal Depression* Churchill Livingstone: Edinburgh

Cunningham F G, MacDonald P C and Gant N F (1989) *William's Obstetrics (18th edn)* Prentice Hall: London

Dalton K (1971) 'Prospective study of puerperal depression' *British Journal of Psychiatry* 118: 689–92

Davison J M (1984) 'Renal disease' in M de Swiet (ed) *Medical Disorders in Obstetric Practice* Ch 7 p 192–259 Blackwell Scientific: Oxford

Department of Health (1989) *Report on Confidential Enquiries into Maternal Deaths in England and Wales 1982–4* HMSO: London

Department of Health (1991) *Confidential Inquiry into Maternal Deaths in the United Kingdom 1985–7* HMSO: London

de Swiet M (1985) 'Thromboembolism' *Clinics in Haematology* 14(3): 643–60

Farrell S J, Andersen H F and Work B A (1980) 'Cesarean section: indications and postoperative morbidity' *Obstetrics and Gynecology* 56: 696

Gordon R E and Gordon K K (1960) 'Social factors in prevention of postpartum emotional disorders' *Obstetrics and Gynecology* 15: 433–7

Heap J (1987) 'Too ashamed to tell' *Nursing Times* Community Outlook: 14–18 October.

Hibbard B M (1988) *Principles of Obstetrics* Butterworth: London

Kakker V V (1984) 'Venous thromboembolism' in M Brudenell and P M Wilds (eds) *Surgical Problems in Obstetrics* Ch 13 175–92 Wright: Bristol

Kendell R E, McGuire R J, Connor Y and Cox J L (1981) 'Mood changes in the first three weeks after childbirth' *Journal of Affective Disorders* 3: 317–26

Kerr-Wilson R J H, Thompson S W, Orr J W, Davis R O and Cloud G A (1984) 'Effect of labour on the postpartum bladder' *Obstetrics and Gynecology* 64: 115

Kumar R (1984) 'Motherhood and mental illness' *Midwives Chronicle* March: 70–4

Kumar R (1985) 'Pregnancy, childbirth and mental illness' in J Studd (ed) *Progress in Obstetrics and Gynaecology Vol 5* 146–59 Churchill Livingstone: Edinburgh

Lazarus R S (1966) *Psychological Stress and the Coping Process* McGraw-Hill: New York

Leclerc J R and Hirsh J (1988) 'Venous thromboembolic disorders' in G N Burrow and T F Ferris (eds) *Medical Complications During Pregnancy* (3rd edn) 204–23 W B Saunders: Philadelphia

Ledger W J (1988) 'A historical view of pelvic infections' *American Journal of Obstetrics and Gynecology* 158: 687

Letsky E A (1985) *Coagulation Problems During Pregnancy* Ch 3 29–61 Churchill Livingstone: Edinburgh

Margison F and Brockington I F (1982) 'Psychiatric mother and baby units' in I F Brockington and R Kumar (eds) *Motherhood and Mental Illness* 223–38 Academic Press: London

Martin C J, Brown G W, Goldberg D P and Brockington I A (1989) 'Psycho-social stress and puerperal depression' *Journal of Affective Disorders* 16: 283–93

Nicolson P (1986) 'Developing a feminist approach to depression following childbirth' in S Wilkinson (ed) *Feminist Social Psychology* Open University Press: Milton Keynes

Nuckolls K B, Cassel J and Kaplan B H (1972) 'Psychosocial aspects' *American Journal of Epidemiology* 95: 431

Oakley A (1980) *Women Confined: Towards a sociology of childbirth* Oxford University Press: Oxford

Oakley A (1986) *Telling the Truth about Jerusalem* Blackwell: London

Oakley A, Rajan L and Grant A (1990) 'Social support and pregnancy outcome' *British Journal of Obstetrics and Gynaecology* 97: 155–62

Parker M T (1977) 'Neonatal streptoccocal infections' *Postgraduate Medical Journal* 53: 598–600

Pines D (1972) 'Pregnancy and motherhood: interaction between fantasy and reality' *British Journal of Medical Psychology* 45: 333–43

Pitt B (1973) 'Maternity blues' *British Journal of Psychiatry* 122: 431–5

Price J (1988) *Motherhood: What it does to your mind* Pandora: London

Raphael-Leff J (1991) *Psychological Processes of Childbearing* Chapman and Hall: London

Rehu M and Nilsson C G (1979) 'Risk factors for febrile morbidity associated with cesarean section' *Obstetrics and Gynecology* 53: 354

Rich A (1986) *Of Woman Born* Virago: London

Romito P (1989) 'Unhappiness after childbirth' in I Chalmers, M Enkin and M J N C Kierse (eds) *Effective Care in Pregnancy and Childbirth* 1433–46 Oxford Medical: Oxford

Royal College of General Practitioners (1967) 'Oral contraception and thromboembolic disease' *Journal of the Royal College of General Practitioners* 13: 267–79

Semmelweis I P (1981) 'Childbed fever: classics in infectious diseases' *Reviews of Infectious Diseases* 3(4): 53–5

Simpson F G, Robinson P J, Bar J and Lowsky M J (1980) 'Prospective study of thrombophlebitis and 'pseudo thrombophlebitis' *Lancet* i: 331–3

Simpson M L, Gaziano E P, Lupo V R and Petersen P K (1988) 'Bacterial infections during pregnancy' in G N Burrow and T F Ferris (eds) *Medical Complications During Pregnancy (3rd edn)* 345–71 W B Saunders: Philadelphia

Sleep J and Grant A (1987) 'Pelvic floor exercises in postnatal care' *Midwifery* 3(4): 158–64

Sneddon J (1987) 'Postnatal illness' *Midwives Chronicle* Nov: 342–7

Stein A, Cooper P J, Campbell E A, Day A and Altham P M E (1989) 'Social adversity and perinatal complications: their relation to postnatal depression' *British Medical Journal* 298: 1073–4

Wood E G and Dillon H C (1981) 'A prospective study of group B streptoccocal bacteruria in pregnancy' *American Journal of Obstetrics and Gynecology* 140: 515–20

World Health Organization (1989) *AIDS Series 3. Guidelines for Nursing Management of People Infected with Human Immunodeficiency Virus* WHO: Geneva

30   Family planning

Contraception refers to the intentional control of fertility by natural or artificial means (Collins 1989). The term 'natural family planning' is used to describe methods such as celibacy, periodic abstinence and ovulation assessment, to distinguish them from 'artificial' methods (Flynn and Brooks 1984). Giving family planning advice involves more than contraception. It includes fertility awareness, pregnancy spacing and the timing of conception (Guillebaud 1985). Access to family planning is regarded as a basic human right.

This chapter considers the history of family planning, reasons for its use, the concept of the 'perfect method' and influences on choice. The individual methods will be discussed including their modes of action, advantages and disadvantages. The role of the midwife, other professionals and agencies in the giving of advice will be considered.

History of contraception

Over most of its history, the human race has sought to control conception (Himes 1970). In many cases, the wish was to encourage pregnancy (Himes 1970). There are biblical references to family planning as in the case of Onan who 'spilt his seed upon the ground' (coitus interruptus) (Genesis 38 : 9). Knowledge of the menstrual cycle, ovulation and conception was often rudimentary, undermining the effectiveness of any measures adopted. For example, in Tudor and Stuart England it was assumed that the man's sperm contained all the necessary ingredients for fetal life. All that was required was to 'plant' this in the woman's uterus which acted solely as the host (Eccles 1982). Historical records of the use of pessaries (which were often herbal), intrauterine devices to prevent pregnancy in animals (stones placed in the uterus of a camel) and condoms (made of leather, fabric or animal intestines) show that modern methods are far from original (Himes 1970). A society's attitude to premarital sex and the age of marriage also influences family size, as can be seen today in the People's Republic of China where the 'one child' policy is maintained, sometimes using coercion to gain permission for an abortion and financial penalties should the couple have more than one child (Lorraine 1985).

Overpopulation was not a problem up until the industrialisation of society in the nineteenth century. In agricultural communities, high infant and maternal mortality rates allied to famine and infectious disease required large families simply to maintain the population and to provide a large enough workforce (Macfarlane 1986). The social reforms of the last century, most notably the work in the United Kingdom of Edwin Chadwick to ensure a clean water supply and safe disposal of sewage led to population growth (Wohl 1983). The rise in literacy (although still low amongst the labouring classes in the late nineteenth century) and the burdens of child care following prohibition of the use of child labour made limitation of family size an attractive proposition (Wohl 1983).

The attitude of the churches in the last century was that sexual intercourse could not be separated from procreation, that fertility was divinely ordained and therefore not to be interfered with. This led to public censure of individuals who sought to publicise the rudimentary methods of birth control then available (Himes 1970). In the United States in 1873, the Comstock Act declared that information relating to the avoidance of conception was obscene (Lehfeldt 1987). The fall in the infant mortality rate, together with increasing literacy amongst the female population, resulted in moves for women to do more with their lives than constant child-bearing and nursing (Llewellyn-Davies 1978). Advice on avoiding pregnancy was available to the middle and upper classes through (often imported) books and pamphlets (Himes 1970). In the United Kingdom Dr Albutt, a Leeds physician, was removed from the medical register for writing a pamphlet in 1887, *The Wife's Handbook*, in which he gave instructions for the use of the diaphragm (Himes 1970).

The first family planning clinic was established in Amsterdam in 1882 by Aletta Jacobs (Lehfeldt 1987). The first clinic in the United States was established in Brooklyn in 1916, but it was not until 1921 that Marie Stopes opened the first family planning clinic in England (Lehfeldt 1987). This gave practical help (such as the cervical cap) and advice to poor working-class women. Llewellyn-Davies (1978) highlighted the plight of these women, worn down by years of repeated childbearing and hard physical labour undertaken to supplement the family income. Their husbands were rarely in secure employment. Overcrowding and lack of privacy only increased family stress (Llewellyn-Davies 1978).

In 1930, the British Government gave permission for local authorities to provide family planning advice for couples, where a further pregnancy would be detrimental to health. Very few authorities provided such a service. In the same year, the voluntary agencies (with the exception of the Stopes Clinics) combined to become the National Birth Control Council, in 1939 becoming the Family Planning Association (Tacchi 1989). Despite the formation of the National Health Service in 1948, family planning was not included as part of the service (Tacchi 1989). Its provision remained the responsibility of local councils, who then ran most community health services (with the exception of general practitioners) including domiciliary midwifery. Voluntary agencies filled the gaps left by the lack of local authority provision. It was not until 1966 that the Government reminded local authorities of the necessity of providing facilities in their area.

The introduction of oral contraception brought family planning into the sphere of doctors, due to the need for medical supervision of its use (Guillebaud 1984). The 1974 NHS reorganisation brought family planning into the NHS with the Government accepting the financial responsibility of the service (Tacchi 1989). Single women have been able to obtain birth control since 1970. Family planning clinics, although less expensive per client than GP services, are becoming increasingly beleaguered in these times of economic stringency (Chamberlain 1989; Tacchi 1989). Chamberlain (1989) is critical of the rundown of clinics which provide family planning advice, screening, pregnancy testing and sexual and abortion counselling. They provide a service for many who would either not visit their GP (due to inconvenient surgery times or personal preference) or require facilities not available at their local surgery (Snowden 1985). In addition, the clinics are a valuable educational resource for family planning nurses, midwives and doctors (Tacchi 1989).

Internationally, the acceptability and provision of family planning advice is variable (Lorraine 1985). In some countries, contraception is illegal and there can be programmes to encourage population growth (as in prerevolutionary Romania). In other countries, religious prohibition means that provision is restricted.

Politically sanctioned sterilisation strategies such as those used in India have been superseded by the 'one child' policy and prohibition of early marriage, as practised in the People's Republic of China (Lorraine 1985). Too many couples in the world do not have access to family planning advice because of poverty, isolation or illiteracy. However high mortality rates and large ideal family size in many developing countries has led to continual rises in population (Lorraine 1985). The average size of a family in Kenya is eight children (Lorraine 1985). After the third pregnancy and birth, the rate of maternal mortality increases significantly with each successive delivery (Royston and Armstrong 1989). In Western countries, access to medical care and education, together with increased consumerism and an improvement in women's position in society, have resulted in a restriction of family size (Lorraine 1985). In some cases, this is at such a low level that the population was not being maintained, as in West Germany before unification.

In Great Britain, it is unlawful for a male to have sexual intercourse with a girl before she is 16 years old (17 years in Northern Ireland) (Sexual Offences Act 1956).

The age of majority is 18, although young people are permitted to give consent to medical treatment once they are 16 (Family Law Reform Act 1969). This includes family planning advice, examinations and the prescribing of contraceptives. A controversy still rages surrounding the giving of contraceptive advice and treatment to people under the age of 16. A court case was brought in the early 1980s in the United Kingdom by Mrs Victoria Gillick against her local health authority. In it, she sought assurances that none of her daughters (then all aged less than 16 years old) would be given contraceptive advice without her knowledge and consent (Timmins 1984). The authority could not give her these assurances and the court ruled that existing guidelines permitting assistance for underage girls were not unlawful. At the Appeal Court, the first ruling was overruled. Advice or treatment could only be given without parental consent in an 'emergency' situation (Seymour 1986). This term was not defined. Following this case, most contraceptive services and sexual and general health education classes for the under 16s were stopped. In 1985 the House of Lords finally ruled that:

> A girl under 16 of sufficient understanding and intelligence may have the legal capacity to give valid consent to contraceptive advice and treatment including necessary medical examinations.
>
> Giving such advice and treatment to a girl under 16 without parental consent does not infringe parental rights.
>
> Doctors giving such advice in good faith are not committing a criminal offence of aiding and abetting unlawful intercourse with girls under 16 (Lobb 1987).

Revised guidance from the Department of Health and Social Security is that the girl should be encouraged to inform her parents or allow the GP to do so. If she refuses, the doctor or other professional can give advice, provided that they are satisfied that the young person understands their advice, that they will begin or continue to have sexual intercourse with or without contraceptive treatment and that, without such advice, their physical or mental health could suffer (Lobb 1987).

This allows discretion to be used in cases of young women who are not well supported by their parents and are at high risk of pregnancy. It takes great courage and maturity for a young person to seek family planning advice. They require much tact and understanding to encourage their mature attitude (Bowen-Simpkins 1988). A censorious approach will possibly alienate the young women, placing them at risk of pregnancy (Bowen-Simpkins 1988).

Choice of contraceptive method

The perfect contraceptive would be 100% effective, rapidly reversible, have no side-effects, be cheap and easily available, be obtainable independent of the medical professions, should not interfere with sexual intercourse and it should be acceptable to all religions and cultures (Guillebaud 1984). Unfortunately, no such state of perfection exists. The choice of method is a compromise between acceptability of mode of action, effectiveness and side-effects (Guillebaud 1984). The effectiveness of any method is calculated by measuring the number of failures if 100 women were to use the technique for 1 year. It must be remembered that if these 100 women used no contraception at all, the 'failure' or pregnancy rate would be 80–90/100 women years (Guillebaud 1985) (see Table 30.1).

The choice of contraceptive method is a very individual one. It depends whether the couple have any children and whether they want any more (Guillebaud 1985). Those without a regular partner may prefer a method which can be used when the need arises, such as the sheath or cap, rather than a continuous method, such as hormonal contraception. The age of the woman is important because fertility declines over the age of 31 (van Noord-Zaadstra *et al.* 1991), making some of the less reliable methods (in periods of peak fertility) more acceptable (Bowen-Simpkins 1988). Older couples may prefer the more permanent solution of sterilisation, but the poor rate of reversibility necessitates a need for caution with younger couples in this age of common marital breakdown (Calvert 1987). The couple's feelings about their sexuality must be taken into consideration. The fitting of a diaphragm will be unacceptable to a woman unwilling to touch her own genitalia

Table 30.1 User failure rates for different methods of contraception/100 woman years

Sterilisation	
Male	0–0.2
Female	0–0.5
Injectable Hormones	0–1
Combined pills	
50µg oestrogen	0.1–1
< 50µg oestrogen	0.2–1
IUCD	
Lippes loop C	0.3–4
Copper 7	0.3–4
Progestogen only pill	0.3–5
Diaphragm	2–15
Condom	2–15
Coitus interruptus	8–17
Spermicides alone	4–25
Natural family planning	
Pre-plus post ovulation	15–30
Post ovulation alone	1–6
Contraceptive sponge	9–25
No method, young women	80–90
No method at age 40	40–50
No method at age 45	c10–20
No method at age 50	c0–5

(Source: Prescriber's Journal (1987) p. 13)

(Hickerton 1985). Many ethnic and religious groups have prohibitions against certain contraceptive techniques; in a society where the left hand is regarded as unclean, the necessity of using two hands to insert a diaphragm makes this method unacceptable (Warren and Masil 1988). In societies where men are especially dominant, they may wish to be in charge of the family planning method, making condoms the only acceptable technique. In societies which view women as unclean during menstruation, techniques such as an intrauterine contraceptive device (IUCD) which increases bleeding would be unacceptable (Hickerton 1985). Before offering advice, it is vital to consider the couple's social, religious and cultural background, as well as their desired family size. It is important to determine whether the contraception is being used to prevent a pregnancy or to space the family (Guillebaud 1984).

Provision of family planning services

Family planning clinics are still available in most areas in the United Kingdom although their location and clinic hours may no longer be as convenient (Tacchi 1989). These clinics are staffed by specially trained doctors, nurses and sometimes midwives (Tacchi 1989). The personnel can give full advice and prescribe all types of contraception for both men and women including the IUCD and the diaphragm (Snowden 1985). In addition they can carry out 'well person' screening, offer pregnancy testing, psychosexual abortion and presterilisation counselling (Snowden 1985). Clinics offer an anonymous service with the person's doctor only being informed with the individual's consent.

In some UK cities there are domiciliary services which provide help for those unable to attend clinics. However, general practitioners give most advice and treatment (Department of Health and Social Security 1988). This usually involves prescribing the oral contraceptive pill (Snowden 1985). There are lists of GPs with post-registration training in family planning (who can fit IUCDs and diaphragms) available for consultation through local family practitioner committees. Because the scheme of payment costs each item separately, it is possible to visit a doctor with whom one is not registered for advice (Tacchi 1989). GPs cannot, however, provide free condoms, which are only available free through family planning clinics (Snowden 1985).

Midwives give much family planning advice during the postnatal period, but are unable to give any practical help. In other countries (such as the United States) midwives receive family planning teaching as part of their midwifery education (Silverton 1988). They are allowed to fit diaphragms and, by observing strict locally agreed protocols, to prescribe oral contraception. Such skills would mean British midwives would not have to send recently delivered mothers to their local clinic or GP for treatment. With shorter stays in hospital after the birth, women are less likely to receive contraceptive advice and treatment under medical supervision (Murphy-Black 1989).

Contraceptive methods

Natural methods

Natural methods are commonly used world-wide and there are few religious prohibitions against their use (Flynn and Brooks 1984).

Breast feeding

In poor countries prolonged breast feeding is vital to maintain birth intervals and to give the baby the best possible start in life (Thapa *et al*. 1988). This effect is increased in areas where sexual intercourse does not recommence until feeding has stopped (Jelliffe and Jelliffe 1978). Howie *et al*. (1982) have shown that the first ovulation is delayed where the mother is breast feeding. To maintain this effect, she must continue to feed frequently (especially during the night) for a total time exceeding 1 hour each day (McNeilly *et al*. 1983). In the West, lactation is not a sufficiently reliable form of family planning (Dewart and Loudon 1987). Combining its use with other natural methods can improve its effectiveness (Thapa *et al*. 1988).

Coitus interruptus

This is withdrawal of the penis from the vagina prior to ejaculation. This method is widely practised, since it involves little preparation (Guillebaud 1985). It is reliant on a high degree of control by the male partner. Since semen leakage can occur prior to ejaculation and also sperm deposited on the vulva can reach the uterus, its failure rate is between 8 and 17/100 woman years (Prescribers Journal 1987).

Periodic abstinence

The technique relies on abstaining from sexual intercourse during the fertile period in the menstrual cycle (Flynn and Brooks 1984). It requires commitment and motivation from both partners. The effectiveness is dependent upon the woman's knowledge of her own fertility (Flynn and Brooks 1984). Because sperm can survive in the genital tract for on average 3–4 days, intercourse prior to ovulation is always riskier than that after (Flynn and Brooks 1984). It is thought that the ovum is capable of fertilisation for 12–24 hours. Conception is most likely to occur when the motile sperm are already present in the fallopian tubes at ovulation (Eddy and Pauerstein 1980).

The most accurate way to determine fertility is by the assessment of cervical mucus. When menstruation ends, low oestrogen levels produce a thick mucus which blocks the cervical os (Flynn and Brooks 1984). As the cycle continues, oestrogen levels rise. The mucus becomes thinner, sticky and opaque. When oestrogen reaches its peak prior to ovulation, the mucus is clear, slippery and copious (Flynn and Brooks 1984). This facilitates the passage of sperm through the cervix into the uterine cavity. This mucus is very stretchy and it can be pulled between thumb and forefinger (Flynn and Brooks 1984). Following ovulation, the mucus again becomes thick and sticky and the vagina relatively dry (Norman 1986). By avoiding intercourse from the last 'dry' day (approximate by 20 days before the next menstrual period for a short cycle) until 4 days after the peak of mucus production, the fertile period will be avoided (Norman 1986). These techniques can also be reversed to facilitate conception.

Recordings of basal body temperature are often used in conjunction with observations of cervical mucus. These are unreliable alone, since they detect the onset of progesterone production following ovulation (Guillebaud 1985). If intercourse has continued until this time, conception may occur, since sperm may be present in the uterine cavity at ovulation (Flynn and Brooks 1984). Progesterone causes a rise of $0.2°C$ in basal body temperature over the level before ovulation, which is maintained until menstruation. The woman should take her temperature at the same time each morning before rising from bed. Easy-to-read fertility thermometers are available for this purpose. After 3 days of raised temperature, the couple can resume intercourse. Care should be taken when using this method alone, since mild illness, tiredness, stress or getting up during the night can interfere with accuracy (Flynn and Brooks 1984).

Barrier methods

Condoms

The most commonly used method in this category is the sheath or condom (Tayob and Guillebaud 1990). It is cheap to buy, easy to obtain and can be used with limited knowledge (Guillebaud 1985). Its safe use requires that the thin rubber sheath be applied to the erect penis before any contact occurs with the woman's vulva and vagina to avoid the risk of pregnancy from sperm in the pre-ejaculatory fluid (Guillebaud 1985). A space must be left in the tip of the condom without a teat to prevent bursting on ejaculation. The condom must be held in place during withdrawal to prevent spillage of semen. Spermicides increase the effectiveness of condoms (Tayob and Guillebaud 1990). Some condoms are impregnated with the spermicide nonoxynol-9, which can also protect against HIV infection (Hicks et al. 1985). Lubricated sheaths do not necessarily contain spermicide.

Condoms made to British Standard are rigorously tested, although even they are not guaranteed to be 100% free of holes. The effectiveness of a condom depends upon its correct use and also upon the length of time that the couple have been using the method (Vessey et al. 1976). Prescriber's Journal (1987) quotes a failure rate of 2–15/100 woman years.

The use of condoms has increased following the advent of HIV infection and the 'safe sex' health education campaigns. Whilst not offering total protection against infection, the condom does reduce the risk of transmission. The use of a condom is advisable for any man where either partner in the relationship has a history of intravenous drug usage, where the relationship is not of long standing or where there are multiple partners.

Diaphragms

The diaphragm is a dome of thin rubber attached to a metal spring circle. It is placed in the vault of the vagina between the posterior fornix and the back of the symphysis pubis, forming a physical barrier between the cervix and sperm (Tayob and Guillebaud 1990). The diaphragm requires expert fitting to ensure a close fit without causing discomfort or exerting pressure on the bladder (Guillebaud 1985). The fit must take account of the increase in size of the upper vagina during sexual arousal (Johnson *et al.* 1974). The woman must be motivated to use this method which many find inconvenient, premeditated and messy if used as directed with spermicides (Guillebaud 1985). As the woman's shape alters with changes in her weight and after pregnancy, the cap size may need to be changed (Guillebaud 1985). For increased effectiveness, the diaphragm should be used with a spermicide, which can make it rather slippery to insert.

The woman inserts the diaphragm prior to intercourse and then checks that the cervix is fully covered (Guillebaud 1985). If intercourse occurs later that 3 hours after its insertion, more spermicide should be applied. The diaphragm should be left in place for 6 hours after intercourse, then removed, washed and dried (Guillebaud 1985).

Spermicides usually containing Nonoxynol-9 are available as creams, foam and pessaries (Tayob and Guillebaud 1990). If more than one type is used, care should be taken that they are of the same pH, to avoid any chemical reactions which can neutralise their action.

Diaphragms are contra-indicated where the woman has a vaginal prolapse; for such women a vault cap may be used (Tayob and Guillebaud 1990). If recurrent cystitis occurs, the fit should be checked. If it is correct, the woman may need to change her contraceptive technique.

The failure rate of the diaphragm is similar to that for the condom. Failures are few in older women or amongst conscientious users (Stott 1988). Research is continuing into the use of barrier methods of contraception with and without spermicides to assess the effect on the failure rate.

Cervical and vault caps can also be used, although they are more easily dislodged during intercourse if the suction with which they adhere to the cervix is broken (Tayob and Guillebaud 1990). They are less commonly used than diaphragms.

The vaginal sponge

These were originally introduced as an over-the-counter equivalent to the condom. The sponge, which is impregnated with spermicide, is moistened with water before being placed high in the vaginal vault (McEwan 1986). It can remain *in situ* for 24 hours. There is a tape attached to the underside of the sponge to aid removal. It should not be removed until 6 hours after the last episode of intercourse (McEwan 1986). The American manufacturers claim a much lower failure rate than that which has been achieved in British studies, which was recorded at 24.5/100 woman years (Bounds and Guillebaud 1984). This is unacceptable for most women, but it could be used for older age groups where fertility is already lowered (Bowen-Simpkins 1988), or in those who are delaying rather than totally avoiding pregnancy. In addition, it could be used to supplement the contraceptive effects of lactation (McEwan 1986).

Femshield

Newly available in the UK is the Femidom or 'female condom'. This consists of a polyurethane sheath which is designed to cover the vagina and external genitalia (Tayob and Guillebaud 1990). Early studies showed that the method was acceptable to half of couples in the sample and that it caused less loss of sensation to women than occurred to men with the condom (Bounds *et al.* 1988).

Intrauterine contraceptive device (IUCD)

The intrauterine contraceptive device (IUCD) or coil is a small device usually made of plastic, often surrounded with coils of copper which is inserted into the uterine cavity (Van Os 1983). The IUCD requires expert insertion and removal. The popularity of the coil has reduced, following scares about pelvic infection and subsequent infertility (Salih 1987). One design of coil previously used extensively in the United States (the Dalkon Shield) has given rise to a series of successful legal claims for damage following its use (Salih 1987).

The mode of action of the IUCD is unclear, but the following mechanisms have been suggested (Moyer and Shaw 1980):

1. It speeds the passage of the ovum through the fallopian tube, interfering with its process of maturation.
2. Raised osmolality (solute concentration) in the uterine cavity causes death of the blastocyst.
3. It changes the motility of the uterus.
4. It changes the composition of the endometrium.
5. It induces an inflammatory reaction, which prevents implantation (Moyer and Shaw 1980).

The effect of copper which is used on some coils is similarly unclear (Van Os 1983).

The use of the IUCD is contra-indicated in woman with a history of pelvic inflammatory disease and in those who already experience heavy periods (Salih 1987). IUCDs can be difficult to fit in nulliparous women and are often contra-indicated, due to the risk of pelvic inflammatory disease and subsequent subfertility (Salih 1987). Care should also be taken following uterine surgery, such as a caesarean section.

The IUCD is inserted, usually by a doctor, during the latter part of menstruation or immediately after (Potts 1988). The uterine condition and position is determined by bimanual examination. The woman is then placed in lithotomy, dorsal or lateral Sims position and a speculum is inserted to visualise the cervix. The cervix is cleaned with an antiseptic solution before the introduction of a uterine sound to measure the size of the uterine cavity. If necessary, a small cervical dilator may be used. The IUCD is introduced; when it is in the correct position, the introducer is removed, leaving the device *in situ* (Potts 1988). The nylon threads are then cut to the required length, so the woman can check after each period that the coil is still in place.

Once inserted, the coil can be left in place for 2–5 years, depending upon the type and requires little attention. The disadvantages of the coil are that it needs skilful fitting to avoid damaging the uterus (Guillebaud 1985). Some women find the coil painful or suffer from menorrhagia necessitating its removal (Potts 1988). Infections can lead to pelvic inflammatory disease. Ideally IUCDs should be used only where both partners in the relationship are monogamous, reducing the risk of pelvic infections (Salih 1987).

The IUCD can be inserted post-coitally up to 5 days after unprotected intercourse (before implantation) (Rowlands 1983). The coil is unacceptable to some groups, who state that it procures an early abortion rather than preventing conception.

IUCDs have a failure rate of 0.3–4/100 woman years (Prescriber's Journal 1987). These are usually due to expulsion of the coil during a menstrual period (Salih 1987). If the pregnancy occurs with the coil *in situ*, there is a 38% risk of spontaneous abortion (Vessey *et al.* 1976, 1982). Although there is no evidence regarding an increase in fetal abnormality, should a pregnancy occur, there is no evidence of the technique's safety (Salih 1987).

Experiments are continuing with coils containing slow-release hormones, which can decrease the adverse effects and increase reliability (Drife 1989).

Hormonal contraception

This section includes the various types of oral contraception, injectable hormones and those being developed for slow release by implants or vaginal rings.

Combined oral contraception (COC)

This consists of a combination of oestrogen and a synthetic progesterone (Guillebaud 1984). These are taken daily for 21 days, followed by a 7 day break, during which a withdrawal bleed occurs (Rowlands 1987). Biphasic and triphasic preparations are similar, although the dosages of the 2 hormones are altered to approximate those in a natural menstrual cycle. Progestogen levels start low and increase at 7 day intervals; oestrogen is increased in the second week and reduced in the third to mirror physiology (Guillebaud 1984, 1985).

The mode of action includes the prevention of ovulation by suppression of follicle stimulating and luteinising hormones (Guillebaud 1984). In addition, progesterone makes the cervical mucus impenetrable to sperm, creates an endometrial lining not appropriate for implantation and slows down motility of the fallopian tubes

(Guillebaud 1984). The latter delays entry of the ovum (if ovulation occurs) into the uterine cavity.

The effectiveness of oral contraception depends on the maintenance of hormone levels. If a tablet is forgotten, it must be taken as soon as its omission is discovered (Guillebaud 1987). If the delay is more than 12 hours, other contraceptive techniques must be used for the next 7 days (Guillebaud 1987). Gastric disturbances can affect absorption, necessitating the use of other measures to prevent conception (Rowlands 1987).

The current low-dosage pills cause fewer side-effects (Guillebaud 1985). Minor disorders include weight gain, breakthrough bleeding, nausea, altered libido, mild depression and amenorrhoea (Guillebaud 1984). More serious effects are cardiovascular disorders including cerebral-vascular accidents, hypertension and thromboemboli together with a possible increased risk of cancers of the breast and cervix (McEwan 1985a, 1985b). The risks of cardiovascular complications are significantly greater amongst women who smoke (Croft and Hannaford 1989). Combined oral contraception is contra-indicated in women with:

Hypertension	Obesity
Over 45 if a non-smoker	Over 35 if a smoker
Previous thromboembolism	Presence of cardiac anomalies
Diabetes mellitus with complications	Liver disorder
Lactation (oestrogen inhibits prolactin production)	Pregnancy (Nicholas 1987)

Care should also be taken by those women with bad varicose veins.

Before prescribing contraception, the doctor must check the woman's history for the presence of risk factors, and measure her weight and blood pressure. The woman should be seen again in 3 months to remeasure these parameters (Guillebaud 1984). On discontinuation of use, there may be a 2–3 month delay before ovulation resumes (Guillebaud 1985). Indeed a couple who wish to start a family are advised to use an alternative contraceptive method for 3 months after discontinuing oral contraception.

Progesterone-only pill (also known as the mini pill)

This pill should be taken at the same time each day with no omissions. The progesterone-only pill does not inhibit ovulation (Guillebaud 1985); it relies on the uterine lining being inappropriate for the fertilised ovum, preventing passage of sperm through the cervix. Effects on the menstrual cycle vary from none to amenorrhoea (Guillebaud 1984).

The effect of progesterone on cervical mucus is at a maximum 4 hours after the dose is taken and lasts approximately 20 hours (Fotherby 1982). It is therefore vital that the pill is taken at the same time each day, usually in the early evening (Rowlands 1987). Progesterone-only pills are useful for breast-feeding mothers, as there is no inhibition of prolactin production (Dewart and Loudon 1987). In those women at risk of cardiovascular disturbances with the combined pill, this pill may be appropriate (Elstein and Nuttall 1982). The failure rate is 0.3–5 pregnancies/100 woman years as compared to 0.2–1/100 woman years for the combined pill (Prescriber's Journal 1987).

Post-coital contraception

This involves the woman taking 100 mg of ethinyloestradiol with 500 mg of levonorgestrel within 72 hours of unprotected intercourse and repeating the dosage after 12 hours (Yuzpe and Lancee 1977). Using a progestogen in combination with the oestrogen reduces the incidence of nausea (Bromwich 1985). The treatment is for use in an emergency only (for example, following breakage of a sheath, or rape) and not for routine use. In the United Kingdom the 'morning-after' pill is available on prescription from general practitioners and family planning clinics.

Slow-release injectable progesterone

This acts in a similar way to the mini pill but the fact that it is a slow-release, intramuscular injection means that it is long-lasting (up to 3 months) and minimises the risk of conception (Wilson 1988). Depo-provera is the main type licensed for use in the United Kingdom. It is used where conception would be hazardous (for example, following rubella immunisation) or in those who have failed with other methods (Wilson 1988). The effect on the menstrual cycle is variable, with amenorrhoea and irregular bleeding being common (Wilson 1988). The return of fertility may be delayed by up to 8–12 months after use (Pardthaisong 1984).

There has been much controversy over the use of depo injections with the mentally handicapped and for women whose full informed consent has not been obtained. It has also been used controversially in some poor countries as part of government-sponsored population control measures (Lorraine 1985).

The future

Experiments are progressing with new delivery systems for hormonal contraceptives, usually providing a slow release of progestogen. These include subdermal implants which are placed on the underside of the upper arm (Drife 1989). The implant is designed to last for five years, although it is easily removed at any time (Drife 1989). Another development is the use of hormone-impregnated vaginal rings. These are designed to stay *in situ* for three weeks, to be removed for one and then replaced in a pattern similar to that used for the combined pill (Drife 1989). Current trials involve a mixture of oestrogen with a synthetic progestogen. A multicentre trial of the rings is underway (Drife 1989). Research into male methods of hormonal contraception is continuing, although most simple methods of stopping spermatogenesis have an effect on the libido.

Sterilisation

There has been a rise in the number of men and women asking to be sterilised, having decided that they have completed their family (Wellings 1986). It is not something to be undertaken lightly. The difficulty of successful reversal necessitates careful counselling for the couple, in case they would be better suited by a reversible method of contraception (Drife 1988). The techniques carry a very small risk of failure, about which the couple should be warned (Drife 1988). Many couples experience an increase in their level of sexual satisfaction once the fear of pregnancy has been removed.

Female sterilisation (bilateral tubal ligation) involves the clipping, diathermy or surgical division of the fallopian tubes during a laparoscopy, usually carried out under general anaesthesia (Drife 1988). The removed portion of the tube is usually sent for histological examination to ensure that it is the tube and not a portion of the broad ligament which has been divided. The operation can be performed while the woman is menstruating, so that her non-pregnant state can be confirmed (Drife 1988).

Should the women be delivered by caesarean section for obstetric reasons, the sterilisation can be performed at that time. Otherwise it is usually left until at least 3 months after the birth, when the risk of thromboembolic disturbances is less. Since many couples wanting sterilisation have a small family, this delay is advised until the period of high risk for a sudden infant death has passed.

Vasectomy involves the division and suturing of both the man's vas deferens. This is performed under local anaesthetic and it is a less invasive procedure than female sterilisation (Drife 1988). The scrotum may remain oedematous for 48 hours or more, but discomfort usually clears rapidly. Fourteen percent of men experience scrotal swelling and pain in the first fortnight after the operation (Drife 1988). It is important for the couple to continue to use other forms of contraception (and to have regular intercourse) until two successive sperm counts are negative. This can take up to 4 months; samples are usually tested at 3 and 4 months after surgery. Following a vasectomy, spermatozoa continue to be produced. They are absorbed by phagocytosis. In 50% of cases, antisperm antibodies develop; it is the existence of these which severely limits the successful rate of pregnancy following reversal should anastomosis be achieved (Drife 1989).

References

Bounds W and Guillebaud J (1984) 'Randomised comparison of the use-effectiveness and patient acceptability of the colltex (Today) contraceptive sponge and the diaphragm' *British Journal of Family Planning* 10: 69–75

Bounds W, Guillebaud J, Stewart L and Steele S J (1988) 'A female condom (Femshield): A study of its user acceptability' *British Journal of Family Planning* 14: 83–7

Bowen-Simpkins P (1988) 'Contraception by age group' *Practitioner* 232(Jan): 15–20

Bromwich P (1985) 'Post-coital contraception' *The Practitioner* 229: 427–9

Calvert J P (1987) 'Reversal of female sterilisation' *British Medical Journal* 294: 140–1

Chamberlain G (1989) 'Obstetrics after the White paper' *British Medical Journal* 298: 702–3

Collins (1989) *Concise Dictionary Plus* Collins: London

Croft P and Hannaford P C (1989) 'Risk factors for acute myocardial infarction in women: evidence from the Royal College of General Practitioner's oral contraception study' *British Medical Journal* 298: 165–8

Department of Health and Social Security (1988) *Contraceptive Trends in Great Britain 1974–86* DHSS: London

Dewart P J and Loudon N B (1987) 'Contraception and lactation' *Midwife, Health Visitor and Community Nurse* 23(8): 333–4

Drife J O (1988) 'Sterilisation–the before and after' *Practitioner* 232: 39–43

Drife J O (1989) 'New developments in contraception' in J Studd (ed) *Progress in Obstetrics and Gynaecology Vol 7* 245–62 Churchill Livingstone: Edinburgh

Eccles A (1982) *Obstetrics and Gynaecology in Tudor and Stuart England* Croom Helm: London

Eddy C A and Pauerstein C J (1980) 'Anatomy and physiology of the fallopian tube' *Clinical Obstetrics and Gynecology* 23: 1177

Elstein M and Nuttall I D (1982) 'Progestogen-only contraception' in J Studd (ed) *Progress in Obstetrics and Gynaecology Vol 2* 167–83 Churchill Livingstone: Edinburgh

Flynn A M and Brooks M (1984) *A Manual of Natural Family Planning* George Allen and Unwin: London

Fotherby K (1982) 'The progestogen-only contraceptive pill' *British Journal of Family Planning* 8: 7–10

Guillebaud J C (1984) *The Pill* Oxford University Press: Oxford

Guillebaud J C (1985) *Contraception: Your Questions Answered* Pitman: London

Guillebaud J C (1987) 'The forgotten pill–and the paramount importance of the pill-free week' *British Journal of Family Planning* Suppl 12: 35–43

Hickerton M (1985) 'Cultural influence and contraception' *The Practitioner* 229: 393–4

Hicks D R, Martin L S and Getchell J P (1985) 'Inactivation of HTLV–III/LAV infected cultures of normal human lymphocytes with nonoxynol-9 in vitro' *Lancet* ii: 1422

Himes N E (1970) *Medical History of Contraception* Schoken Books: New York

Howie P W, McNeilly A S, Houston M J, Cook A and Boyle H (1982) 'Fertility after childbirth: postpartum ovulation and menstruation in bottle and breast feeding methods' *Clinical Endocrinology* 17: 3323–32

Jelliffe D B and Jelliffe E F P (1978) *Human Milk in the Modern World* Oxford University Press: Oxford

Johnson V, Masters M and Cramer Lewis K (1974) in M L Calderone (ed) *Manual of Family Planning and Contraceptive Practice* 237–8 Williams and Watkins: Baltimore, Cited by Tayob and Guillebaud (1990)

Lehfeldt H (1987) '60 years of contraception' *Midwife, Health Visitor and Community Nurse* 23(7): 282–5

Llewellyn-Davies M (1978) *Maternity: Letters From Working Women* Virago: London

Lobb M O (1987) 'Teenage pregnancies' *Update* 1 Oct: 622–8

Lorraine J A (1985) 'Family planning: the global challenge' *Practitioner* 229: 407–12

Macfarlane A (1986) *Marriage and Love in England 1300–1840* Blackwell: Oxford

McEwan J (1985a) 'Hormonal contraception methods' *The Practitioner* 229: 415–23

McEwan J (1985b) 'Hormonal methods of contraception and their adverse effects' in J Studd (ed) *Progress in Obstetrics and Gynaecology Vol 5* 259–75 Churchill Livingstone: Edinburgh

McEwan J (1986) 'Contraceptive sponges' *Maternal and Child Health* 11(10): 338–41

McNeilly A S, Glasier A F, Howie P W, Houston M J, Cook A and Boyle H (1983) 'Fertility after childbirth: pregnancy associated with breast feeding' *Clinical Endocrinology* 18: 167–73

Moyer D L and Shaw S T (1980) 'Mode of action of intrauterine devices' in E S E Hafetz (ed) *Human Reproduction, Conception and Contraception (2nd edn)* 661–81 Harper and Row: New York

Murphy-Black T (1989) *Postnatal Care at Home: A Descriptive Study of Mothers' Needs and the Maternity Services* Department of Nursing Studies: University of Edinburgh

Nicholas N S (1987) 'What pill?' *Maternal and Child Health* 12(11): 316–20

Norman C (1986) *Charting the Fertility Cycle* Natural Family Planning Centre: Birmingham

Pardthaisong T (1984) 'Return of fertility after use of the injectable contraceptive Depo-Povera: 'Updated data analysis' *Journal of Biosocial Science* 16: 23–4

Potts M (1988) 'The IUD' *The Practitioner* 232(Jan): 23–8

Prescriber's Journal (1987) 'User failure rates for different methods of contraception/100 woman-years' *Prescriber's Journal* 13

Rowlands S (1983) 'Postcoital contraception' *Maternal and Child Health* 8(12): 468–70

Rowlands S (1987) 'Pill-taking regime' *Midwife, Health Visitor and Community Nurse* 23(12): 531–2

Royston E and Armstrong S (1989) *Preventing Maternal Deaths* WHO: Geneva

Salih D (1987) 'Complications of intra-uterine contraceptive devices' *Maternal and Child Health* 12(12): 355–59

Seymour J (1986) 'No longer beyond the pill' *Nursing Times* 82(26 Mar): 19–20

Silverton L I (1988) *Midwifery Education in the USA* School of Social Sciences, University College of Swansea

Snowden R (1985) *Consumer Choices in Family Planning* Family Planning Association: London

Stott P (1988) 'Rediscovering the diaphragm' *British Medical Journal* 296: 377–8

Tacchi D A (1989) 'The future of family planning clinics' *Maternal and Child Health* 14(10): 338–40

Tayob Y and Guillebaud J (1990) 'Barrier methods of contraception' in J Studd (ed) *Progress in Obstetrics and Gynaecology Vol 8* 371–90 Churchill Livingstone: Edinburgh

Thapa S, Short R V and Potts M (1988) 'Breast feeding, child spacing and their effects on child survival' *Nature* 335(10): 679–82

Timmins N (1984) 'Victory for Gillick' *The Times* Dec 11: 1

Van Os W A A (1983) 'Intrauterine devices' in J Studd (ed) *Progress in Obstetrics and Gynaecology Vol 3* 293–304 Churchill Livingstone: Edinburgh

van Noord-Zaadstra B M, Looman C W N, Alsbach H, Habbema J D F, te Velde E R and Karbaat J (1991) 'Delaying childbearing: effect of age on fecundity and outcome of pregnancy' *British Medical Journal* 302: 1361–5

Vessey M, Doll E, Peto R, Johnson B and Wiggins P (1976) 'A long-term follow-up study of women using different methods of contraception' *Journal of Biosocial Science* 8: 375–427

Vessey M, Lawless M and Yeates D (1982) 'Efficiency of different contraceptive measures' *Lancet* i: 841–2

Warren V M C and Masil J R (1988) 'Cultural and religious attitudes in family planning' *Midwife, Health Visitor and Community Nurse* 24(9): 381–3

Wellings K (1986) 'Sterilisation trends' *British Medical Journal* 292: 1029–30

Wilson E (1988) 'Injectable contraception' *The Practitioner* 232(Jan): 32–6

Wohl A S (1983) *Endangered Lives: Public Health in Victorian Britain* J M Dent and Sons: London

Yuzpe A A and Lancee W J (1977) 'Ethinyl estradiol and d-norgestrel as a post-coital contraceptive' *Fertility and Sterility* 28: 932–6

31   Loss and grief in midwifery practice

'Grief is a normal reaction to the loss of something or someone that/who is loved.' (Davies 1988, p. 4)

This chapter will first describe some of the emotions experienced by the bereaved, with mention of both the stages and tasks of grieving. Specific situations in which grief is encountered in midwifery will be discussed, together with the role of the midwife and the place of voluntary agencies. Finally the epidemiology, prevention and management of sudden infant death syndrome (SIDS) will be considered.

Grief

The processes surrounding the psychological effects of grief have been well described, beginning with the work of Lindemann (1944), a Freudian psychoanalyst. It was however the writings of Kubler-Ross (1970) which gained popularity, as she described the grief process in easily accessible terms. It must be remembered that grief is a perfectly normal and necessary reaction to loss (Worden 1982). The emotions involved are so intense that they can overwhelm all other feelings. Because each episode of loss is as different as our relationship with the person or object lost, every grief episode is different (Davies 1988). We are not able to practise grieving or to 'get good at it'. Events which can provoke grief include the death (or departure) of a loved person, the loss of an idea or a hope (as in the case of infertility), and the loss of material goods (such as following a burglary or a fire) (Davies 1988).

Worden (1982) refers to the tasks of mourning which the bereaved person must undertake in order to resolve or come to terms with their loss successfully. This does not mean, however, that the deceased is forgotten but that the bereaved individual is able to live without the person who has died. The tasks of mourning are:

1. To accept the reality of the loss.
2. To experience the pain of grief.
3. To adjust to an environment from which the deceased is missing.
4. To withdraw emotional energy and to reinvest it in another relationship (Worden 1982).

It could be argued that Worden's (1982) tasks of grief are more appropriate than Kubler-Ross's (1970) stages of grief which imply a stepwise progression from one stage to the next. The content of the stages: denial and isolation, anger, bargaining, depression and acceptance (Kubler-Ross 1970) are incorporated within the tasks to be undertaken, but they may be present as part of more than one task.

To accept the reality of the loss. When a death, however much it was anticipated, actually occurs, there is always a sense of unreality. Kubler-Ross (1970) refers to this as 'denial' but the term 'shock' as suggested by Lindemann (1944) is often more appropriate, since it implies disbelief rather than an active act of denial (Karl 1987). While accomplishing this task of acceptance, the bereaved person may seek out the loved one. Worden (1982) states that accepting that the person in the crowd who resembles the deceased is someone else is the beginning of accepting the reality of the loss.

When this task is not completed, denial can occur. This can take the form of 'denying the facts of the loss' by retaining the person's belongings or bedroom to await their return (Worden 1982). This is normal behaviour in the early weeks, but it becomes denial if it continues for months or years. Following the death of a young child, the nursery and toys may be kept as a shrine, inhibiting acceptance of the reality of the loss (Worden 1982).

Another form of denial is to minimise the meaning of the loss by reducing the deceased person's importance. This may be by removing every trace of the deceased, as much a sign of denial as mummification of their belongings (Davies 1988). An additional way of reducing the meaning of the loss is to employ 'selective memory' (Worden 1982). This results in a blocking of memories, both abstract and visual. The final form of denial is not to accept that the death is irreversible. The actions taken may include talking to the deceased or a continued reliance on spiritualism (Worden 1982). This is not the same as looking forward to a reunion with the deceased after the bereaved person's own death.

To experience pain and grief. The pain can be physical, emotional or behavioural. Parkes (1972) comments that anything which interferes with feeling the pain (avoidance or suppression), will increase the time taken to resolve the grief. The use of alcohol or prescribed medication to numb the pain will only prolong the time taken to complete this task (Davies 1988). In addition, the unacceptability of showing grief in some sections of our society can cause the bereaved person to feel that they should not need to grieve (Worden 1982). Amongst cultures where there are specific behaviours designed to release the grief, it appears that this task may be easier (but not easy) to accomplish. Feelings experienced at this time may include painful yearning, anger at the bereaved for having left and guilt (especially following sudden death) for acts of omission and commission.

In addition to suppressing the pain felt by internalising their emotions, some people may keep themselves very busy with frenetic activity or travelling extensively to find relief from their grief (Davies 1988). Because the pain has to be felt at some time, completion of this task is delayed (Worden 1982).

To adjust to an environment in which the deceased is missing. This is a particularly difficult task, because it is only at this stage that the bereaved person comes to appreciate fully the roles filled by the deceased (Parkes 1972). The actions required to undertake this task depend on the role of the deceased (Worden 1982). A widow may have to learn how to manage household accounts or a widower to cook or to care for children. With the death of a baby or a young child, the changes involve not doing things (such as bathing or reading to the child) rather than undertaking different activities. When the person does not adjust, he/she promotes personal helplessness, may neglect themself and withdraw from the world (Worden 1982).

To withdraw emotional energy and reinvest it in other relationships. This does not mean that the deceased is forgotten or in any sense dishonoured (Worden 1982). Bereaved parents may be anxious later about embarking on another pregnancy, in case that baby should also die (Lewis 1989). They may also feel that a new baby will be seen by others as a replacement for the one they have lost (Bourne 1983). This task is probably the most difficult (Worden 1982). Progress through it can be disrupted by meeting people who do not know of the bereavement. This can cause acute embarrassment on both sides and prevent the bereaved person going out and renewing social contacts (Davies 1988).

To assist people to accomplish their tasks of grief are professional and voluntary agencies. In the case of perinatal death, there may be a bereavement counselling midwife, who the parents can contact if they feel the need. There are also specific local initiatives involving midwives, psychologists, nurses, health visitors and general practitioners, who either run support groups or provide counselling. Voluntary agencies provide support groups in most areas. The scope of each agency's responsibility depends on which groups have local representation. Major groups are the Stillbirth and Neonatal Death Society (SANDS), the Society After Termination for Abnormality (SATFA) and the Society for Compassionate Friends.

Maternity and loss

This section will consider events related to childbirth which can give rise to grief.

They will be approached in chronological order from subfertility through to infant death. The intention is to alert midwives to areas in which a sensitive approach is required and to suggest some possible course of action. Suggestions for more detailed reading regarding the events included (other than those referred to in the text) will be given at the end of this chapter.

Subfertility

Where a couple are having problems conceiving, one or both may experience grief over the baby that they cannot have (Borg and Lasker 1981). It is not unknown for some women to grieve at the start of every menstrual period. Where the woman has had a hysterectomy, she may experience grief that her ability to have a(nother) child is now at an end. Coming to terms with infertility may cause the couple to seek to adopt a baby or to lavish their affections on an animal. In some cultures where male babies are more acceptable than female, the woman may grieve if she produces a daughter (Samil 1989). Although midwives rarely care for women having subfertility treatment (except those for whom it is successful), it is necessary that they are aware of the desperation of some couples and of the emotional energy they invest whenever treatment (such as IVF) is given (Bryar and Silverton 1988).

Miscarriage

This is now recognised as an emotionally traumatic event (Jolly 1987). Whether the pregnancy was planned or not, the woman may feel guilt about whether her actions precipitated events (Borg and Lasker 1981; Moulder 1990). However early the miscarriage occurs, most couples will have already begun to plan for their new baby (Moulder 1990). The couple may feel themselves to be failures (Borg and Lasker 1981). Because miscarriage is a common event which is rarely mentioned, there is little 'folk knowledge' passed on which would help couples in this situation (Borg and Lasker 1981). Some professionals' attitude is that the couple should forget past events and simply 'try again'. It is, however, important to resolve the grief from this pregnancy before embarking upon another (Lewis 1989; Forrest *et al.* 1982). Medical staff are embarrassed by the woman's grief and, if she has been admitted to hospital, they may discharge her home as soon as possible (Moulder 1990). Where the miscarriage happens at an advanced stage of pregnancy, it is possible for the couple to see and hold their baby should they wish to do so (Lewis 1989). Although the hospital will usually arrange 'disposal' of the body, the couple can request to do this themselves. They are rarely informed of this right (Morris 1988).

Because the pregnancy was not far enough advanced, the couple may receive no visits after the miscarriage (for example, from a midwife). Also there may be no grave for them to visit and they may not have an image of the fetus which they can use when grieving (Moulder 1990). There is no legal recognition that the pregnancy ever occurred. Since miscarriages occur before the legal limit for birth notification of 24 weeks, there is no stillbirth certificate. For further information on the effect of miscarriage upon the woman, see Oakley *et al.* (1984).

Termination of pregnancy

Whatever the grounds, termination of pregnancy can give rise to feelings of grief. It was previously thought that termination of pregnancy on the grounds of fetal abnormality would be easier to accept. However guilt and shame are common emotions surrounding such procedures (Kenyon 1988). Many couples reported that the procedures to confirm abnormality were often delayed, information was not always readily given and that there was no way of commemorating the pregnancy (Kenyon 1988). A support group (SATFA) has been established to offer help to couples after termination for abnormality. In some areas, nurses and midwives offer a counselling service for affected parents.

Having a termination of pregnancy for 'social' reasons is sometimes accompanied by guilt about having 'killed' a normal baby (McAll 1982). Having to keep the pregnancy secret from family and friends, together with religious considerations and publicity from anti-abortion pressure groups can lead to suppression of grief (Bryar and Silverton 1988). Guilt and grief may be reawakened during a later pregnancy or birth (Forrest 1989). This can be especially traumatic where the woman's partner is not aware of the previous pregnancy. The mother will grieve for the baby she did not have (Jolly 1987). In a similar way, women whose baby is adopted will grieve for their loss, knowing that the baby is alive somewhere (Jolly 1987). On every birthday their grief is particularly reawakened by imagining what their child is doing at that time. For all these women, the midwife must have great sensitivity when taking a history in a subsequent pregnancy. She must respect the mother's right to privacy regarding her obstetric history. During labour and birth, the midwife should always be aware of the possibility of reawakening previously unresolved grief (Forrest 1989). The mother may wish to talk about past events and the midwife must be available to listen. Where the partner is unaware of the previous pregnancy, support from the midwife must be given with great tact and diplomacy.

Stillbirth

The role of the midwife in caring for parents following a stillbirth has received most attention in recent years. In 1984, a joint Health Education Council and Royal College of Midwives Workshop was held to consider the impact of stillbirth on midwifery practice (Kohner 1985). In this chapter, consideration will be given to the care of a couple with a known intrauterine death, rather than a death occurring during labour. To have a stillbirth is an especially traumatic event (Bourne 1983; Giles 1985). Although each case must be managed according to individual circumstances, stillbirth is never anticipated. However much the mother has been anxious about a cessation of fetal movements, there is always the possibility that the baby is all right (Borg and Lasker 1981).

Preparations for the birth and care at home of the new baby will be well advanced. Friends and relatives will be eagerly anticipating the new arrival. The way in which the discovery and the diagnosis of a stillbirth are managed sets the tone for the whole event. Mothers often suspect that all is not well and hope that they will be proved wrong (Thomson 1988). The midwife must be aware of her non-verbal communication at this time. The mother is very sensitive to any signals, such as those of anxiety, given by the midwife. Although non-detection of the fetal heart does not confirm the diagnosis, the mother will be aware that all is not well. Neilson (1986) recommends that ultrasonography is available around the clock to save women in this situation having to wait for confirmation of the diagnosis overnight or even until after the weekend. It is important to ask the woman whether she wishes to summon her partner or a friend to stay with her until the tests can be performed. There is always disagreement about whether the woman should return home alone to tell her partner or if he should be summoned by telephone. If this is the case, what should he be told? Is knowing nothing more upsetting than knowing the truth? The mother may be unable (in her shocked state) to make a decision. The midwife must consider the particular circumstances, in discussion with the mother if the latter is unable to decide.

Once the diagnosis has been made, the next decision is whether or not to induce labour. It may be be necessary for obstetric reasons, such as the presence of ruptured membranes, with the risk of intrauterine infection, or severe antepartum haemorrhage with risks of coagulation disturbances (Tindall and Reid 1989). In the absence of obstetric complications, women can be given the choice whether to wait for spontaneous labour or to have it induced. Some women cannot wait for things to be over (Bourne 1983) whereas others want time to adjust to their loss (Jolly 1987). If the woman chooses to wait, she will experience the sensation of the fetus 'moving' inside her in response to changes in posture. Where 69 women were given the choice, Kellner et al. (1984) found that 32 (46%) chose immediate delivery whereas 37 (53%) preferred to wait. Spontaneous labour will occur within 2 weeks of intrauterine death in 80% of women, with only 10% being undelivered after 3 weeks (Kellner et al. 1984).

It may be possible to offer the mother choice in the place of delivery. Most labour wards are busy places, where babies can be heard crying. Parents should be warned of this (Kohner 1985). Depending on the mother's gestation and the state of her cervix, induction of labour is usually by extra-amniotic prostaglandin (Tindall and Reid 1989). If oxytocin is used, there is an argument as to whether the membranes should be ruptured (Tindall and Reid 1989). Since labour can be long, due to early gestation and a softer than usual presenting part, there is a risk of developing infection if delivery is delayed (Tindall and Reid 1989). However, tonic contractions may result following oxytocin administration when spontaneous rupture of the membranes occurs (Keirse and Chalmers 1989). Caesarean section would only be considered in cases of gross cephalopelvic disproportion, uterine rupture or where the mother has had two or more previous operative deliveries (Tindall and Reid 1989).

It was accepted practice to give the mother an epidural to relieve her from the physical pain, accompanied by intramuscular narcotics to keep her unaware of what was happening (Thomson 1988). This often resulted in a mother who was unaware of what had transpired, together with a feeling of unreality. Thomson (1988) questions whose grief are we dealing with, that of the parents or that of the midwife? The conduct of the birth should be discussed with the parents if possible before, or if not during, the labour. It is important that the father is included as much as possible. Since it is difficult to know when the fetus died, the couple should be prepared for the fact that the baby's skin may be peeling (Thomson 1988). One practice which has been reported is to deliver the baby onto warm drapes which are placed at the end of the bed until the placenta has been delivered (Thomson 1988). The midwife can then quickly examine the baby for obvious abnormalities; the baby is then wrapped up and given to the parents in such a way that they see first what is normal (Thomson 1988; Forrest 1989). They can then hold their baby and if they wish, unwrap him/her and examine his/her body (Forrest 1989). Any abnormality is less serious than the deformities imagined if the couple have not seen their child. Should the couple not wish to see their baby, the child should be dressed and photographs taken which minimise any abnormality (Forrest 1989). These should then be kept in the case notes, in case the parents request them (Brierley 1988).

Sometimes the couple change their minds and the baby can be brought to them so that they can see him/her (Brierley 1988). In some hospitals, there is a family room in the mortuary where the couple (and their other children if they so wish) can be alone with the baby (Brierley 1988). A keepsake, such as a name band or a lock of hair, can be offered to the parents, along with the photograph. They should be allowed as much time and privacy as they wish with their baby (Forrest 1989). Some hospitals have a room set aside on the postnatal or labour ward where the family can see their baby without the necessity of visiting the mortuary.

Most hospitals in the United Kingdom now have facilities to allow the partner to stay overnight. This can lessen the need for night sedation for the mother (Kohner 1985). In some areas, they have a room with a double bed. The couple should be given the choice as to where they would prefer to be cared for: in a postnatal, antenatal or gynaecological ward (Thomson 1988) and either in an open ward, with the advantage of support from other women but little privacy, or in a single room, where the woman can feel very lonely and it is easy for the staff through embarrassment to isolate her. The length of stay depends on individual needs (Kohner 1985). The mother may prefer to stay longer in hospital until she feels more settled. Some mothers gain comfort from cuddling a live baby, which can help prevent 'empty arm syndrome' (Borg and Lasker 1981; Forrest 1989).

With respect to the formalities after a stillbirth, the parents (usually the father) will be asked if they give permission for a post-mortem examination. Although this may help to discover the cause of death, it is not acceptable to some religious groups and also to some others who cannot bear the thought of further injury to their baby (Forrest 1989). In the United Kingdom the stillbirth must be registered. A certificate of stillbirth is required before a burial can be arranged.

The funeral can be arranged (at no cost) by the health authority in a communal grave, although most authorities now maintain a book of remembrance or have a monument at the cemetery. Since a funeral is part of the way in which society recognises that someone has died, many parents prefer to arrange their own (Engel 1964). This can be expensive, depending whether or not the baby has his/her own grave. If the parents do attend the funeral they should be forewarned about the small size of the coffin (Thomson 1988).

When the mother goes home, she should be prepared for the onset of lactation, if it has not already occurred (Forrest 1989). In some cases, stilboestrol may be used for the suppression of lactation, although stilboestrol is not without its risks. The return home is traumatic, as the couple will have to face friends and relatives (Bourne 1968). It is not advisable to clear away any preparations made for the baby without prior discussion with the parents as this may increase their sense of unreality (Thomson 1988). Some couples view the putting away of the baby's possessions as a part of the process of saying goodbye. The community midwife will visit as normal, but it is important that other professionals are alerted to what has happened so that they do not call unnecessarily or unprepared (Forrest 1989). The couple should be referred to local bereavement counselling services or to voluntary agencies as appropriate. They should be warned that friends and acquaintances will be embarrassed and may avoid them (Bourne 1968).

Other children in the family may also be grief-stricken (Lewis 1989). They can tell that their parents are upset and that their routine has been disrupted, but they may not know why (Cain *et al.* 1964). They may even blame themselves for the loss of the baby, if they were not looking forward to the new arrival (Lewis 1989). Where one twin is stillborn and the other living, the parents may find it hard to grieve while caring for their surviving baby.

Professionals find it very hard to cope with such an abnormal event (Kohner 1985). Midwives are accustomed to delivering live babies and to working in a positive environment. Caring for a bereaved couple can be an emotionally draining experience for the midwife. She must be able to show her own distress (this can be helpful to the couple) and also to obtain support from her colleagues (Kohner 1985; Thomson 1988). In some areas, staff support groups have been established (Roch 1987). Staff can experience stress from having to provide support and care for grieving and rejoicing couples at the same time.

Maternal death

Although this is thankfully a rare event, its occurrence can put great strain on the partner and any children in the family. If the baby survives, the father is faced with the reality of caring for a small infant and continuing in paid employment (Dunn 1987). The occurrence of a maternal death also causes stress and unhappiness to those professionals involved, who may blame their actions for the outcome.

Handicap

The birth of a handicapped baby is particularly traumatic for his/her parents (Bicknell 1983). They can experience guilt over the effects of their past behaviour on the baby, whether this caused the abnormality or not (Clifford 1985). While they are grieving for the loss of the normal baby whose birth they were anticipating, they must also care for and nurture the baby they do have. They will also grieve for what they perceive as the loss of normal parenthood and a normal future (Bicknell 1983). Guilt and grief can manifest themselves in behaviour as disparate as overprotective caring or neglect (see Chapter 38 for more details).

Sudden infant death syndrome

The death of a child who is known as a person by his/her parents and siblings gives rise to severe grief (Jolly 1987). Even where the child has been ill, for example in a Neonatal Intensive Care Unit, the loss of hope is accompanied by grieving (Jolly 1987). This section will concentrate on sudden infant death syndrome (SIDS). SIDS is the

> 'sudden death of any infant or young child which is unexpected by history and which a thorough post mortem examination fails to demonstrate an adequate cause of death'. (Beckwith 1983, p. 15)

SIDS is the leading cause of death in children aged between 1 month and 1 year (Office of Population Censuses and Surveys 1988). It occurs in the United Kingdom in approximately 2.24 : 1000 live births (Office of Population Censuses and Surveys 1988). Over 80% of infant deaths from SIDS occur between 1 and 6 months of age, with 42% in babies aged 2 or 3 months (Office of Population Censuses and Surveys 1988). Sixty-six per cent of the deaths occur during the winter months of October to March (Office of Population Censuses and Surveys 1988). Boys are at greater risk than girls, as are preterm and low birthweight infants, multiple births and children of mothers of high parity, those who smoke and those who bottle feed (Limerick 1985b).

Much time has been spent analysing the epidemiological and aetiological aspects of SIDS. It has been described as a syndrome because it is not a discrete disease entity (Emery 1989). The causes of SIDS are far from clear. Suggested causes include infant botulism infection (Lancet 1986); overheating due to overwrapping in warm rooms (Sunderland and Emery 1981); the fear paralysis reflex, which can cause apneoa in animals in response to separation from parents or physical restraint (Murphy *et al.* 1986); cardiovascular (Southall *et al.* 1977) and respiratory control abnormalities (Fleming and Levine 1983); metabolic disorders (Howat *et al.* 1984); deficiencies of surfactant, similar to changes seen in the presence of lower respiratory tract infection (Morley *et al.* 1982); and developmental abnormalities (Quattrochi *et al.* 1980).

Initiatives to reduce infant deaths have involved devising a scoring system to assess the presence of risk factors. The factors included are high maternal parity, short duration of the second stage of labour and young maternal age (Taylor *et al.* 1983). A further score is made at 1 month, taking into account the presence of apnoeaic or cyanotic attacks while in hospital, problems with feeding and short interval since the previous birth (Taylor *et al.* 1983). Children categorised as being at high risk received extra visits from health visitors, including assessment of weight gain. This helps to reduce the numbers of children showing minor signs of illness or behaviour in the days prior to sudden death (Taylor *et al.* 1983). Using the combined system there was a 50% reduction in cases of SIDS (Carpenter and Emery 1977). In the United Kingdom the Government has launched a campaign to discourage parents from putting their baby down to sleep on its front. They are advised to place their baby on its back or side.

In another scheme, it was noted that intense health surveillance by health visitors, with special attention to weight loss, static weight or poor weight gain, reduced the occurrence of SIDS (Powell 1985). The use of weight centile charts is an important part of the system. Parents were also instructed about the recognition of early signs of illness or changes in their child's behaviour. They were encouraged to seek medical assistance whenever they were worried (Powell 1985). GPs were informed about the identity of babies at high risk in their practice, so they could identify priorities. Additional information on the maintenance of the baby's temperature without overheating was also given to parents (Powell 1985).

Madeley (1988) argues that there has been a fall in the incidence of SIDS which is unrelated to the surveillance schemes. The fall in birthrate, especially amongst families of manual workers, and improved birth intervals may be contributory factors (Madeley 1988). He states that the scoring systems were a very crude tool which was inaccurate in identifying at-risk babies. He suggested that greater attention should be paid to managing respiratory tract infections, especially during the winter, and to the raising of health standards generally (Madeley 1988). One factor currently under investigation is the baby's sleeping position; it has been suggested that the prone position is more likely to predispose to SIDS (de Jonge *et al.* 1989).

Although SIDS is also known as 'cot death', death can occur at any time, not just when the baby is asleep. Barker (1987) suggests that keeping the baby in close physical contact with an adult continuously stimulates the baby's senses and minimises the risks of apnoea. It could also reduce the risks of overheating. When the baby is discovered, parents often attempt resuscitation measures which are occasionally successful (Catchpole 1984). If their efforts are unsuccessful, there then follows the trip to hospital in a private car or ambulance or the calling of a general practitioner. The parents' distress (and that of other family members) is heightened by the fact that, as this is a sudden death, both the police and the coroner have to be informed (Limerick 1985b). It is also usual for a post-mortem to be performed before a certificate of burial can be obtained. Most authorities are becoming more sensitive to the needs of the parents and it is not unusual for the visit by the police (to inspect the place of death) to be undertaken out of uniform and in an unmarked car. Visits by the GP and health visitor can be of comfort to the parents and can also help in explaining some of the practicalities.

Because this is a sudden death, the parents will not have experienced any anticipatory grief; they may initially be shocked and numb (Worden 1982). They may need help to make arrangements; support will also be needed for siblings and grieving grandparents. Following the post-mortem, the coroner will decide if there needs to be an inquest. If not, the funeral can be arranged. The parents will also need to come to terms with memories of their baby in every room of the house. Once the results of the post-mortem (if any) are known, this can help the parents to realise that they are not to blame. Sensitive counselling is necessary, especially regarding subsequent pregnancies. The whole question of using an apnoea alarm (which sounds an alarm if the baby fails to breathe within a set time interval) for the next baby is contentious (Simpson 1987). Although the parents need to be instructed in resuscitation techniques for the alarms to be fully effective, they are useful in putting the parent's mind at rest and allowing them to sleep at night (Simpson 1987). The Foundation for the Study of Infant Deaths is undertaking a study of infants born to families who have had a previous sudden infant death. In the care of subsequent babies, the Foundation is comparing the effectiveness of regular assessment of weight gain against the use of apnoea alarms (Limerick 1985a).

References

Barker W (1987) 'Close encounters of a preventive kind' *Senior Nurse* 7(1): 13–5

Beckwith J B (1983) 'Sudden death in infancy' in B Knight (ed) *The Cot Death Syndrome* 15–41 Faber and Faber: London

Bicknell J (1983) 'The psychopathology of handicap' *British Journal of Medical Psychology* 56: 167–78

Borg S and Lasker J (1981) *When the Pregnancy Fails* Beacon: Boston

Bourne S (1968) 'The psychological effects of stillbirth on women and their doctors' *Journal of the College of General Practitioners* 16: 103

Bourne S (1983) 'Psychological impact of stillbirth' *The Practitioner* 227(1): 53–60

Brierley J (1988) 'Management of perinatal death' *Midwife, Health Visitor and Community Nurse* 24(3): 80–1

Bryar R M and Silverton L I (1988) *Bereavement in Pregnancy: A Workshop Report* School of Social Studies: University College of Swansea

Cain A C, Fast I and Erikson M E (1964) 'Children's disturbed reactions to the death of a sibling' *American Journal of Orthopsychiatry* 34: 741–52

Carpenter R G and Emery J L (1977) 'Multistage scoring system for identifying infants at risk of unexpected death' *Archives of Disease in Childhood* 52: 606–12

Catchpole A (1984) 'Near-miss sudden infant death' *Nursing Times* 16 May: 35–6

Clifford S (1985) 'The guilt factor' *Midwife, Health Visitor and Community Nurse* 21(10): 364–7

Davies R (1988) 'The grief process' in R M Bryar and L I Silverton (eds) *Bereavement in Pregnancy: A Workshop Report* 4–15 School of Social Studies: University College of Swansea de Jonge G A, Engleberts A C, Koomen-Liefting A J M and Kostense P J (1989) 'Cot death and prone sleeping position in The Netherlands' *British Medical Journal* 298: 722

Dunn S E (1987) 'Suddenly at home' *Midwives Chronicle* May: 132–4

Emery J L (1989) 'Is sudden infant death syndrome a diagnosis?' *British Medical Journal* 299: 1240

Engel G L (1964) 'Grief and grieving' *American Journal of Nursing* 64: 93–8

Fleming P J and Levine M R (1983) 'The development of stability of control of respiration in newborn infants: implications for the understanding and prediction of sudden infant death syndrome' *Intensive Care Medicine* 9: 43–6

Forrest G C (1989) 'Care of the bereaved after perinatal death' in I Chalmers, M Enkin and M J N C Keirse (eds) *Effective Care in Pregnancy and Childbirth* 1423–32 Oxford Medical: Oxford

Forrest G C, Standish E and Baum J D (1982) 'Support after perinatal death: a study of support and counselling after perinatal bereavement' *British Medical Journal* 285: 1475–9

Giles P F H (1985) 'The psychological response to stillbirth and neonatal death' in J Studd (ed) *Progress in Obstetrics and Gynaecology Vol 5* 134–45 Churchill Livingstone: Edinburgh

Howat A J, Bennett M J and Variend S (1984) 'Deficiency of medium chain fatty acyl co-enzyme A dehydrogenase presenting as sudden infant death syndrome' *British Medical Journal* 288: 976

Jolly J (1987) *Missed Beginnings. Death Before Life has Been Established* Austen Cornish: Reading

Karl G T (1987) 'A new look at grief' *Journal of Advanced Nursing* 12: 641–5

Keirse M J N C and Chalmers I (1989) 'Methods for inducing labour' in I Chalmers, M Enkin and M J N C Keirse (eds) *Effective Care in Pregnancy and Childbirth* 1057–79 Oxford Medical: Oxford

Kellner R, Donnelly H A and Gould S D (1984) 'Parental behaviour after perinatal death' *Obstetrics and Gynecology* 63: 809–14

Kenyon S (1988) 'Support after termination for fetal abnormality' *Midwives Chronicle* June: 190–1

Kohner N (1985) *Midwives and Stillbirth* Health Education Council: London

Kubler-Ross E (1970) *On Death and Dying* Tavistock: London

Lancet (1986) 'Editorial: Infant botulism' *Lancet* ii: 1256–7

Lewis E (1989) 'The grief of pregnancy loss' *Maternal and Child Health* 14(8): 275–7

Limerick S (1985a) 'Cot deaths: is prevention possible?' *Self Health* 6 March: 26–7

Limerick S (1985b) 'Cot deaths: where does the GP stand?' *Maternal and Child Health* 10(10): 294–8

Lindemann E (1944) 'Symptomology and management of acute grief' *American Journal of Psychiatry* 101(3): 141–8

Madeley R (1988) 'Preventing sudden infant death syndrome: future strategies' *Health Visitor* 61(8): 241–3

McAll K (1982) *Healing the Family Tree* Sheldon: London

Morley C J, Brown B D, Hill C M, Barson A J and Davies J A (1982) 'Surfactant abnormalities in babies dying from sudden infant death syndrome' *Lancet* i: 1320–3

Morris D (1988) 'Disposal arrangements for second trimester foetuses' *British Journal of Obstetrics and Gynaecology* 95(6): 545–6

Moulder C (1990) *Miscarriage: Women's Experiences and Needs* Pandora: London

Murphy M F G, Campbell M J and Jones D R (1986) 'Increased risk of sudden infant death syndrome in older infants at weekends' *British Medical Journal* 294: 364–5

Neilson J P (1986) 'Indications for ultrasonography in obstetrics' *Birth* 13(1): 16–20

Oakley A, McPherson A and Roberts H (1984) *Miscarriage* Fontana: London

Office of Population Censuses and Surveys (1988) *Sudden Infant Deaths 1985–7* Monitor DH3 88/3 OPCS: London

Parkes C M (1972) *Bereavement: Studies of Grief in Adult Life* International Universities Press: New York

Powell J (1985) 'Keeping watch' *Nursing Times* Community Outlook Jan: 15–19

Quattrochi J, Baba W, Liss L and Adrion W (1980) 'Sudden infant death syndrome; a preliminary study of reticular dendritic spines in infants with SIDS' *Brain Research* 181: 245–9

Roch S (1987) 'Sharing grief' *Nursing Times* 8 April: 52–3

Samil A R (1989) 'Obstetrics and Pakistani women' *British Medical Journal* 298: 1248–9

Simpson H (1987) 'Infantile apnoea and home monitoring' *British Medical Journal* 294: 1367

Southall D P, Arrowsmith W A, Oakley J R, McEnery G, Anderson R H and Shinebourne E A (1977) 'Prolonged QT interval and cardiac arrhythmias in two neonates: sudden infant death syndrome in one case' *Archives of Disease in Childhood* 190: 677–9

Sunderland R and Emery J L (1981) 'Febrile convulsions and cot death' *Lancet* ii: 176–8

Taylor E, Emery J L and Carpenter R G (1983) 'Identifying children at risk of unexpected death' *Lancet* ii: 1033–4

Thomson A M (1988) 'Midwives and stillbirth' in R M Bryar and L I Silverton (eds) *Bereavement in Pregnancy: A Workshop Report* 16–23 School of Social Studies: University College of Swansea

Tindall V R and Reid G D (1989) 'The management of intrauterine death' in J Studd (ed) *Progress in Obstetrics and Gynaecology Vol 7* 199–215 Churchill Livingstone: Edinburgh

Worden J W (1982) *Grief Counselling and Grief Therapy* Tavistock: London

Further reading

Dominica F (1987) 'Reflections on death in childhood' *British Medical Journal* 294: 108–10

Hughes P (1987) 'The management of bereaved mothers; what is best?' *Midwives Chronicle* Aug: 226–9

Lewis E (1987) 'Coping with the death of a twin' *Midwife, Health Visitor and Community Nurse* 23(4): 158–61

Robinson J (1987) 'A basket instead of a crib' *Senior Nurse* 7(1): 16–8

32   Adaptation of the newborn to extra-uterine life

This chapter considers the initiation of respiration by the newborn (neonatal resuscitation has been described in Chapter 21), circulatory and cardiac changes after birth, control of temperature, birth injuries and neonatal reflexes.

Initiation of respiration

Whilst in utero, the fetus has received freshly oxygenated blood from the placenta via the umbilical vein (Kelnar and Harvey 1987). Pressure on the right side of the fetal heart was greater than on the left, producing a right-to-left movement of blood through the foramen ovale (oval window) in the atrial septum (Assali *et al.* 1968). Little blood circulated through the lungs (Assali *et al.* 1968). Once the baby is born, it has to expand its lungs with air, increase greatly its pulmonary blood flow, initiate its gastrointestinal tract to function, maintain its body temperature and dispense with the temporary circulatory structures necessary for intrauterine life (for further details concerning fetal circulation see later).

The initiation of respiration relies on various interrelated factors:

1. Maturity. The baby requires a mature respiratory centre in the brain, developed lung tissue and the presence of surfactant to reduce surface tension, preventing alveolar collapse (Henderson-Smart 1986).

2. The respiratory centre is stimulated by raised serum carbon dioxide levels detected by chemoreceptors in the carotid artery and the aorta (Krauss *et al.* 1975). During the second stage of labour, expulsive uterine contractions inhibit placental gaseous exchange, increasing fetal carbon dioxide level. If this is too high, as occurs in cases of acute hypoxia, respiration is depressed (Roberton 1986).

3. During intrauterine life, the fetal lungs contain a mixture of amniotic fluid and plasma filtrate (Walters and Olver 1978). During vaginal delivery, the thorax is squeezed expelling up to 40 ml of this fluid (Saunders 1978). The remainder is absorbed by capillaries and lymphatics after birth (Strang 1977). When the thorax is released from the vagina, the compressed ribs and intercostal muscles recoil, causing 10–40 ml of air to be drawn into the lungs. Preterm babies and those delivered by caesarean section do not have the same degree of compression and recoil (Milner *et al.* 1978). They can suffer from retention of lung fluid, which can give rise, amongst other conditions, to transient tachypnoea of the newborn.

4. Response to stimuli. In utero, the fetus has been maintained in a stable environment. He has been protected from bumps, kept warm, dark and has heard noises through liquid. Once delivered he/she is assailed by bright light, the full force of gravity, loud clear noises, a marked drop in temperature and he/she is being touched.

The vast majority of babies breathe spontaneously and require no assistance (Roberton 1986). Within 1 minute of delivery 90–95% of babies are breathing well (Chamberlain *et al.* 1975). The baby's first few breaths are huge, with pressures up to 100 cm of water pressure (Karlberg *et al.* 1962); they are necessary to expand the lung field and pulmonary circulation (Henderson-Smart 1986). It is important to dry the baby well to prevent excess heat loss from evaporation. Although babies weighing more than 750 g have been shown to be able to maintain their temperature, this is at the expense of increased energy expenditure (Gandy *et al.* 1964). The baby should be given straight to mother, as the period of alertness following delivery lasts only about 2 hours (Desmond 1966). If there is an overhead heater, the baby can be given naked to mother, otherwise a warmed blanket can be placed over the two of them taking special care to cover the baby's head, or the baby can be wrapped in a warmed towel or blanket.

To assess the condition of the baby in the minutes immediately after birth, the Apgar score may be used. This was devised by an American paediatrician Virginia Apgar (1953) and it assesses neonatal well-being by determining neonatal heart rate, respiratory effort, muscle tone, colour and response to stimulation. The Apgar score, has not been shown, however, to be predictive of future outcome (Fields *et al.* 1983), although it does have the advantage of encouraging staff to keep a close eye on the baby. The score is normally determined at 1 minute and 5 minutes after birth. Where there are problems establishing respiration a score may be taken at 10 minutes. For further information see Chapter 21.

Fetal circulation and changes at birth

During intrauterine life, the fetus obtained its oxygen supply via the placenta. To facilitate the transfer of oxygen from maternal to fetal circulations, the fetus had a different type of haemoglobin, HBF. This is capable of carrying more oxygen at low pressures of available oxygen (from the placenta) than is adult haemoglobin (Kelnar and Harvey 1987). In addition, the fetus has a haemoglobin level in excess of that for an adult at 17–18 g/100 ml (Walker and Turnbull 1953).

In the fetus oxygenated blood comes from the placenta via the umbilical vein (see Figure 32.1). The umbilical vein divides just below the liver, most blood passes via the ductus venosus to join blood from the lower limbs in the inferior vena cava, the remainder enters the portal vein and passes to the liver. The mainly oxygenated blood in the inferior vena cava enters the right atrium of the heart at such an angle that it is directed across the atrium, and through the foramen ovale (a flap in the atrial septum) into the left atrium (Dawes 1963). Oxygenated blood in the left atrium (which came through the foramen ovale), passes to the left ventricle and leaves the heart via the aorta. In this way, most oxygenated blood passes straight to the brain, which is very oxygen-dependent. Deoxygenated blood from the head and the superior vena cava enters the right atrium and passes to the right ventricle, leaving the heart via the pulmonary artery (Assali *et al.* 1968). Little blood passes through the lungs in intrauterine life, the majority going through the ductus arteriosus to the descending aorta (Assali *et al.* 1968). Blood from the descending aorta returns to the placenta via the hypogastric vessels and the umbilical arteries.

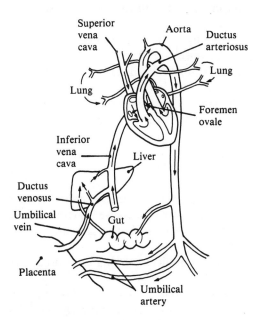

Figure 32.1 Diagrammatic representation of fetal circulation.

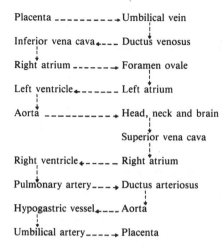

Figure 32.2 Diagrammatic representation of fetal circulation.

To recapitulate (see Figure 32.2):

1. Oxygenated blood enters the fetus via the umbilical vein.
2. Most of this blood bypasses the liver and joins the inferior vena cava via the ductus venosus.
3. Oxygenaged blood passes through the foramen ovale to the left side of the heart and the aorta.
4. Due to pressures being higher in the right side of the heart than in the left, the foramen ovale is kept open.
5. Deoxygenated blood from the head leaves the right side of the heart in the pulmonary artery. Due to high pulmonary resistance, most of this blood avoids the lungs, going to the descending aorta via the ductus arteriosus.
6. Deoxygenated blood returns to the placenta via the two umbilical arteries.

Changes in circulation at birth

1. When the neonate takes his first breath, resistance in the pulmonary vessels is reduced and blood flow is vastly increased (Assali *et al.* 1968).
2. There is a corresponding increase in the pressure of blood entering the left atrium via the pulmonary vein.
3. Once blood flow in the umbilical vein has decreased, there is a reduction of pressure in the right atrium.
4. This pressure differential pushes closed the valve of the foramen ovale, causing it to be functionally closed. It is not permanently closed (anatomically closed) until 4–6 months of age (Barclay *et al.* 1939).
5. The umbilical vein contricts due to exposure of the umbilical cord to air, blood

stagnates in the umbilical vein. The ductus venosus collapses and by 3–7 days of life is fibrosed to become a ligament.

6. The ductus arteriosus is very sensitive to oxygen levels and closes shortly after birth (within 10–96 hours) becoming fibrosed by 2 to 3 weeks of life (Clymann and Heymann 1981). In preterm infants and those suffering from hypoxia it can remain patent.

These circulatory changes occur over a period of time, diagnosis of congenital heart disease is frequently delayed until the second week of life (see Chapter 38).

Thermoregulation

It has been known for many years that low neonatal body temperature is associated with poor rates of survival (Day *et al.* 1964). The neonate loses heat to the environment in four ways:

1. *Convection*: This is the loss of heat from a body surface to the cooler surrounding air. Heat loss is increased as the air temperature drops, by low levels of humidity and as the speed of air movement rises (Rutter 1986).
2. *Radiation*: This is the transfer of heat from the body to a cooler solid surface with which it is not in direct contact, such as the walls of an incubator (Rutter 1986).
3. *Evaporation*: When fluid evaporates to vapour, it utilises heat. The newborn who is born wet or is being bathed can lose much heat unless dried quickly. Movement of air and low levels of humidity increase evaporation (Rutter 1986).
4. *Conduction*: By direct contact with a cooler solid object such as a plastic-covered mattress (Rutter 1986).

Man is homeothermic; that is, he is able to maintain his body temperature despite great variations in the temperature of external surroundings (Rutter 1986). By regulating production and loss of heat, a balance can be achieved. Heat is produced by metabolism (the breakdown of fats and sugars) and by activity, including shivering (Rutter 1986). Heat loss is reduced by insulation, such as fat and clothing. The neonate is at a disadvantage in both heat loss and production. The surface area/volume ratio of the neonate is much larger than that of the adult; to some extent, the flexed posture of the well term-baby can reduce this effect (Hey 1975). The baby is born wet, moving from an ambient temperature of 37.7°C to a delivery room ideally at 25°C (Rutter 1986). Some babies, especially if preterm or small for gestational age, have limited fat stores to provide insulation (Jung 1982).

For heat production, the newborn baby is totally reliant on metabolism, as he is unable to shiver (Smales and Kime 1978). Metabolic heat production requires a ready store of energy and a good supply of oxygen. The term baby has stores of brown fat on his back, shoulders, upper chest and surrounding internal organs, which are readily mobilised to provide heat (Hull 1966). The low-birthweight baby is often deficient in brown fat. Heat production is impaired where an energy source is not available (due to delayed feeding or with a small baby), or where oxygen supply is limited (hypoxia of whatever cause). For each birthweight, gestational age and age after birth, there is a range of environmental temperatures where heat production is a minimum, body temperature is normal and the baby does not need to sweat (Hey 1975). This is referred to as the thermoneutral temperature for that particular baby. As the baby gets older, this ideal temperature becomes less.

Guidelines for maintaining neonatal temperature

1. The temperature should be measured after delivery and on reception in the postnatal ward. In some United Kingdom maternity units, if these are normal, the temperature is not taken again while the baby remains in hospital. Others measure and record temperature daily. There has been no research conducted into the effectivness of either scheme of management. Once at home the community midwife may measure the baby's temperature if he or the room in which he is being cared for feel cold. Local guidelines should be observed. As a quick guide to temperature, if the back of the baby's head below the occiput is warm, then the baby is not chilled.

2. The newborn baby should be dried properly after delivery, and then wrapped in warmed dry towels or blankets. When bathing the baby, the room should be warm, free of draughts and the baby should be exposed for the shortest possible time (Smales and Kime 1978).

3. Several thin layers of clothing trap more air and keep the baby warmer than one thick garment (Hey 1983). Remembering to cover the head (Stothers 1981), hands and feet is important to reduce heat loss. Skin-to-skin contact between mother and baby is another useful way of maintaining the baby's temperature.

4. Try to reduce draughts. A padded cot guard is useful to reduce air flow around the baby.

5. Maintain the neonate in a warm environment day and night. Ideally the newborn's room temperature should not fall below 20°C (68°) for the first 3 or 4 weeks of life.

6. Cool surfaces such as the carry-cot mattress should be covered to insulate the baby against conduction.

It is important not to put the newborn near any unprotected form of heat such as an unguarded fire or a hot water bottle. The latter is useful for keeping the cot warm while the baby is being fed, but should be removed when the baby is returned to the cot. (Mittens and bootees must be checked inside for any loose threads which can be wrapped around little fingers or toes. Cases of amputation have been reported (Mathews 1986).)

Neonatal cold injury

Severe neonatal hypothermia occurs where the baby has a rectal temperature of less than 34°C (Rutter 1986). Once the recording is below 32°C, there is serious chilling; this is referred to as neonatal cold injury. Such a low temperature is a result of persistent cooling and can lead to neonatal death (Rutter 1986). The baby is placid, sleepy and reluctant to feed. The baby feels cold to the touch and oedema especially of the periphery is common. In certain cases the oedema becomes 'woody' (hard) and is known as sclerema. These babies appear well and healthy due to redness of their face and extremities (Rutter 1986).

Such babies require slow warming to avoid the surface temperature being greater than the core, which can cause severe hypotension (Rutter 1986). This is achieved by nursing the infant in an incubator with a temperature 1–2°C higher than that of the core temperature. An increase in temperature of 1°C/hour can be achieved (Rutter 1986). It is also necessary to determine that the baby is not hypoglycaemic and to feed the baby by the best route (Rutter 1986). For very ill or small babies, this may include intravenous or nasogastric feeding.

The urge to care

The newborn baby requires total care by his parents. He is dependent upon them for food, shelter, warmth and protection from harm. The psychologist Lorenz (1981) has commented that the features of human babies and other animal young appear 'cute' to encourage adults to pick them up and to care for them. This 'cuteness' takes the form of an infant with small features, combined with an overlarge head and a small body; indeed depictions of a baby with adult proportions (as appear in some medieval paintings) appear odd. Lorenz (1981) postulates that this 'cuteness' helps to ensure survival of the young by encouraging the giving of care by adults. Preterm babies do not have such a well-developed 'cute' appearance making it difficult for some adults to relate to them.

Birth injuries

With improved obstetric care, birth injuries are thankfully rare. Injury is caused by trauma or hypoxia; the latter can cause neurological disturbance and intraventricular haemorrhage which are discussed elsewhere.

Soft tissue trauma includes caput succedaneum and cephal haematoma, as described in Chapter 33. In addition abrasions can be caused to the presenting part by a scalp electrode; accidental incisions may occur during caesarean section and forceps blades can cause indentation, bruising and minor skin abrasions.

Trauma to muscle

Excessive rotation or extension of the neck, for example in cases of shoulder dystocia, can cause a sternomastoid tumour. This is noticeable a few days after birth as a swelling and a torticollis (wry neck). Passive movements and massage of the swelling with warm oil after feeds can help prevent permanent shortening of the muscle.

Nerve injury

The most common nerve injuries produce only temporary paralysis. These are caused by pressure or excessive stretching of the nerves. A facial nerve palsy can be caused by pressure of forceps blades or of the midwife's or obstetrician's hands on the side of the baby's face. The incidence of this condition has been recorded as 7.5 : 1000 births (Levene *et al.* 1984). A third of cases followed spontaneous vaginal birth (Levene *et al.* 1984). This condition usually resolves spontaneously. Eye care may be required to prevent damage, where the eye is open. The infant should be nursed, with the affected side uppermost. Overstretching of the neck or pressure on the shoulder can cause damage to the brachial plexus, resulting in an Erb's palsy (the so-called 'waiter's-tip' hand) where the arm hangs limply with the palm of the hand directed backwards. This occurs in 1:500 births (Levene *et al.* 1984). An orthopaedic opinion is necessary to decide the best treatment (Kelnar and Harvey 1987).

In addition to the above, internal tissue damage and fractures are occasional results of assisted deliveries, such as vaginal breech delivery. One of the most common is a fracture of the clavicle which occurs in 2:1000 births (Levene *et al.* 1984).

Neonatal reflexes

The baby is born with a number of primitive neurological reflexes, which disappear in early infancy. Their presence or absence is used by paediatricians to determine neurological function and gestational age.

The Moro reflex

This reflex can be elicited with the baby laying supine and the head and trunk held from below; allowing the shoulders and head to fall back 'startles' the baby (Peiper 1963). The lower limbs are rapidly abducted and extended before being more slowly flexed and abducted. The baby may cry when this reflex is elicited. This reflex persists until 2–3 months of age (Illingworth 1986).

Rooting reflex

If the edge of the baby's mouth is stroked, the baby will open its mouth and move it to the site of the stimulus. This can be used to advantage when breast feeding.

Grasp reflexes

The fingers and toes will flex in response to a finger or pencil being placed on the palmar surface of the hand or on the plantar surface of the foot. This reflex disappears when the baby is about 2 months old (Peiper 1963).

Placing reflex

If the infant is held upright and a foot is brought up under the edge of a solid surface, the baby will flex its leg and bring the foot up and onto the surface (Peiper 1963). This reflex is not seen after 6–8 weeks of age (Illingworth 1986).

Primitive walking

When the sole of the baby's foot comes into contact with a firm surface, the infant will appear to walk (Peiper 1963). As with the placing reflex, this reflex disappears after 6–8 weeks (Illingworth 1986).

Traction reflex

Pulling the baby up from a supine position by holding onto her wrists results in the flexion of neck and arms. This lasts until the baby has developed head control by approximately 6 weeks after birth.

References

Apgar V (1953) 'A proposal for a new method of evaluation of the newborn infant' *Current Research in Anesthesia and Analgesia* 32: 260

Assali N S, Berkey J A and Morrison L W (1968) 'Fetal and neonatal circulation' in N S Assali (ed) *Biology of Gestation Vol II: The Fetus and Neonate* Academic Press: New York

Barclay A E, Barcroft J, Barron J H and Franklin K J (1939) 'Radiographic demonstration of circulation through heart in adult and fetus, and identification of ductus arteriosus' *British Journal of Radiology* 12: 505

Chamberlain R, Chamberlain G, Howlett B and Claireaux A (1975) *British Births Vol 1* Heinemann: London

Clymann R J and Heymann M A (1981) 'Pharmacology of the ductus arteriosus' *Pediatric Clinics of North America* 28: 77

Dawes G S (1962) 'The umbilical circulation' *American Journal of Obstetrics and Gynecology* 84: 1634

Day R L, Caliguiri L, Kamenski C and Erlich F (1964) 'Body temperature and survival of premature infants' *Pediatrics* 34: 171–81

Desmond M M (1966) 'The transitional care nursery: A mechanism for preventive medicine in the newborn' *Pediatric Clinics of North America* 13: 651–8

Fields L M, Entman S S and Boehm F H (1983) 'Correlation of one minute Apgar score and the pH value of umbilical arterial blood' *Southern Medical Journal* 76: 1477

Gandy G, Adamsons K, Cunningham N, Silverman W and James I (1964) 'Thermal environment and acid base homeostasis in human infants during the first few hours of life' *Journal of Clinical Investigation* 43: 751–8

Henderson-Smart D J (1986) 'Pulmonary disease of the newborn. Part 1: Neonatal respiratory physiology' in N R C Roberton (ed) *Textbook of Neonatology* 259–73 Churchill Livingstone: Edinburgh

Hey E N (1975) 'Thermal neutrality' *British Medical Bulletin* 31: 69–74

Hey E N (1983) 'Temperature regulation in sick infants' in J Tinker and M Rapin (eds) *Care of the Critically Ill Patient* 1013–29 Springer Verlag: Berlin

Hull D (1966) 'The structure and function of brown adipose tissue' *British Medical Bulletin* 22: 92–6

Illingworth R S (1986) *The Normal Child (9th edn)* Churchill Livingstone: Edinburgh

Jung R (1982) 'The brown fat story' *Hospital Update* Sept: 1157–63

Karlberg P, Cherry R B, Escardo F and Koch G (1962) 'Respiratory studies in newborn infants. II, Pulmonary ventilation and mechanics of breathing in the first minutes of life including the onset of respiration' *Acta Paediatrica Scandanavica* 51: 121–36

Kelnar C J H and Harvey D (1987) *The Sick Newborn Baby (2nd edn)* Balliere Tindall: London

Krauss A N, Klain D B, Waldman S and Auld P A M (1975) 'Ventilatory response to carbon dioxide in newborn infants' *Pediatric Research* 9: 46–50

Levene M G, Holdroyde J, Woods J R, Siddiqi T A, Scott M and Miodovnik M (1984) 'Birth trauma: Incidence and predisposing factors' *Obstetrics and Gynecology* 63: 792

Lorenz K (1981) *The Foundations of Ethology* Springer-Verlag: New York

Mathews M G (1986) 'Autoamputation of infant's finger by knitted mitten: a forgotten hazard' *British Medical Journal* 292: 1107

Milner A D, Saunders R A and Hopkins I E (1978) 'The effect of delivery by caesarean section on lung mechanics and lung volume in the human neonate' *Archives of Disease in Childhood* 53: 545

Peiper A (1963) *Cerebral Function in Infancy and Childhood* Pitman: London

Roberton N R C (1986) 'Resuscitation of the newborn' in N R C Roberton (ed) *Textbook of Neonatology* 239–56 Churchill Livingstone: Edinburgh

Rutter N (1986) 'Temperature control and its disorders' in N R C Roberton (ed) *Textbook of Neonatology* 148–61 Churchill Livingstone: Edinburgh

Saunders R A (1978) 'Pulmonary volume relationships during the last phase of delivery and the first postnatal breaths in human subjects' *Journal of Pediatrics* 93: 667

Smales O R C and Kime R (1978) 'Thermoregulation in babies immediately after birth' *Archives of Disease in Childhood* 53: 58–61

Stothers J K (1981) 'Head insulation and heat loss in the newborn' *Archives of Disease in Childhood* 56: 530–4

Strang L B (1977) *Neonatal Respiration* Blackwell: Oxford

Thacker K E, Lim T and Drew J H (1987) 'Cephalhaematoma: a 10 year review' *Australia and New Zealand Journal of Obstetrics and Gynaecology* 27: 210

Walker J A and Turnbull E P N (1953) 'Haemoglobin and red cells in the human foetus and their relation to the oxygen content of the blood in the vessels of the umbilical cord' *Lancet* ii: 312

Walters D V and Olver R E (1978) 'The role of catecholamines in lung liquid absorption at birth' *Pediatric Research* 12: 239–42

33   Care of the normal newborn baby

The midwife in the United Kingdom is responsible for the well-being of both mother and baby for a minimum of 10 days and a maximum of 28 days (United Kingdom Central Council 1986). The newborn baby, following its initial adaptation to extrauterine life, requires intermittent observation to ensure continued well-being. Once born, the baby is rapidly colonised by thousands of microorganisms, very few of which are pathogenic (Walker and Champion 1986). Should infection occur, the sites most commonly affected are the eyes, skin and the umbilical cord (Pearce and Roberton 1986). In addition to infection, the skin is easily damaged by contact with new substances such as fabric softeners, baby wipes and prolonged contact with urine (Walker and Champion 1986). By daily examination of the newborn baby and instruction of the mother in how to recognise and report abnormalities, the midwife can institute corrective treatment before the situation becomes too serious. This chapter will consider the daily examination of the normal newborn baby, care of the umbilical cord, prevention and treatment of sore buttocks, weight gain, the external and internal anatomy of the foetal skull, screening tests and neonatal sleeping patterns.

Daily examination of the newborn baby

The value of the individual elements of this examination has not yet been

504

demonstrated by research. The examination is usually performed daily until the tenth day after birth. It should be carried out in a warm area, free from draughts and in a good light (Berger 1989). The mother should be encouraged to observe, as she can be shown what is and what is not normal.

1. Skin colour. Before disturbing the baby skin colour should be observed. Soon after birth, the neonate is a healthy pink colour (although the extremities may remain a little blue for the first 12–24 hours), becoming slightly paler in the next few days, due to breakdown of surplus erythrocytes not required for extrauterine life (Walker and Champion 1986). A close watch should be kept for signs of jaundice (see Chapter 35) which can be seen in up to 50% of normal babies on the second or third day after birth (Mowat 1986). Babies of non-white races develop their skin pigmentation from 5 days after birth. Any cyanosis, jaundice or undue paleness should be referred to the paediatrician or general practitioner.

2. Activity. The well baby has good muscle tone, with vigorous movements in all limbs (Nelms and Mullins 1982). When awake, he/she is alert and interested in his or her environment (Gandy 1986). Sudden movement and loud noise can startle and cause the baby to cry (Gandy 1986).

3. Temperature. As mentioned in Chapter 32, temperature control is crucial for the well-being of the neonate (Rutter 1986). It is customary to measure the baby's rectal temperature daily during the early days of life and thereafter as required, depending on the baby's well-being and local policy. Mothers can be advised that by feeling the back of their baby's head just below the occiput, an easy check can be made on their baby's temperature. If the occiput feels warm the baby is not too cold; however the test cannot detect overheating. Liquid crystal display thermometers which can be placed on the child's forehead are becoming increasingly popular with parents.

4. The mother should be asked how many times the baby has had his/her bowels open and has passed urine (approximately 10% of normal babies do not pass urine until 24 hours after birth (Pynnonen et al. 1972).) A brick-red deposit seen sometimes on the nappy is caused by urate crystals in the urine. This is more commonly seen in boys, who produce a more concentrated stream of urine on one area of the nappy. The first stool passed by the newborn is the greenish-black meconium (the colour is due to the large amount of bilirubin which the meconium contains), which has a consistency like tar. This changes after 2 or 3 days to a transitional pale/green/yellow stool before becoming a normal milk-fed stool by the end of the first week of life (Nelms and Mullins 1982). The stool of the breast-fed baby is often bright yellow and semiformed; it should not have a noxious odour (Illingworth 1986). Stools may be passed with a frequency from once at each feed to once a day or less (Illingworth 1986). Because breast milk is easily digested, the quantity of stool passed is less than for the bottle-fed baby. The stool of the artificially-fed baby is a yellow-brown colour and more formed than for the breast-fed baby. Due to the presence of potentially pathogenic bacteria (such as *E. coli* and *Strep. faecalis*)

in the gut of the artificially-fed baby the stool often has a disagreeable odour.

5. The baby's skin should be observed in a systematic manner for spots or rashes. Particular attention should be taken with skin folds in the axilla and groin where infection can otherwise go unnoticed (Walker and Champion 1986) (see Chapter 37 for further details on neonatal infection). Dry flaking skin is often seen in post-mature and growth-retarded babies (Berger 1989). It is easily treated by adding baby oil to the bath water or applying it directly to the skin.

   Normal skin phenomena include erythema toxicum, a fluctuating erythematous rash in the first week of life caused by eosinophil-filled vesicles (Walker and Champion 1986). About half of newborn babies have milia or hypertrophic sebaceous glands, most commonly seen on the nose (Walker and Champion 1986).

   Most non-white babies together with many of Mediterranean origin have a Mongolian blue spot (Illingworth 1986). This is an area of slate-grey blue pigmentation of the skin, most commonly seen over the lower back, thighs or buttocks. It is of no significance, becoming less noticeable with time. In some unfortunate cases, Mongolian blue spot has been mistaken for bruising caused by non-accidental injury (Illingworth 1986).

   Between 30 and 50% of babies have a simple naevus (mole) on the upper face and below the occiput. It is often known as a stork's beak mark. This capillary haemangioma usually fades from the eyelids, forehead, upper lip and the bridge of the nose by the end of the first year of life (Walker and Champion 1986). Those on the neck are usually permanent, but are hidden by the hairline.

6. The mouth should be carefully examined for signs of infection, especially thrush which can be mistaken for milk curds (Pearce and Roberton 1986). A cluster of white spots on the roof of the mouth are epithelial pearls, which occur in the midline at the junction of the hard and soft palates, and are normal (Nelms and Mullins 1982). Sucking pads or callouses are often seen on the lips. They are dry thickened areas of epithelium which can be present at birth and in the absence of any oral feeding. Natal teeth (usually a lower incisor) occur in 1:2000 newborns; they cause few problems but if loose are usually removed (Illingworth 1986).

7. Hormonal effects. Babies of both sexes can demonstrate gyaenocomastia, an enlargement of breast tissue. This is seen in over 80% of babies born at term (McKiernan and Hull 1981). It is thought to be caused by the withdrawal of placental hormones, which inhibit the action of prolactin whilst in utero (Illingworth 1986). The breasts should not be handled and the situation resolves in a few days. In some cases, lactation may occur. Female babies may experience a slight discharge of blood and mucus from the vagina. Again, this is caused by the withdrawal of placental hormones which produces a shedding of the hypertrophic vaginal epithelium (Illingworth 1986). Mothers become very anxious at this and require an explanation which provides reassurance.

The umbilical cord

In the early days after delivery, the cord has a fleshy translucent appearance (Gandy 1986). It separates 5–10 days after birth by a process of dry gangrene or it may leave a residual moist base. Because of the proximity of blood vessels giving direct access to the general circulation, any infection is potentially serious (Pearce and Roberton 1986). Treatment regimes for the cord vary, but they include the application of powders (with or without antiseptics) and the cleaning of the base of the cord with water or spirit swabs (Salariya and Kowbus 1988). The use of a disposible cord clamp is now almost universal in the United Kingdom, with the clamps usually being removed after the third day. In some areas, especially in the community, as opposed to the hospital, cord ligatures are occasionally employed. Comparing treatments applied to the cord, Mugford et al. (1986), in a randomised controlled trial, demonstrated that separation time and the degree of healing were influenced by the type and frequency of their application. Use of an antiseptic powder independent of other cleaning methods led to a shortened time before separation, but lengthened the period of healing (Mugford et al. 1986). The use of alcohol swabs for cleaning produced a small delay in separation, but the difference was not as marked as had been previously reported (Mugford et al. 1986). In a later study, Salariya and Kowbus (1988) concluded that minimal handling of the cord (cleaning the area with tap water only when it was soiled) produced earlier separation and the use of alcohol wipes with frequent handling and intervention delayed events. They recommend that mothers be instructed to wash their hands before giving any cord care (Salariya and Kowbus 1988).

Sore buttocks

The skin of the newborn is delicate and easily damaged (Walker and Champion 1986). One of the most common areas to experience soreness or rashes is the buttocks (Illingworth 1986). Ammonia, from breakdown of urea in the urine, can produce severe excoriation if soiled nappies remain in contact with the skin for prolonged periods (Illingworth 1986). Other factors which can cause problems include inadequate rinsing of soap or cleanser residues, incomplete drying of the skin (especially if moist baby wipes are used) and the use of biological washing powders and fabric softeners for terry nappies. Infection with thrush can also produce characteristic soreness which, unlike nappy rash, is present in the skin folds (Barrie 1987). As with many disorders, prevention is better than cure. Leaving a baby with a moist nappy covered with plastic pants encourages the growth of bacteria (Illingworth 1986). Terry towelling nappies should ideally be used with one-way liners which keep the area next to the skin dry. Disposable nappies have these liners included. When washing nappies they should be soaked first in a special solution to kill bacteria, then washed at high temperature and thoroughly rinsed to cleanse them of any residues.

At each nappy change, the area should be thoroughly washed and dried with a fluffy towel or cotton wool. Leaving the buttocks exposed to the air (if the room is warm) can help remove any remaining moisture (Illingworth 1986). Barrier creams, such as zinc and castor oil or petroleum jelly, are good preventative measures, but cannot be used with water-repellent liners as they block the pores in the mesh (Barrie 1991). If infection does arise, antifungal or antibacterial creams may need to be prescribed (Barrie 1987). Herbal remedies containing chamomile or calendula (English marigold) are growing in popularity. They have anti-inflammatory and soothing properties.

Weight

In the recent past, it was common practice to weigh the baby on at least alternate days. This is happily no longer the case, since pressure was placed upon already anxious mothers, especially those who were establishing breast feeding. The newborn baby loses up to 10% of its birthweight in the first few days of life, usually regaining its birthweight by 7–10 days of life (Illingworth 1986). Much of the weight loss consists of extracellular fluid (Tuck 1986). Average weekly weight gain in the first 3 months of life is 196 g (Illingworth 1986). This, however, conceals huge variations (Hindmarsh and Brook 1988). Growth charts used by most child welfare clinics were drawn up using data supplied from artificially-fed babies who have more consistent patterns of growth than do the breast fed (Paul and Whitehead 1986). Some breast-fed babies gain far in excess of the bottle fed, whereas others have much slower growth. There is certainly a case for using different growth charts for the different babies, those for the breast fed having a much wider range of acceptable rates of growth (Paul and Whitehead 1986).

It is now common to weigh normal babies at birth and then not to reweigh until the baby is old enough to be taken to the child welfare clinic. This eliminates inaccuracies caused by using different sets of scales. Where the midwife is concerned about the baby's weight, she should obviously check the situation.

The fetal skull

Unlike most bones, which develop from cartilage, those of the fetal skull are formed from membranes. Ossification begins in five centres on the membrane from as early as 5 weeks after conception. As calcium is laid down, the skull bones develop out from the ossification sites (see Figure 33.1). If the baby is born prematurely, the skull bones are not as ossified as those of a baby born at term (Kelnar and Harvey 1987). Babies who are post-mature have more rigid skulls which may not mould as well. The gaps in the membranes not yet ossified are known as sutures; these permit the skull bones to overlap during labour. Where two or more sutures meet, a fontanelle occurs.

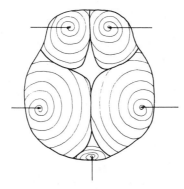

Figure 33.1 Vault of the fetal skull showing ossification sites.

A knowledge of the fetal skull is important for the midwife, because the vast majority of fetuses present head first (Cunningham *et al.* 1989). Information which is important includes:

1. A knowledge of skull measurements for comparison with those of the pelvis.
2. Determining the fetal position in the pelvis by recognition of suture lines and fontanelles.
3. Detection of malpositions.
4. Assessing the extent of moulding during and after delivery.

The fetal skull is divided into three regions:

1. The face: this extends from the junction of the chin and the neck to the supraorbital ridges. It is made up of 14 fused bones and is incapable of moulding during labour.
2. The base: from where the chin joins the neck to just below the occipital protuberance. These bones are also firmly fixed. The base is pierced by the foramen magnum and articulates with the cervical vertebrae.
3. The vault: this is of major importance in childbirth. It extends from the supraorbital ridges to just below the occipital protuberance.

The vault of the fetal skull is divided into two main areas:

1. The vertex: this is bounded anteriorly by the anterior fontanelle, posteriorly by the posterior fontanelle and laterally by the parietal eminences (see Figure 33.2).
2. The sinciput (or brow) extends from the coronal suture lines to the supraorbital ridges. Other important landmarks outside the vault of the skull are the mentum (chin) and the glabella (bridge of the nose).

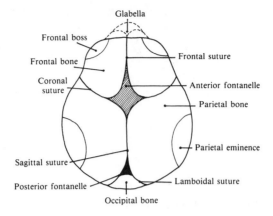

Figure 33.2 Vault of the fetal skull.

The vault of the fetal skull consists of five bones, with two further bones forming part of the lateral walls (see Figure 33.3). There are two frontal bones (with bosses), two parietal bones (with eminences), one occipital bone (with its protuberance) and two temporal bones (which help form the side walls of the fetal skull). The bones are separated by unossified membranes known as sutures. The width of these sutures reduces with increasing maturity (Kelnar and Harvey 1987). These sutures allow overlapping of the fetal skull bones during labour; this is known as moulding. The main sutures are:

- Frontal suture: this separates the two frontal bones.
- Coronal suture: this divides the frontal from the parietal bones.
- Sagittal suture: this lies between the two parietal bones.
- Lambdoidal suture: this separates the parietal and occipital bones.

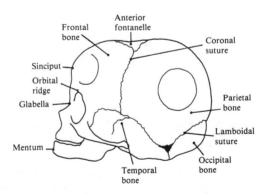

Figure 33.3 Side view of the fetal skull.

Where two or more suture lines meet there is a membraneous area known as a fontanelle; the two most important in midwifery are the anterior and posterior fontanelles.

The anterior fontanelle (or bregma) is formed at the junction of the frontal, coronal and sagittal sutures. It is diamond-shaped, measuring approximately 3.5 cm long × 2.5 cm wide. If this fontanelle is felt on vaginal examination, then the fetal head is deflexed. After birth, this fontanelle can help indicate the state of the baby's hydration; it will be sunken if the baby is dehydrated. In cases of cerebral oedema, it may feel tense; this also occurs when the baby cries. This fontanelle is ossified by about 18 months after birth.

The posterior fontanelle or lambda is formed by the junction of the sagittal and lambdoidal sutures. It is small and triangular. Feeling this fontanelle during a vaginal examination indicates that the fetal head is well flexed. The lambda is ossified by 6–8 weeks after birth.

Diameters of the fetal skull

A knowledge of the measurements of the fetal skull can assist the midwife in her conduct of delivery and in the care of the woman's perineum during the second stage of labour, by using flexion to encourage the smallest diameters to deliver first (see Figures 33.4 and 33.5). The following are average diameters:

1. Diameters in a well-flexed head.
   The suboccipito-bregmatic measures on average 9.5 cm. The biparietal is measured between the two eminences and averages 9.5 cm. When this diameter has passed through the pelvic brim, the head is said to be engaged. The circumference of a well-flexed head is 28 cm.
2. Diameters in a poorly flexed head.
   Suboccipito-frontal, from the suboccipital region to the glabella. This measures 10 cm and is also the diameter which sweeps the perineum in a well-flexed vertex presentation.

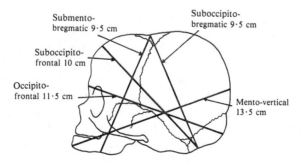

Figure 33.4 Diameters of the fetal skull.

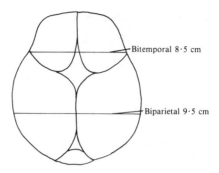

Figure 33.5 Diameters of the fetal skull.

3. Diameters is a deflexed head.
   Occipito-frontal – from the occipital protuberance to the glabella. This measures 11.5 cm and is oval rather than round.
   Biparietal – 9.5 cm.
   The circumference of this presentation is 35 cm.
4. Diameters in a face presentation.
   Submento-bregmatic – from under the chin to the anterior fontanelle, this measures 9.5 cm.
   Bitemporal diameter – 8.5 cms.
   The perineum is distended on flexion of the head by the submento-vertical diameter – 11 cms.
5. Diameters in a brow presentation.
   Mento-vertical – from the point of the chin to just above the posterior fontanelle. This measures 13.5 cm and is therefore too large to pass through the normal gynaecoid pelvis. A preterm baby may manage to deliver in this presentation. The circumference of a brow presentation is 38 cm.

Internal anatomy of the fetal skull

The skull provides protection for the internal structures of the brain. The brain consists of two cerebral hemispheres (the cerebrum), made up of lobes which correspond to the bones which cover them. The cerebrum consists of the outer cerebral cortex and an inner area containing the basal ganglia. Between and below the cerebral hemispheres lie the ventricles which secrete cerebro-spinal fluid (CSF) and connect with the subarachnoid space and the spinal cord. The brain, spinal cord and nerve roots are covered by a three-membrane layer known as the meninges. The layer closely applied to the brain is the pia mater; next to this is the arachnoid mater with CSF flowing between the two. The final covering is the dura mater, which is next to the bones of the skull and fuses with the suture lines and fontanelles. A double fold of the dura mater dips down between the two cerebral hemispheres to form the falx cerebri. This is attached anteriorly to the root of the nose and posteriorly to the occiput. Another fold of dura mater runs horizontally between the occipital lobes of the cerebrum and the cerebellum. This crescent-shaped structure is known as the tentorium cerebelli (see Figure 33.6).

Sinuses, with considerable blood flow, run along the margins of the falx cerebri and over the tentorium at its junction with the falx. At the anterior junction of the tentorium and the falx runs the great vein of Galen. The sinuses, the falx and the tentorium can survive the stresses of normal labour but, should moulding be excessive or very rapid, great strain on the junction between the structures can occur, causing tears (Wigglesworth and Pape 1986). Neonatal death or residual neurological disorder usually result.

Moulding

Moulding is the process of overriding of the skull bones at the suture lines during labour and delivery. The engaging diameters are reduced whilst those at right angles are increased (see Figures 33.7–33.10). The shape of the head appears distorted. By examining the head after delivery, it is possible to determine the position and

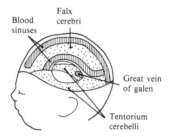

Figure 33.6 Internal anatomy of the fetal skull.

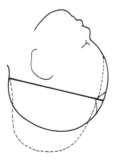

Figure 33.7 Moulding in a well-flexed head. Reduced suboccipito bregmatic diameter and increased mentovertical.

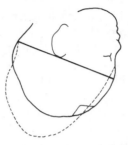

Figure 33.8 Moulding in a poorly flexed head. Reduced suboccipito-frontal diameter.

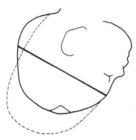

Figure 33.9 'Sugar loaf' moulding with a deflexed head. Reduced occipito-frontal diameter.

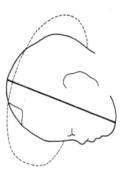

Figure 33.10 Moulding for a brow presentation. Reduced mentovertical diameter, increased suboccipito-bregmatic.

presentation of the fetus in the pelvis (Cunningham *et al.* 1989). Slowly achieved moulding is of no danger to the fetus. However, should moulding be rapid (as during a precipitate birth) excessive (as can occur in obstructed labour) or where the fetus is very premature, care should be taken, due to the risk of cerebral haemorrhage (Wigglesworth and Pape 1986). The baby's head returns to its usual rounded shape within 24–36 hours following delivery.

The scalp

The scalp consists of five layers of tissue (see Figure 33.11).

> **Skin**
> Sub **Cutaneous layer**
> **Aponeurosis** of the occipito-frontalis muscle
> **Loose** connective tissue
> **Periosteum** of the skull bones

There are two conditions involving the scalp present during or after labour; both cause a swelling on the baby's head.

Caput succedaneum

This is a collection of fluid in the subcutaneous tissues of the scalp. It is an oedema which pits on pressure (Cunningham *et al.* 1989). Caput succedaneum is caused by pressure exerted on the presenting part by the cervix resulting in impedence of venous return. The resulting congestion produces oedema. Because caput succedaneum occurs in the superficial tissues of the scalp, it is able to occur on both sides of a suture line. During labour, the extent of caput formation can be assessed on vaginal examination Caput succedaneum can occur on any presenting part, including the buttocks. By 24–48 hours after birth, caput succedaneum should have disappeared completely. Delivery using the ventouse will create an artificial caput known as a chignon on the site of application of the cup (Malmstrom 1954).

Cephalhaematoma

As its name suggests, this is a collection of blood, a haematoma. It feels hard to the touch and does not pit on pressure. Because the bleeding occurs between the skull bones and the periosteum, the swelling cannot cross a suture line, although bilateral haematoma may occur. Cephalhaematoma is caused by trauma when the periosteum is sheared off the skull bones. This can occur in cases of mild

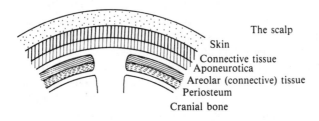

Figure 33.11 The scalp.

cephalopelvic disproportion or as a result of a forceps delivery (Cunningham *et al*. 1989). Cephalhaematoma, by definition, only occurs on the skull, never on other presentations. It can take up to 3 months for the haematoma to resolve; no specific treatment is necessary except for giving vitamin K (0.5–1 mg intramuscularly) to aid blood clotting (Kelnar and Harvey 1987) and minimise the size of the haematoma. Dangers of this condition include anaemia and jaundice, due to the breakdown of erythrocytes within the haematoma. In addition, the haematoma occasionally becomes calcified to form a permanent lump. Parents find the haematoma disfiguring, especially if bilateral; a bonnet can help restore a more 'normal' appearance.

Screening tests

A number of tests are performed on the newborn baby to detect the presence of specific conditions, including congenital dislocation of the hip (see Chapter 38), inborn errors of metabolism and hearing tests. Between the sixth and the tenth days of life, following at least 48 hours of oral feeds), blood is obtained from the baby via a heel stab for chromatographic analysis to test for inborn errors of metabolism. The disorders most commonly screened for include phenylketonuria and hypothyroidism (this subject is covered in more detail in Chapter 38). Babies in at-risk groups are also screened for thalassaemia and sickle cell disease (see Chapter 15).

   The auditory response cradle has been developed to test the hearing of the neonate (Battacharya *et al*. 1984). Research is continuing to evaluate its potential (Curnock 1989). It is thought that by early detection of hearing impairment, the intellectual, social and emotional development of the baby can be helped before deprivation has had its effects (Curnock 1989). The cradle works by analysing the baby's reactions to sounds; these include movement, changes in breathing and being startled (McCormick 1986).

Sleep

In Western society, it is expected that a newborn baby will sleep between feeds. In addition, he will often sleep alone in his own room (Condor 1988). In other societies, babies are carried with their mother and sleep with their family at night (Condor 1988). Even newborn babies have some periods when they are awake, either after feeds or sometimes staying awake between feeds. The newborn baby is awake in the first week of life for approximately 11% of the time, rising to 21% by the end of the first month (Wolff 1965). As with all other human beings, they like attention and entertainment. Habits established in the early weeks are not easily broken (Illingworth 1986). New babies are not usually disturbed (unless they are already awakening) by normal household noises such as doorbells, radios and vacuum cleaners. If the baby becomes accustomed to a very quiet house this may cause problems in later years (Illingworth 1986). To assist in developing a day/night pattern, it is helpful if whichever parent attends to the child during the night does so as quietly as possible. In this way, the baby learn the appropriate time to play after feeds and when he should sleep. This is easier to achieve with a breast-fed baby, since the baby can be fed in bed and kept in bed after the feed or placed back in his cot with the minimum of disturbance. Many breast-fed babies do not need 'winding' after feeds.

Crying

Baby's crying cause the new mother much concern. Until she 'knows' her baby, it is difficult for her to differentiate one type of cry from another (Illingworth 1986). Babies cry because they are hungry, thirsty, uncomfortable, in pain or bored (Illingworth 1986). Most crying is easily resolved by feeding, changing, cuddling and/or talking to the baby. There are great differences between individual babies in the amount of time they spend crying (Kirkland 1985). Excessive crying, however that is defined, can place considerable strain on the families concerned (Schmitt 1985). New parents should be supported and assured that they will not be spoiling the child by picking him up when he is crying (Kirkland 1985).

One major cause of episodic crying, usually occurring at the same time each day is 'colic' (Schmitt 1985). This is a collection of behaviours exhibited by a significant minority of babies under the age of 3 months. The symptoms include inconsolable crying for more than 30 minutes (usually in the early evening) which is not eased by normal soothing techniques (Wessel *et al.* 1954). The baby may go red in the face and draw up his knees as if suffering from abdominal pain. Weissbluth (1984) believes that the abdominal pain is as a result of air swallowed during crying, rather than being a direct result of the cause. Other explanations for crying include an allergy to cow's milk or to the metabolites of cow's milk ingested by the mother and passed on in breast milk. Another explanation is overfeeding with dilute milk, which can result from feeding from both breasts and not allowing the baby to have the richer, more satisfying hind milk (Woolridge and Fisher 1988).

Whatever the cause, colic results in considerable disruption and stress in affected households (Kirkland 1985). The only reassurance which can be given is that, by 3 months of age, most babies have stopped exhibiting these symptoms. However this does not help the parents who have to care for an inconsolable and distressed baby (Schmitt 1985).

Baby care

Most first-time mothers require assistance in learning the techniques of childcare; for many of them it will be the first time that they have given direct care to a newborn baby (Simkin and Enkin 1989). The midwife must assess what the woman and her partner already know and what they want to learn. First-time mothers are often unaware of the robustness of their baby and tend to treat him as if he were made of fine china. The midwife's role in instruction involves direct teaching of the parents (for example, bathing and feeding), observing them performing these tasks, giving feedback and teaching by example.

Whilst many mothers are competent carers, some require reminding of some key points, especially if they are artificially feeding (Jones and Belsey 1978). The midwife should offer instruction in an open and non-patronising manner so that the parents do not feel embarrassed by gaps in their knowledge. There are many different ways of caring for a baby. It is important that the midwife should impart to the parents the key points relating to safe practice. The parents can then adapt, within these guidelines, to find those techniques which best suit them. This can help to prevent lack of confidence and uncertainty when new parents think that they may not be acting correctly.

References

Barrie H (1987) 'Infection with thrush' *Midwife, Health Visitor and Community Nurse* 23(6): 248–50

Barrie H (1991) 'Getting to the cause of nappy rash' *Midwife, Health Visitor and Community Nurse* 27(3): 74–6

Battacharya J, Bennett M J and Tucker S M (1984) 'Long term follow up of newborn tested with the auditory response cradle' *Archives of Disease in Childhood* 59: 504–11

Berger H (1989) 'Clinical examination of the newborn infant' in I Chalmers, M Enkin and M J N C Keirse (eds) *Effective Care in Pregnancy and Childbirth* Ch 83 1403–16 Oxford Medical: Oxford

Condor K (1988) 'Sleep in child rearing–a cross cultural perspective' *Midwife Health Visitor and Community Nurse* 24(4): 126–38

Cunningham F G, MacDonald P C and Gant N F (1989) *Williams' Obstetrics (18th edn)* Prentice Hall: London

Curnock D A (1989) 'The senses of the newborn' *British Medical Journal* 299: 1478–9

Gandy G M (1986) 'Examination of the neonate including gestational age assessment' in N R C Roberton (ed) *Textbook of Neonatology* 131–47 Churchill Livingstone: Edinburgh

Hindmarsh P C and Brook C G D (1988) 'Screening for growth' *Maternal and Child Health* 11(2): 39–42

Illingworth R S (1986) *The Normal Child (9th edn)* Churchill Livingstone: Edinburgh

Jones R A K and Belsey E M (1978) 'Common mistakes in infant feeding: survey from a London borough' *British Medical Journal* 2: 112–5

Kelnar C J H and Harvey D (1987) *The Sick Newborn Baby (2nd edn)* Balliere Tindall: London

Kirkland J (1985) *Crying Babies* Croom Helm: Kent

Malmstrom T (1954) 'The vacuum extractor, an obstetrical instrument' *Acta Obstetrica et Gynaecologica Scandanavica* 4(Suppl): 33

McCormick B (1986) 'Screening for hearing impairment in the first year of life' *Midwife, Health Visitor and Community Nurse* 22(6): 199–202

McKiernan J F and Hull D (1981) 'Breast development in the newborn' *Archives of Disease in Childhood* 56: 525

Mowat A P (1986) 'Disorders of the liver and biliary system' in N R C Roberton (ed) *Textbook of Neonatology* 394–406 Churchill Livingstone: Edinburgh

Mugford M, Somchiwong M and Waterhouse I L (1986) 'Treatment of umbilical cords' *Midwifery* 2(4): 177–86

Nelms B C and Mullins R G (1982) *Growth and Development* Prentice Hall: Englewood Cliffs

Paul A and Whitehead R (1986) 'The weighting game' *Nursing Times* Community Outlook July: 11–17

Pearce R G and Roberton N R C (1986) 'Infection in the newborn' in N R C Roberton (ed) *Textbook of Neonatology* 725–81 Churchill Livingstone: Edinburgh

Pynnonen A L, Kouvalvalainen K and Jaykka S (1972) 'Time of the first urinations in male and female newborn' *Acta Paediatrica Scandanavica* 61: 303

Rutter N (1986) 'Temperature control and its disorders' in N R C Roberton (ed) *Textbook of Neonatology* 148–61 Churchill Livingstone: Edinburgh

Salariya E M and Kowbus N M (1988) 'Variable umbilical cord care' *Midwifery* 4(2): 70–6

Schmitt B D (1985) 'Colic: Excessive crying in newborns' *Clinics in Perinatology* 12(2): 441–51

Simkin P and Enkin M (1989) 'Antenatal classes' in I Chalmers, M Enkin and M J N C Keirse (eds) *Effective Care in Pregnancy and Childbirth* Ch 20 318–34 Oxford Medical: Oxford

Tuck S (1986) 'Fluid and electrolyte balance in the neonate' in N R C Roberton (ed) *Textbook of Neonatology* 163–77 Churchill Livingstone: Edinburgh

United Kingdom Central Council (1986) *Midwives' Rules* UKCC: London

Walker N P J and Champion R H (1986) 'Neonatal dermatology' in N R C Roberton (ed) *Textbook of Neonatology* 677–88 Churchill Livingstone: Edinburgh

Weissbluth M (1984) *Cry Babies: Coping With Colic* Croom Helm: Kent

Wessel M A, Cobb J C and Jackson E B (1954) 'Paroxysmal fussing in infancy sometime called "colic"' *Pediatrics* 14: 421–4

Wigglesworth J S and Pape K E (1986) 'Pathophysiology of intracranial hemmorrhage in the newborn' *Journal of Perinatal Medicine* 8: 119

Wolff P H (1965) 'The development of attention in young infants' *Annals of the New York Academy of Science* 118: 815–30

Woolridge M W and Fisher C (1988) 'Colic, "overfeeding" and symptoms of lactose malabsorption in the breastfed baby: a possible artifact of feed management?' *Lancet* ii: 382–4

34   Infant feeding

This chapter will review the subject of infant feeding. This is very important for the midwife, because much of her time in parent education and in the puerperium is spent assisting the mother in the feeding of her child. The definition of the role of the midwife includes the point that she should promote the uptake of breast feeding (United Kingdom Central Council 1986). The advantages of breast feeding will be described, then the constituents of breast milk. The choice of feeding method will be discussed in relation to the influences on this of the media and the attitudes of society. The characteristics of the woman most likely to breast feed will be described. The physiology and management of breast feeding will then be discussed. In the section on artificial feeding, the history and methods will be described. Included in this section will be a discussion of the effects of introducing artificial milks in developing countries. Finally, there will be an introduction to the subject of weaning. This has been included because midwives receive many requests from mothers for information on this subject.

Advantages of breast feeding

Neonatal advantages

In addition to the flexibility of the composition of breast milk to suit the needs of the growing child (Department of Health and Social Security 1988), it has other benefits. Breast-fed babies are less likely to be overweight than bottle-fed infants in the days of unmodified milks (Hall 1975). It is thought, however, that breast feeding has a protective effect against the occurrence of obesity in adolescence (Kramer and Moroz 1981). The fat content increases as the feed progresses, to act as an appetite regulator (Hall 1975). Also, unlike artificial feeds, breast milk cannot be too concentrated, nor can anything be added to it.

Infections, especially of the gastrointestinal tract, are less common in breast-fed infants (Victoria *et al.* 1987). They are protected from these in many ways. White cells in the milk, such as neutrophils and macrophages, destroy harmful bacteria in the gut; growth of pathogens is inhibited by the acid environment of the gut and by the growth of gram-positive organisms, such as lactobacilli (Lucas 1983).

Lactoferrin binds to enteric iron, making it unavailable for the growth of *E. coli*, and breast milk contains immunoglobulins (mainly immunoalphaglobulin (IgA) which prevent passage of enteroviruses and pathogens through the gastric mucosa (Bullen *et al.* 1972; Goldman and Smith 1973).

Delaying the introduction into the diet of foreign proteins by breast feeding has been shown to reduce, rather than totally protect against, the incidence of allergies in infancy.

Maternal advantages

Breast feeding helps the mother to use the fat stores laid down in pregnancy in preparation for feeding, although lactating women become more energy-efficient and do not need to increase their dietary intake as much as was previously thought (Illingworth *et al.* 1986). Prolonged and regular feeding (especially during the night) delays the return of ovulation (Howie *et al.* 1982). In the developing world, this is an important aid to birth spacing. Breast feeding requires no preparation or the purchase of any equipment. It can cause less disruption during the night or when travelling. Society's attitudes to breast feeding, especially in public, may create some difficulties (Newson and Newson 1965) although, in practice, discrete feeding can usually be accomplished. If nursing mothers continue to be isolated from the rest of society, there will be little chance of breast feeding becoming an acceptable public activity (McIntosh 1985). Many women find breast feeding to be a very pleasurable activity, which promotes a feeling of closeness and intimacy between the mother and child (Messenger 1982). Some mothers also experience an increase in libido (and may on occasions even reach orgasm) during feeding, which may give rise to embarrassment especially if unexpected (Masters and Johnson 1966).

Constituents of breast milk

As more research is carried out on the properties of breast milk, scientists are becoming increasingly aware of its uniqueness. The composition of human breast milk varies with the time of day, the length of lactation, the nutritional status of the mother (if severely malnourished), individual differences and as each feed progresses (Hytten 1954a). Early research into the composition of milk examined 'drip' milk, which consists of fore-milk from the start of the feed which is dilute, low in fat and therefore low in calories (Lucas *et al.* 1978). The hind-milk which is produced during the feed, once the fore-milk has been removed, has higher levels of fat and is much more concentrated (Lucas *et al.* 1979).

The first milk produced by the breasts after birth is colostrum, and is produced in small quantities. It is a thick yellow fluid which is high in proteins, mainly in the form of antibodies which help guard the baby against infection and prevent absorption of foreign proteins from the digestive tract (Lucas 1986a). Colostrum also has a laxative effect which encourages the passage of meconium. On day 2 or 3 there is a change to mature milk, which is mixed with colostrum. By 10 days, the mother is producing mature milk, which often appears thin and watery. The composition of this milk is perfect for the baby (Department of Health and Social Security 1977).

Protein

Human babies grow slowly and therefore require lower protein levels than other mammals, such as calves (Bernhart 1961). The protein which makes up approximately 1.1% of the total feed (Department of Health and Social Security 1988) is 60% lactalbumin or whey protein, which is easily digested (Hambraeus 1977). This is different from cow's milk protein which is almost entirely caseinogen (77%) which forms a solid, slow-to-digest curd in the stomach (Hambraeus 1977).

Fat

The fat composition of breast milk reflects maternal dietary fat (Department of Health and Social Security 1977). It is low at the start of the feed, increasing three or fourfold by the end (Hytten 1954a). The milk contains a high proportion of unsaturated fatty acids and much more cholesterol than cow's milk (Lucas 1986a). This cholesterol may protect the individual from high blood cholesterol in later life. Breast milk contains the enzyme lipase, which aids absorption, preventing fat being lost in the stools; pancreatic lipases are produced in small quantities in the neonate (Lucas 1986b).

Carbohydrates

Breast milk is very high in lactose, making up 7% of total volume (Department of Health and Social Security 1988). This is metabolised to glucose and galactose in the presence of the enzyme lactase (Lucas 1986b). Lactose is important for calcium absorption and for encouraging the growth of lactobacilli, which increase gut acidity and inhibit the proliferation of pathogenic organisms (Lucas 1986a; Department of Health and Social Security 1988).

Vitamins

These are present in plentiful amounts, as long as the mother has good nutritional status (Department of Health and Social Security 1988). Particular care should be taken with vitamin D, where the mother's diet is deficient (Rudolph *et al.* 1980). Both water-soluble (a trace) and fat-soluble forms of this vitamin are present in breast milk (Lucas 1986a).

Iron

Babies born at term have iron stores in their livers, which are supplemented with recycled iron from the breakdown of excess haemoglobin not required after birth. The neonate is born with a haemoglobin level of 18–22 g/100 ml which was necessary to maintain oxygenation in utero. This store should provide sufficient iron for the next 3–6 months (Department of Health and Social Security 1988). Breast milk contains small quantities of iron, of which 80% is absorbed (Saarinen and Siimes 1979). This is a much larger proportion of iron than that absorbed from artificial milk (Lucas 1986a).

Minerals

Levels of sodium, potassium, phosphorus and calcium are low, to prevent placing a strain on the neonate's kidneys, which are unable to produce concentrated urine in response to a large solute load (Hambraeus 1977, Lucas 1986a; Department of Health and Social Security 1988).

Who are the breast feeding mothers?

The 1988 report by Martin and White, *Infant Feeding 1985*, showed that, as in previous reports, there were geographical and social variations in the United Kingdom in the women who chose to breast feed. It must be remembered that these figures apply to a mother who may have put the baby to the breast on only one occasion, as well as to those who establish feeding. Social class has an influence on choice of feeding method. In 1985, 81% of all babies born to mothers in non-manual classes (I, II, IIINM) were breast fed as opposed to 58% in manual groups and 44% in unclassified groups (including students, the unemployed and the armed forces) and in the absence of a partner (Martin and White 1988). Social class is defined by the occupation of the male breadwinner and takes no account of the woman's occupation, if any. The overall breast-feeding rate was 64% (Martin and White 1988). Education level was also important with, better-educated women being most likely to feed, as are older women, with 42% of under-20's feeding initially, as opposed to 86% of those aged over 30 (Martin and White 1988).

There are geographical variations in breast feeding, with the rate falling moving North and West from the South-East of the United Kingdom (Martin and White 1988). Rates were 81% in London and the South-East and 53% in Scotland (Martin and White 1988). It is interesting that the situation in the developed world is almost the opposite of that in poorer countries. In the latter, it is the rural poor who are most likely to feed and the urban professionals who are least likely (Jelliffe and Jelliffe 1978). This is similar to the United Kingdom at the turn of the century. When groups which previously breast fed emigrate to this country, they quickly adopt the practices of the majority and in most cases stop feeding. Research amongst the Chinese in Glasgow and the Bengali community in Tower Hamlets, London shows that women who previously would feed for a year or more in their own country, are bottle feeding within a year or two of arrival in the United Kingdom (Goel *et al.* 1978; Ahmet 1989).

As would be expected, having fed a previous child for more than 6 weeks increases the chances of the mother feeding again (Martin and White 1988). Despite the effect of previous experience, women having their first baby are more likely to feed than mothers of later babies, 69% against 59%. An interesting point is that mothers on maternity leave, whether paid or unpaid, are more likely to feed than those who have to return to work after 6 weeks and, more surprisingly, than those who are not working (Martin and White 1988). This is possibly related to social class and educational achievement. Where the mother smokes, she is less likely to begin feeding. This imbalance is maintained, even within groups where smoking is more common (Martin and White 1988). Hally *et al.* (1981) in Newcastle looked at choice of feeding method and type of housing. Although, as one would expect, this is related to socio-economic status, an interesting point was that mothers in privately rented accommodation were almost as likely to feed as were owner-occupiers. This could be related to lack of privacy and overcrowding in publically rented housing (McIntosh 1985).

Factors influencing choice of feeding method

Raphael (1973) stated that, by the time a woman has reached adulthood, she has decided how she would feed any baby. Two other studies are in support of this. Both Hally *et al.* (1981) (75% of women in their survey) and Thomson (1989) (84% of primiparae in her study) showed that the majority of women had decided on feeding method before attending their first antenatal clinic, most of whom adhered to their choice. The mother who chooses to bottle feed tends to make her decision later in pregnancy (Beske and Garvis 1982).

Since so few women have actually seen a baby being breast fed (Eastham *et al.* 1976), letting the woman see a baby being fed can be a useful experience in assisting the making of an informed choice (Coombes 1979). This would be best placed as a part of the teaching about health which takes place in schools (Eastham *et al.* 1976).

Brack (1975), a feminist writer in the United States, suggested that the choice of feeding method is not as free as we would like to think. The influence of social factors, such as society's attitude to the breasts and the lack of realistic portrayal of breast feeding in the media, has served to convince many women that they are incapable of feeding (Hewat and Ellis 1986) or that it is not the 'done thing' (Brack 1975). Attitudes, once formed, may be very resistant to change.

Recent work by Gregg (1989) reported the results of a questionnaire given to 14 and 15 year olds in Liverpool, a city where the rate of breast feeding is only 30–35%. Only 18% had themselves been breast fed and few had ever witnessed a baby being fed (40% of girls and 28% of boys). Although three-quarters of the sample thought that breast feeding was more natural and healthier than bottle feeding, 60% said the latter was more convenient and 36% more modern (Gregg 1989). When they were questioned about their feelings on seeing a woman feeding, 15% stated that it would remind them of the photographs of 'topless' women featured in some of the more popular but downmarket newspapers and this made them feel embarrassed. Eleven per cent thought breasts were 'rude' and 8% that breast feeding was 'rude' (Gregg 1989).

To prevent the perpetuation of such opinions, it is necessary to approach children before puberty. Ray (1985) suggests that showing a mother feeding her baby to infant and young junior school children as part of a health education package is necessary. At this early age, children are (hopefully) not yet so sexually aware and are therefore better able to appreciate how natural it is for a woman to feed her child (Ray 1985). Such input may not work if the child has been raised in a repressed atmosphere or where the family members are uncertain about their own sexuality. Children are very sensitive to the prevailing atmosphere and can quickly internalise feelings of confusion and disquiet just as readily as a positive, natural and relaxed attitude to health and human behaviour. Emphasis within a family of the sexual rather than the nutritive functions of the breast will continue to deter young women from breast feeding (Jelliffe and Jelliffe 1978). More research is required into the way that attitudes on feeding are formed and into the influence of the media, family members and close friends.

Research undertaken in the late sixties and early seventies showed that negative feelings about breast feeding were so strong that they amounted almost to a taboo (Newton and Newton 1967). Since an important factor in the choice of method is how the woman was fed herself as a child (Sloper *et al.* 1975), we are now caring for a generation of mothers, very few of whom were themselves breast fed (Thomson 1989). In addition, the (until recent) prevalence of advertisements for artificial milks and their presumed equivalence (in the minds of the general public) to breast milk (Scowen 1989) have militated against an increased uptake and continuation of breast feeding. It has now reached the stage when many

Table 34.1 Reasons given by mothers for choice of feeding method

Breast feeding	Thomson	Martin and White
Best for baby	76%	78%
More convenient	19%	33%
Natural	38%	17%
Cheaper	10%	16%
Closer bond between mother and baby	26%	21%
Previous experience	N/A	15% (30% of multiparous women only)
Best for mother		6%
Always wanted to	7%	N/A
Bottle feeding		
Others can feed baby/ convenience	32%	38%
Previous experience	N/A	31% (47% of multiparae)
Do not like the idea of breast feeding	25%	23%
Embarrassment	75%	6%
Can see how much baby has had	19%	6%
Medical contra-indications	N/A	4%
Early return to work	N/A	4%
Awareness of personal tension and effect on breast feeding	12%	N/A
Put off by other people's bad breast feeding experience	12%	N/A

(Thomson 1989, p. 231–2; Martin and White 1988, p. 24)

women think that they are no longer physically capable of breast feeding (Palmer 1989).

When the reasons for choosing a particular method of feeding were explored for primiparous women only by Thomson (1989) and by Martin and White (1988), it was apparent that the rationale for breast feeding concentrated on the advantages for the baby, whereas that for bottle feeding related almost entirely to social reasons, or to reasons for not breast feeding (see Table 34.1).

Anatomy of the breasts and changes in pregnancy

At puberty, under the influence of increasing levels of oestrogen secreted by the ovaries, growth and development of the breasts occurs (Foley 1952). The breasts are attached to the pectoralis major muscles on the anterior chest wall. They extend from the second to the sixth ribs and from the sternum to the midaxilliary line. They are hemispherical in shape, with the addition of an axilliary tail which drains lymph into the nodes in the axillae. Each breast is divided into 15–25 segments, which are separated from each other by bands of fibrous tissue which radiate out from the nipple like the spokes of a wheel (Applebaum 1970) (see Figure 34.1). Each lobe is divided into many lobules; these consist of alveoli lined with acini cells, which produce the milk, and lactiferous ducts along which it is transported. Each alveolus is surrounded by myo-epithelial cells, which contract under the influence of oxytocin to squeeze the milk out of the lobule (Richardson 1947). The lactiferous ducts from each lobule combine to form a larger lactiferous tubule, then pass towards the nipple. Behind the areolar, the lactiferous ducts widen to form ampullae or reservoirs. The baby obtains milk by compressing these ampullae between his hard palate and his tongue (Woolridge 1986a). Milk reaches the ampullae due to contractions of the myo-epithelial cells in each alveolus (Woolridge 1986a).

There are considerable variations in size of the mature breast, but this has no bearing on the ability of the breast to produce milk (Messenger 1982). Similarly, there are differences in the size of the nipple and the areolar which surrounds it. The nipple is composed of erectile tissue, which causes it to stand out when the woman is aroused in some way. This can occur due to touch, sexual arousal, by exposure to cold or on contact with a baby. Each lobe has an opening on the surface of the nipple. Muscle fibres in the nipple act as a type of sphincter to prevent leakage of milk (Woolridge 1986a).

Surrounding each nipple is the areola, the pigmented area onto which open a series of small glands, the Montgomery's tubercles, appearing as small nodules on the areolar from 14 weeks gestation. These are openings of sebaceous glands, which secrete a lubricant substance during pregnancy and lactation to keep the area soft and supple (Newton 1952).

Great changes can occur in the breast during pregnancy. Tingling, tenderness and darkening of the areolar are early signs of pregnancy. In brunettes, this increased pigmentation can extend to an area surrounding the areolar, sometimes called the secondary areolar. Oestrogen, prolactin and human placental lactogen (HPL)

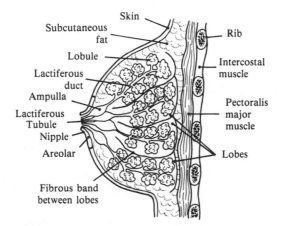

Figure 34.1 The breast (shown in cross-section).

stimulate the growth of the breasts in the first half of pregnancy, while progesterone encourages development of the ductile system and the secretory apparatus in the latter half (Foley 1952). Colostrum may leak from 20 weeks onwards; this is produced under the influence of human placental lactogen (from the placenta) and small amounts of prolactin (from the anterior pituitary gland). High oestrogen and progesterone levels in pregnancy interfere with the action of prolactin and adrenal hormones, so lactation is inhibited (Cunningham *et al.* 1989).

Since the breasts can increase in size during pregnancy by one or two bra sizes, all women are advised to obtain an adequate supporting bra which can help to maintain a good posture and prevent the development of stretch marks. No other specific preparation for breast feeding is required during pregnancy. Indeed, some techniques recommended in the past have been harmful (Inch 1989). Where the mother has flat or inverted nipples she may be given 'shells' to wear which are supposed to increase their prominence. The need for their use has been questioned. Hytten (1954b) found that only 14% of his sample of primparae had flat nipples and in only 2% (of the total) did they cause difficulty in feeding, whereas 3.5% of mothers with 'normal' nipples experienced problems. Changes in the shape of the nipple which help in feeding occur in late pregnancy and during the early postnatal period (Hytten and Baird 1958). These 'shells' are currently under investigation in a large multicentre trial in the United Kingdom.

Educational input for mothers intending to feed (and their partners) is vital during pregnancy (Wiles 1984). For all parents, but especially those who have never seen a baby being fed, being able to see a mother feeding and having the opportunity to question her about it is an invaluable experience (Coombes 1979).

Physiology of breast feeding

There are two aspects to the physiology of lactation, milk production and milk ejection. These will be discussed separately.

Milk production

Following delivery of the placenta, circulating levels of oestrogen and progesterone fall and the action of prolactin is no longer suppressed (Neifert *et al.* 1981). Prolactin causes nutrients to be selectively withdrawn from maternal blood surrounding the alveoli and milk is produced by the acini cells (Laycock and Wise 1983). Other hormones important for milk production include insulin, thyroxine and the glucocorticoids (Laycock and Wise 1983).

To establish, maintain and increase the milk supply, it is necessary that the baby should suckle frequently at the breast. This sends nervous impulses to the anterior lobe of the pituitary gland, more prolactin is released and therefore more milk is produced (Applebaum 1970). This neurohormonal reflex is responsible for controlling the milk supply. If the baby requires more milk, as happens at the time of a periodic growth spurt, which occurs at about 10–14 days, 6 weeks and 3 months

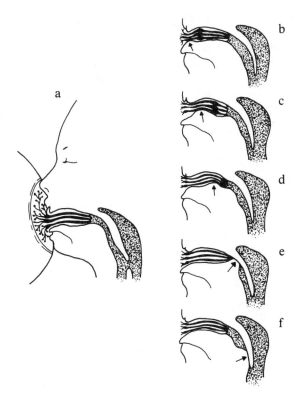

Figure 34.2 Shows a complete 'suck' cycle; the baby is shown in median section. The baby exhibits good feeding technique with the nipple drawn well into the mouth, extending back to the junction of the hard and soft palate (the lactiferous sinuses are depicted within the teat though these cannot be visualised on scans). (a) 'Teat' is formed from the nipple and much of the areola, with the lacteal sinuses, which lie behind the nipple, being drawn into the mouth with the breast tissue. The soft palate is relaxed and the nasopharynx is open for breathing. The shape of the tongue at the back represents its position at rest, cupped around the tip of the nipple. (b) The suck cycle is initiated by a welling up of the anterior tip of the tongue. At the same time, the lower jaw, which had been momentarily relaxed (not shown), is raised to constrict the base of the nipple, thereby 'pinching off' milk within the ducts of the teat (these movements are inferred as they lie outside the sector viewed in ultrasound scans). (c) The wave of compression by the tongue, moves along the underside of the nipple in a posterior direction, pushing against the hard palate. This roller-like action squeezes milk from the nipple. The posterior portion of the tongue may be depressed as milk collects in the oropharynx. (d) and (e) The wave of compression passes back past the tip of the nipple and pushes against the soft palate. As the tongue impinges on the soft palate, the levator muscles of the palate contract raising it to seal off the nasal cavity. Milk is pushed into the oropharynx and is swallowed if sufficient has collected. (f) The cyle of compression continues and ends at the posterior base of the tongue. Depression of the back portion of the tongue creates negative pressure, drawing the nipple and its milk contents once more into the mouth. This is accompanied by a lowering of the jaw which allows milk to flow back into the nipple. In ultrasound it appears that compression by the tongue, and negative pressure within the mouth, maintain the tongue in close conformation to the nipple and palate. Events are portrayed here rather more loosely to aid clarity (Woolridge 1986a). Reproduced with permission of Churchill Livingstone Ltd.

of age), he will suckle more frequently (Messenger 1982), more prolactin will be released and milk production will increase (Short 1984). During a growth spurt, the baby will commonly feed every 2–3 hours for 24–36 hours until the supply is sufficient to meet the demand. When the baby is being introduced to solid foods at 4–6 months of age, the frequency of feeds may reduce and milk production will be less (Morse and Harrison 1988). The same outcome occurs if complementary or supplementary feeds are introduced, especially when lactation is being established (Inch and Garforth 1989).

Milk ejection

The baby obtains milk by compressing the ampullae of the breast between his tongue and the hard palate, a peristaltic movement of the pressure from the tip of the tongue backwards to its base strips milk from the ampullae (Woolridge 1986a) (see Figure 34.2). Early in the feed, the milk which is in the alveoli and ampullae is removed; this fore-milk makes up about a third of the quantity of the whole feed (Applebaum 1970). Suckling stimulates nerves in the nipple, which send impulses to the posterior lobe of the pituitary gland causing the release of oxytocin (Ely and Petersen 1924). This causes the myo-epithelial cells surrounding the alveoli to contract and milk is squeezed down the lactiferous tubules towards the nipple (Applebaum 1970). The baby, when suckling, squeezes the ampullae and removes this hind-milk from the breast. Because the milk is being actively propelled into the ampullae, the baby needs to suck less frequently than at the start of the feed (Woolridge 1986a). The mother often perceives this let-down reflex as a tingling sensation in the breasts; in some cases it causes a transitory feeling of pain (Applebaum 1970).

In the early days of breast feeding, it may take 2 or 3 minutes for let-down to occur (Ely and Petersen 1924); for this reason it is vital not to restrict suckling time. Once lactation is established, let-down occurs more swiftly and, as a conditioned reflex, it can also occur when the mother thinks about her child or hears a baby cry (Applebaum 1970). Let-down, especially in the early days, is inhibited by maternal anxiety or discomfort (Newton and Newton 1962).

Early in the feed, the baby will have two or three jaw movements for every swallow. Once the let-down occurs, the reverse may be true with two or three swallows for each movement of the jaw (Woolridge 1986a). The milk ejection may be so strong that the milk is propelled out of the nipple at some force (Woolridge 1986a). The pattern of suckling should be explained to mothers, so they do not misinterpret a reduction in the baby's activity as showing that the baby has had enough. Once the baby is satisfied he will come off the breast unprompted (Woolridge and Fisher 1988).

Management of breast feeding

Before discussing the management of feeding, it is necessary to consider events which inhibit the establishment of breast feeding. In 1985, in the United Kingdom, of mothers who started to breast feed, only 73% were feeding completely on discharge from hospital (Martin and White 1988), 12% were giving both breast and bottles and 15% had given up completely (Martin and White 1988). Nineteen per cent of all those who started feeding, including those who put the baby to the breast only once, had ceased feeding within 2 weeks of birth (Martin and White 1988). The use of general anaesthesia reduces the mother's chances of success. Of those who received a general anaesthetic, 27% gave up before 2 weeks, compared with 19% who had regional or no anaesthetic (Martin and White 1988). The giving of small doses of analgesics to the mother in labour has been shown (in a small study of 38 mothers) to delay effective feeding by on average 6 hours and in one case by 52 hours (Mathews 1989). This supports work by Richards and Bernal (1972), who showed that pethidine freely crosses the placenta, diminishing the infant's sucking ability in the first 24–48 hours.

Where the mother was able to put the baby to the breast immediately or within an hour of birth, as occurred in 59% of cases, only 14% had stopped feeding by 2 weeks after birth, compared with 24% between 4 and 12 hours and 31% with a first feed occurring later than 12 hours (Martin and White 1988). This does not demonstrate cause and effect, since a delay can occur due to complications in maternal and/or neonatal conditions. Where the baby is admitted to the Special Care Baby Unit it appears that delays in feeding are better tolerated. This could be related to the use of a breast pump to maintain lactation, or to the greater motivation of mothers whose baby is in such a unit, or to the fact that expressing milk is the only thing the mother can do for her child. The use of a breast pump is usually insufficient to maintain lactation, unless supplemented by occasional episodes of breast feeding (Howie 1985). Where delays of over 24 hours occurred before the baby was put to the breast, 23% of mothers whose baby was admitted to Special Care Baby Unit gave up in 2 weeks, compared to 46% whose baby was in the ward (Martin and White 1988). Giving expressed breast milk via a bottle only confuses the baby, who has to learn two different feeding techniques. There is little advantage in using bottles, since feeding from the breast is easier and less tiring (Meier and Cranston-Anderson 1987). Where the baby is unable to take the whole feed from the breast, the remainder should be given via a nasogastric tube.

Both rigid frequency and duration of feeds are associated with early discontinuation of feeding (Illingworth and Stone 1952; Martin and White 1988; Inch and Garforth 1989). Both these policies interfere with the establishment of lactation and the regulation of supply and demand (Applebaum 1970). A similar effect occurs where the baby is routinely or regularly given extra feeds, whether expressed breast milk, artificial milk or clear fluids (Houston et al. 1983; Martin and White 1988).

As Applebaum (1970) commented, successful feeding depends on the mother and child discovering what suits them and sticking to it. Although breast feeding is natural, it does not mean that it is innate, both mother and child have skills to learn before feeding is properly established (Woolridge 1986a). The keys to success are:

● The baby should be correctly fixed onto the breast.

- Feeding should begin as soon as possible after birth.
- No restrictions should be imposed on either the length or frequency of feeds.
- No supplementary or complementary feeds should be given to normal babies.
- One or both breasts should be used at each feed, depending on the baby's needs.

Attachment to the breast

The mother's position for feeding should be one in which the baby is facing the breast with his neck slightly extended and mouth at the level of the nipple (Royal College of Midwives 1988). The baby's head and shoulders should be firmly supported. The Royal College of Midwives (1988) booklet *Successful Breast Feeding* advises that support can be given to a large breast by placing a hand under the breast raising the nipple and keeping the area around the baby's nose clear. Common positions are sitting upright possibly supported by cushions, or laying on one side. The latter position is useful where the mother has a painful perineum or caesarean section wound, and for feeds during the night.

The baby must take enough of the areolar into his mouth so that the ampullae lie behind the gums and the nipple extends back as far as the soft palate (Woolridge 1986a) (see Figure 34.2). The baby can be encouraged to open his mouth by stroking his cheek with the nipple to elicit the rooting reflex. The baby will open his mouth and move towards the nipple. When correctly fixed, the baby's mouth should be wide open and his chin pressed against the breast (Woolridge 1986a). The bottom lip should be placed at least half inch (1.5 cm) below the lower edge of the nipple, so that enough of the areolar below can be taken into the mouth (Woolridge 1986a). The mother (looking from above) cannot see this and she may be tempted to try to put in too much of the upper areolar, which results in the baby being unable to compress the ampullae adequately (Fisher 1983).

When the baby is correctly attached, there should be no sounds of sucking. Because the baby is exerting no pressure on the nipple, there should be no soreness (Woolridge 1986b). The presence of any pain indicates that the baby is not correctly fixed (Woolridge 1986b). Where a baby has received some bottle feeds (for example, while in Special Care Baby Unit) it may take a little time re-educating the baby from the sucking action used to feed from a bottle to the suckling action used on the breast (Royal College of Midwives 1988).

The first feed

Depending on the well-being of both mother and baby, the first feed should take place as soon as possible after delivery, ideally in the labour ward (de Chateau *et al.* 1977; Martin and White 1988). Even where it was hospital policy to encourage mothers to feed as soon as possible after the birth, Garforth and Garcia (1989), in their observation of the labour ward, showed that the average time before the first feed was 98 minutes. Widstrom *et al.* (1987), in an observational study of ten newly born infants put in the prone position between their mothers' breasts, have shown that, following 15 minutes of rest, the infants began rooting and sucking. By an average time of 55 minutes after birth, the infants had each found the nipple and begun to suckle (Widstrom *et al.* 1987). The mothers of the babies in this study had not received analgesia during labour. Whilst some babies are wide awake and ready to feed soon after delivery, others become alert during the first hour, whereas those whose mother had received narcotic analgesia may sleep for some time (Mathews 1989). This should be explained to the mother, so that she does not worry unduly.

If the room is warm enough, the newborn baby can be covered with a blanket and put to the breast in such a way that mother and child can enjoy skin-to-skin contact. The first feed should not be rushed, as it provides an ideal opportunity for explanation of the physiology and management of breast feeding (Royal College of Midwives 1988). Once the mother fully understands the processes involved, she is then able to develop a feeding pattern to suit herself and her baby (Jones *et al.* 1986). Wherever possible and needed by the mother, a midwife should be available to be present during feeds in the first 24 hours after delivery. If this is not feasible, the mother must know how and where to summon assistance.

Frequency of feeds

Following the first feed, the baby may sleep for up to 8 hours (Desmond 1966). For the well baby who is feeding properly this is quite normal and allows the mother to rest. Babies should be allowed to feed as often as they wish, which will speed their rate of growth and prolong the duration of breast feeding (Illingworth and Stone 1952; Martin and White 1988). The length of feeds should not be restricted, as this will interfere with establishment of the let-down reflex (Applebaum 1970). The rate at which babies obtain their milk varies greatly and there are similar variations in the length of feeds (Howie *et al.* 1981). Once the milk supply commences on the second or third day, most babies will feed at least six times daily (Inch and Garforth 1989). Since breast milk is easily digested by babies (Lucas 1986a), it is common for them to want feeding more often than at three-hourly intervals, at least for part of the day (Hewat and Ellis 1986). Older female relatives who have experience of feeding a baby with cow's milk formula may interpret frequent feeds as showing a deficiency in the milk supply (McIntosh 1985). These feeds, which were similar to 'doorstep' milk, formed a tough resistant curd in the baby's stomach, which took a long time to digest (Hambreaus 1977). Today's highly modified formulae produce a feeding pattern similar to that of the breast-fed baby (Lucas 1986a). Where the feeds occur very frequently or are prolonged, it is important to check that the baby is correctly fixed on the breast and that the let-down reflex is occurring (Applebaum 1970; Royal College of Midwives 1988; Inch and Garforth 1989).

Complementary or supplementary feeds

The use of complementary or supplementary feeds is contra-indicated in the establishment of successful breast feeding (Houston *et al.* 1983, Martin and White 1988).

The use of one or both breasts at each feed

Babies are all individuals; some always feed off both breasts, whereas others will only feed off one (Woolridge and Fisher 1988). It is important that the baby is allowed to finish the first breast, after which the second one should be offered. If the baby is not permitted to finish the first breast he may take too much of the dilute fore-milk and insufficient of the more satisfying hind-milk (Hytten 1954a; Applebaum 1970; Woolridge and Fisher 1988). This can result in a baby having a sufficient volume of milk but still being hungry (Woolridge and Fisher 1988). The changing composition of milk as the feed progresses should be explained to the mother, so she does not become concerned if her baby refuses the second breast. As long as the mother ensures that she begins the next feed on the other breast she will not become lop-sided.

Problems while feeding

Problems with feeding take up a considerable amount of the midwife's time. Good teaching by the midwife in the early days not only increases maternal confidence, but can also prevent problems occurring (Jones and West 1985, 1986). Martin and White (1988) found that 30% of mothers had problems in hospital (39% for first births and 21% for later births) and 34% at home. The major difficulties, together with those which resulted in the mothers ceasing feeding in both Martin and White's (1988) (at 2 weeks after birth) and Thomson's (1989) study, are shown in Table 34.2.

Breast engorgement

Following delivery of the placenta, the action of prolactin is no longer inhibited. This leads to stimulation of milk production and a great increase in blood supply to the breasts (Applebaum 1970). The appearance of vascular engorgement depends on the amount of this increase (Waller 1946). It will often settle without any treatment. Milk engorgement occurs when milk is being produced at a rate faster than the baby's ability to remove it, causing severe distension of the alveoli (Waller 1946). Restriction of suckling time only serves to increase the problem (Illingworth and Stone 1952). As a result, the breasts are swollen and hot (Gunther 1973). It may be necessary to express a small amount of milk or to warm the breasts with warm water before the baby can fix. None of these remedies was demonstrated to be effective in a randomised controlled trial (Inch and Renfrew 1989). Prevention of milk engorgement by early unrestricted feeding is always better than trying to treat it (Inch and Renfrew 1989). Fluid restriction is of no benefit and will only make the

Table 34.2 Problems experienced by breast feeding mothers and reasons given for discontinuing feeding at 2 weeks (Martin and White (1988) and 6 weeks (Thomson 1989) after birth

	Problems		Reasons for stopping	
	Hospital	Home	Martin and White	Thomson
Sore/cracked nipples	28%	22%	28%	14%
Not latching on	20%	4%	16%	14% (not sucking)
Baby hungry	19%	50%	50%	52%
Baby ill	15%	6%	4%	
Baby did not like milk	9%	6%		
Baby vomiting	4%	7%		
Too much/too little wind	2%	10%		
Too much milk				9%
Abscess				5%
Mother ill		15%	5%	
Breast feeding too tiring		7%		

(Martin and White 1988, p. 29, 34 and 35; Thomson 1989, p. 234)

mother dehydrated (Dearlove and Dearlove 1981). The breasts should, for comfort, be well supported, taking care not to apply pressure, which can lead to stasis and possible mastitis. Mild analgesics, such as paracetamol, may be prescribed.

Sore nipples

This is another complication which is easier to prevent than to cure (Inch and Renfrew 1989). The cause is almost invariably incorrect positioning on the breast, which gives rise to soreness and even damage (Woolridge 1986a, 1986b). In the early hours, observation by the midwife of the mother's feeding technique can detect any problems. The mother should be aware of how the baby both looks and feels when correctly attached (Woolridge 1986a). There is no scientific basis for the use of creams, sprays or lotions to either prevent or treat sore nipples (Inch and Renfrew 1989). Resting the nipple is as effective as repositioning the baby at encouraging nipple healing, but it has the disadvantage that the milk supply will be reduced (Nicholson 1985).

Insufficient milk supply

This is often a problem of incorrect expectations and misunderstanding of physiology. Inch and Renfrew (1989) highlight the problems inherent in confirming adequacy of milk supply. They comment upon the importance of differentiating between an insufficient volume of milk and those babies who are receiving an imbalance of fore-milk to hind-milk (Woolridge and Fisher 1988; Inch and Renfrew 1989). Growth spurts result in frequent feeding for 24–36 hours in order to increase milk supply, which can be misinterpreted as insufficient milk. Introducing complementary or supplementary feeds only reduces stimulation and therefore milk production (Houston *et al.* 1983). Where the baby is not properly fixed he may be unable to elicit the let-down reflex (Woolridge 1986a). The baby should be well attached and allowed to finish the first breast before being offered the second one (Woolridge and Fisher 1988). Mothers should be warned that an increase in physical activity can diminish milk supply. All that is required is that she should eat and drink as her appetite instructs and her milk supply will not suffer (Dearlove and Dearlove 1981; Illingworth *et al.* 1986).

Mothers worry whether or not their baby is getting enough milk. The way to check is whether the baby settles between feeds and has frequent wet and dirty nappies (Royal College of Midwives 1988). Monthly visits to the child welfare clinic, where the child can be weighed and the weight compared with the appropriate growth charts, is the best way to assess infant well-being (Wood *et al.* 1988).

Mastitis

This is usually caused by stasis of milk in the lobes and ducts, due to engorgement or pressure from clothing (Inch and Renfrew 1989). The affected area, which is usually wedge-shaped, appears red and swollen (Gunther 1973). The mother may have a pyrexia and feel generally unwell (Gunther 1973). The resolution of this non-infective mastitis is helped by encouraging the mother to continue feeding and to empty each breast at each feed (Thomsen *et al.* 1984). Very gentle massage of the affected lobe (if this does not cause the mother too much discomfort) can often result in the production of a thin strand of solidified fat. If the mother's condition does not improve quickly, she is at risk of developing infective mastitis (Devereux 1970).

Infective mastitis can result when bacteria enter the breast via damage to the nipple from incorrect fixing. It can also follow unresolved non-infective mastitis (Devereux 1970). Thomsen *et al.* (1984) defined infective mastitis as existing where a woman had more than 1 000 000 leucocytes and more than 1000 bacteria/ml of breast milk. A sample of milk should be sent for bacterial and leucocyte counts. An antibiotic suitable for breast-feeding mothers needs to be prescribed and expression of the breasts continued to ensure a satisfactory outcome (Thomsen *et al.* 1984). If untreated there is a severe risk of abscess formation (Thomsen *et al.* 1984).

Breast abscess

This is a serious complication. Infection in a lobe results in a discrete, painful swelling. It usually occurs as a result of untreated infective mastitis (Thomsen *et al.*

1984). Medical attention is required with appropriate antibiotic therapy and possible surgical incision and drainage of the abscess (Cunningham *et al.* 1989). Where possible, feeding should continue on the affected side as this will speed resolution and healing (Benson and Goodman 1970).

Contra-indications to breast feeding

These are fortunately few, but include women on contra-indicated medications and those who are drug abusers. In the United Kingdom, where there is a safe alternative to breast feeding, women who are HIV-positive are advised not to feed as the virus can be transmitted in breast milk (Department of Health and Social Security 1988; Weinbreck *et al.* 1988). Women who have had breast surgery involving resiting of the nipple are usually unable to breastfeed (Royal College of Midwives 1988)

Stopping feeding

It is important that the mother be allowed to continue feeding her baby for as long as they both wish. Western society does not have an especially favourable attitude towards prolonged feeding (after 6–9 months) (Hewat and Ellis 1986). This may lead to pressure on the mother to give up or to her being evasive when questioned on the subject (Silverton, personal communication). When the mother does wish to stop feeding once lactation is established, she should not do so suddenly, as severe engorgement can result. A preferable approach is to gradually discontinue particular feeds, leaving those in the early morning and late at night until last. This allows the supply to decrease slowly as stimulation of the breasts is reduced (Morse and Harrison 1988).

Whatever reason the mother gives for stopping feeding in the early weeks, it is difficult to tell if it is the real cause or one thought to be more socially acceptable (McIntosh 1985). In the case of 'difficult' babies, it is rarely demonstrated that a change in feeding method leads to an improvement in the baby's behaviour (Illingworth 1986). How far unrealistic expectations or pressure from relatives based on out-of-date information are to blame is impossible to tell. Insufficient milk was the main cause of stopping feeding for babies under 4 months old, when having breast fed as long as the mother intended became the major reason (Martin and White 1988). Physical problems, such as sore breasts or nipples, and problems fixing the baby on the breast are only of major importance for the first 2–4 weeks (Martin and White 1988) (see Figure 34.2). It appears that if the early difficulties can be overcome, either by support for the mother from family members, friends, midwives or breast-feeding counsellors, or through better parent education, feeding stands a chance of becoming established (Houston 1982; Hewat and Ellis 1986). With the problem of insufficient milk, better knowledge regarding the control of milk supply and the individual differences of babies should go a long way to preventing early cessation of feeding (Kapilowitz 1983). Houston (1982) showed that home support of breast-feeding mothers reduced the numbers who stopped feeding in the first 12 weeks.

Artificial feeding

History of artificial feeding

Throughout history women have sought alternatives to the breast feeding of their own child. There are references to wet nursing in the Bible (Fildes 1986). Wet nurses were in demand for thousands of years to nurture the infants of the nobility and to give sustenence to foundlings (Fildes 1986). They were usually required to have impeccable standards of demeanour and morality (Dick 1987). In the nineteenth century, demand for their services increased amongst the growing numbers of middle-class parents (Phillips 1978). Instead of the baby being sent to the country to be nursed, the wet nurse was by now more likely to leave her home in the poor area of the town to live in the house of her employers (Phillips 1978). This resulted in the infants of wet nurses being removed from the breast at a very early age and raised by strangers on concoctions based on bread and cow's milk (Phillips 1978). Not surprisingly, the incidence of infection and infant mortality were catastrophically high (Dick 1987).

The use of the milk of domesticated animals was initially less popular than the employment of a wet nurse, because it was thought that the child would inherit the characteristics of the person (or animal) who suckled him (Fildes 1986). When animals were used as the source of milk, this often took the form of direct suckling of the infant by the animal, especially where foundlings and orphans were being cared for (Fildes 1986). Early feeding bottles made of horn, hide, pottery and glass were also in use. Teats were usually made of leather or fabric (Fildes 1986). The difficulties of adequately cleaning these vessels, together with infection in the milk combined to render artificial feeding a risky activity. Cow's milk was not boiled, since it was thought that this rendered it unsuitable for babies (Fildes 1986). The introduction of pasteurisation at the end of the nineteenth century, and an understanding that boiling could be used to sterilise equipment, did much to reduce infections. There was little understanding that fresh cow's milk was not a suitable food for human babies.

Artificial feeding grew in popularity in the United Kingdom during the twenties and thirties (Spence 1938). The greatest reduction in breast feeding occurred during the Second World War when women were needed to work in the factories (Spiro 1988). Babies were cared for in Government-run nurseries on subsidised National Dried Milk, which was supplied and prepared under strict controls for both hygiene and content.

Modification of milks

In 1920, Wyeth produced the first product aimed at mimicking breast milk. This formula was called Scientific Milk Adaptation (SMA). These early formulae were designed to be fed to the baby at regular intervals and led to the introduction of a similar set regime for breast-fed infants much to their disadvantage (King 1924).

National Dried Milk was available for many years, until phased out following the recommendations of the Committee on Medical Aspects of Food Policy under the chairmanship of Professor Oppe (Department of Health and Social Security 1974). This was an unmodified cow's milk formula (although a half-cream variety was available for very small babies) which was high in protein (mainly indigestible casein) and minerals such as sodium, potassium and phosphorus (Department of Health and Social Security 1974). The concentration of the feed was altered according to the age and weight of the baby and sugar was also added (Scowen 1989). The milk was complicated to make up and there were many instances of overconcentration of feeds, resulting in excess weight gain and metabolic disorders, such as hypernatraemia (Arneil 1967).

The Oppé report (Department of Health and Social Security 1974) recommended that only milks which were highly modified were suitable for use for young infants. There are now two main types of milk available, those based on whey and others containing curd (Department of Health and Social Security 1988).

Demineralised whey formulae

These are the most highly modified feeds, being recommended for use from birth (Department of Health and Social Security 1988). They are based on whey, which is a byproduct of the cheese industry. Minerals are removed to lower the solute load, a small amount of skimmed milk is added to provide casein (curd), fats of vegetable or animal origin and lactose (or malto-dextran) are added to meet energy requirements (Department of Health and Social Security 1980). Vitamins and minerals complete the formula.

Added carbohydrate formulae

These are high in casein. They have a higher total protein content than whey-based formulae or breast milk. This is required because the casein is incompletely digested and some protein is lost in the stools (Department of Health and Social Security 1980). Carbohydrate is added and vegetable oil may be substituted for the existing fat. Although the solute load is reduced, it is not as low as that in breast or highly modified milks. Mothers often change to these milks in order to make the baby more settled (Martin and White 1988). There is no evidence that such a change achieves the desired effect (Department of Health and Social Security 1988).

It is recommended that either breast milk or formula feeds be used for at least the first year of life, with 'follow-on' milks being suitable to substitute for highly modified milks from 6 months (Department of Health and Social Security 1988). Pasteurised cow's milk can be used after this time. Reduced-fat milks are not recommended before the age of 5 years as they are too low in calories (Department of Health and Social Security 1988).

Soya-based formulae

These are designed for use in the small number of infants who have cow's milk or lactose intolerance (Lucas 1986a). Their use in the prevention of allergies is debatable (Taitz 1982). Because of difficulties related to their differing solute load (high zinc and low chloride and iodine levels), they should only be used under medical supervision (Wells 1988).

Special formulae

These are used under medical supervision for infants with inborn errors of metabolism such as phenylketonuria.

Management of artificial feeding

Mothers who are intending to bottle feed their infants should be shown how to prepare feeds. This can be done in the antenatal period, but is better remembered when done in the ward or at home. In a small study by Jacob (1985), 11 out of the 30 mothers in his sample could not remember receiving any instruction in the techniques of bottle feeding. Bottle feeding is not as simple as it seems and there is plenty of scope for error. Jones and Belsey (1978) survey showed that very few mothers exactly followed the manufacturer's instructions and that the number of errors increased with maternal parity. In all, 49% of mothers were making 'important' mistakes which compares with findings by Oates (1973), who showed that only 42% of mothers were following the manufacturer's instructions. Jeffs (1989) assessed the variation in weight of milk powder measured by 28 mothers, using scoops provided by the manufacturers. The smallest amount measured was 2.8 g and the largest 5.6 g. The author suggests that accuracy could be improved by supplying the milk powder in premeasured sachets (Jeffs 1989). It is important that the midwife should give the experienced mother a refresher course in preparing feeds and that this is done in such a way that the mother does not feel patronised.

The equipment used should all be thoroughly sterilised. This can be achieved by covering with water and boiling rapidly for 5 minutes, but hypochlorite sterilising solutions are more commonly used. The manufacturer's instructions regarding mixing the solution and the amount of time needed to sterilise the items should be followed carefully. Jacob (1985) found that 53% of mothers in his survey were not sterilising the bottles and teats correctly. Metal containers and cutlery cannot be dealt with in this way and should be boiled. Hands should be washed before removing the clean equipment. It is advised that the bottles are well rinsed with cool boiled water to remove the sterilant (Devlin 1984). Microwave ovens are not recommended for the sterilising of feeding bottles (Biela and McGill 1985).

Since most hospitals use ready-to-feed prepared bottles, the first time a mother has to prepare a feed is when she returns home. Instructions on the tin of feed should be closely followed (Department of Health and Social Security 1988).

Slightly cooled boiled water should be poured into the bottle to the required amount. One loose scoop of formula is then added to the bottle for each fluid ounce of water (Department of Health and Social Security 1980). The top is screwed on the bottle and the whole mixed well by shaking. Prepared feeds can be stored in a refrigerator for up to 24 hours after mixing. There is no need to reheat the feed before giving it to the baby, although many mothers continue to do this. Microwave ovens should not be used, as the milk is easily overheated and scalding can occur (Sando *et al*. 1984). Any milk remaining at the end of a feed must be discarded.

When the baby is fed he should be held close, in the same way as a mother would breast feed her child. Care should be taken that the hole in the teat is not too large (to prevent choking) nor too small, so that the child tires before eating his fill. The bottle should be removed every 5 minutes so the baby can be sat up to encourage the passage of wind. The whole feed usually takes no more than 20 minutes in all. Artificially fed infants, like those who are breast-fed, should be fed on demand (Department of Health and Social Security 1988).

Advertising of infant milks

In 1981, the World Health Organization produced a voluntary code of conduct for the marketing of breast milk substitutes. This was aimed at encouraging mothers to breast feed and discouraging early weaning. In developing countries, aggressive marketing of artificial milks and implying their alleged superiority over breast milk has caused a huge toll in infant mortality and morbidity (Chetley 1979; Dobbing 1988). The key points of the World Health Organization's code are as follows:

1. There should be no advertising of baby milk products, bottles and teats direct to the public.
2. Free samples should not be given to mothers by anyone especially not health professionals.
3. No gifts should be given to mothers or to health workers by milk manufacturers or advertising agencies.
4. There should be no pictures of babies on the milk packets. There should be a statement on the packet that breast milk is best for the baby. All information contained should be purely factual in nature.
5. Health workers should encourage breast feeding (World Health Organization 1981).

Weaning

The 1988 Department of Health and Social Security report recommends that weaning (the introduction of semi-solid foods) should not take place before the age of 3 months and that the majority of infants should be on a mixed diet by 6 months (Department of Health and Social Security 1988). Because of the risks of developing allergies to foreign proteins, it is recommended that puréed fruit or sieved vegetables cooked without added sugar or salt are ideal weaning foods (Department of Health and Social Security 1988). Cereals containing gluten are no longer given early because of the risk of coeliac disease, although rice-based cereals are growing in popularity (Stevens *et al.* 1987).

References

Ahmet L (1989) 'A model for midwives-support for ethnic breast-feeding mothers' *Midwives Chronicle* Jan: 5–7

Applebaum R M (1970) 'The modern management of successful breast feeding' *Pediatric Clinics of North America* 17(1): 203–25

Arneil G C (1967) *Dietary study of 4,365 Scottish infants* Scottish Health Service Studies, No 6, Scottish Home and Health Department

Benson E A and Goodman M A (1970) 'An evaluation of the use of stilboestrol and antibiotics in the early management of acute puerperal breast abscess' *British Journal of Surgery* 57: 258

Bernhart F W (1961) 'Correlation between growth rate of the suckling of various species and the percentage of total calories from protein in milk' *Nature* 191: 358–60

Beske E J and Garvis M S (1982) 'Important factors in breastfeeding success' *Maternal and Child Nursing* 7: 174–9

Biela A and McGill A E J (1985) 'Can baby feeding equipment be sterilised in the domestic microwave oven?' *Journal of the Royal Society of Health* 4: 131–2

Brack D C (1975) 'Social forces, feminism and breastfeeding' *Nursing Outlook* 23(8): 556–61

Bullen J J, Rogers H J and Leigh L (1972) 'Iron-binding proteins in milk and resistance to Escherichia coli infection in infants' *British Medical Journal* 1: 69

Chetley A (1979) *The Baby Killer Scandal* War on Want: London

Coombes S (1979) 'Breast-feeding, a problem conquered' *Nursing Times; Community Outlook* Vol 75: 13.12.79 387–9

Cunningham F G, MacDonald P C and Gant N F (1989) *William's Obstetrics (18th edn)* Prentice Hall: London

Dearlove J C and Dearlove B M (1981) 'Prolactin, fluid balance and lactation' *British Journal of Obstetrics and Gynaecology* 88: 652–4

de Chateau P, Holmberg H, Jakobsson K and Winberg J (1977) 'A study of factors promoting and inhibiting lactation' *Developmental Medicine and Child Neurology* 19: 575–84

Department of Health and Social Security (1974) *Present Day Practice in Infant Feeding* HMSO: London

Department of Health and Social Security (1977) *The Composition of Mature Human Milk* HMSO: London

Department of Health and Social Security (1980) *Artificial Feeds for the Young Infant* HMSO: London

Department of Health and Social Security (1988) *Present Day Practice in Infant Feeding: Third Report* HMSO: London

Desmond M M (1966) 'The transitional care nursery: A mechanism for preventive medicine in the newborn' *Pediatric Clinics of North America* 13: 651–8

Devereux D P (1970) 'Acute puerperal mastitis' *American Journal of Obstetrics and Gynecology* 108: 78

Devlin R (1984) 'The great sterilising debate' *Nursing Times* Community Outlook 80 (July 11): 246

Dick D (1987) *Yesterday's Babies* Bodley Head: London

Dobbing J (ed) (1988) *Infant Feeding: Anatomy of a Controversy* Springer Verlag: London

Eastham E, Smith D, Poole D and Nelligan G (1976) 'Further decline of breastfeeding' *British Medical Journal* 1: 305–7

Ely R and Petersen W E (1924) 'Factors involved in the ejection of milk' *Journal of Dairy Science* 24: 211 Cited by Applebaum (1970)

Fildes V A (1986) *Breasts, Bottles and Babies* Edinburgh University Press: Edinburgh

Fisher C (1983) 'Positions of success' *New Generation* 2(2): 20–1

Foley S J (1952) 'Lactation' in A S Parkes (ed) *Marshall's Physiology of Reproduction Vol II (3rd edn)* 525–647 Longmans, Green and Co.: London

Garforth S and Garcia J (1989) 'Breast feeding policies in practice—No wonder they get confused' *Midwifery* 75–83

Goel K M, House F and Shanks R A (1978) 'Infant feeding practises among immigrants in Glasgow' *British Medical Journal* 2: 1181–3

Goldman A S and Smith C W (1973) 'Host resistance factors in human milk' *Journal of Pediatrics* 82: 1082–90

Gregg J E M (1989) 'Attitudes of teenagers in Liverpool to breast-feeding' *British Medical Journal* 299: 147–8

Gunther M (1973) *Infant Feeding* Penguin: Harmondsworth

Hall B (1975) 'Changing composition of human milk and early development of appetite control' *Lancet* i: 779–81

Hally M R, Bond J, Crawley J, Gregson B A, Philips P and Russell I (1981) *A Study of Infant Feeding* Report No 21 Health Care Research Unit University of Newcastle upon Tyne

Hambraeus L (1977) 'Proprietary milk versus human breast milk in infant feeding' *Pediatric Clinics of North America* 24(1): 17–36

Hewat R J and Ellis J (1986) 'Similarities and differences between women who breastfeed for short and long duration' *Midwifery* 2(1): 37–43

Houston M J (1982) *Requirements for Successful Breastfeeding* PhD thesis CNAA

Houston M J, Howie P W and McNeilly A S (1983) 'Factors affecting the duration of breast-feeding; 1 Measurement of breastmilk intake in the first week of life' *Early Human Development* 8: 49–54

Howie P W (1985) 'Breastfeeding – A new understanding' *Midwives Chronicle* July: 184–92

Howie P W, Houston M J, Cook A, Smart L, McArdle T and McNeilly A S (1981) 'How long should a breastfeed last?' *Early Human Development* 5: 71–7

Howie P W, McNeilly A S, Houston M J, Cook A and Boyle H (1982) 'Fertility after childbirth: post partum ovulation and menstruation in bottle and breast feeding methods' *Clinical Endocrinology* 17: 3323–32

Hytten F E (1954a) 'Clinical studies in lactation; II: Variation in the major constituents during a feed' *British Medical Journal* 1: 176–9

Hytten F E (1954b) 'Clinical studies in lactation; IX: Breast-feeding in hospital' *British Medical Journal* 2: 1447–52

Hytten F E and Baird D (1958) 'The development of the nipple in pregnancy' *Lancet* i: 1201–4

Illingworth R S (1986) 'Why change feed?' *Midwife, Health Visitor and Community Nurse* 22(2): 42–6

Illingworth P J, Jung R T, Howie P W, Leslie P and Isles T E (1986) 'Diminution in energy expenditure during lactation' *British Medical Journal* 292: 437–41

Illingworth R S and Stone D G (1952) 'Self-demand feeding in a maternity unit' *Lancet* ii: 683–7

Inch S (1989) 'Antenatal preparation for breastfeeding' in I Chalmers, M Enkin and M J N C Keirse (eds) *Effective Care in Pregnancy and Childbirth* 335–42 Oxford Medical: Oxford

Inch S and Garforth S (1989) 'Establishing and maintaining breastfeeding' in I Chalmers, M Enkin and M J N C Keirse (eds) *Effective Care in Pregnancy and Childbirth* 1359–74 Oxford Medical: Oxford

Inch S and Renfrew M J (1989) 'Common breastfeeding problems' in I Chalmers, M Enkin and M J N C Keirse (eds) *Effective Care in Pregnancy and Childbirth* 1375–89 Oxford Medical: Oxford

Jacob F (1985) 'Getting it right' *Nursing Times* Community Outlook 81(Dec): 20–1

Jeffs S G (1989) 'Hazards of scoop measurement in infant feeding' *Journal of the Royal College of General Practitioners* 39(3): 113

Jelliffe D B and Jelliffe E F P (1978) *Human Milk in the Modern World* Oxford University Press: Oxford

Jones D A and West R R (1985) 'Lactation nurse increases duration of breast feeding' *Archives of Disease in Childhood* 60: 772–4

Jones D A and West R R (1986) 'Effect of a lactation nurse on the success of breast feeding: A randomised controlled trial' *Journal of Epidemiology and Community Health* 40: 45–9

Jones D A, West R R and Newcombe R G (1986) 'Maternal characteristics associated with duration of breastfeeding' *Midwifery* 2: 141–6

Jones R A K and Belsey E M (1978) 'Common mistakes in infant feeding: a survey from a London borough' *British Medical Journal* 2: 112–5

Kapilowitz D D (1983) 'The effect of an education programme on the decision to breastfeed' *Journal of Nutrition Education* 15: 61–5

King F T (1924) *The Expectant Mother and Baby's First Month* Macmillan: London

Kramer M S and Moroz B (1981) 'Do breast feeding and the delayed introduction of solid foods protect against subsequent atopic eczema?' *Journal of Pediatrics* 98: 546–50

Laycock J and Wise P (1983) *Essential Endocrinology (2nd edn)* Oxford University Press: Oxford

Lucas A (1983) 'Human milk and infant feeding' in R Boyd and F C Battaglia (eds) *Perinatal Medicine* 172–200 Butterworths: London

Lucas A (1986a) 'Feeding the fullterm infant' in N R C Roberton (ed) *Textbook of Neonatology* 193–203 Churchill Livingstone: Edinburgh

Lucas A (1986b) 'Nutritional physiology: dietary requirements of term and preterm infants' in N R C Roberton (ed) *Textbook of Neonatology* 178–92 Churchill Livingstone: Edinburgh

Lucas A, Gibbs J A H and Baum J D (1978) 'The biology of drip breast milk' *Early Human Development* 2: 351–61

Lucas A, Lucas P J and Baum J D (1979) 'Pattern of milk flow in breast fed babies' *Lancet* ii: 57–8

Martin J and White A (1988) *Infant Feeding 1985* HMSO: London

Masters W H and Johnson V E (1966) *Human Sexual Response* Little Brown: Boston

Mathews M K (1989) 'The relationship between maternal labour analgesia and delay in the initiation of breastfeeding in healthy neonates in the early neonatal period' *Midwifery* 5(1): 3–10

McIntosh J (1985) 'Barriers to breast feeding: Choice of feeding method in a sample of working class primiparae' *Midwifery* 1(4): 213–24

Meier P and Cranston-Anderson J (1987) 'Responses of small preterm infants to bottle and breast feeding' *Maternal and Child Nursing* 12(2): 97–105

Messenger M (1982) *The Breastfeeding Book* Century: London

Morse J M and Harrison M J (1988) 'Patterns of mixed feeding' *Midwifery* 4(1): 19–23

Neifert M, McDonough S and Neville M (1981) 'Failure of lactogenesis associated with placental retention' *American Journal of Obstetrics and Gynecology* 140: 477–8

Newson J and Newson E (1965) *Patterns of Infant Care in an Urban Community* Pelican: London

Newton N (1952) 'Nipple pain and nipple damage' *Journal of Pediatrics* 41: 411–23

Newton N and Newton M (1962) 'Mothers' reactions to their newborn babies' *Journal of the American Medical Association* 181: 206

Newton N and Newton M (1967) 'Psychological aspects of lactation' *New England Journal of Medicine* 277(22): 1179–88

Nicholson W (1985) 'Cracked nipples in breastfeeding mothers: a randomized trial of three methods of management' *Nursing Mothers of Australia Newsletter* 21: 7–10

Oates R K (1973) 'Infant feeding practices' *British Medical Journal* 2: 763

Palmer G (1989) *Politics of Breastfeeding* Pandora: London

Phillips V (1978) 'Children in early Victorian England: Infant feeding in literature and society, 1837–57' *Tropical Pediatrics and Environmental Child Health* Aug: 158–66

Raphael D (1973) *The Tender Gift* Prentice Hall: Englewood Cliffs, New Jersey

Ray G (1985) 'Psychology of choice' *Nursing Mirror* Mar 20 25–8

Richards M P M and Bernal J F (1972) 'Effects of obstetric medication on mother-infant interaction and infant development' *Psychosomatic Medicine in Obstetrics and Gynaecology* 303–7 Proceedings of the Third International Congress 1971 Karger: Basel

Richardson K C (1947) 'Some structural features of mammary tissues' *North Carolina Medical Journal* 5: 123

Royal College of Midwives (1988) *Successful Breastfeeding* RCM: London

Rudolph M, Arulantham K and Greenstein R M (1980) 'Unsuspected nutritional rickets' *Pediatrics* 99: 192–6

Saarinen L M and Siimes M A (1979) 'Iron absorption from breast milk, cow's milk and iron supplemented formula.' *Pediatric Research* 13: 143–7

Sando W C, Gallagher K J and Rodgers B M (1984) 'Risk factors for microwave scald injuries in infants' *Journal of Pediatrics* 105: 864–6

Scowen P (1989) 'Twenty-five years of infant feeding 1964–89' *Midwife, Health Visitor and Community Nurse* 25(7): 293–305

Short R V (1984) 'Breast feeding' *Scientific American* 250(4): 23–9

Sloper K, McKean L and Baum J D (1975) 'Factors influencing breastfeeding' *Archives of Diseases in Childhood* 50: 165–70

Spence J C (1938) 'The modern decline of breastfeeding' *British Medical Journal* 2: 729–33

Spiro A (1988) 'Fads and fashions' *Nursing Times* Community Outlook 84(Jan): 12–15

Stevens F M, Egan-Mitchell B, Cryan E, McCarthy C F and McNichol B (1987) 'Decreasing incidence of coeliac disease' *Archives of Disease in Childhood* 62: 465–8

Taitz L S (1982) 'Soya feeding in infancy' *Archives of Disease in Childhood* 57: 814–5

Thomsen A C, Espersen T and Maigaard S (1984) 'Course and treatment of milk stasis, non-infective inflammation of the breast and infectious mastitis in nursing women' *American Journal of Obstetrics and Gynecology* 149: 492–5

Thomson A M (1989) 'Why don't women breast feed?' in S Robinson and A M Thomson (eds) *Midwives, Research and Childbirth Vol 1* 215–40 Chapman and Hall: London

United Kingdom Central Council (1986) *Midwives' Rules* UKCC: London

Victoria C G, Smith P G, Vaughan P J, Nobre L C and Lombardi C (1987) 'Evidence for protection by breastfeeding against infant deaths from infectious diseases in Brazil' *Lancet* ii: 319–22

Waller H (1946) 'Early failure of breastfeeding' *Archives of Disease in Childhood* 21: 1–12

Weinbreck P, Lonstaud V and Denis F (1988) 'Postnatal transmission of HIV infection' *Lancet* i: 482

Wells J (1988) 'Soya based infant formulas and the dietary management of cow's milk intolerance' *Maternal and Child Health* (6): 145–8

Wiles L S (1984) 'The effect of prenatal breastfeeding education on breastfeeding success and maternal perception of the infant' *Journal of Obstetrical, Gynecological and Neonatal Nursing* 13: 253–7

Woolridge M W (1986a) 'The "anatomy" of infant suckling' *Midwifery* 2: 164–71

Woolridge M W (1986b) 'Aetiology of sore nipples' *Midwifery* 2: 172–6

Woolridge M W and Fisher C (1988) 'Colic, "overfeeding" and symptoms of lactose malabsorption in the breastfed baby: a possible artifact of feed management?' *Lancet* ii: 382–4

Wood C S, Isaacs P J, Jensen M and Hilton H G (1988) 'Exclusively breastfed infants: growth and calorie intake' *Paediatric Nursing* 14(2): 117–25

World Health Organization (1981) *International Code of Marketing of Breast-milk Substitutes* WHO: Geneva

35 Jaundice

Jaundice is one of the commonest abnormal signs in the newborn (Mowat 1986). When neonatal bilirubin levels are compared with those for a normal adult, all newborn babies have a degree of jaundice (Maisels *et al.* 1971). Its severity cannot be assessed simply by the amount of yellowing of the baby's skin, but is related to serum bilirubin levels, the ratio of fat to water-soluble bilirubin (on blood analysis), gestation, birthweight and the time of onset (Schaffer and Emery 1977). It is vital to detect and treat jaundice, since bilirubin is toxic to all cells, especially those in the central nervous system (Karp 1979). Severe hyperbilirubinaemia causes a toxic encephalopathy called kernicterus. Where death results from this condition, yellow staining of cells in the central nervous system (especially in the basal ganglia) can be seen on post-mortem examination (Haymaker *et al.* 1961). At its most extreme, kernicterus can cause an early death or severe brain damage, resulting in delayed development, cerebral palsy or deafness. Initial signs of toxicity are drowsiness, lethargy and poor feeding; later effects include convulsions and opisthotonus, which is hyperextension of back and limbs (Poland and Ostrea 1986).

Physiology

Most bilirubin comes from the breakdown of red blood cells (Wennberg 1986).

547

Neonates have a more rapid turnover of red cells than adults, since the mean red cell lifespan of 45–70 days is significantly less than the adult figure of 120 days (Letsky 1986). Bilirubin production in the newborn is, for her size, twice that of the adult at 8–10 mg/kg/day (Maisels *et al.* 1971). The newborn is therefore breaking down erythrocytes at a faster rate than an adult. Destruction of red cells occurs in the spleen to produce:

- Globin – a protein which is reused.
- Haem – the iron pigment which is reused.
- Biliverdin – a waste product requiring excretion (Wennberg 1986).

Biliverdin is changed by enzymes in the spleen into bilirubin which is soluble in fat (Wennberg 1986). One gram of haemoglobin produces approximately 35 mg (600 μmol) of bilirubin (Wennberg 1986). Bilirubin, because it is fat-soluble, requires a mechanism to transport it to the liver for metabolism, which is achieved by its attachment to binding sites on the protein albumin (Odell 1959). The newborn, especially if preterm, may have low levels of the albumin in the serum (Wennberg 1986). Albumin binding sites are not specific to bilirubin, but are used by other substances such as drugs in the sulphonamide and salicylate groups (Wennberg *et al.* 1977). Once in the liver, the process can begin to make the bilirubin water-soluble and therefore capable of being excreted in the stools or urine (see Figure 35.1). For this to occur, the baby requires glucose to produce glucuronic acid, together with oxygen and the enzyme glucuronyl transferase for the chemical reaction (Wennberg 1986). Neonatal glucuronyl transferase has a reduced level of activity than with the adult enzyme (Goldstein *et al.* 1980). It can take 14 weeks for glucuronyl transferase levels in the baby to reach those of the adult (Wennberg 1986).

The conjugated bilirubin produced is water-soluble and can therefore be excreted in the stools and urine. Conjugated bilirubin does not cause kernicterus, as it is not soluble in the fatty cells of the central nervous system (Mowat 1986).

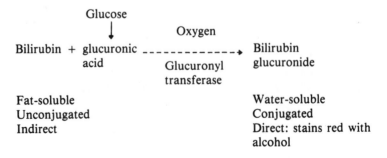

Figure 35.1 The conjugation of bilirubin which occurs in the liver.

Causes of jaundice

1. Due to excess red cell breakdown:
   (a) rhesus incompatibility;
   (b) ABO incompatibility;
   (c) red cell abnormality;
   (d) infection.
2. Hepatic causes:
   (a) deficiencies of glucuronyl transferase;
   (b) hepatocellular damage;
   (c) obstruction.
3. Thyroid deficiency.
4. Breast milk jaundice.
5. Physiological jaundice.

Jaundice due to excess red cell breakdown

Rhesus incompatibility

The rhesus antigen was first demonstrated by Landsteiner and Weiner in 1940. It is present on the red blood cells of 83% of the population in the United Kingdom. People who lack this antigen are known as rhesus-negative. In 1941 Levine *et al.* showed that some cases of erythroblastosis fetalis were due to the presence of maternal isoimmunisation. There are three genotypes for rhesus D groupings:

DD   Homozygous rhesus-positive
Dd   Heterozygous rhesus-positive
dd   Homozygous rhesus-negative (Bowman 1986).

Rhesus antigens are inherited in the same way as other dominant genes. If two heterozygous people have children their possible offspring are shown in Figure 35.2.

When rhesus-positive blood enters the circulation of a rhesus-negative person, antibodies are produced (Kleihauer *et al.* 1957). The antibody is referred to as anti-

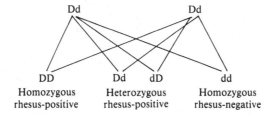

Figure 35.2 Possible outcomes of offspring of two parents who are heterozygous for the rhesus factor.

D, and will destroy any rhesus-positive cells in the circulation (Bowman 1986). The anti-D antibody is small and can cross the placenta from mother to fetus. Should the fetus be rhesus-positive, its cells will be haemolysed causing varying degrees of anaemia (Bowman 1986). A rhesus-negative woman can be immunised in two ways:

1. By transfusion of rhesus-positive blood. This is unlikely with efficient cross-matching, but can occur in less developed countries or where very large quantities of blood are required, for example following acute trauma.
2. Feto-maternal haemorrhage. Where the fetus is rhesus-positive fetal blood can enter the maternal circulation spontaneously – this occurs in at least 50% of pregnancies (Zipursky et al. 1963) – or following a therapeutic or spontaneous abortion, amniocentesis, antepartum haemorrhage or at delivery, especially by caesarean section. Freda (1973) has demonstrated that 2% of rhesus-negative women will be immunised if untreated following a spontaneous abortion and 5% following a termination of pregnancy. A rhesus-negative woman with a rhesus-positive baby has a 16% chance of immunisation with each pregnancy (Bowman 1985); 2% will be immunised by the time of birth, 7% more by 6 months postpartum and a further 7% by the time of the next pregnancy (Bowman 1985). Fetal blood cells can be demonstrated in the maternal circulation using the Kleihauer test. This utilises the differing effects of washing them with acid on adult and fetal cells (Kleihauer et al. 1957).

If the fetal blood is incompatible with the mother's for ABO grouping, the cells will be destroyed by existing anti-A and anti-B before the antigenic response to the D-positive cells has occurred (Bowman 1986). There is only a 2% chance of rhesus-isoimmunisation occurring where the mother and baby are ABO-incompatible (Bowman 1986). The most common time for feto-maternal haemorrhage is at delivery and, due to the time lag in antibody production, the baby from that pregnancy is usually unaffected (Bowman 1986).

It is not possible to prevent immunisation in all cases, especially where an early spontaneous abortion has occurred and the maternal blood group is unknown. A rhesus-negative woman should have blood taken for a Kleihauer test after delivery. If she is positive and the baby is rhesus-negative, prophylactic anti-D is given, the dose being determined by the level of fetal cells present in the maternal blood (Cunningham et al. 1989). Anti-D produces the destruction of fetal rhesus-positive cells before antibodies are formed (Bowman 1986). Anti-D should be given as a precautionary measure to all rhesus-negative women after amniocentesis, abortion or APH; the fetus in such cases is presumed to be rhesus-positive (Freda 1973; Bowman 1985). The usual dose is 250 iu (50 μg) before 20 weeks and 500 iu (100 μg) thereafter (Tovey 1988). Where an especially large number of fetal cells are seen on the Kleihauer test, a larger dose is given, with a repeat test after 24–48 hours to check that all the fetal cells have been destroyed (Cunningham et al. 1989). The anti-D commercially available is obtained from the plasma of people (usually men) sensitised to rhesus-positive cells. It is heat-treated to remove any risk of infection (Centers for Disease Control 1985).

Experiments have taken place, giving prophylactic anti-D at 28 and 34 weeks gestation to rhesus-negative women, which have been successful in reducing the incidence of isoimmunisation (Bowman and Pollock 1978; Thornton *et al.* 1989). Bowman and Pollock (1978) report that a single dose of 300 μg given at 28 weeks gestation is almost as effective as the two doses. Thornton *et al.* (1989) had good results with doses of 100 μg.

Haemolytic disease of the newborn

There are three manifestations of haemolytic disease, depending on its severity.
Hydrops fetalis. This is the most severe effect of rhesus isoimmunisation, resulting in cases of stillbirth or early neonatal death, although some babies do now survive (Bowman and Pollock 1965). Excess intrauterine haemolysis results in severe anaemia, producing generalised oedema with marked ascites and heart failure (Etches 1986). The ascites produces portal hypertension which interferes with placental transfer of nutrients (Etches 1986). If an X-ray is performed, such fetuses have a characteristic appearance with a Buddah-like posture (presenting by the breech due to the presence of ascites which prevents complete flexion of the hips) and a halo of oedema between the skull and scalp (Gordon 1971). Polyhydramnios is common (being present in 75% of cases in one study) and there is an increased incidence of proteinuric hypertension (Hutchison *et al.* 1982). The baby may be double its expected weight, due to oedema, whilst the placenta is very large and overhydrated (Etches 1986). The baby, if born alive, develops severe jaundice very soon after birth (Bowman 1986).
Icterus gravis neonatorum. This is the most commonly seen form of haemolytic disease of the newborn (Poland and Ostrea 1986). During labour and delivery, there are signs of the effects: the liquor is a greenish-gold colour from bilirubin, Wharton's jelly in the cord is stained green and any vernix may appear yellow (Poland and Ostrea 1986). The baby is rarely jaundiced at birth, although pale from anaemia, since any bilirubin has been excreted via the placenta while in utero (Bowman 1986). Jaundice develops rapidly, its severity being related to speed of onset (Bowman 1986). If untreated, respiratory distress (due to anaemia and prematurity), tachypnoea (due to an enlarged oedematous liver) and convulsions (from kernicterus) can occur, with later sequelae of brain damage and mental retardation (Bowman and Pollock 1965).
Haemolytic anaemia. This is a mild but rare form of the disease (Poland and Ostrea 1986). The baby does not develop jaundice, although her low haemoglobin (6–8 g/100 ml) makes her prone to infection (Bowman 1977). Top-up blood transfusions can help to counteract the anaemia, but care must be given not to overtransfuse and suppress the neonatal bone marrow (Bowman 1977). Oral iron supplementation is usually required (Bowman 1977). Antenatal management of the rhesus-negative woman is considered in Chapter 18.

ABO incompatibility

The disorder produced by this condition is normally much milder than haemolytic disease of the newborn (Bowman 1986). The disorder usually arises when a group O mother has a group A or B infant (Bowman 1986). Naturally occurring anti-A and anti-B antibodies are present in the blood of individuals of blood group O without the necessity for prior sensitisation. In 20% of pregnancies, the baby is ABO-incompatible with her mother (Bowman 1977). Problems only occur in the small number of mothers whose isoagglutinins are on IgG which crosses the placenta, rather than the usual larger IgM which does not (Bowman 1986). All-ABO incompatible babies can be affected including the firstborn. There is a recurrence rate of 87% in a subsequent pregnancy (Katz *et al.* 1982). The baby usually presents with mild jaundice, although occasional cases can be more severe (especially in less mature babies); management depends on the severity of the jaundice (Bowman 1986).

Red cell abnormalities

Red cell abnormalities can result in excessive haemolysis and jaundice. These include congenital spherocytosis, a disorder of the cell membrane, causing premature ageing of the red blood cell (Lux and Glader 1981), sickle cell disease, thalassaemia and enzyme abnormalities such as glucose-6-phosphate dehydrogenase deficiency (G6PD), where the cells are fragile and liable to damage (Letsky 1986). In all these disorders, the red blood cells have abnormally short lifespans. Damaged or old cells are removed from the circulation by the spleen, which can become enlarged (Letsky 1986).

Severe infection

Severe infection especially of the urinary tract, can give rise to haemolysis (Poland and Ostrea 1986). Newborn babies suffering from sepsis are often lethargic and poor feeders. Bacteria can produce haemolysins which increase red cell destruction; dehydration worsens the increase of the serum concentration of bilirubin (Pearce and Roberton 1986). In some newborn babies, the only sign of infection is the presence of prolonged jaundice (Pearce and Roberton 1986). For this reason, some units recommend screening all babies with jaundice for the presence of infection (Mowat 1986).

Hepatic causes of jaundice

Deficiencies of glucuronyl transferase production

Causes of this include Crigler-Najjar syndrome, an inherited absence (type one) or deficiency of the enzyme glucuronyl transferase (type two) (Mowat 1986), and the administration of drugs which require glucuronyl transferase for their metabolism and compete for the limited production, such as chlorpromazine and large doses of vitamin K (Mowat 1975).

Hepatocellular damage

Causes of this include infection by bacteria, viruses or protozoa. Infection with hepatitis A or B is rare in the newborn (Pearce and Roberton 1986). A protracted jaundice may be the first clinical sign of galactosaemia, an inborn error of metabolism caused by an inability to metabolise galactose, a constituent of the disaccharide lactose, which causes liver damage (Danks and Brown 1986).

Obstruction

Congenital absence of the bile duct is rare but serious, with persistent jaundice, which rarely appears before the end of the first week of life (Mowat 1986). On examination of the serum, it is found that, unlike physiological jaundice, where most of the bilirubin is unconjugated (or indirect), there is a high level of conjugated (or direct) bilirubin present (Mowat 1986). Clinical signs include a green/golden skin colour and pale bulky stools (Poland and Ostrea 1986). If untreated, the liver will be irreparably damaged. Some cases of extrahepatic atresia are amenable to surgery (Mowat 1986). Atresia of ducts within the liver is inoperable. In neonates with cystic fibrosis, thick mucous secretions may cause temporary blockage of the biliary tree, which can be mistaken for true obstruction.

Hypothyroidism

A persistent jaundice in the first month of life is a clinical feature of hypothyroidism. The jaundice is caused by the slowdown in all metabolic pathways, including the activity of the liver (Barnes 1986).

Breast milk jaundice

This is a persistent jaundice usually appearing in the second week of life. It occurs in a baby whose mother secretes pregnanediol, a metabolite of progesterone, in her milk (Mowat 1986). This competes for glucuronyl transferase for its metabolism, resulting in a jaundice which can last for up to 10 weeks (Mowat 1986). Poland and Ostrea (1986) suggest that the condition is related to the presence of non-esterified fatty acids in the milk which act as 'in vitro inhibitors' of glucuronyl transferase and also compete with bilirubin for intrahepatic binding proteins. Stopping feeding for 1 day, followed by a reduction in the level of jaundice, is the only method of diagnosis (Mowat 1986). Recommencing feeding causes the bilirubin to rise and the jaundice to recur (Mowat 1986). The condition is worsened by low fluid intakes, but has never been shown to cause kernicterus (Maisels 1979). There is no indication to discontinue breast feeding.

Physiological jaundice

This is by far the most common form of jaundice, occurring in about half of babies both term and preterm (Mowat 1986). It is rarely seen before 24 hours after birth (Mowat 1986). The baby is born with a haemoglobin level of 18–20 g/100 ml, which was required to ensure adequate oxygenation in utero. Now that the baby derives her oxygen from the air via her lungs, she does not require such a high level of haemoglobin; the excess red cells are broken-down, putting a strain on a relatively immature liver (Goldstein *et al.* 1980). The situation is worsened by the presence of extensive bruising, which increases haemolysis (Mowat 1986), a delay in clamping the cord after giving an oxytocic drug or milking the cord, which both increase the baby's blood volume (Saigel *et al.* 1972). Delay in passing meconium can lead to reabsorption of bile salts from the meconium, which worsens any jaundice (Odell 1980).

The use of certain drugs also increases the risks of jaundice, for example sulphonamides, salicylates and benzodiazepines which compete for albumin binding sites (Wennberg *et al.* 1977) and vitamin K (if present in excess) and chlorpromazine, which require glucoronyl transferase for their metabolism.

Dehydration and delay in feeding can also increase serum bilirubin levels (Mowat 1986). Physiological jaundice does not appear in the first 24 hours of life and should have resolved by 7–10 days after birth (Mowat 1986). The baby has a variable level of yellowing of the skin and may appear drowsy (Poland and Ostrea 1986). Jaundice worries mothers, who are concerned for the well-being of their baby and fearful of the baby being detained in hospital. Full and clear explanations of the situation are vital to allay unfounded concerns.

Physiological jaundice is in most cases a self-limiting condition. Since skin colour is a poor guide to serum bilirubin levels, blood should be obtained for analysis via a heel stab or a machine used to assess transcutaneous recordings in order to avoid toxicity (Mowat 1986).

Management of jaundice

The management of jaundice involves assessing serum bilirubin levels and deciding on the severity of the condition (Schaffer and Avery 1977). Table 35.1 gives an example of a scheme to determine management.

In cases of physiological jaundice, it is very important to prevent dehydration (thus reducing bilirubin excretion), which may result if the baby is drowsy and reluctant to feed (Mowat 1986). Depending on local procedures, blood for serum bilirubin levels will be obtained via a heel stab by a midwife, paediatrician or general practitioner. Should the midwife undertake this task, she should inform the relevant

Table 35.1 Guidelines for the management of hyperbilirubinaemia by phototherapy and exchange transfusion

Birthweight (g)					
Bilirubin (μmol/1)	< 1000	1000 – 1500	1500 – 2000	2000 – 2500	> 2500
100	PT	OR	0	0	0
150		PT	OR	0	0
200	XT		PT	OR	0
250		XT		PT	OR
300			XT		PT
350				XT	
400					XT

Key: O = observe,   OR = observe   and   repeat   bilirubin,
PT = phototherapy, XT = exchange transfusion.
Source: G M Gandy and N R C Roberton (1987) *Lecture Notes on Neonatology* 257, Blackwell Scientific: Oxford.

doctor about her actions. The midwife, while awaiting results, should ensure adequate feeds, either frequent breast feeds or three-hourly artificial feeds. Supplementing the breast-fed baby can inhibit establishment of lactation and have no positive effects on the jaundice (Nicoll 1982). If the baby is too sleepy to feed (which is unusual), expressed breast milk or bottled milk can be given via a nasogastric tube (Poland and Ostrea 1986). Should the serum bilirubin be above a certain level (see Table 35.1), treatment is instituted; the level is usually above 300 μmol/l in the term baby with much lower levels for ill, preterm or small for gestational age infants (Schaffer and Avery 1977).

The treatment of choice for physiological jaundice is phototherapy (Mowat 1986). This was developed in the 1960s following observations that sunshine affected bilirubin levels in serum samples left on a windowsill and that neonatal jaundice is much commoner in the winter than in the summer in Scandinavia, where there are great variations in day length and natural light levels (Cremer *et al.* 1958). The effective component is light at a wavelength of 450 nm in the visible blue part of the spectrum (Cremer *et al.* 1958). This acts upon bilirubin in the skin and surface blood vessels, breaking it down into non-toxic compounds which the baby can excrete (Lucey *et al.* 1968). Unfortunately the light makes the baby appear blue, which can mask the presence of cyanosis.

Management of phototherapy is the treatment of choice for physiological jaundice; it is also used in cases of ABO and rhesus incompatibility in conjunction with other therapies (Mowat 1986).

1. Preferably the baby should be nursed by her mother's bedside, avoiding separation wherever possible (Kelnar and Harvey 1987).
2. Eye pads should be used to prevent possible eye damage. Although this has

only been demonstrated in animals, it is thought desirable to take precautions (Messner *et al.* 1979). This should be carefully explained, as parental anxiety may occur. The eye pads should be removed whenever the baby is receiving care or is being fed.

3. The baby should be nursed naked to increase the surface area covered by the light and be repositioned three to six hourly (Mowat 1986).

4. To maintain temperature, an incubator or a cot with a heatshield or lid should be used. The baby's temperature should be measured three hourly for hypothermia or hyperthermia; a skin probe can be employed to minimise disturbance (Mowat 1986).

5. A side-effect of phototherapy is the production of loose stools (Drew *et al.* 1976). Bilirubin in the gut attracts water to lower the osmolality; this, together with increased insensible fluid loss (which occurs when the baby is nursed naked), increases the risk of dehydration, so extra fluids may be required (Mowat 1986). An additional intake of 25 ml/kg/day is normally sufficient (Poland and Ostrea 1986).

6. The mother should be encouraged to switch off the lights, remove the eye pads and to feed her baby as normally as possible. Intermittent phototherapy has been shown in some studies to be as effective as continuous phototherapy (Cremer *et al.* 1958).

7. Serum bilirubin levels are determined eight to twelve hourly (Mowat 1986). Phototherapy slows the increase in bilirubin level before a fall occurs. On stopping treatment, monitoring should continue for a further 12–24 hours, because the bilirubin level may rise again (Mowat 1986).

8. The baby should be observed for the signs of any infection which may worsen the situation.

Involving the parents in the care of their baby and keeping them fully informed of all developments is vital to prevent unnecessary worry. Phototherapy may be used for other more severe causes of jaundice to reduce the need for repeat exchange transfusions (Bowman 1986).

Management of rhesus disease

Immediately after a birth where the mother is rhesus-negative, it is usual to carry out early cord clamping. The maternal end of the cord can be drained to help prevent backflow of fetal blood into the maternal sinuses and possible iso-immunisation (Bowman 1986). A sample of cord blood is sent to the laboratory for blood grouping and Coombs's test (Bowman 1986). This is a test for the presence of antibodies which can coat red blood cells. It is most commonly used to detect rhesus antibodies in maternal serum; when mixed with the antiglobulin, clumping occurs if the antibody is present (Coombs *et al.* 1945). If the baby is rhesus-negative, no further action is taken; if positive, maternal blood will be sent to the laboratory for a Kleihauer test to detect the presence of fetal cells (Kleihauer *et al.* 1957). In the situation where the baby is already known to be affected by rhesus isoimmunisation, cord blood is also tested for haemoglobin and bilirubin levels (Bowman 1986). Following analysis of cord blood, such a baby is usually put under immediate phototherapy until the results are available (Bowman 1986). Phototherapy helps to control bilirubin levels, although antibodies remain in the neonatal circulation haemolysing rhesus-positive cells (Bowman 1986). In severe cases, exchange transfusion may be required in the first few hours after delivery (Bowman 1986).

Management of exchange transfusion

In cases of rhesus disease, or where physiological or ABO incompatibility are severe, an exchange tranfusion may be performed (Wallerstein 1946). This has the effect of removing antibodies and sensitised red blood cells, replacing them with donor blood compatible with both neonatal and maternal serum, i.e. rhesus-negative ABO compatible blood (Bowman 1985). By exchanging most of the plasma, the serum bilirubin level is also reduced, but by only 25%, because most of the bilirubin is contained in the extracellular tissues (Bowman 1985). The bilirubin level at which an exchange is carried out is dependent upon gestation, size and age at onset of jaundice (Shaffer and Avery 1977). Kelnar and Harvey (1987) suggest the following as the danger levels for kernicterus at various gestational ages, at which time exchange transfusion should be performed (see Table 35.2).

If the baby is in a poor condition, an exchange may be carried out at lower levels (Kelnar and Harvey 1987). By using twice the neonatal blood volume in the exchange, an 80% exchange of neonatal blood can be achieved (Veall and Mollison 1950). To calculate the quantity of blood required, 170 ml of fresh blood is used per kilogram of body weight (Veall and Mollison 1950). The exchange transfusion is carried out by a paediatrician using a long-line catheter via the umbilical vein into the inferior vena cava (Poland and Ostrea 1986). The blood must be at body temperature to avoid causing shock; overheating should be avoided, due to the risk of haemolysis (Bowman 1977). The blood should for preference be less than 48 hours old (Bowman 1977). Careful monitoring of skin temperature, heart rate,

Table 35.2 Bilirubin levels at which exchange tranfusion is recommended by gestational age of the baby

Gestation	Bilirubin (μmol/l)
39 weeks or more	380
35–38 weeks	350
31–34 weeks	250
30 weeks or less	240

(Kelner and Harvey 1987, p. 246)

blood gases and glucose levels is necessary during the procedure (Bowman 1977). It may be necessary to measure blood gases and urea and electrolyte levels during the transfusion (Poland and Ostrea 1986). Blood is first withdrawn from the neonate before the donor blood is slowly given; 10–20 ml amounts are usually exchanged each time (Poland and Ostrea 1986). The whole procedure can take more than 2 hours to complete (Poland and Ostrea 1986). The first and last samples withdrawn are sent to the laboratory for bilirubin, haemoglobin, calcium and electrolyte level tests and for possible future cross-matching (Bowman 1977). After the procedure, phototherapy is continued, which may help reduce the need for further transfusions (Bowman 1977). The nurse or midwife assisting with the procedure must maintain careful records, including observations of the baby's condition. The parents are usually very anxious about such a procedure. When obtaining permission, the paediatrician must give full, honest explanations, keeping the parents aware of all developments.

References

Barnes N D (1986) 'Endocrine disorders' in N R C Roberton (ed) *Textbook of Neonatology* 623–4 Churchill Livingstone: Edinburgh

Bowman J M (1977) 'Neonatal management' in J T Queenan (ed) *Modern Management of the Rh problem (2nd edn)* 200–39 Harper and Row: Maryland

Bowman J M (1985) 'Controversies in Rh management: Who needs Rh immune globulin and when should it be given?' *American Journal of Obstetrics and Gynecology* 151: 289

Bowman J M (1986) 'Haemolytic disease of the newborn (Erythroblastosis fetalis)' in N R C Roberton (ed) *Textbook of Neonatology* 469–83 Churchill Livingstone: Edinburgh

Bowman J M and Pollock J M (1965) 'Amniotic fluid spectrophotometry and early delivery in the management of erythroblastosis fetalis' *Pediatrics* 35: 815–35

Bowman J M and Pollock J M (1978) 'Antenatal Rh prophylaxis: 28 week gestation service program' *Canadian Medical Association Journal* 118: 622

Centers for Disease Control (1985) 'Lack of transmission of human immunodeficiency virus through Rh immune globulin (human)' *MMWR* 36: 728 Cited by Cunningham *et al.* (1989)

Coombs R R A, Mourant A E and Race R R (1945) 'A new test for the detection of weak and "incomplete" Rh antigens' *British Journal of Experimental Pathology* 26: 255–66

Cremer R J, Perryman P W and Richards D H (1958) 'Influence of light on hyperbilirubinaemia in pregnancy' *Lancet* i: 1094

Cunningham F G, MacDonald P C and Gant N F (1989) *William's Obstetrics (18th edn)* Prentice Hall: London

Danks D M and Brown G K (1986) 'Inborn errors of metabolism' in M R C Roberton (ed) *Textbook of Neonatology* 644–58 Churchill Livingstone: Edinburgh

Drew J H, Marriage K, Bayle B V, Bajraszewske E and McNamara (1976) 'Phototherapy-short and long-term complications' *Archives of Disease in Childhood* 51: 454–8

Etches P C (1986) 'Hydrops fetalis' in N R C Roberton (ed) *Textbook of Neonatology* 484–94 Churchill Livingstone: Edinburgh

Freda V J (1973) 'Hemolytic disease' *Clinical Obstetrics and Gynecology* 16: 72

Gandy G M and Roberton N R C (1987) *Lecture Notes of Neonatology* 257 Blackwell Scientific: Oxford

Goldstein R B, Vessey D A and Zakim D (1980) 'Perinatal developmental changes in hepatic UDP-Glucuronyltransferase' *Biochemical Journal* 186: 841

Gordon H (1971) 'The diagnosis of hydrops fetalis' *Clinical Obstetrics and Gynecology* 14: 548–60

Haymaker W, Margoles C, Pentschew A, Jacob H, Lindberg R and Arroyo L S (1961) 'Pathology of kernicterus and posticteric encephalopathy' in C A Swinyard (ed) *Kernicterus and its Importance in Cerebral Palsy* 21 Charles C Thomas: Springfield

Hutchison A A, Drew J H, Yu V Y H, Williams M L, Fortune D W and Beischer N A (1982) 'Nonimmunologic hydrops fetalis: a review of 61 cases' *Obstetrics and Gynecology* 59: 347–52

Karp W B (1979) 'Biochemical alterations in neonatal hyperbilirubinaemia and bilirubin encephalopathy' *Pediatrics* 64: 361

Katz M A, Kanto W P and Korotkein J H (1982) 'Recurrence rate of ABO hemolytic disease of the newborn' *Obstetrics and Gynecology* 59: 611

Kelnar C J H and Harvey D (1987) *The Sick Newborn Baby (2nd edn)* Balliere Tindall: London

Kleihauer E, Braun H and Betke K (1957) 'Demonstration von Fetalem Haemoglobin in den Erythrozyten eines Blutausstriches' *Klinsches Wosenschrift* 35: 638

Landsteiner K and Weiner A S (1940) 'An agglutinable factor in human blood recognised by immune sera for rhesus blood' *Proceedings of the Society for Experimental Biology and Medicine* 43: 223

Letsky E A (1986) 'Anaemia in the newborn' in N R C Roberton (ed) *Textbook of Neonatology* 449–64 Churchill Livingstone: Edinburgh

Levine P, Katzin E M and Burnham L (1941) 'Isoimmunization in pregnancy: its possible bearing on the etiology of erythroblastosis fetalis' *Journal of the American Medical Association* 116: 825–7

Lucey J, Ferreiro M and Hewitt J (1968) 'Prevention of hyperbilirubinaemia of prematurity by phototherapy' *Pediatrics* 41: 1047

Lux S E and Glader B E (1981) 'Disorders of the red cell membrane' in D G Nathan and F A Oski (eds) *Hematology of Infancy and Childhood* 492–532 W B Saunders: New York

Maisels M J (1979) 'Neonatal jaundice: III. Breast milk jaundice' *Perinatal Press* 3: 19

Maisels M J, Pathak A, Nelson N M, Nathan D G and Smith C A (1971) 'Endogenous production of carbon monoxide in normal and erythroblastotic newborn infants' *Journal of Clinical Investigation* 50: 1

Messner K H, Maisels M J and Leure du Pree A E (1979) 'Phototoxicity to a newborn primate retina' *Investigative Ophthalmology* 17: 178–88

Mowat A P (1975) 'Obstetrical causes of neonatal jaundice' Proceedings of the 3rd Study Group Royal College of Obstetricians and Gynaecologists *Management of Labour* 257–67 RCOG: London

Mowat A P (1986) 'Disorders of the liver and biliary system' in N R C Roberton (ed) *Textbook of Neonatology* 394–406 Churchill Livingstone: Edinburgh

Nicoll A (1982) 'Supplementary feeding and jaundice in newborns' *Acta Paediatrica Scandanavica* 71: 759–61

Odell G B (1959) 'Studies in kernicterus: I. The protein binding of bilirubin' *Journal of Clinical Investigation* 38: 823

Odell G B (1980) *Neonatal Hyperbilirubinaemia* Grune and Stratton: New York

Pearce R G and Roberton N R C (1986) 'Infection in the newborn' in N R C Roberton (ed) *Textbook of Neonatology* 725–81 Churchill Livingstone: Edinburgh

Poland R L and Ostrea E M (1986) 'Neonatal hyperbilirubinaemia' in M H Klaus and A A Fanaroff (eds) *Care of the High Risk Neonate (3rd edn)* 239–61 W B Saunders: Philadelphia

Saigel S, O'Neil A, Surainder Y, Chua L B and Usher R (1972) 'Placental transfusion in hyperbilirubinemia in the premature' *Pediatrics* 49: 406–19

Schaffer A J and Avery M E (1977) *Diseases of the newborn (4th edn)* 644 W B Saunders: London

Thornton J G, Page C, Foote G, Arthur G R, Tovey L A D and Scott J S (1989) 'Efficacy and long term effects of antenatal prophylaxis with anti-D immunoglobulin' *British Medical Journal* 298: 1761–4

Tovey L A D (1988) 'Anti-D and miscarriages' *British Medical Journal* 297: 977–8

Veall N and Mollison P L (1950) 'The rate of red cell exchange in replacement transfusion' *Lancet* ii: 792–7

Wallerstein H (1946) 'Treatment of severe erythroblastosis by simultaneous removal and replacement of blood of the newborn' *Science* 103: 583–4

Wennberg R P (1986) in N R C Roberton (ed) *Textbook of Neonatology* 383–93 Churchill Livingstone: Edinburgh

Wennberg R P, Rasmussen L F and Ahlfors R C (1977) 'Displacement of bilirubin from human albumin by three diuretics' *Journal of Pediatrics* 90: 647–50

Zipursky A, Pollock J M, Neelands P, Chown B and Israels L G (1963) 'The transplacental passage of fetal red blood cells and the pathogenesis of Rh immunisation during pregnancy' *Lancet* ii: 489–93

36   The low-birthweight baby

Low birthweight is the term used to describe babies weighing less than 2.5kg who are preterm or small-for-gestational-age (Stewart 1986). Infants weighing less than 2.5 kg at birth account for 66% of deaths occurring in the first week of life (Wallis and Harvey 1986). Such babies often require treatment in neonatal intensive care or Special Care Baby Units.

The forerunner of such units was established by the French obstetrician Budin in Paris in the late nineteenth century (Budin 1907). He recognised the plight of the small, sick, premature and often unwanted baby, being especially aware that the cold could be lethal to these infants; he devised the first incubator which surrounded the well-wrapped baby with warmed air (Klaus *et al.* 1986). The first premature baby unit in the United Kingdom was opened at the Sorrento Hospital in Birmingham in 1931. At that time, the majority of babies were born at home; if sick or preterm they usually remained there, as few other facilities were available. Techniques were developed for feeding small babies and for keeping them warm. One of the latter was the Sorrento cot, which used a system of hot water bottles refilled in rotation to surround the cot, maintaining a steady temperature.

Classification of low birthweight

Preterm is used to describe any baby born before completion of the thirty-seventh week of gestation (World Health Organization 1977; Gandy 1986). The difficulties experienced by these babies relate to immaturity of the various body systems (Kelnar and Harvey 1987). The causes of preterm birth are still poorly understood. There is a multifactorial element, involving social factors (House of Commons Social Services Committee 1980). Some result from elective early delivery, due to maternal illness such as hypertensive disease in pregnancy or antepartum haemorrhage (Hibbard 1987). Other causes include multiple pregnancy, fetal abnormality, acute onset polyhydramnios and cervical incompetence (Hibbard 1987).

Small-for-gestational-age (SGA), the birthweights of babies at a particular gestational age conform to a normal distribution (see Figure 36.1). The majority (80%) of babies have birthweights appropriate for their gestational age, but 10% are larger and 10% smaller than anticipated (Wallis and Harvey 1986). In some centres, only the smallest 5% at each gestational age are classified as being SGA (Wallis and Harvey 1986). It is in the smallest 10% that problems are most likely to occur. These babies are growth-retarded as a result of congenital abnormality or poor placental perfusion, which reduces transfer of oxygen and nutrients, producing reduced growth (Wallis and Harvey 1986). Causes include smoking in pregnancy (Scott *et al.* 1981), malnutrition (Stein *et al.* 1978), hypertensive disease in pregnancy (Lunell *et al.* 1982), infection and predisposing social factors such as unemployment or poor housing (Wallis and Harvey 1986). If growth is deficient from early in pregnancy when cell division is at its most rapid, the whole baby will be small, as occurs in some cases of chromosomal abnormality (Winick and Noble 1966). This is called symmetrical growth retardation. If the rate of growth is compromised only in late pregnancy, brain development is usually the last area to be affected (Gruenwald 1974). The baby appears long and thin; this is known as assymetrical growth retardation (Wallis and Harvey 1986). In the United Kingdom 7% of all babies weigh less than 2.5 kg at birth and a third of them are small-for-

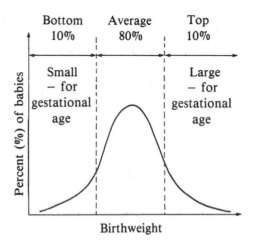

Figure 36.1 Graph of birthweights at a given gestation showing normal distribution.

gestational-age (Wallis and Harvey 1986). The factors involved in determining size at birth include race, geography (altitude) and socio-economic status (Wallis and Harvey 1986).

Whilst babies can be either preterm or SGA, a significant number are in both categories (Stewart 1986). Their management is complex, requiring expert neonatal care. For the purposes of this chapter, the two types of low-birthweight baby will be considered separately.

The preterm baby

Prematurity is a major cause of neonatal death. Yu *et al.* (1986) in Australia reported 1 year survival rates of 7% for babies born at 23 weeks gestation and 75% at 28 weeks. In the United Kingdom Marlow *et al.* (1987) had no survivors born at less than 25 weeks gestation with a 48% survival rate at 28 weeks.

The baby, whose only problem is prematurity, has grown to the correct size for its gestation, but its body systems are immature (Kelnar and Harvey 1987). Such babies appear to have a large head and abdomen, a small chest and underdeveloped genitalia (Gandy 1986). Before 27 weeks gestation, the skin looks red and translucent with visible veins due to the lack of subcutaneous fat; lanugo may be present (Gandy 1986). Before 33 weeks, due to lack of cartilage development, the ear pinna may be composed solely of skin. On examining the hands and feet, the skin creases may be absent prior to 32 weeks gestation (Gandy 1986). Medical staff use a combination of physical and neurological examination of the infant, together with the mother's history to determine gestational age (Gandy 1986). A commonly used scheme is that devised by Dubowitz *et al.* (1970). Components of this scheme include assessment of the physical maturity of the infant, such as skin fold thickness, presence of lanugo and maturity of genitalia, together with neurological observations related, for example, to body posture (Dubowitz *et al.* 1970). The healthy preterm baby, should be active, with free limb movements, she should be alert when awake, although her cry may be high pitched and feeble (Gandy 1986).

The overall aim of care is to achieve maximal rates of growth; when planning care for the preterm baby it is helpful to remember that the care given should seek to mimic the functions of the placenta, liquor and the uterus to which the neonate no longer has access. These are:

1. Temperature control.
2. Oxygenation.
3. Nutrition.
4. Excretion.
5. Protection from infection or injury. ·

Preterm babies do not grow as quickly as they would have done if still in utero (D'Souza *et al.* 1985). The decisions about where and how to care for such a baby are made with reference to condition at birth and gestational age (Yu 1987a). Expert resuscitation is vital, so a paediatrician should be present at each preterm delivery (Dear 1984); hypoxia and hypothermia are a great danger to the preterm infant in its first minutes of life (Yu *et al.* 1982). After resuscitation, a well baby weighing over 2 kg can be nursed by her mother's bedside in a warm single room; this has the effect of limiting separation, encouraging breast feeding and preventing complications, such as infection (Boxall *et al.* 1989). In addition, Special Care Baby Unit staff are freed to care for the most sick babies (Dear and McCain 1987). However the transitional care unit must have sufficient staff to care for its babies, without detracting from the care given to other mothers and babies. Any baby who is ill should be admitted to Special Care Baby Unit for observation and treatment. Babies admitted to neonatal intensive care or Special Care Baby Units are usually put in an incubator for the first 12–24 hours, which has the advantage of a stable environment allowing easy observation (Kelnar and Harvey 1987). If her condition is satisfactory, the baby may later be transferred to a cot.

Temperature control

Preterm babies lose heat rapidly; they have a high surface area-to-volume ratio and little subcutaneous fat. The wet, newly-born baby will cool rapidly, unless dried well and placed in warm wraps (Rutter 1986). Exposure to cold increases the baby's risks of mortality and slows the rate of growth (Glass *et al.* 1969). All newborn babies are poor at generating heat, especially the preterm or ill baby (Bruck *et al.* 1962, Chellapah 1980). For every baby there is a specific external temperature which allows her to maintain her temperature with minimal oxygen and energy consumption and no sweating. This is known as the thermoneutral environment; the temperature reduces with gestation and the age of the infant (Rutter 1986). Very low-birthweight babies (below 1.5 kg) can require an external temperature of 35–36°C when nursed in an incubator (Hey 1975). Perspex heat shields can minimise heat loss and facilitate observation (Rutter 1986). In some areas, double-walled incubators have been shown to reduce heat loss (Marks *et al.* 1981). Hats and bootees are helpful (Stothers 1981). As soon as the baby does not require such close observation he can be dressed and the incubator temperature reduced (Rutter 1986). Many ill babies have their temperatures monitored with a skin probe, which minimises disturbance and limits manual recordings to six-hourly (Rutter 1986). Babies being nursed in cots require adequate clothing; thin layers which trap air are preferred to one thick covering (Hey 1983). Cot lids are available, which are especially useful on the postnatal ward or for the baby receiving phototherapy. Some units use radiant heaters over infants in open cradles or cots rather than incubators (Rutter 1986). Heat is gained by radiation but lost by convection to the circulating air. This method facilitates access to the baby, although insensible fluid loss is increased (Williams and Oh 1974).

Oxygenation

Depending on the maturity of lung tissue and neurological control, major respiratory problems can occur in the preterm baby (Henderson-Smart 1986). The simple effort of breathing can be too exhausting for some babies. One of the most frequent disorders is respiratory disease of the newborn (RDN), also referred to as idiopathic respiratory distress syndrome and hyaline membrane disease (Morley 1986). Signs of RDN usually present within 4 hours of birth (even with good Apgar scores at delivery) and include tachypnoea of more than 60 breaths/minute for at least 1 hour, grunting on expiration and sternal recession (Morley 1986). Hypoxia and cyanosis develop if the condition is untreated (Morley 1986). On chest X-ray a characteristic 'ground glass' appearance is seen, due to multiple areas of atelectasis (Kelnar and Harvey 1987).

The major cause of RDN is a lack of surfactant (Adams et al. 1970), a phospho-lipid which reduces surface tension within the alveoli, preventing them from closing totally on expiration (Watkins 1968). Without sufficient surfactant, the alveoli collapse on expiration and great effort is needed to reflate the lungs, resulting in sternal retraction and intercostal recession, due to increased lung resistance (Morley 1986). In an effort to prevent the alveoli collapsing, the glottis is partially closed during expiration, producing an audible grunt (Kelnar and Harvey 1984). Hypoxia and carbon dioxide retention occur, as the infant is unable to ventilate the lungs adequately (Morley 1986). RDN is most common before 34 weeks gestation after which surfactant production improves. The infant of a diabetic mother is more likely to experience RDN at later gestations, due to alterations in surfactant production (Speidal 1983).

Antenatal use of steroids when a preterm baby is anticipated can speed production of surfactant (Liggins and Howie 1972) (see Chapter 23 for more details). A multicentre randomised controlled trial of the effectiveness of administering artificial surfactant to babies born between 23 and 28 weeks gestation has shown improvements in survival (Ten Centre Group 1987). One hundred milligrams of artificial surfactant were given via an endotracheal tube at birth and, if artificially ventilated, on up to three further occasions; the control group received 1 ml of normal saline. The treated group had a mortality of 14% compared with 27% in the control group. There was a reduction in periventricular haemorrhage from 24% to 16% and also in the severity of RDN with the experimental group, requiring on average 19 fewer hours in more than 30% oxygen, 20 hours less ventilation and 17 fewer hours of supplemental oxygen (Ten Centre Study Group 1987).

In otherwise well babies with mild RDN, for example where the only symptom is tachypnoea, the only treatment required may be oxygen supplementation (Morley 1986). This can be given directly into the incubator (for concentrations up to 35%), or using a headbox (up to 60%) (Kelnar and Harvey 1987). When caring for such babies, the oxygen analyser should be placed near the baby's face but away from the oxygen supply. Infants with moderate RDN can require treatment with continuous positive airways pressure (CPAP) (Gregory et al. 1971), also known as continuous distending pressure. This imitates the action of a surfactant by maintaining a small positive pressure (approximately 5 cm H_2O) in the lungs on expiration, preventing alveolar collapse while the baby breathes spontaneously (Morley 1986). CPAP (a positive pressure flow of air, supplemented with oxygen which is often humidified) can be given through an endotracheal tube, a face mask or with nasal prongs (Morley 1986). An open nasogastric tube should be *in situ* to remove any air blown into the stomach and to reduce the risk of aspiration. Arterial blood gas analysis is performed at least four-hourly with the aim of maintaining the reading in the following range:

PaO_2 6–12 kPa
$PaCO_2$ 5–7 kPa
pH 7.25–7.5 (Morley 1986).

Babies with severe RDN usually need intermittent positive pressure ventilation (IPPV) given via an endotracheal tube (Morley 1986). Modern ventilators are highly flexible, allowing variations of respiratory rate, inspiratory/expiratory ratios and pressures to be employed (Morley 1986). Pressures should be sufficient to ventilate the baby without damaging the preterm lung structure, causing a pneumothorax (Morley 1986). Very occasionally, the baby will require paralysing with pancuronium to prevent it fighting the ventilator (Stark *et al*. 1979). For all infants with RDN, close observation of blood gas levels is maintained; oxygen is a drug requiring careful administration; too little causes hypoxia, too much increases the risk of retinopathy of prematurity (Morley 1986). Medical staff can assess blood gas levels from arterial blood obtained from peripheral lines, or more readily via an umbilical arterial catheter (Morley 1986). Transcutaneous monitoring of CO_2 and O_2 levels is possible. This does not give recordings as accurate as an intravascular oxygen electrode mounted on the tip of the arterial catheter (Morley 1986). Oxygen levels should be maintained at 8–12 kPa (Morley 1986). As the condition of the infant receiving IPPV improves, treatment may be changed to CPAP (Kelnar and Harvey 1987). All infants receiving ventilation require neonatal intensive care including physiotherapy, some units use an insulated electric toothbrush to achieve the required chest wall vibration (Kelnar and Harvey 1987). Minimal handling is important, as disturbance increases the baby's oxygen requirements (Long *et al*. 1980). Feeding is usually parenteral (Yu 1976). Oral feeding is always stopped where the baby is ill and also for a period after extubation, to reduce the risk of aspiration.

The other main respiratory problem is transient tachypnoea of the newborn (TTN) (Vyas and Milner 1986). This is commoner in older infants, especially where they have been delivered before labour by caesarean section. Malan (1966) gave the frequency of TTN for vaginal births as 5% of those born at term and 16% if at low birthweight, but following a caesarean section, it was 9% at term and 22% if low birthweight. TTN is caused by retention of fluid in the alveoli, resulting in tachypnoea and possible grunting (Milner *et al*. 1978). Low levels of oxygen therapy can be of assistance, the condition usually resolving itself within 48 hours (Vyas and Milner 1986).

Nutrition

The preterm baby is capable of rapid growth, although optimum rates are rarely achieved (Brook 1984; D'Souza 1988). Most newborn babies lose 5–10% of their bodyweight after delivery, but the sick preterm baby can lose more than this (Lorenz et al. 1982). It can take over 4 weeks to regain birthweight (Reichman et al. 1981). The fit preterm infant can be commenced on oral feeds within 4 hours of birth.

The timing and frequency of feeds must take into account maturity of the sucking and swallowing reflex (before 32 weeks gestation these are not integrated (Lucas 1986)), and the stomach capacity. In addition the preterm infant may be deficient in some enzymes necessary for digestion (Lucas 1986). Infants weighing less than 1.8 kg often require initial tube feeding with a nasogastric tube; if carefully anchored, this can remain in place for a number of days without interfering with respiration (Kelnar and Harvey 1987). Before any feed is given, the tube must be aspirated, to check that it is in the stomach (Kelnar and Harvey 1987); preterm gastric secretions tend to be less strongly acid than those of a term baby. Feeds can be given one to three-hourly, depending on stomach capacity or via a continuous pump with aspiration of all stomach contents three-hourly to assess absorption rates. The stomach will empty better if the infant is nursed prone or on her right side (Kelnar and Harvey 1987).

Gandy and Roberton (1987) recommend starting all babies on 60 ml/kg/day, increasing by 30 ml/kg increments, depending on tolerance, to a maximum of 200 ml/kg/day by 2 weeks (Yu 1987a). For infants with an increased fluid requirement, receiving phototherapy or using radiant heaters, and for SGA babies, this maximum can be increased to 225–250 ml/kg/day (Tuck 1986). Discussion has occurred as to which is the best milk to give preterm babies (Morgan 1988). The milk of a mother delivered preterm has a higher protein content than mature milk, but still does not provide sufficient protein for growth (Morgan 1988). There are also a number of proprietary preterm milk formulae with raised protein, mineral and carbohydrate contents (Morgan 1988). Most preterm infants receive multivitamin and folic acid supplements (Lucas 1986); iron therapy is usually delayed until haemoglobin levels are low, to avoid depressing red cell production in the bone marrow, or until at least 6–8 weeks after birth (Lucas 1986).

Parenteral nutrition may be required for the ill preterm baby, where oral or tube feeding is impossible, inadequate or hazardous due to malformation, disease or immaturity (Yu 1986). Nutrition is initially with a glucose and electrolyte solution, but later with amino acid and lipid preparations (Brook 1984). The amounts given depend on the baby's gestational age and urea and electrolyte balance (Yu 1986). Early intravenous therapy is necessary to avoid dehydration and hypoglycaemia, which can worsen respiratory and temperature control problems (Yu 1987a). Oral feeding is rarely used for ill babies as, should hypoxia develop, the gut can become ischaemic; bacteria in the gut feeding off static milk can invade the gut wall, causing necrotising enterocolitis (NEC) (Yu et al. 1977). NEC results in inflammatory and haemorrhagic changes in the gut, which can later become necrotic, giving rise to possible perforation and peritonitis (Yu et al. 1977). This is a life-threatening condition, requiring surgical resection (Yu 1987a). When an infant is receiving total parenteral nutrition, careful monitoring is required; for instance, the lipid solution, if overtransfused, can cause hyperlipaemia (Yu 1987a). The infusion site should be observed for tissuing of the infusion with attendant risks of localised necrosis and tissue ulceration (Ramamurthy *et al.* 1975) and the quantities transfused via the syringe pump need observing to prevent overinfusion or underinfusion. All giving sets and tubing should be changed daily to prevent infection; asepsis is vital to avoid septicaemia (Yu 1987a).

Excretion

Careful observation of urinary output is necessary for the ill baby, as kidney failure can occur with respiratory disorders (Tuck 1986). To obtain accurate recordings in an ill baby, nappies may be weighed to calculate output. Total fluid output can be calculated by estimating insensible fluid loss and adding this to the volume of urine produced (Tuck 1986). Urine collecting bags are seldom used for long-term measurement of output, since the skin can become damaged by repeated removal of the adherent surface.

Protection from harm

Good hygiene standards must be employed to protect the vulnerable baby (with an immature immune response) from infection (Pearce and Roberton 1986). The use of plastic aprons and gloves is common but, it is important to use new ones every time the baby is given care, to minimise cross-infection. Infection screens are regularly performed on the infant, (including eye, nose, throat and umbilical swabs and specimens of stool and urine), incubators and cots are changed weekly and bacterial swabs are obtained from taps, sinks, wastebins and the heating system at set intervals (Kelnar and Harvey 1987). The unit should be kept clean by regular damp dusting of surfaces and mopping of the floors (Kelnar and Harvey 1987).

A sick newborn baby does not like being disturbed or handled; she can be startled by sudden jolts and movements (Long *et al.* 1980). Noise levels are quite high in incubators, although there have been no confirmed reports of hearing damage from this (Yu 1987b). Mann *et al.* (1986) have shown that the healthy preterm baby grows faster, feeds for shorter times and sleeps longer when day/night regimes are established. In their study, lighting and noise levels were cut by using low-intensity lights, switching off the radio and reducing staff noise levels between 7 pm and 7 am.

The small-for-gestational age baby

The small-for-gestational age (SGA) infant presents a different physical picture from the preterm baby (Wallis and Harvey 1986). These babies are usually long and thin, with sparse subcutaneous fat and dry loose skin which hangs in folds, especially over the backs of the thighs and the buttocks (Gandy 1986). In very severely growth-retarded babies, the head circumference may be below the tenth centile (Wallis and Harvey 1986), but brain growth is usually spared in intrauterine starvation (Gruenwald 1974). SGA babies are usually very alert, voracious feeders; problems are related to lack of oxygen and nutrients in utero (Wallis and Harvey 1986).

Perinatal asphyxia

For a fetus with an already compromised utero-placental circulation, the strain of labour may be too much (Hutchins 1980). Chronic intrauterine hypoxia gives little spare capacity to cope with the usual reduction in oxygen supply during contractions (Hutchins 1980). Fetal distress during labour is more common; meconium may be passed and, should intrauterine gasping occur, meconium aspiration can lead to pneumonitis and secondary bacterial infection (Miller 1985). If meconium is present or an SGA baby is anticipated, a paediatrician must be standing by at delivery (Wallis and Harvey 1986). During resuscitation, a laryngoscope should be passed and suction performed under direct vision (Miller 1985). If any meconium is visible below the vocal cords, bronchial lavage may be performed.

Hypothermia

Hypothermia occurs due to lack of both subcutaneous fat and of a readily available energy source (Wallis and Harvey 1986). Such babies cool easily and need to be quickly dried after birth (Rutter 1986).

Hypoglycaemia

As SGA babies are mature, they have higher calorie requirements than a preterm baby of the same weight and postnatal age (Wallis and Harvey 1986). They have active brains and poor glycogen stores, so hypoglycaemia can easily occur (Wallis and Harvey 1986). Blood glucose levels should be measured for at least the first 24 hours and this, together with early feeding, can usually prevent problems (Wallis and Harvey 1986).

Infections

SGA babies are susceptible to infection, especially of the chest and skin. They have low levels of gamma globulins (Wallis and Harvey 1986). Their cracked peeling skin provides an easy entry route and haven for microorganisms. Baby oil massaged onto the skin or added to the bath can help. Careful observation for septic spots and other foci is vital.

Sequelae of low birthweight

Survival rates of preterm infants are improving with improved technology and understanding, but the effects on morbidity are less well known (Yu *et al*. 1986). It is documented that sudden infant death syndrome occurs more commonly in preterm babies (Kelnar and Harvey 1987). Some other children are left with mental retardation or behavioural and learning problems (Stewart 1986). Retinopathy of prematurity (ROP) is still a problem. In this condition, there is proliferation of the capillaries and dilation of the retinal arteries and veins. Oedema occurs which can lead to partial or total retinal detachment and blindness (Mushin and Roberton 1986). It is caused in part by high levels of oxygen used in the care of extremely preterm infants (Mushin and Roberton 1986). ROP is the commonest cause of blindness in the neonatal period (Mushin and Roberton 1986).

Ventilated babies are susceptible to chest infections and chronic lung disorders (Yu 1987a). Brain damage following intraventricular haemorrhage requires long-term assessment through child welfare clinics (Stewart 1986).

There are many ethical dilemmas as to how long treatment should be continued and at what point does one decide that the situation is hopeless. Kuhse and Singer (1987) have explored this issue by asking whether life itself has a value, or whether it is only life of a certain quality which is valuable. If so, where does one draw the line between acceptable and unacceptable quality (Kuhse and Singer 1987)? Who should make the decision? In a time of economic stringency, neonatal intensive care has to argue for a share of resources against such causes as kidney dialysis and hip replacements (Kuhse and Singer 1987).

Working in a neonatal intensive care unit is a very stressful experience for staff who require much support to avoid 'burn-out' (Vas Dias 1987).

Involving the parents

The birth of a low-birthweight baby is a time of great anxiety for the parents (Ludman 1989). Plans have been disrupted and arrangements surrounding the birth have had to be changed (Richards 1986).

Parents feel that they are somehow to blame (Kaplan and Mason 1960) and this feeling is not helped by the frightening appearance of Special Care Baby Units (Slade 1988). The parents are concerned for the future of their baby while everyone rushes around looking efficient and busy (Richards 1986). Preterm babies do not look like the picture parents have of healthy neonates; some find their baby hard to love (Burdeau 1989); they do not have the 'cute' features which encourage caring and attachment (Lorenz 1981). If a small baby is anticipated, a visit to the Intensive Care Unit prior to the birth can be a great help. If this is not possible, a visit from the paediatrician during labour, to explain what will happen after birth is reassuring (Richards 1986).

If possible after the birth the parents should see and hold their baby before her transfer to the neonatal unit (Richards 1986). At all times, full explanations should be given to foster an atmosphere of trust. In a descriptive study of mothers of babies in a Special Care Baby Unit, McHaffie (1989) found that the mothers obtained most support from their partners. Midwifery staff in the unit were helpful, but there could be difficulties establishing new relationships when the staff changed. Other family members were not especially useful, tending to want to reassure, which did not assist the mother (McHaffie 1989). Slade (1988) found that she gained most support and encouragement from the mothers of babies who were at the same stage as her own.

Photographs can be taken for the parents to keep, and some units use closed circuit television to limit feelings of separation (McIntosh et al. 1985). Free visiting is common in most units, with parents being encouraged to stay as long as they want (Richards 1986). In some hospitals, there are facilities for fathers to stay overnight. As the infant's condition improves, parents are encouraged to help in the care, which makes them feel that they are 'doing something' (Richards 1986). When the mother goes home, a breast pump can be loaned so that her milk can be brought in for the baby. For families on low incomes, there may be help available towards the cost of visiting. Some units have a support network of parents whose babies have been treated there, which can be a great help. Parental anxiety is high for all babies in special care; this can be reduced by avoiding unnecessary admissions (Richards and Roberton 1978). Before the baby goes home, parents are encouraged to return to the unit to stay for 24–48 hours, giving complete care under the supervision of neonatal staff.

References

Adams F H, Fujiwara T, Emmanouilides G C and Raiha N (1970) 'Lung phospholipids of human fetusus and infants with and without hyalin membrane disease' *Journal of Pediatrics* 77: 833–43

Boxall J F, Whitby C, Lawrence C and Tripp J (1989) 'Who is holding the baby?' *Midwives Chronicle* Feb: 32–6

Brook O G (1984) 'Low birthweight and feeding' in G Chamberlain (ed) *Contemporary Obstetrics* 236–44 Butterworth: London

Bruck J, Adams F H and Bruck M (1962) 'Temperature regulation in infants with chronic hypoxemia' *Pediatrics* 30: 350–60

Budin P (1907) *The Nursling* Caxton Publishing: London

Burdeau G (1989) 'The perceived attractiveness of preterm infants with cranial moulding' *Journal of Obstetrical, Gynecological and Neonatal Nursing* 18(1): 38–44

Chellapah G (1980) *Aspects of Thermoregulation in Term and Preterm Newborn Babies* PhD Thesis, University of Nottingham

Dear P R F (1984) 'Low birthweight-hospital care' in G Chamberlain (ed) *Contemporary Obstetrics* 227–35 Butterworth: London

Dear P R F and McCain B I (1987) 'Establishment of an intermediate care ward for babies and mothers' *Archives of Disease in Childhood* 62: 597–600

D'Souza S W (1988) 'Outcome of modern intensive care for low birthweight infants' *Midwife, Health Visitor and Community Nurse* 24(11): 484–8

D'Souza S W, Vale J, Simms D G and Chiswick M L (1985) 'Feeding, growth and biochemical studies in very low birthweight infants' *Archives of Disease in Childhood* 60: 215–8

Dubowitz L M S, Dubowitz V and Goldberg C (1970) 'Clinical assessment of gestational age in the newborn infant' *Journal of Pediatrics* 77: 1–10

Gandy G M (1986) 'Examination of the neonate including gestational age assessment' in N R C Roberton (ed) *Textbook of Neonatology* 131–47 Churchill Livingstone: Edinburgh

Gandy G M and Roberton N J C (1987) *Lecture Notes on Neonatology* Blackwell Scientific: Oxford

Glass L, Silverman W A and Sinclair J C (1969) 'Relationship of the thermal environment and caloric intake to growth and resting metabolism in the late neonatal period' *Biology of the Neonate* 14: 324–40

Gregory G A, Kitterman J A, Phibbs R H, Tooley W H and Hamilton W K (1971) 'Treatment of idiopathic respiratory distress syndrome with continuous positive pressure' *New England Journal of Medicine* 284: 1333–40

Gruenwald P (1974) 'Pathology of the deprived fetus and its supply line' in K Elliot and J Knight (eds) *Size at Birth* Ciba Symposium No 27 3–9 Associated Scientific Publishers: Amsterdam

Henderson-Smart D J (1986) 'Pulmonary disease of the newborn. Part 1: Neonatal respiratory physiology' in N R C Roberton (ed) *Textbook of Neonatology* 259–73 Churchill Livingstone: Edinburgh

Hey E N (1975) 'Thermal neutrality' *British Medical Bulletin* 31: 69–74

Hey E N (1983) 'Temperature regulation in sick infants' in J Tinker and M Rapin (eds) *Care of the Critically Ill Patient* 1013–29 Springer Verlag: Berlin

Hibbard B M (1987) 'Aetiology of preterm labour' *British Medical Journal* 294: 594–5

House of Commons Second Report From the Social Services Committee (1980) *Perinatal and Neonatal Mortality* 96–105 HMSO: London

Hutchins C J (1980) 'Delivery of the growth retarded baby' *Obstetrics and Gynecology* 56: 683–6

Kaplan D M and Mason E A (1960) 'Maternal reactions to premature birth viewed as an acute emotional disorder' *American Journal of Orthopsychiatry* 30: 539–52

Kelnar C J H and Harvey D (1987) 'Respiratory distress syndrome' in G Chamberlain (ed) *Contemporary Obstetrics* 267–80 Butterworth: London

Kelnar C J H and Harvey D (1987) *The Sick Newborn Baby (2nd edn)* Balliere Tindall: London

Klaus M H, Fanaroff A A and Martin R J (1986) 'The physical environment' in M H Klaus and A A Fanaroff (eds) *Care of the High Risk Neonate (3rd edn)* 96–112 W B Saunders: Philadelphia

Kuhse H and Singer P (1987) 'Ethical issues raised by treatment of extremely preterm infants' in V Y H Yu and E C Wood (eds) *Prematurity* 257–73 Churchill Livingstone: Edinburgh

Liggins G C and Howie R N (1972) 'A controlled trial of antepartum glucocorticoid treatment for the prevention of respiratory distress syndrome in premature infants' *Pediatrics* 50: 515

Long J G, Phillips A G S and Lucey J F (1980) 'Excessive handling as a cause of hypoxemia' *Pediatrics* 65: 203–7

Lorenz J M, Kleinman L I and Kotagul U R (1982) 'Water balance in very low birthweight infants: relationship to water and sodium intake and effect in outcome' *Journal of Pediatrics* 101: 423

Lorenz K (1981) *The Foundations of Ethology* Springer-Verlag: New York

Lucas A (1986) 'Nutritional physiology: dietary requirements of term and preterm infants' in N R C Roberton (ed) *Textbook of Neonatology* 178–92 Churchill Livingstone: Edinburgh

Ludman L (1989) 'The psychological care of mothers with very sick neonates' *Maternal and Child Health* 14(7): 197–9

Lunell N O, Nylund L E, Lewander R, Sarby B and Thornstrom S (1982) 'Uteroplacental blood flow in pre-eclampsia measurements with indium-113m and a computer linked gamma camera' *Clinical and Experimental Hypertension* B1: 105–17

McHaffie H E (1989) 'Mothers of low birthweight babies: who supports them?' *Midwifery* 5(3): 113–21

McIntosh N, Berger M and Jay L (1985) 'Facilitating attachment by television' *Maternal and Child Health* 10(3): 74–6

Malan A F (1966) 'Neonatal tachypneoa' *Australian Paediatric Journal* 3: 159–63

Mann N P, Haddow R, Stokes L, Goodley S and Rutter N (1986) 'Effect of day and night on preterm infants in a newborn nursery' *British Medical Journal* 293: 1265–7

Marks K A, Lee C A, Bolan C D and Maisels J M (1981) 'Oxygen consumption and temperature control of premature infants in a double-wall incubator' *Pediatrics* 68: 93–8

Marlow N, D'Souza S W and Chiswick M L (1987) 'Neurodevelopmental outcome in babies weighing less than 2001 gms at birth' *British Medical Journal* 294: 1582–6

Miller F C (1985) 'The significance of meconium in amniotic fluid' in J Studd (ed) *Management of Labour* 188–94 Blackwell Scientific: Oxford

Milner A D, Saunders R A and Hopkin I E (1978) 'Effects of delivery by caesarean section on lung mechanics and lung volume in human neonates' *Archives of Disease in Childhood* 53: 545–8

Morgan J B (1988) 'Nutrition and feeding of low birthweight infants' *Midwife, Health Visitor and Community Nurse* 24(8): 324–5

Morley C J (1986) 'The respiratory distress syndrome' in N R C Roberton (ed) *Textbook of Neonatology* 274–311 Churchill Livingstone: Edinburgh

Mushin A S and Roberton N R C (1986) 'Neonatal ophthalmology' in N R C Roberton (ed) *Textbook of Neonatology* 721–4 Churchill Livingstone: Edinburgh

Pearce R G and Roberton N R C (1986) 'Infection in the newborn' in N R C Roberton (ed) *Textbook of Neonatology* 725–81 Churchill Livingstone: Edinburgh

Ramamurthy R S, Harris V and Pildes R S (1975) 'Subcutaneous calcium deposition in the neonate associated with intravenous administration of calcium gluconate' *Pediatrics* 55: 802–6

Reichman B L, Chessex P and Putet G (1981) 'Diet, fat accretion and growth in premature infants' *New England Journal of Medicine* 305: 1495

Richards M P M (1986) 'Psychological aspects of neonatal care' in N R C Roberton (ed) *Textbook of Neonatology* 20–34 Churchill Livingstone: Edinburgh

Richards M P M and Roberton N R C (1978) 'Admission and discharge policies for for special care units' in F S W Brimblecombe, M P M Richards and N R C Roberton (eds) *Separation and Special Care Baby Care Units* Clinics in Developmental Medicine No 68 82–110 Heinemann: London

Rutter N (1986) 'Temperature control and its disorders' in N R C Roberton (ed) *Textbook of Neonatology* 148–61 Churchill Livingstone: Edinburgh

Scott A, Moar V and Ounstead M (1981) 'The relative contributions of different maternal factors in small-for-gestational-age pregnancies' *European Journal of Obstetrics and Gynaecology* 12: 157–65

Slade P (1988) 'A psychologists view of a special care baby unit' *Maternal and Child health* 13(8): 208–12

Speidal B (1983) 'Infant of the diabetic mother' *Medicine International* 1(35): 1641–2

Stark A R, Bascom R and Franz I D (1979) 'Muscle relaxation of mechanically ventilated infants' *Journal of Pediatrics* 94: 439–43

Stein Z, Susser M and Rush D (1978) 'Prenatal nutrition and birthweight: experiments and quasi-experimental in the past decade' *Journal of Reproductive Medicine* 21: 287–99

Stewart A L (1986) 'Follow-up studies' in N R C Roberton (ed) *Textbook of Neonatology* 42–59 Churchill Livingstone: Edinburgh

Stothers J K (1981) 'Head insulation and heat loss in the newborn' *Archives of Disease in Childhood* 56: 530–4

Ten Centre Study Group (1987) 'Ten centre trial of artificial surfactant (artificial lung expanding compound) in very premature babies' *British Medical Journal* 294: 991–6

Tuck S (1986) 'Fluid and electrolyte balance in the neonate' in N R C Roberton (ed) *Textbook of Neonatology* 163–77 Churchill Livingstone: Edinburgh

Vas Dias S (1987) 'Psychotherapy in special care baby units' *Nursing Times* 83(10): 50–2

Vyas H and Milner A D (1986) 'Other respiratory diseases in the neonate' in N R C Roberton (ed) *Textbook of Neonatology* 312–39 Churchill Livingstone: Edinburgh

Wallis S M and Harvey D (1986) 'Fetal growth, intrauterine growth retardation and small for dates babies' in N R C Roberton (ed) *Textbook of Neonatology* 119–28 Churchill Livingstone: Edinburgh

Watkins J C (1968) 'The surface properties of pure phospholipids in relation to those of lung extracts' *Acta Biochemica Physica* 152: 293–306

Williams P R and Oh W (1974) 'Effects of radiant warmer on insensible water loss in newborn infants' *American Journal of Diseases in Childhood* 128: 511–4

Winick M and Noble A (1966) 'Cellular response in rates during malnutrition at various ages' *Journal of Nutrition* 89: 300–6

World Health Organization (1977) 'Recommended definitions, terminology and format for statistical tables related to the perinatal period and use of a new certificate for cause of perinatal deaths' *Acta Obstetrica and Gynaecologica Scandanavia* 56: 247–53

Yu V Y H (1976) 'Cardiorespiratory response to feeding in newborn infants' *Archives of Disease in Childhood* 51: 305–9

Yu V Y H (1986) 'Parenteral nutrition in the neonate' in N R C Roberton (ed) *Textbook of Neonatology* 211–21 Churchill Livingstone: Edinburgh

Yu V Y H (1987a) 'Neonatal complications in preterm infants' in V Y H Yu and E C Wood EC (eds) *Prematurity* 148–69 Churchill Livingstone: Edinburgh

Yu V Y H (1987b) 'Survival and neurodevelopment outcome of preterm infants' in V Y H Yu and E C Wood (eds) *Prematurity* 223–45 Churchill Livingstone: Edinburgh

Yu V Y H, Loke H L, Symoniwitz W, Orgill A A and Astbury J (1986) 'Prognosis for infants born at 23–28 weeks gestation' *British Medical Journal* 293: 1200–3

Yu V Y H, Tudehope D I and Gill G (1977) 'Neonatal necrotizing enterocolitis: clincal aspects' *Medical Journal of Australia* 1: 685–8

Yu V Y H, Zhao S M and Bajuk B (1982) 'Results of intensive care for 375 very low birthweight infants' *Australian Paediatric Journal* 18: 188–92

37   The newborn requiring extra care

This chapter considers those babies at high risk of complications or poor outcome, whose care is not considered elsewhere in this book. The subjects included are the infant of the diabetic mother, the neurologically disturbed baby including the infant of the drug-addicted mother, and infections occurring before, during and after birth.

The infant of the diabetic mother

In recent times the outlook for the infant of the diabetic mother (IDM) has improved greatly (Ballard *et al*. 1984). Closer surveillance of all pregnant women detects most women with gestational diabetes. The known insulin-dependent diabetic is better stabilised by new insulin regimes and high-fibre diets (Vaughan 1987).

The grossly overweight plethoric infant is now a rare occurrence, although for the IDM, perinatal mortality and morbidity rates are still higher than for their peers (Brudenell and Wills 1984). Whilst good control of diabetes has helped to reduce the rate of congenital anomalies (most commonly musculo-skeletal or cardiac Cousins 1983), careful neonatal assessment is still vital (Lewis and Steyger 1985). Excess fetal growth (macrosomia) is still found (Dandona *et al*. 1984). This may be due to an increased production of growth factors, in addition to the excess laying-down of fat which occurs in hyperglycaemia. Even with good diabetic control, glucose concentrations in amniotic fluid have been found to be higher than for the infant of a non-diabetic mother (Tchobrobtsky *et al.* 1980). In some mothers with diabetes of long standing, placental insufficiency can result in a growth-retarded baby (Pederson and Pederson 1979).

As with most at-risk infants, the IDM requires expert care immediately after birth (Aynsley-Green and Soltesz 1986). Early cord clamping can prevent overtransfusion of an already plethoric baby (Dewhurst 1981). IDMs may be delivered prematurely, due to maternal complications. For these babies, especially those born by caesarean section, expert resuscitation is vital, since respiratory disease of the newborn (RDN) is more common in the IDM, as lung maturity is often delayed (Stubbs and Stubbs 1978). The plasma glucose level in cord blood should be determined and used as a baseline for later recordings (Aynsley-Green and Soltesz 1986). Glucose levels fall rapidly after birth, staying low (1.1–1.7 mmol/l) until the resolution of the high circulating insulin levels, caused by intrauterine hyperglycaemia. Early feeding is helpful in preventing hypoglycaemia (Lewis and Steyger 1985). Should this condition develop in an already ill baby, care should be taken not to give too much glucose, as insulin production will be further stimulated, compounding the problem. For the well baby who develops hypoglycaemia, glucagon (0.03–0.1 mg/kg) will promptly increase blood glucose level (Aynsley-Green and Soltesz 1986).

Depending on the gestation and condition of the infant she can be nursed with her mother or admitted to a Special Care Baby Unit (Lewis and Steyger 1985). One compromise is transitional care. This allows the baby's mother and postnatal ward staff to care during the day, the baby being transferred to Special Care Baby Unit overnight.

For the first 12 hours after birth, a close watch is kept on blood glucose levels (two to four-hourly); if satisfactory and the infant is feeding well, problems are unlikely (Aynsley-Green and Soltesz 1986). Early feeding (either breast or artificial), has reduced the need for parenteral glucose with all its attendant risks of rebound hypoglycaemia and inflammation at the drip site. The sensitivity of current blood glucose-measuring techniques and the purity of human insulin, which is now commonly used, have allowed the nursing mother to control her diabetes while breast feeding her child (Alban Davies *et al.* 1989). However the baby's need for early feeding before the milk supply has commenced has to be balanced against the necessity of stimulating the mother's milk supply. For this reason, the baby should be put to the breast whenever hungry and then, if necessary, 'topped-up' with EBM (Lewis and Steyger 1985). This should be discontinued as soon as the mother's lactation begins. There is no evaluative research on the need to give extra-expressed breast milk to breast-fed IDMs in the early days before lactation is established. Mothers used to managing their own diabetes may express concern at the relatively low blood glucose levels of the neonate (Lewis and Steyger 1985). Careful explanation can help the mother understand that readings of 2–3 mmols/l are quite normal for her baby.

Given the increased occurrence of respiratory distress syndome and transient tachypnoea of the newborn (TTN), heart and respiratory rates are measured (usually three to four-hourly) for the first 12–24 hours, depending on the baby's condition at birth (Lewis and Steyger 1985). Some babies may require additional oxygen or even assisted ventilation for a time. Where the diabetes was poorly controlled, the IDM may present with a raised packed cell volume and polycythaemia, haemoglobin levels can be in excess of 20 g/100 ml (Brudenell and Wills 1984). Resulting problems include heart failure and respiratory distress, although the most common is jaundice (Lewis and Steyger 1985). The IDM who develops jaundice is doubly disadvantaged, as the baby (often preterm) becomes lethargic and difficult to feed, upsetting her energy balance. Treatment is by the early use of phototherapy. In rare severe cases, exchange transfusion may be required (Lewis and Steyger 1985).

The parents will be very concerned for the welfare of their baby. Detailed explanations should be given as to the causes of the problems and their management. Preparation before delivery and an awareness that the baby might require special care can help ease the situation. The parents should be encouraged to care for their child as much as possible, whether in the postnatal ward or Special Care Baby Unit. The mother may feel guilty that it is she who has caused the problems for their baby. Such a situation requires skilful and tactful handling. With regard to longer-term effects, Persson (1986) found that 3% of a sample of 73 children of diabetic mothers themselves developed diabetes by the age of 10 years, compared to a rate of 0.1% for the general population.

The neurologically disturbed baby

This is a term used to describe a baby showing abnormal neurological signs affecting its level of alertness, including hypotonia and convulsions (Volpe 1981). In the newborn, most neurological disorders are secondary to metabolic, circulatory, infectious, physical or environmental disturbances. Disorders originating in the central nervous system, such as cerebral aqueduct stenosis, account for a small proportion of cases (Arniel-Tison et al. 1986).

Major causes of cerebral dysfunction in the neonatal period include:

Antepartum:	Chronic fetal distress.
	Acute fetal distress (possibly due to maternal or fetal haemorrhage).
	Chromosomal anomalies.
	Congenital malformations.
	Infections, e.g. CMV, rubella.
	Drugs, e.g. narcotics.
	Vascular changes, e.g. cerebral ischaemia, haemorrhage.
Intrapartum:	Birth injury.
	Cerebrovascular compromise – acute fetal distress or extra stress upon an already compromised fetus.

Postpartum: Acute respiratory disease (usually in low-birthweight babies).
Infections, especially meningitis.
Metabolic disturbances: hypoglycaemia, hypocalcaemia,
hypomagnesaemia, hyponatraemia and hypernatraemia,
hyperbilirubinaemia, hypothyroidism.
(Adapted from Arniel-Tison *et al.* (1986), p. 357.)

There are four main types of seizure which occur in the neonate, listed in order of increasing severity:

1. Subtle manifestations. These include deviation or jerking of the eyes, repeated blinking and tonic posturing of the limbs (Tarby and Volpe 1986). There may be apnoeic episodes. Such signs are easily missed.
2. Focal clonic. Well-localised clonic jerking of one or more limbs (Tarby and Volpe 1986).
3. Multifocal clonic. Clonic movements of one or more limbs, which migrate in a non-ordered fashion to other areas of the body. These may progress to a more generalised clonic seizure (Tarby and Volpe 1986).
4. Tonic. Characterised by extension of the limbs, stenortorous (noisy) breathing, eye jerking and apnoea. The baby may lie rigid and be hypertonic (Tarby and Volpe 1986). This type of convulsion is often present in cases of severe brain damage and has a poor prognosis (Kelnar and Harvey 1987).

It is important for the midwife to distinguish the more subtle types of seizure from jitteriness, which is common in many newborn babies (Tarby and Volpe 1986). In jitteriness, the movements are fast, of equal rate and synchronous (Arniel-Tison *et al.* 1986). Bending a jittery limb stops it moving; jitteriness returns when the limb is straightened. The movements in a fit, however, have fast and slow phases; in the latter, where relaxation takes over from active contraction.

Medical diagnosis

A detailed history, including the medical history of the mother and the progress of the pregnancy, labour and birth will need to be taken to search for causative events (Casaer *et al.* 1986). The following investigations will also be performed:

1. Blood gases, to detect hypoxia and acidosis.
2. Blood electrolyte levels, to detect metabolic disturbances.
3. Full blood count.
4. Full infection screen including blood culture.
5. Lumbar puncture, to exclude meningitis.
6. Head circumference.
7. Cranial ultrasound, to demonstrate intracranial or intraventricular bleeding.
8. A CT scan.

A full physical and neurological examination will also be carried out.

Medical treatment involves removing the cause, if known or, if not, giving supportive and symptomatic care. For short-term control of convulsions, diazepam (IM or IV) or, less commonly, paraldehyde (deep IM or rectally) are used, but care should be taken as respiratory depression or apnoeic episodes can occur (Arniel-Tison *et al.* 1986). Where more prolonged therapy is required, phenobarbitone can be used with an initial IM dose, thereafter six-hourly orally; as the rate of metabolism in the neonate is variable, monitoring of blood levels is necessary (Arniel-Tison *et al.* 1986).

Midwifery management

1. Admit to Special Care Baby Unit.
2. Involve the parents, who will be very worried.
3. Put the baby into an incubator for observation, providing a stable environment and ensuring minimal handling. The incubator may need to be sited away from direct light.
4. As an aid to observation, an apnoea alarm, a temperature probe and a heart-rate monitor should be used. These also minimise disturbance when observations of the baby's condition are being made.
5. Observations. The following are the minimum observations required. Depending on the infant's condition, some or all may need to be recorded more frequently:

   Hourly – heart and respiratory rate.
   Three-hourly – colour, skin temperature, incubator temperature, muscle tone, reaction to stimuli. Care of intravenous site if present.
   Six-hourly – rectaloraxilla temperature. Blood glucose.

   A detailed record of all fits, their focus, duration and time of occurrence should be kept.
6. Nutrition must be maintained, the route depending on neonatal well-being. The mother who wishes to breast feed, but whose baby is unable to suckle should be encouraged to express milk, which could be fed via a nasogastric tube or stored until the baby is fit enough to receive it.
7. All the normal care given to a newborn baby should be continued if at all possible.

Volpe (1981) has noted an improvement in the outcome for babies with neurological disturbances since the mid 1960s, but this is still dependent upon the underlying cause. Kelnar and Harvey (1987) give the prognoses for various causes of convulsion as follows:

- Good prognosis – fits due to mild birth asphyxia, subarachnoid haemorrhage and hypocalcaemia.

- Guarded prognosis – fits due to severe birth asphyxia, intraventricular haemorrhage, prolonged hypoglycaemia, meningitis and hyponatraemia or hypernatraemia.
- Poor prognosis – in cases of cerebral malfunction or any infant suffering prolonged neurological abnormality.

The hypotonic (floppy) baby

Hypotonia is the most common abnormal neurological sign in the newborn (Lou and Volpe 1986). Hypotonia can be a natural occurrence for a short time after a difficult delivery, but the most common cause is intrauterine asphyxia, especially if complicated by prematurity. Assessment of neonatal muscle tone is difficult, but it is important to differentiate between weak movements and paralysis (Carroll 1986). It is unusual for an otherwise well baby to be floppy, but there are some rare causes such as neonatal myaesthenia gravis (Carroll 1986).

The hypotonic infant requires close observation of movement (especially those made against gravity) and the ability to suck and swallow (Arniel-Tison et al. 1986). Diagnostic techniques are similar to those used to investigate the baby suffering with convulsions. If the cause was a traumatic delivery, the baby, unless suffering cerebral damage, should recover with tender loving care. Where possible, the underlying cause should be treated, other problems being dealt with symptomatically. Where hypotonia persists, the prognosis is poor. The parents will require much support at this time and they should be made aware of the gravity of the situation.

The infant of the drug-dependent mother

The most commonly reported fetal response to maternal drug abuse is intrauterine growth retardation (Stern 1984). It is, however, difficult to demonstrate cause and effect, given the chaotic lifestyle adopted by many abusers (Cohen 1982). Alcohol and tobacco may have been used, which inhibit fetal growth in addition to suppressing maternal appetite. Narcotics themselves may interfere with transfer of nutrients and gases between mother and fetus (Lindo 1987). It appears that growth retardation occurs more commonly where the mother is using heroin than when she is on methadone (Zelon 1973). Preterm delivery is more common amongst drug abusers (Lindo 1987). Where the drugs are given intravenously, there is risk of transfer of hepatitis B (Harper et al. 1974) and HIV, necessitating both antenatal and neonatal screening (Brooklyn Health Action Committee 1986). Sudden withdrawal of drugs in pregnancy has been associated with fetal distress and stillbirth, possibly due to the increase in maternal oxygen requirements at the time of withdrawal, resulting in intrauterine hypoxia (Chappel 1972).

A baby who has become accustomed to drugs in utero will, on or after delivery, show signs of withdrawal (Lindo 1987). These may not be anticipated, as, for many addicted women, there are few obvious signs of abuse. Given the increasing popularity of smoking, sniffing or ingesting drugs, outward signs such as needle marks are not always apparent (Phillips 1986). Signs of withdrawal exhibited by the baby in order of decreasing frequency are as follows:

1. Tremors
2. Irritability
3. Hypertonicity
4. Vomiting
5. High-pitched cry
6. Sneezing
7. Respiratory distress
8. Fever
9. Diarrhoea
10. Sweating
11. Mucus secretion
12. Convulsions
13. Yawning (Kelnar and Harvey 1987).

The time of onset of these symptoms depends upon the type of substance used and the timing of the last dose taken by the mother (Phillips 1986). The average time of the onset of symptoms is 72 hours, with a range from 24 hours to 32 days (the latter for methadone, which has a range for the onset of symptoms of 10–32 days (Kandall and Gartner 1974). Where a 'cocktail' of drugs has been taken, withdrawal may be prolonged (Williams 1983). The infant of the drug-dependent mother tends to be irritable, fretful and not easily comforted. Sucking may appear adequate, but feeding is often poor, due to lack of coordination of sucking and swallowing and the poor strength of sucking.

Treatment of babies in withdrawal is aimed at reducing irritability and preventing convulsions (Kelnar and Harvey 1987). Drugs employed include phenobarbitone, chlorpromazine and diazepam, although none is ideal (Phillips 1986). Phenobarbitone depresses the central nervous system and causes withdrawal symptoms, chlorpromazine produces drowsiness while diazepam, which is poorly metabolised in the neonate, can, in addition to sedation, exacerbate jaundice. The doses of the various drugs are reduced every other day, but can be increased should symptoms recur.

The baby requires close observation in addition to peace and quiet (to prevent irritability). Some infants find swaddling a comfort, whereas others prefer being left in a darkened, quiet corner (Phillips 1986). A number of babies obtain relief of symptoms by being carried in a sling, the closeness to another human being bringing comfort. Depending on the condition of the child, nasogastric tube feeding may be necessary; breast feeding is contra-indicated where the mother is taking methadone which, due to its small molecular size, is excreted (although only in small quantities) in breast milk. Parents should be encouraged to visit and care for their child. All babies need screening for HIV and hepatitis B virus; for the latter immunoglobulin can be given to help prevent chronic infection (Lindo 1987). Even with proper care, the child of the drug-dependent mother has an increased perinatal mortality rate and a higher incidence of sudden infant death syndrome.

The future for the child is hard to predict. It is dependent on the parents' home environment, lifestyle, whether addiction continues and upon the presence of a non-addicted, responsible adult (Williams 1983). In some cases, the newborn has been placed under court protection or in the care of the social services from birth. The child care system in the United Kingdom is cumbersome, cannot see into the future and can only assess the effectiveness of its actions in hindsight (Jones *et al*. 1987). All the midwife can do is to prepare the parents both antenatally and postnatally for the responsibility they are to assume.

Infection in the newborn

A fetus can develop infection at any time between conception and birth. Most resist infection by the use of defence mechanisms and are born unaffected, some die in utero and others are born handicapped (Morgan-Capner and Griffiths 1984). Due to the immaturity of its immune system, the newborn is susceptible to infection, especially if ill or preterm (Pearce and Roberton 1986).

Defences against infection:

1. *Physical*. These include intact skin and mucus membranes, acting as a barrier to organisms wishing to reach the tissues beneath.
2. *Humoral*. Immunoglobulins.
   (a) Immunoglobulin G (IgG) can, due to its small molecular size, cross the placenta, especially in the last 3 months of pregnancy. Preterm babies are likely to have low levels of IgG (Cates *et al*. 1983) At birth, IgG levels are the same as maternal but these passively acquired antibodies are gradually destroyed up until 3 months of age. The infant's production of antibodies is only in response to exposure to infection. Adult levels of IgG are reached again at 3 years of age (Pearce and Roberton 1986).
   (b) Immunoglobulin M (IgM) is unable to cross the placenta. IgM is necessary to counteract gram-negative bacteria. The fetus produces small amounts of IgM; high levels at birth indicate the presence or history of intrauterine infection (Pearce and Roberton 1986). Small quantities of IgM are found in breast milk (Pearce and Roberton 1986).
   (c) Immunoglobulin A (IgA) is synthesised by the neonate from birth. This is the immunoglobulin present in the greatest amounts in colostrum and breast milk (Pearce and Roberton 1986). In the latter, it acts with lactoferrin to prevent the growth of *E. coli*, protecting the neonate from gastroenteritis (Kelnar and Harvey 1987).
3. *Cellular immunity*. The newborn has lower than adult levels of lymphocytes and leucocytes (Pearce and Roberton 1986). This, in conjunction with low levels of immunoglobulins, partly explains the neonate's impaired ability to attack pathogens.

Timing of infection:

1. Prenatal or transplacental.
2. Intranatal.
3. Neonatal.

Transplacental infections

In utero, the fetus is protected from most infections by intact amniotic membranes and by the placenta, which forms a barrier to most bacteria (Larsen *et al*. 1974). The fetus can become infected by viruses (rubella, HIV and cytomegalovirus (CMV), by spirochaetes (syphilis) or protozoa (toxoplasmosis).

Rubella

If acquired in utero, rubella has serious consequences for the developing fetus (Gregg *et al*. 1945). The earlier in pregnancy the infection is acquired, the worse the outlook (Peckham 1972). During the major period of organogenesis (3–6 weeks) there is a 50% risk of damage, which is usually widespread (Peckham 1972). The most common results of rubella infection are congenital heart disease, cataracts or microophthalmia, mental retardation, microcephaly, boney abnormalities and deafness (Pearce and Roberton 1986). Infection in late pregnancy results in a highly infectious neonate. Many babies may be growth-retarded, anaemic and actively excreting the virus. The virus can be cultured from excretions for up to 1 year after birth (Pearce and Roberton 1986).

As a preventative measure, schoolgirls are encouraged to be immunised against rubella, but many slip through the net and the lack of immunity amongst boys and younger children has maintained the pool of infection. Babies in the United Kingdom are now offered vaccination against measles, mumps and rubella in the first year of life. All pregnant women are screened for immunity. If necessary, vaccine is offered after delivery (after ensuring adequate contraception for the next 3 months) (Morgan-Capner and Griffiths 1984). Pregnant women are advised to avoid contact with anybody with a rash, in case the woman is not immune; detailed antibody profiles can be performed if contact does occur. If the pregnancy is found to be at risk of damage from rubella, a termination of pregnancy will be offered (Cunningham *et al*. 1989).

Cytomegalovirus (CMV)

This is a virus similar to herpes which can cause microcephaly, mental retardation, deafness, epilepsy, spasticity, jaundice and hepatosplenomegaly (Preece *et al*. 1984). The neonate may also be growth-retarded and develop respiratory distress. Infection with CMV at any stage in pregnancy can cause problems, but episodes of infection are often unrecognised (Cunningham *et al*. 1989). Screening programmes are of limited help, as they could only be used early when therapeutic abortion could be offered (Morgan-Capner and Griffiths 1984). Not all babies are affected, even in severe cases of infection (Pearce and Roberton 1986). Most authorities favour delaying a full-blown screening programme until the development of a vaccine (Best 1987).

Syphilis

Congenital syphilis is now rare in the United Kingdom, although it is common in some developing countries (Adler 1984). The spirochaete *Treponema pallidum* crosses the placenta in the second half of pregnancy, spreading through the fetal tissues, resulting, in some cases, in stillbirth (Cunningham *et al.* 1989). Early signs of infection in the newborn include failure to thrive, skin rashes (syphilitic pemphigus), fever, snuffles (associated with infection of the nasal bones) and jaundice. Diagnosis is by testing serum at the Venereal Disease Reference Laboratory or the *Treponema pallidum* haemoglutination tests which should be repeated, as passive transfer of antibodies from an infected mother to a non-affected fetus can occur (Kelnar and Harvey 1987). All antenatal women are screened for syphilis at the first antenatal visit. The later signs of congenital syphilis include abnormal teeth (the upper incisors are barrel-shaped and notched), scarring in the eyes and boney abnormalities (Kelnar and Harvey 1987). Treatment of an infected newborn is with procaine penicillin (Kelnar and Harvey 1987).

Toxoplasmosis

This is a world-wide infection caused by a protozoa which is thought to be acquired from eating inadequately cooked meat (Harper and Jing 1974). It is also known to affect domestic cats, which excrete it in their faeces. Few cases of infection in pregnancy have been reported, as infection is usually subclinical (Ho-Yen and Joss 1988). The main effects in the fetus are central nervous system abnormalities, including hydrocephalus, microcephalus, microophthalmia and jaundice (Ho-Yen and Joss 1988). Diagnosis is by detecting a high level of antibody in neonatal serum (Pearce and Roberton 1986). Although infection with toxoplasmosis is comparatively rare in pregnancy, the risks to the fetus are enormous (Ho-Yen and Joss 1988). As maternal antibody titres are rarely assessed, it is not known how useful advice to eat only well-cooked meat and to avoid handling cat litter in pregnancy can be.

Listeria

This is a bacterial infection which can be acquired through eating inadequately reheated cook–chill meals and from certain varieties of soft cheese (Acheson 1989). Pregnant women are advised to avoid these types of food (Acheson 1989). The bacteria is also present in the environment. The infection is seen as a mild non-specific flu-like pyrexial illness, which may be missed (Khong *et al.* 1986). It is estimated to affect 1 : 20 000 births in the United Kingdom (Spencer 1987). Fetal infection can cause abortion, stillbirth or preterm delivery, with meconium-stained liquor. The results of neonatal infection includes septicaemia and meningitis (Spencer 1987).

Hepatitis B

Although clinical hepatitis in the neonatal period is rare, infants of chronic carriers may well be excreting the virus. Maternal-fetal spread of hepatitis B is common, in many areas of the world being the major means of virus spread (Morgan-Capner and Griffiths 1984). Injections of hepatitis B immunoglobulins to an affected neonate can help prevent the chronic carrier state. For more information see Chapter 17.

Intrapartum infections

Prolonged rupture of the membranes can permit ascending infection from the vulva and vagina, causing amnionitis with the attendant risks of neonatal pneumonia and septicaemia. Particularly virulent is infection caused by Group B streptococci (Cunningham *et al.* 1989). The fetus can also become infected during its passage through the birth canal (Pearce and Roberton 1986). *Gonoccocci* and chlamydia (causing ophthalmia neonatorium) and herpes are most commonly involved (Pearce and Roberton 1986). Transplacental passage of herpes is rare, but, should the mother have active herpes at the time of delivery, a severe infection can result (Pearce and Roberton 1986). Mortality is given as 60% (Adler 1984), surviving babies being severely brain-damaged. For this reason, any mother with primary or recurring herpes infection who has active lesions on her cervix or vulva, or who is shedding the virus from 36 weeks gestation onwards, should be delivered by caesarean section (Pearce and Roberton 1986).

Neonatal infections

The response of the neonate to infection is subtle and hard to detect (Kelnar and Harvey 1987). Temperature may be raised, normal or low; the baby may seem lethargic, reluctant to feed or fretful; vomiting may occur and this, combined with poor feeding, can lead to weight loss; jaundice can be present and may be prolonged (Speck *et al.* 1986). In severe cases of infection, apnoea attacks and convulsions can occur (Speck *et al.* 1986). Infection spreads rapidly, so delays in taking action can be serious (Pearce and Roberton 1986).

Diagnosis involves taking a detailed history from the mother and/or midwife, obtaining a full infection screen, as well as a detailed physical examination.

Infection screen: • Swabs – Eyes.
                             Nose.
                             Throat.

> Any septic focus.
> Umbilical cord.
- Stool sample.
- Urine sample (may be obtained using a urine bag or via a suprapubic aspiration performed by the paediatrician).
- Blood culture.
- (Possibly a sample of cerebrospinal fluid).

A full blood count is taken to assess white cell response. Treatment may be commenced before the results are known, due to the risk of a rapid deterioration in neonatal condition (Kelnar and Harvey 1987). Medical staff usually prescribe either a range of antibiotics or a broad spectrum one. The initial doses may be given intramuscularly, changing to oral therapy to complete the course. Some drugs, such as gentamycin, require monitoring of blood levels to avoid toxicity (Kelnar and Harvey 1987).

Ophthalmia neonatorum

This is defined as a purulent discharge from the eyes of an infant within 21 days of birth. It should not be confused with the more common 'sticky eye'. This latter is caused by a blockage of the tear duct. It is improved by bathing with saline and massaging the tear duct to prevent infection. As a precautionary measure, swabs should be taken, as ophthalmia neonatorum may develop. Organisms implicated in causing ophthalmia neonatorum are *E. coli*, chlamydia and *Gonococcus* (Pearce and Roberton 1986). If untreated, blindness can result. Swabs need to be taken, using the specific culture medium for growth of chlamydia, although a specific test for the presence of antibodies is more accurate (Thomas *et al.* 1984). Most eye infections are cleared by the use of chloramphenical eye drops, but neomycin is required to control chlamydia. Should the causative organism be *gonococcus*, an intensive regime of penicillin eye drops and systemic therapy is necessary (Kelnar and Harvey 1986). In all cases with an eye discharge, the baby should be nursed with the affected eye downmost to prevent spread to the other eye.

Omphalitis

The umbilical cord separates by a process of dry gangrene, assisted by the presence of microorganisms. Infection of the umbilical cord is rare in the United Kingdom, given the widespread use of antiseptic solutions, powders and sprays. They do, however, increase the time period until cord separation occurs (Salariya and Kowbus 1988). If severe infection results, pus may be seen and an erythema can develop, with possible cellulitis. As infection spreads easily through the umbilical vein to the liver, then on to a generalised septicaemia, prompt treatment of infection is vital (Pearce and Roberton 1986). This is usually with antibiotics and intravenous fluids. The baby should be barrier-nursed to prevent spread of infection to weak newborns.

Infection of the alimentary tract

Thrush. This is a common infection acquired during birth or from infected handlers and equipment. It is caused by a yeast-like organism candida albicans, a common inhabitant of the vagina and intestine (Barrie 1987). Infection can also occur when broad spectrum antibiotics kill off normal skin flora. Oral thrush resembles areas of white milk curd within the mouth. They are not easily removed, but if this is done a red raw patch remains. The baby may be reluctant to feed due to discomfort.

Infection of the vulva or scrotum and perianal region can occur. This is differentiated from nappy rash, due to contact with urine soaked nappies which release ammonia, by the fact that it is present in the skin folds (Barrie 1987). Ill babies, especially if preterm, are susceptible to thrush which can lead to candida septicaemia which is often fatal (Barrie 1987). Treatment of all types of thrush is with the antifungal agent nystatitin, which can be given orally after feeds or applied topically (Barrie 1987). Good standards of hygiene are vital to prevent reinfection (Barrie 1987). Care should be taken that non-disposable nappies are properly sterilised.

Gastroenteritis. This is rare amongst the solely breast-fed baby who is protected by immunoglobulins and whose gut is colonised by non-pathogenic flora (Pearce and Roberton 1986). Amongst bottle-fed babies, the most common organism involved is *E. coli* (Pearce and Roberton 1986). Deterioration in the neonatal condition and dehydration can be sudden and the spread of infection rapid, unless mother and baby are isolated and good hygiene observed (Pearce and Roberton 1986). Treatment involves sending stool specimens for culture, rehydration (usually intravenously) and a course of an appropriate antibiotic, if necessary (Pearce and Roberton 1986). Gastroenteritis is entirely preventable by simple techniques such as hand washing and the correct preparation, storage and disposal of unused artificial feeds (Pearce and Roberton 1986).

Urinary tract infections

These are difficult to diagnose; often the only signs are jaundice, vomiting or poor weight gain (Pearce and Roberton 1986). The neonatal period is the only time when such infections are more common in boys than in girls (Abbott 1972). Localised infection can quickly spread to the kidneys, giving rise to pyelonephritis. Diagnosis is often made from the infection screen of an unwell baby without an obvious focus of infection (Pearce and Roberton 1986). Suprapubic urine samples may be taken to avoid the problems of contamination associated with the use of collecting bags. Management is with antibiotics, but care should be taken, as the infection may return when treatment stops, especially if there are anatomical abnormalities (Pearce and Roberton 1986).

Infections of the skin

These are frequent in the neonate and it is difficult, especially for mothers, to differentiate between a heat or starch rash and an infection.

Pyodermia. Small spots or pustules, usually due to staphylococcus, most frequently occurring around the neck or axilla. Infection can spread rapidly, especially in an ill baby, so isolation is required (Kelnar and Harvey 1987). Local treatment with chlorhexidine spirit or hexachlorophane powder, especially around the umbilicus, may be sufficient, although serious cases will require systemic antibiotic therapy (Kelnar and Harvey 1987).

Pemphigus neonatorum. Untreated pyodermia can develop into this serious and lifethreatening condition. Large vesicles full of yellow fluid develop; the blisters then burst, leaving a raw surface and spreading the infection (Kelnar and Harvey 1987). As the blisters coalesce, large areas of tissue are affected, the babies becoming very ill, with possible collapse (Walker and Champion 1986). Strict isolation of both mother and baby is necessary to avoid a spread which would require closure of the unit. Staphylococci can be cultured from the exudate. Treatment is by antibiotics, rehydration and supportive care. The baby's hands should be covered to prevent spread of infection, especially to the eyes.

Prevention of infection

Good hygiene and commonsense are vital for the prevention of neonatal infection in the home, postnatal ward or Special Care Baby Unit (Kelnar and Harvey 1987). Hand-washing, careful disposal of soiled paper towels are of great help (Davies 1982). Any member of the family or staff with an active infection should avoid contact with the baby (Pearce and Roberton 1986).

In hospital, each baby's equipment should be kept separate and facilities made available for the safe disposal of soiled nappies and linen (Kelnar and Harvey 1987). Breast feeding helps prevent infection, but if this is not possible, feeds should be aseptically prepared and stored at the correct temperature, if not commercially prepacked. Facilities should be available for the disposal of partly used feeds. The baby's cots or incubators should not be placed too close together (at least 4–6 feet apart) (Goldman *et al*. 1981) and mothers in postnatal wards should be dissuaded from picking up each other's babies.

All newborn babies are examined daily by the midwife, both at home and in hospital, to look for signs of infection. Prompt action should be taken if infection is suspected. If the baby requires admission to hospital, she should be isolated until the infection screen is clear (Kelnar and Harvey 1987). It has not been shown that unrestricted visiting by healthy adults and children increases infection rates, even in Special Care Baby Units as long as they observe basic precautions, such as hand-washing (Kelnar and Harvey 1987). Anyone with an active infection, however minor, should be dissuaded from visiting (Pearce and Roberton 1986).

References

Abbott G D (1972) 'Neonatal bacteruria: a prospective study of 1460 infants' *British Medical Journal* 1: 267–9

Acheson D (1989) 'Listeriosis' *Midwives' Chronicle* April: 129

Adler M W (1984) 'ABC of sexually transmitted diseases. Pregnancy and the neonate' *British Medical Journal* 288: 624–7

Alban Davies H, Clark J D A, Dalton K J and Edwards O M (1989) 'Insulin requirements of diabetic women who breast feed' *British Medical Journal* 298: 1357–8

Arniel-Tison C, Korobkin R and Klaus M H (1986) 'Neurological problems' in M H Klaus and W B Fanaroff (eds) *Care of the High Risk Neonate (3rd edn)* 356–86 Saunders: Philadelphia

Aynsley-Green A and Soltesz G (1986) 'Disorders of blood glucose homeostasis in the neonate' in N R C Roberton (ed) *Textbook of Neonatology* 605–21 Churchill Livingstone: Edinburgh

Ballard J L, Holroyde J and Tsang R C (1984) 'High malformation rates and decreased mortality in infants of diabetic mothers' *American Journal of Obstetrics and Gynecology* 148: 1111–7

Barrie H (1987) 'Infection with thrush' *Midwife, Health Visitor and Community Nurse* 23(6): 248–50

Best J M (1987) 'Congenital cytomegalovirus' *British Medical Journal* 294: 1440–1

Brooklyn Health Action Committee (1986) 'Statement on drug abuse – the undeclared public health emergency' Cited by Lindo (1987)

Brudenell M and Wills P L (1984) *Medical and Surgical Problems in Obstetrics* Wright: Bristol

Carroll J E (1986) 'Muscle disorders in the newborn' in N R C Roberton (ed) *Textbook of Neonatology* 586–7 Churchill Livingstone: Edinburgh

Casaer P, Eggermont E and Volpe J J (1986) 'Neonatal clinical neurological assessment' in N R C Roberton (ed) *Textbook of Neonatology* 527–32 Churchill Livingstone: Edinburgh

Cates K L, Rowe J C and Ballow M (1983) 'The premature infant as a compromised host' *Current Problems in Pediatrics* 13: 1–63

Chappel J N (1972) 'Treatment of morphine type dependence' *Journal of American Medical Association* 221: 1516

Cohen M S (1982) 'Drug abuse in pregnancy: fetal and neonatal effects' *Drug Theraputics* 165–79

Cousins L (1983) 'Congenital anomalies amongst infants of diabetic mothers' *American Journal of Obstetrics and Gynecology* 147: 333–8

Cunningham F G, MacDonald P C and Gant N F (1989) *Williams' Obstetrics (18th edn)* Prentice Hall: London

Dandona P, Besterman H S and Freedman D B (1984) 'Macrosomia despite well controlled diabetic pregnancy' *Lancet* i: 737

Davies P A (1982) 'Please wash your hands' *Archives of Disease in Childhood* 57: 647–48

Dewhurst C J (1981) *Integrated Obstetrics and Gynaecology (3rd edn)* Blackwell: Oxford

Goldmann D A, Durban W A and Freeman J (1981) 'Nosocomial infections in a neonatal intensive care unit' *Journal of Infectious Diseases* 144: 449–59

Gregg N M, Beavis W R, Heseltine M and Macklin A E (1945) 'Occurrence of congenital defects following maternal rubella during pregnancy' *Medical Journal of Australia* ii: 122–6

Harper R G and Jing J Y (1974) *Handbook of Neonatology* Yearbook Publishers: Chicago

Harper R G, Solish G I, Purow H M, Sang E and Panepinto W C (1974) 'The effects of methadone treatment program upon pregnant heroin addict and the newborn infants' *Pediatrics* 54: 300

Ho-Yen D O and Joss A W L (1988) 'Toxoplasma and cytomegalovirus in pregnancy' *Maternal and Child Health* 13(8): 225–7

Jones D N, Pickett J, Oates M R and Barbor P (1987) *Understanding Child Abuse (2nd edn)* Macmillan: Basingstoke

Kandall S R and Gartner L M (1974) 'Late presentation of drug withdrawal symptoms in the newborn' *American Journal of Diseases in Childhood* 127: 58

Kelnar C J H and Harvey D (1987) *The Sick Newborn (2nd edn)* Balliere Tindall: London

Khong T Y, Frappell J M, Steel H M, Stewart C M and Burke M (1986) 'Perinatal listeriosis. A report of six cases' *British Journal of Obstetrics and Gynaecology* 93: 1083–7

Larsen B, Snider I S and Galask R P (1974) 'Bacterial growth inhibition by amniotic fluid' *American Journal of Obstetrics and Gynecology* 119: 492

Lewis P and Steyger J (1985) 'Caring for the infant of the diabetic mother' *Midwifery* 1(4): 207–12

Lindo M (1987) 'Drug addiction: its effects on mother and baby' *Midwifery* 3(2): 82–91

Lou H and Volpe J J (1986) 'Pathogenesis of hypoxic-ischaemic encephalopathy and germinal matrix haemorrhage' in N R C Roberton (ed) *Textbook of Neonatology* 543–5 Churchill Livingstone: Edinburgh

Morgan-Capner P and Griffiths G (1984) 'Fetal and neonatal infection' *Nursing Times* 80(76): 28–32

Pearce R G and Roberton N R C (1986) 'Infection in the newborn' in N R C Roberton (ed) *Textbook of Neonatology* 725–81 Churchill Livingstone: Edinburgh

Peckham C (1972) 'Clinical and laboratory study of children exposed in utero to maternal rubella' *Archives of Disease in Childhood* 47: 571–7

Pederson J and Pederson K (1979) 'Early growth retardation in diabetic pregnancy' *British Medical Journal* 278: 18–19

Persson B (1986) 'Long term morbidity in the offspring of diabetic mothers' *Acta Endrocrinlogica* 277(Suppl): 150–5

Phillips K (1986) 'Neonatal drug addicts' *Nursing Times* 28(19 Mar): 36–8

Preece P M, Pearl K N and Peckham C (1984) 'Congenital cytomegalovirus infection' *Archives of Disease in Childhood* 59: 1120–6

Salariya E M and Kowbus N M (1988) 'Variable umbilical cord care' *Midwifery* 4(2): 70–6

Speck W T, Aronoff S C and Fanaroff A A (1986) 'Neonatal infections' in M H Klaus and W B Fanaroff (eds) *Care of the High Risk Neonate (3rd edn)* 262–85 Saunders: Philadelphia

Spencer J A D (1987) 'Perinatal listeriosis' *British Medical Journal* 295: 349

Stern L (1984) 'Drug abuse in pregnancy' *Aids Health Science Press* Saunders: Philadelphia

Stubbs W A and Stubbs S M (1978) 'Hyperinsulinism, diabetes mellitus and respiratory disease of the newborn: a common link?' *Lancet* i: 308–9

Tarby T J and Volpe J J (1986) 'Neonatal seizures' in N R C Roberton (ed) *Textbook of Neonatology* 533–42 Churchill Livingstone: Edinburgh

Tchobrovtsky G, Heard H, Tchobrovtsky C and Eschwege W (1980) 'Amniotic fluid C-peptide in normal and insulin dependent pregnancies' *Diabetologia* 18: 289

Thomas D F M, Fernie D S, Bayston R and Spitz L (1984) 'Clostridial toxins in necrotizing enterocloitis' *Archives of Disease in Childhood* 59: 270–3

Vaughan N J A (1987) 'Treatment of diabetes in pregnancy' *British Medical Journal* 294: 558–60

Volpe J J (1981) *Neurology of the Newborn* Saunders: Philadelphia

Walker N P J and Champion R H (1986) 'Neonatal dermatology' in N R C Roberton (ed) *Textbook of Neonatology* 677–88 Churchill Livingstone: Edinburgh

Williams M J H (1983) 'The problems of children born of drug addicts' *Maternal and Child Health* 8(6): 258–63

Zelon C (1973) 'Infant of the addicted mother' *New England Journal of Medicine* 28: 1393

38   The malformed baby

Congenital abnormalities occur fairly frequently, but the vast majority of these are minor (Donnai 1986). Approximately 2% of all babies born in the United Kingdom have some kind of malformation, in some cases affecting more than one system (Office of Population Censuses and Surveys 1987). The defect may be fatal, or at best result in permanent handicap, but some are amenable to treatment. Congenital abnormalities are the cause of 20% of perinatal and 30% of neonatal deaths in the United Kingdom (Mutch *et al.* 1980; Office of Population Censuses and Surveys 1982). When spontaneously aborted first trimester fetuses are examined, they have an abnormality rate of the order of 50% (Lauritsen 1976). It has been suggested that the figure for very early abortions, where chromosomal analysis is not possible, may be even higher. Careful screening of at-risk populations and the availability of genetic counselling are vital to help reduce these figures (Fitzsimmons 1985).

Causes of abnormalities

In many cases the cause is difficult to determine. It is necessary to have a detailed knowledge of family history, environmental conditions and personal health.

Chromosomal abnormalities

These are present in about 0.5% of neonates and about 50% of first trimester spontaneous abortions (Donnai 1986). Abnormalities include those where there are either too many chromosomes or faults in their structure (Baraister and Winter 1986). All humans have 22 pairs of chromosomes (known as autosomes) and 2 sex chromosomes, XY for a male, XX for a female. Half of the chromosome pair is derived from each parent (Baraister and Winter 1986); the exception to this is Turner's syndrome, XO, a monosomy of the sex chromosomes. Incorrect division of genetic material during oogenesis or spermatogenesis can, on fertilisation, produce a zygote with a missing or an extra chromosome (most commonly numbers 21, 18 or 13) (Baraister and Winter 1986). Where a chromosome is missing, the defect is usually lethal. The age of the parents, especially that of the mother, is related to rates of chromosomal anomaly (Donnai 1988). Donnai (1988) states that the risk of a child with trisomy 21 (Down's syndrome) is 1:1205 for a mother aged 20 years, rising to 1:32 at age 45.

Spermatogenesis is affected by age, but genetically abnormal sperm are less capable of fertilisation (Friedman 1981).

The second type of chromosomal abnormality is translocation (Donnai 1986). Part of one chromosome has either been exchanged with part of another – reciprocal translocation – or an arm of one has been attached to another – Robertsonian translocation (Baraister and Winter 1986) (see Figure 38.1). In all cases, the person has the correct quantity of genetic material and is known as a balanced translocation carrier, a situation which occurs in about 1:600 individuals (Donnai 1986). Children of such a parent with reciprocal translocation have the correct numbers of chromosomes but some genes are expressed singly and others in

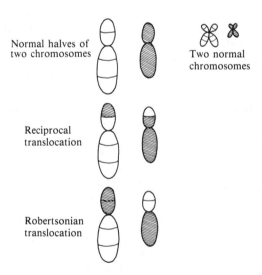

Figure 38.1 Balanced chromosome translocations.

triplicate – partial trisomy (Baraister and Winter 1986). With Robertsonian translocation, some offspring will have only 45 chromosomes and others will have a partial trisomy (Baraister and Winter 1986). Parents with a chromosomal abnormality often experience high abortion, stillbirth and neonatal death rates (Sant-Cassia and Cooke 1981).

Single gene disorders

These are also known as disorders of Mendelian inheritance (Cunningham *et al.* 1989). Abnormalities result from an abnormal (mutuant) gene on any of the 22 pairs of autosomes or on the X sex chromosome (Baraister and Winter 1986). As the knowledge of genetics improves, it is possible in the case of some disorders to identify the faulty gene, thus detecting carriers or affected fetuses (Goldstein and Brown 1987). New mutations can occur spontaneously, producing abnormalities in previously unaffected families (Baraister and Winter 1986).

Autosomal dominant conditions

The dominant gene expresses itself, if present, because it dominates the normal gene (Baraister and Winter 1986) (see Figure 38.2). Males and females are equally likely to be affected. Conditions inherited in this way include achondroplasia (short limbs, large head and lumbar lordosis) and Huntington's chorea (Donnai 1986).

Fifty per cent of children will be affected; those unaffected cannot pass on the disorder to their offspring unless their partner is a carrier (Baraister and Winter 1986). Some autosomal conditions, such as Huntington's chorea, are only apparent in later life after the reproductive years. A predictive test for those with a family history can be of help in preventing the birth of affected children.

Autosomal recessive conditions

For these to occur, two abnormal genes must be present. If only one gene is abnormal, it is not expressed, although the individual can pass the gene to their offspring (Baraister and Winter 1986). The children of two carriers of the gene

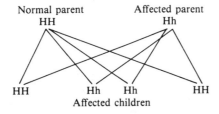

Figure 38.2 Autosomal dominant inheritance. H = normal gene; h = dominant abnormal gene (Huntington's chorea).

have a 25% chance of inheriting two abnormal genes and having the disorder (see Figure 38.3).

Other autosomal recessive conditions include haemoglobinopathies (thalassaemia and sickle cell disease) and inborn errors of metabolism (phenylketonuria and Tay Sachs disease). Screening for carrier states and affected fetuses is possible for some disorders, for example sickle cell disease (World Health Organization 1972) and cystic fibrosis (Goldstein and Brown 1987).

X-linked recessive disorders

Where the X chromosome carries an abnormal recessive gene, this is expressed in affected males, females being asymptomatic carriers (Baraister and Winter 1986) (see Figure 38.4). Disorders inherited in this way include Duchenne muscular dystrophy, red/green colour blindness and haemophilia.

If the mother is a known carrier, unless the specific gene is detectable, abortion of male fetuses is offered, although 50% of these will be genetically normal (Baraister and Winter 1986). The testing of embryos developed using *in vitro* fertilisation has permitted the implantation of female embryos only, removing any necessity for later testing. The ethical issues surrounding the aborting of all male fetuses or the selective implantation of only female fetuses have yet to be resolved.

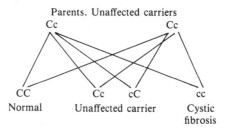

Figure 38.3 Autosomal recessive inheritance. C = normal gene; c = cystic fibrosis gene.

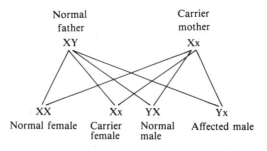

Figure 38.4 X-linked recessive inheritance.

Multifactorial inheritance

The greatest number of congenital abnormalities fall into this group (Fraser 1959). Several genetic factors with one or more events relating to the intrauterine environment combine to produce the anomaly (Wilson 1959). Environmental factors include maternal infections, drugs (therapeutic or abused), alcohol, lead and maternal disease, such as diabetes (Shepard 1986). Several factors have to operate, together with a genetic predisposition, to cross the threshold between normality and abnormality (Wilson 1959). This complex relationship between the differing sensitivity to the risk factors and the timing of their effect goes some way to explaining why a particular circumstance (e.g. alcohol) will affect one woman's pregnancy more than another (Wilson 1959).

Prevention of congenital abnormalities

Individuals with a family history may seek advice from a genetic counsellor who will help them to assess the risk of the particular disorder before embarking on a pregnancy (Fitzsimmons 1985). Certain genes can be detected in both partners prior to embarking upon a pregnancy. Preconception care can also assist in reducing abnormalities by encouraging women to be assessed for rubella immunity. Advice about preconception diet, smoking and alcohol consumption can also be given (see Chapter 4 for more details).

Detection of abnormalities

For the majority of people, screening for the presence of abnormality begins with careful history-taking at the first antenatal clinic visit.

Blood

Blood is taken to assess rubella immunity, presence of phenylktonuria and infection with syphilis. Women from particular ethnic groups can be screened for the presence of sickle cell trait (Tuck and White 1981) or thalassaemia (Perkins 1971). At 16 weeks gestation, blood can be taken for alpha feto protein (AFP) levels, which are raised in the presence of open neural tube defects. AFP is secreted in the fetal urine, some of which crosses the fetal membranes and is detectable in the maternal circulation (Cunningham *et al.* 1989). A high level indicates an increased risk of a neural tube defect; if this is found, the period of gestation is checked and the blood test repeated or a high-definition ultrasound scan performed to visualise the fetal spine. If the second level is raised, amniocentesis will be performed and the AFP level of amniotic fluid determined (American College of Obstetricians and Gynecologists 1986, 1987). Low levels of serum AFP occur in cases of trisomy, such as Down's syndrome (Simpson *et al.* 1986; Palomaki and Haddow 1987). Where the fetus is abnormal, the parents then need to consider whether they want a therapeutic abortion to be performed.

Amniocentesis

This test would be performed in women deemed to be at high risk through family or personal history, such as a previously abnormal baby or maternal age (usually over 37 or 38 years). Liquor is obtained by amniocentesis from 16 weeks gestation, as there is insufficient before this time (Cunningham *et al.* 1989). However Hanson *et al.* (1987) report only a 1.7% rate of fetal loss where the test is performed before 15 weeks. It can be used for the following tests.

Chromosomal analysis

Skin squames in the liquor are grown in culture and the chromosomes examined (Daker and Bubrow 1989). Enzymes which recognise particular combinations of bases in the DNA are applied to the chromosomes. These combinations are called gene probes; they are a group of genes rather than an individual gene (Daker and Bubrow 1989). The sex of the fetus can be determined (for sex-linked conditions), trisomy can be seen and specific gene probes applied (for cystic fibrosis for example) (Daker and Bubrow 1989).

Chemical studies

These can be performed to detect some inborn errors of metabolism and to assess AFP levels to detect open neural tube defects (American College of Obstetricians and Gynecologists 1986, 1987).

Where an abnormality is present (or in the case of an X-linked condition, the fetus is male), the parents will require counselling prior to deciding whether they wish to have a termination of the pregnancy. There are some pathological sequelae associated with amniocentesis; there is a small risk of spontaneous abortion, 1% in one randomised controlled trial (Tabor *et al.* 1986), feto-placental haemorrhage and fetal trauma (Poreco *et al.* 1983). To prevent isoimmunisation, rhesus-negative women should be given anti-D immunoglobulin as a prophylactic (Blajchman *et al.* 1974). Drawbacks of amniocentesis are that it cannot usually be performed until there is sufficient liquor (16 weeks), although some areas are trying to perform it from 12 weeks. The small number of fetal cells obtained means that they have to be cultured, which is slow and it can take up to 3 weeks to obtain sufficient DNA to study (Daker and Bubrow 1989).

Ultrasound scanning

High frequency sound waves, which are reflected and absorbed by different types of tissue structure at differing rates are used (Chudleigh and Pearce 1986). Scientists have declared the use of ultrasound in pregnancy to be safe (Shearer 1984). Hazards of ultrasound in animal experiments include heating of the cells (Kremkau 1983) and resonance of microscopic gas bubbles present in the tissues (Neilson and Grant 1989). It is thought to be unlikely that ultrasound as commonly used in pregnancy will cause any problems, although it should only be used where there is a specific need (Neilson and Grant 1989). Such randomised controlled trials as have been performed into the safety of ultrasound have been small in size and have failed to demonstrate consistent findings (Neilson and Grant 1989). With a skilled operator, the fetus can be viewed quite clearly at 16 weeks gestation, allowing examination of the spine, limbs, heart and kidneys (Sabbagha et al. 1985). In some areas, a 16 week scan to assess fetal normality has replaced the use of serum AFP level determination in the diagnosis of neural tube defects.

Chorionic villus sampling

This is a new technique currently being evaluated in the United Kingdom by a multicentre randomised controlled trial. Using a fine cannula, which is passed through the cervical os, and gentle suction, fetal tissue from the chorionic villi of the placenta can be obtained (Rodeck et al. 1983). The test is carried out between 8 and 11 weeks gestation (Rodeck et al. 1983). Pathological sequelae are rare, but include puncture of the amniotic sac. With refinement of the technique, the spontaneous abortion risk is reduced (Jackson 1988). Rhesus-negative women should receive anti-D immuniglobulin prophylaxis to prevent them developing isoimmunisation. The advantages of this technique are that a sufficiently large sample of fetal tissue can be obtained, which can be examined directly without the need for cell culture (Daker and Bubrow 1989). There is a risk, though, of contamination with maternal cells, which will affect the accuracy of the findings.

Types of congenital abnormality (structural abnormalities)

Neural tube defects

These occur during embryonic development when there is incomplete fusing of the neural plate (Dyball and Tate 1986) (see Chapter 5). The cause is multifactorial, with a poor diet being implicated (Smithells et al. 1981). The incidence is higher amongst Celtic people (Eurocat Working Group 1987). With the use of screening tests, the incidence of neural tube defects is reducing; independently of this, the prevalence is also dropping; this includes aborted fetus and those abnormalities found at birth (Eurocat Working Group 1987).

Anencephaly

In this condition, there is little development of the cerebral hemispheres and an absence of the vault of the fetal skull (Dyball and Tate 1986). This defect is fatal (Carroll 1986).

Spina bifida occulta

In this condition there is no abnormality of the cord or the meninges, but part of the covering vertebra is missing (James and Lassman 1981). It can be recognised as a hairy patch, a mole or a dimple at the base of the spine (James and Lassman 1981). In a minor case like this, genetic counselling is still required, because there is an increased risk of neural tube defects in parents with spina bifida occulta (Lorber and Levick 1967).

Meningocele

In this condition, the meninges are displaced and protrude onto the surface; they may be covered with skin or with a layer of dura mater (Carroll 1986). As the spinal cord is not involved there is no neurological disturbance (Carroll 1986). This defect can occur at the base of the skull where it is known as an encephalocele. Because the meninges are vulnerable to damage, a surgical repair may be advised (Carroll 1986). This type of defect and spina bifida occulta are not detectable by AFP estimation.

Myelomeningocele

This is the most severe form of spina bifida, where the meninges and spinal cord protrude onto the surface of the back (Carroll 1986). If the cord is completely exposed it may be damaged (Carroll 1986). Sensory loss and paralysis can occur below the level of the lesion. The baby has underdeveloped lower limbs, muscle tone varying from floppy to completely flaccid and commonly has no bladder tone, which results in dribbling of urine (Carroll 1986). The baby may be transferred to a specialist unit where surgical closure may be performed, although this type of management is now controversial (Carroll 1986). In a study to compare conservative *versus* active treatment, Deans and Boston (1988) report that early closure does not carry any advantages in preventing mortality and does not reduce the incidence of hydrocephalus or ventriculitis.

Cleft lip and palate

Cleft lip occurs in 1 : 1000 births, which is the same incidence as cleft palate, although the two occur together in 1 : 1500 deliveries (Young 1986). The incidence of cleft lip and palate increases amongst the babies of mothers with epilepsy (Speidel and Meadows 1972). Cleft lip, which can be unilateral or bilateral, is an obvious and upsetting abnormality, but by itself it does not produce feeding problems (Young 1986). Surgical closure is usually performed in the first week of life or at about 3 months of age (Young 1986). Showing 'before and after' pictures to parents may help to contain their worries (Young 1986). Depending on the size of the cleft palate defect, the mother may be able to breast feed (Bowley 1986). If the defect is large, the baby will be unable to produce sufficient suction for feeding; a dental plate or special teat may be used, although some babies find cup and spoon feeding easier (Bowley 1986). Preliminary surgical repair begins at 3 months of age, with final closure at 12–18 months (Young 1986). This is followed by speech therapy and orthodontic treatment to align the teeth (Bowley 1986).

Abnormalities of the alimentary tract

The most common abnormality occurring in 1 : 3000 births is oesophageal atresia, which in 80% of cases is associated with a fistula between the distal oesophagus and the trachea (Young 1986) (see Figure 38.5). In this disorder, the oesophagus ends blindly. Diagnosis is by the recognition of maternal polyhydramnios and noisy breathing in the neonate. If the baby is fed, the first feed causes choking and cyanosis. A stomach tube gently passed down the oesophagus meets resistance

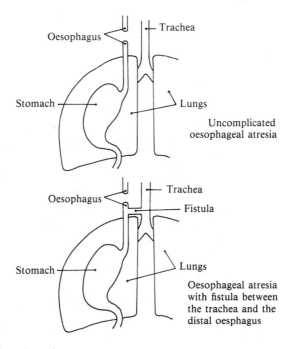

Figure 38.5 Oesophageal atresia.

(Young 1986). Surgical treatment is required to realign the oesophagus, feeding being given intravenously or through a gastrostomy. During transfer to a neonatal surgical unit, it is vital to keep the blind end of the oesophagus free of secretions to prevent aspiration (Young 1986).

Much rarer are small and large bowel obstructions; these are associated with delayed passage of meconium, abdominal distension and vomiting (Young 1986). The first examination of the neonate should exclude the presence of imperforate anus, in which the sphincter itself may be absent or simply covered with a flap of skin (Young 1986).

Exomphalos

This is a group of three conditions of increasing severity (Young 1986). The incidence is 1.9 cases/10 000 births (Office of Population Censuses and Surveys 1987). The first is a rare herniation of the bowel into the base of the umbilicus. Rupture may occur, with secondary infection. Omphalocele is caused by a failure of the embryonic mesoderm to close around the umbilical opening, resulting in a prolapse of bowel and occasionally liver into the omphalocele sac (Young 1986). The most serious of the three conditions is gastroschisis, a defect of the anterior abdominal wall, usually to the right of the umbilicus. The abdominal contents lie completely unprotected outside the abdominal cavity (Young 1986). Surgical repair is required for all these conditions. It is important especially with gastroschisis to keep the area warm and moist, protecting it from damage during transfer to a surgical unit.

Congenital dislocation of the hip

The incidence of congenital dislocation of the hip is 10 : 1000 live births (Manning *et al.* 1982). It occurs six times more frequently in girls than boys and is often found in conjunction with breech presentation or spina bifida (Salter 1968). In this condition, the acetabulum of the pelvis is shallow, the head of the femur small and the joint capsule lengthened (Hensinger and Jones 1986).

Diagnosis is by using the modified Ortolani or Barlow's test. This is performed in the first 24 hours and again within 10 days (Standing Medical and Nursing and Midwifery Advisory Committees 1986). The Committees suggested that local policy should be established to determine who was the most appropriate person to perform this test and that it should only be performed on two occasions (Wilkes 1986). To perform the test, the baby should be relaxed and the examiner's hands warm; gentleness is vital. The baby lies on her back with her feet facing the examiner. Her hips are adducted and fully flexed (the hips can be examined separately or together). To examine both hips, the examiner grasps the upper thigh, with the thumbs on the inside of the thighs, opposite each lesser trochanter. In the first part of the test the examiner tries to reposition a displaced head of femur into the acetabulum. This is achieved by pressing the middle finger upon the greater trochanter and turning the femoral head into the acetabulum. To test for subluxation, the thumb presses backwards on the inside of the thigh, attempting to move the head of femur out of the acetabulum (Standing Medical and Nursing and Midwifery Advisory Committees 1986). If the joint is 'dislocatable', the head can be felt to move a little and there is a 'clunk' (Hensinger and Jones 1986). The presence of this gives rise to the description 'clicky hips'. Any clicks should be referred to a orthopaedic surgeon who may request ultrasound scanning (Berman and Klenerman 1986). Treatment is to splint the hips in abduction and flexion until the joint is stabilised (Hensinger and Jones 1986).

Talipes

This is a common condition which can have multifactorial causes, including positional pressures in utero (Wynne-Davies 1964). The most common type is talipes equinovarus (club foot) which occurs in 1 : 1000 live births (Hensinger and Jones 1986). In this condition, the foot is turned inwards and downwards (Hensinger and Jones 1986). Less common is where the sole of the foot faces out and up (talipes calcaneovalgus). Many cases are resolved through manipulation and strapping followed by stabilisation in a plaster cast; in others, surgery may be necessary (Hensinger and Jones 1986).

Congenital heart disease

This is one of the commonest abnormalities occurring in 8 : 1000 live births (Rheuban 1984). Because of the change from fetal to adult circulation, it may take up to 2 weeks for signs to occur. These include cyanosis, tachypnoea, dyspnoea, tachycardia, murmurs, poor feeding and grunting (Kelnar and Harvey 1987) (see Chapter 32 for details of the fetal circulation).

Left to right shunts

Oxygenated blood passes back to the right side of the heart and circulates through the lungs again. There is no cyanosis.

1. Ventricular septal defect. This is a frequent problem where there is a hole in the septum between the two ventricles (Wilkinson and Cooke 1986). There may be a delay of months before signs occur, as high pressure in the right side of the heart in the neonatal period prevents entry of blood from the left (Wilkinson and Cooke 1986). Only 10% of cases require surgical closure (McNamara and Latson 1982).

2. Patent ductus arteriosus. This is very common in preterm babies because the ductus arteriosus is sensitive to blood oxygen levels. If hypoxia occurs, the ductus stays open (Wilkinson and Cooke 1986). Closure is usually spontaneous, although drugs such as indomethicin, which is effective in the first 2 weeks, may be required (Wilkinson and Cooke 1986). Management depends on the age and size of the infant and the symptoms (Rheuban 1984). The ductus can be surgically ligated.

3. Atrial septal defect. There is a loud murmur and the heart is enlarged. This disorder is usually asymptomatic in infancy (Rheuban 1984). If required, surgical closure is performed before the child is of school age (Rheuban 1984).

Right to left shunts

In these conditions deoxygenated blood returns to the periphery, causing cyanosis (Rheuban 1984). A major deformity is transposition of the great vessels in 5% of cases of congenital heart disease (Rheuban 1984), where the pulmonary artery arises from the left ventricle and the aorta from the right; this requires urgent treatment to prevent death. The baby with this condition is usually symptomatic within 3 days of birth (Wilkinson and Cooke 1986). Deoxygenated blood leaves the heart in the aorta and goes to the brain and oxygenated blood leaves the left side of the heart by the pulmonary artery and returns to the lungs (Wilkinson and Cooke 1986). Some mixing of blood may occur through the foramen ovale and a patent ductus arteriosus (Rheuban 1984). Initial treatment is to widen the foramen ovale to encourage mixing of the blood until the child is old enough to undergo surgery (Rheuban 1984).

Obstruction

Coarctation of the aorta results in a slowing of blood flow. Symptoms include tachypnoea, difficulties with feeding and femoral pulses which are weak or absent (Wilkinson and Cooke 1986). If severe, the whole left side of the heart may be underdeveloped. If untreated, infant mortality is up to 50% (Mitchell *et al.* 1971). Treatment involves the use of anticongestive drugs and aortoplasty (Wilkinson and Cooke 1986).

Chromosomal abnormalities

There are many chromosomal abnormalities, but this chapter will consider only the commonest. Down's syndrome or trisomy 21 occurs in 6.7 : 10 000 live births (Office of Population Censuses and Surveys 1987). It is the commonest cause of severe mental subnormality, with an IQ of less than 50 (Baraister and Winter 1986). There are classical clinical features which are fairly consistent in all races:

- Flat occiput (thin neck).
- Small mouth (protruding tongue).
- Speckling of the iris (Brushfield spots).
- Almond-shaped eyes which slope upwards and outwards.
- Inner epicanthic folds (single palmar crease).
- Wide gap between first and second toes.
- Floppy musculature.
- There may be associated congenital dislocation of the hip and gastrointestinal anomalies (Baraister and Winter 1986).

Children with Down's syndrome have varying degrees of learning difficulties. Because of the association with increasing parental age, such children can become a burden to older parents, who may themselves be frail and worry who will care for their child after their death. In an effort to prevent rejection, some authorities recommend that no-one tries to separate mother and baby. Other trisomies include the rarer Edward's syndrome (trisomy 18) and Patau's syndrome (trisomy 13) (Baraister and Winter 1986).

Abnormalities of sex chromosomes include Turner's syndrome (XO) in women which is characterised by short squat stature with a broad neck, low hair line, broad chest with wide-spaced nipples, streak ovaries, kidney anomalies and low intelligence (Baraister and Winter 1986).

Inborn errors of metabolism

These are a group of inherited biochemical disorders associated with mental subnormality and/or an early death (Danks and Brown 1986). Each disorder is due to a specific gene defect, most conditions being autosomal-recessive, that is, they occur when both the parents are asymptomatic carriers (Danks and Brown 1986). Because of the gene defect, the enzyme necessary for a specific biochemical process is absent (Danks and Brown 1986).

Phenylketonuria (PKU)

In this condition, the enzyme phenylalanine hydroxylase is absent. This enzyme is required for the metabolism of phenylalanine to tyrosine (see Figure 38.6) (Danks and Brown 1986). Phenylalanine builds up to toxic levels, causing damage to the developing brain, while tyrosine levels are low. As the condition is autosomal-recessive, any child of carrier parents will have a 1 : 4 risk of developing the disease (Baraister and Winter 1986). Frequency of occurrence of PKU is 1 : 10–15 000 births, but there are great variations between nationalities (Cunningham et al. 1989).

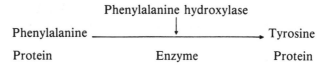

Figure 38.6 The metabolism of phenylalanine.

Diagnosis

Although this section is dealing with diagnosis of PKU, other inborn errors of metabolism are detectable with similar techniques.

1. The Scriver test, using blood (obtained via a heel stab on the tenth day of life) which is put in a capillary tube. The blood is tested by chromatography for phenylalanine levels.
2. The Guthrie test, is performed on the sixth day of life. Blood from a heel stab is used to fill marked circles on a collection card. Originally, the dried blood discs were punched out and put on an agar plate with bacteria (*Bacillus subtilis*) and incubated. If the organism grows, phenylalanine is present. The blood filled circles are now tested using chromatography.

When taking the blood sample it is important not to damage the bone in the heel. If the sample is taken from the side of the heel, damage may be avoided (Moxley 1989). Careful explanations must be given to the parents before they give their permission (Polichroniadis 1989). If the disease is present, treatment is by giving a low phenylalanine diet. This is continued until 8 or 10 years of age when brain growth is complete (Williamson *et al*. 1981). It is necessary for women with PKU to commence the same diet prior to embarking upon a pregnancy, to avoid damaging the fetal brain (Rohr *et al*. 1983).

Galactosaemia

A rare disorder (1 : 40–80 000 births), characterised by the absence of galactose 1 phosphate uridyl transferase (Danks and Brown 1986). The result is an inability to metabolise galactose (a constituent of the milk sugar lactose) to glucose (Danks and Brown 1986). Galactose builds up in the blood, damages the liver and it is excreted in urine. Galactose 1 phosphate build-up in red blood cells is toxic (Danks and Brown 1986). Most signs are apparent in the second week of life. They include vomiting, reluctance to feed, diarrhoea, weight loss, dehydration, hypoglycaemia, hepatosplenonegaly, jaundice and cataracts (Danks and Brown 1986). Diagnosis is by urine testing for the presence of galactose, or the Scriver or Guthrie tests for chromatographic analysis (Bickel *et al*. 1980). In affected families, cord blood can be analysed (Bickel *et al*. 1980). If the diagnosis is positive, all milk feeds must be stopped and a galactose-free diet substituted (Danks and Brown 1986). Dietary restrictions for life are often necessary, although some people develop alternative metabolic pathways or acquire tolerance.

There are other inborn errors of metabolism affecting lipid metabolism (Tay Sachs, Gaucher's and Neimann Pick disease), connective tissue metabolism (Hunter's and Hurler's syndromes) and copper metabolism (Wilson's disease); see Danks and Brown (1986) for more details. Some of these are now detectable antenatally by the use of gene probes.

Cystic fibrosis

This is an autosomal-recessive condition affecting the exocrine glands of the body (Baraister and Winter 1986). It occurs in 1:2500 births in the United Kingdom (British Paediatric Association Working Party on Cystic Fibrosis 1988). In this condition, the mucus-secreting glands are very distended, secreting a thick sticky mucus; sweat glands appear normal, but the sweat has very high electrolyte levels (Weinberger and Weiss 1988). Mothers comment that their baby tastes salty; the pancreas is abnormal, so there is a lack of digestive secretions reaching the intestine, and lung secretions are altered, encouraging growth of bacteria; infections and abcesses can occur (Bray 1984).

In the neonate, there may be a delay in passing meconium, which can be interpreted as intestinal obstruction (Young 1986). The stools of the older child are greasy, bulky and foul smelling (due to poor fat absorption) and respiratory tract infections are common (Bray 1984). Diagnosis is by testing meconium for high levels of albumen or by the sweat test to check electrolyte levels (Bray 1984). If a duodenal aspirate is obtained, there is an absence of pancreatic enzymes.

Long-term management includes the use of prophylactic antibiotics, postural drainage and physiotherapy to prevent chest infections, with high-protein diet with extra vitamins and replacement of pancreatic enzymes to help improve digestion (Bray 1984). Such children can survive into adult life if lung damage is not severe (British Paediatric Association Working Party on Cystic Fibrosis 1988). Some are now receiving heart–lung transplants to replace damaged lungs.

Hypothyroidism

With an occurrence rate of 1:4000 births, this is twice as common as PKU (Grant and Smith 1988). If untreated, severe physical and mental retardation can occur (Hulse 1984).

Hypothyroidism is usually due to absence or underdevelopment of the thyroid gland (Barnes 1986). Signs, which may not appear in the early weeks in an affected baby, include placidity, poor feeding, thick tongue, hoarse cry, jaundice, constipation and a low hair line (Barnes 1986). Blood taken at the same time as the Guthrie test can be used to assess thyroxine levels. Treatment is thyroxine replacement for life (Barnes 1986). With screening, some children with slightly reduced thyroid function are being detected, possibly saving them from mild mental retardation (Grant and Smith 1988).

Effect of malformation upon parents

For the parents who have been anticipating the birth of a normal baby, any abnormality comes as a great shock (Bicknell 1983). They have not only to come to terms with the baby's handicap, but also to grieve for the loss of the normal baby they were expecting (Bicknell 1983). Many parents feel guilty that they have brought this upon their child and can also feel guilty for resenting the changes a handicapped child will impose upon their lives (Clifford 1985). The child may be rejected, as some parents find congenital abnormality impossible to accept and manage. Such babies are placed in foster care and eventually put forward for adoption. Other parents can become overprotective, preventing normal development (Forrest 1989). Caring for a handicapped child requires a team approach and the parents must be consulted at every step (Heavyside 1985). They should also be offered counselling to help them come to terms with the situation. Genetic counselling will be required if the couple are planning to have further children (see Chapter 31 for the grieving process in relation to childbirth).

References

American College of Obstetricians and Gynecologists (1986) *Prenatal Detection of Neural Tube Defects* Technical Bulletin No 99

American College of Obstetricians and Gynecologists (1987) *Antenatal Diagnosis of Genetic Disorders* Technical Bulletin No 108

Baraister M and Winter R (1986) 'Genetics and congenital malformations' in N R C Roberton (ed) *Textbook of Neonatology* 495–526 Churchill Livingstone: Edinburgh

Barnes N D (1986) 'Endocrine disorders' in N R C Roberton (ed) *Textbook of Neonatology* 623–4 Churchill Livingstone: Edinburgh

Berman L and Klenerman L (1986) 'Ultrasound screening for hip abnormalities: preliminary findings in 1001 neonates' *British Medical Journal* 293: 719–22

Bickel D, Guthrie R and Hammerson G (1980) *Neonatal Screening for Inborn Errors of Metabolism* Springer-Verlag: Berlin

Bicknell J (1983) 'The psychopathology of handicap' *British Journal of Medical Psychology* 56: 167–78

Blajchman M A, Maudsley R F, Uchida I and Zipursky A (1974) 'Diagnostic amniocentesis and fetal-maternal bleeding' *Lancet* i: 993

Bowley A J (1986) 'Cleft lip and palate in perspective' *Midwives Chronicle* March: 50–5

Bray P T (1984) 'Cystic fibrosis' *Update* 15 Aug: 271–6

British Paediatric Association Working Party on Cystic Fibrosis (1988) 'Cystic fibrosis in the United Kingdom 1977–85: an improving picture' *British Medical Journal* 297: 1599–1604

Carroll J E (1986) 'Muscle disorders in the newborn' in N R C Roberton (ed) *Textbook of Neonatology* 586–7 Churchill Livingstone: Edinburgh

Chudleigh P and Pearce J M (1986) *Obstetric Ultrasound* Churchill Livingstone: Edinburgh

Clifford S (1985) 'The guilt factor' *Midwife, Health Visitor and Community Nurse* 21(10): 364–7

Cunningham F G, MacDonald P C and Gant N F (1989) *William's Obstetrics (18th edn)* Prentice Hall: London

Daker M and Bubrow M (1989) 'Screening for genetic disease and fetal anomaly during pregnancy' in I Chalmers, M Enkin and M J N C Keirse (eds) *Effective Care in Pregnancy and Childbirth* 368–81 Oxford Medical: Oxford

Danks D M and Brown G K (1986) 'Inborn errors of metabolism' in N R C Roberton (ed) *Textbook of Neonatology* 644–58 Churchill Livingstone: Edinburgh

Deans G T and Boston V E (1988) 'Is surgical closure of the back lesion in open neural tube defects necessary?' *British Medical Journal* 296: 1441–2

Donnai D (1986) 'Genetic aspects' in G Chamberlain and J Lumley (eds) *Prepregnancy Care: A Manual for Practice* 11–29 Wiley: London

Donnai D (1988) 'Genetic risk' in D K James and G M Stirrat (eds) *Pregnancy and Risk* Ch 4 45–80 Wiley: Chichester

Dyball R E J and Tate P A (1986) 'Basic embryology and the embryological basis of malformation syndromes' in N R C Roberton (ed) *Textbook of Neonatology* 109–18 Churchill Livingstone: Edinburgh

Eurocat Working Group (1987) 'Prevalence of neural tube defects in 16 regions of Europe, 1980–1983' *International Journal of Epidemiology* 16(2): 264–51

Fitzsimmons B (1985) 'Counselling for the future' *Nursing Times* 81(11 Dec): 22–4

Forrest G (1989) 'Care of the bereaved after perinatal death' in I Chalmers, M Enkin and M J N C Keirse (eds) *Effective Care in Pregnancy and Childbirth* 1423–31 Oxford Medical: Oxford

Fraser F C (1959) 'Causes of congenital malformations in human beings' *Journal of Chronic Diseases* 10: 97

Friedman J M (1981) 'Genetic disease in the offspring of older fathers' *Obstetrics and Gynecology* 57: 745

Goldstein J C and Brown M S (1987) 'Prevention and treatment of genetic disorders' in *Harrison's Principles of Internal Medicine (11th edn)* 327 McGraw Hill: New York

Grant D B and Smith I (1988) 'Survey of neonatal screening for primary hypothyroidism in England, Wales and Northern Ireland 1982–4' *British Medical Journal* 296: 1355–8

Hanson F W, Zorn F M, Tennant F R, Marioanas S and Samuels S (1987) 'Amniocentesis before 15 weeks gestation: Outcome, risks and technical problems' *American Journal of Obstetrics and Gynecology* 87: 285

Heavyside Y (1985) 'Handicapped babies and their families' *Midwife, Health Visitor and Community Nurse* 21(11): 388–92

Hensinger R N and Jones E T (1986) 'Orthopaedic problems in the newborn' in N R C Roberton (ed) *Textbook of Neonatology* 696–720 Churchill Livingstone: Edinburgh

Hulse J A (1984) 'Outcome for congenital hypothyroidism' *Archives of Disease in Childhood* 59: 23–30

Jackson L (1988) *Chorion Villus Sampling Newsletter* No 24 (14 Feb)

James C C M and Lassman L P (1981) *Spina Bifida Occulta* Academic Press: London

Kelnar C J H and Harvey D (1987) *The Sick Newborn (2nd edn)* Balliere Tindall: London

Kremkau F W (1983) 'Biological effects and possible hazards' *Clinical Obstetrics and Gynecology* 10: 395–405

Lauritsen J G (1976) 'Aetiology of spontaneous abortion' *Acta Obstetrica et Gynecologica Scandanavica* (Suppl) 52: 1–29

Lorber K and Levick K (1967) 'Spina bifida cystica: incidence of spina bifida occulta in parents and controls' *Archives of Disease in Childhood* 42: 171–3

McNamara D and Latson L A (1982) 'Long-term follow-up of patients with malformations for which definitive repair has been available for 25 years or more' *American Journal of Cardiology* 50: 560

Manning D, Hensey O, Lenehan and O'Brien N (1982) 'Unstable hip in the newborn' *Irish Medical Journal* 75: 463–4

Mitchell S C, Korones S B and Berendes H W (1971) 'Congenital heart disease in 56,109 births' *Circulation* 43: 323–32

Moxley S (1989) 'Neonatal heal puncture' *The Canadian Nurse* 85(1): 25–7

Mutch L M M, Brown M J, Speidel D B, and Dunn P M (1980) 'Perinatal mortality and neonatal survival in Avon 1976–9' *British Medical Journal* 282: 119–22

Neilson J and Grant A (1989) 'Ultrasound in pregnancy' in I Chalmers, M Enkin and M J N C Keirse (eds) *Effective Care in Pregnancy and Childbirth* 419–39 Oxford Medical: Oxford

Office of Population Censuses and Surveys (1982) OPCS Series 3 DH 83/1 HMSO: London

Office of Population Censuses and Surveys (1987) *Congenital Malformations and Monitoring System 1986* Monitor No MB3 87/1 HMSO: London

Palomaki G E and Haddow J E (1987) 'Maternal serum alpha fetoprotein, age and Down's syndrome risk' *American Journal of Obstetrics and Gynecology* 156: 460

Perkins R P (1971) 'Inherited disorders of hemoglobin synthesis and pregnancy' *American Journal of Obstetrics and Gynecology* 111: 120–59

Polichroniadis M (1989) 'Parental understanding and attitudes towards neonatal biochemical screening' *Midwives Chronicle* Feb: 42–3

Poreco R, Young P E, Resnik R, Cousins L, Jones O W and Richards T (1983) 'Reproductive outcome following amniocentesis for genetic implications' *American Journal of Obstetrics and Gynecology* 143: 653

Rheuban K S (1984) 'The infant with congenital heart disease: Guidelines for care in the first year of life' *Clinics in Perinatology* 11(1): 199–212

Rodek C H, Gosden C M and Gosden J R (1983) 'Development of an improved technique for first trimester sampling of chorion' *British Journal of Obstetrics and Gynaecology* 90: 1113

Rohr J R, Doherty L B, Waisbren S E and Bailey A V (1983) 'New England maternal PKU project: prospective study of treated and untreated pregnancies and their outcomes' *Journal of Pediatrics* 110: 391

Sabbagha R E, Sheikh Z, Tamura R K, DalCompo S and Simpson J L (1985) 'Predictive value, sensitivity, and specificity of ultrasonic targeted imaging for fetal anomalies in gravid women at high risk for birth defects' *American Journal of Obstetrics and Gynecology* 152: 822

Salter R B (1968) 'Etiology, pathogenesis and possible prevention of congenital dislocation of the hip' *Canadian Medical Association Journal* 98: 933–45

Sant-Cassia L J and Cooke P (1981) 'Chromosomal analysis of couples with repeated spontaneous abortions' *British Journal of Obstetrics and Gynaecology* 88: 52–8

Shearer M H (1984) 'Revelations: A summary and analysis of the NIH Concensus Development Conference on ultrasound imaging in pregnancy' *Birth* 11: 23

Shepard T H (1986) 'Human teratogenicity' *Advanced Pediatrics* 33: 225

Simpson J L, Baum L D, Marder R, Elias S, Ober C and Martin A O (1986) 'Maternal serum alpha feto-protein screening: Low and high values for detection of genetic abnormalities' *American Journal of Obstetrics and Gynecology* 155: 593

Smithells R W, Sheppard S and Scorah C J (1981) 'Apparent prevention of nearal tube defects by periconceptual vitamin supplementation' *Archives of Disease in Childhood* 56: 911–18

Speidel R B and Meadows S R (1972) 'Maternal epilepsy and abnormalities of the fetus and newborn' *Lancet* ii: 839–43

Standing Medical and Nursing and Midwifery Advisory Committees (1986) *Screening for Congenital Dislocation of the Hip* DHSS: London

Tabor R, Madsen M, Obel E B, Philip J, Bang J and Norgaard-Pederson B (1986) 'Randomized controlled trial of genetic amniocentesis in 6406 low risk women' *Lancet* i: 1287–93

Tuck S M and White J M (1981) 'Sickle cell disease' in J Studd (ed) *Progress in Obstetrics and Gynaecology Vol 1* Ch 6 Churchill Livingstone: Edinburgh

Weinberger S E and Weiss S T (1988) 'Pulmonary diseases' in G N Burrows and T F Ferris (ed) *Medical Complications During Pregnancy (3rd edn)* Ch 19 448–84 W B Saunders: Philadelphia

Wilkes J B (1986) 'Screening for congenital dislocation of the hip: Professional guidelines' *Midwives Chronicle* Nov: 260

Wilkinson J L and Cooke R W I (1986) 'Cardiovascular disorders' in N R C Roberton (ed) *Textbook of Neonatology* 340–82 Churchill Livingstone: Edinburgh

Williamson J L, Kock R, Azen C and Chang C (1981) 'Correlates of intelligence test results in treated phenylketonuric children' *Pediatrics* 68: 161

Wilson J G (1959) 'Experimental studies on congenital malformations' *Journal of Chronic Disease* 10: 111

World Health Organization (1972) *Treatment of Haemoglobinopathies* Report Series No 72 WHO: Geneva

Wynne-Davies R (1964) 'Family studies and the cause of congenital club foot' *Journal of Bone and Joint Surgery* 46B: 445–63

Young D G (1986) 'Congenital defects and surgical problems' in N R C Roberton (ed) *Textbook of Neonatology* 407–38 Churchill Livingstone: Edinburgh

39 Child abuse

Background

Defining what constitutes child abuse is difficult, since it encompasses those behaviours towards the child which are viewed by society as unacceptable (Meadow 1989). Society however, is not a homogeneous unit, all of whose members agree with its aims and actions (Meadow 1989). Child rearing practices and the position of children in society have altered throughout history in addition to the presence of cultural diversity (Meadow 1989). That being said, there is a degree of general agreement that every child has the right to be cared for physically and emotionally and being protected from harm (Skuse 1989a). The Royal College of Psychiatrists (1982) defined the needs of the child as follows:

1. Physical care and attention.
2. Affection and approval.
3. Stimulation and teaching.
4. Discipline and controls which are appropriate to the child's age and development.
5. Opportunity and encouragement to acquire gradual autonomy, i.e. to take gradual control over his or her own life (Royal College of Psychiatrists 1982).

Child abuse is not a new phenomenon, although its increasing coverage in the media heightens public awareness (Wild 1986). Reporting of abuse appears to be on the increase, but it is difficult to determine its actual prevalence (Meadow 1989). Publicised cases in the United Kingdom such as the deaths of Maria Caldwell and Tyra Henry result in tighter guidelines for professionals to follow in this area (Gilmour 1985). A midwife or other health worker who observes the family in their own environment may be the first professional to detect that all is not well (Department of Health and Social Security and the Welsh Office 1988). Antenatal visiting to assess the mother's condition can sometimes reveal an older child who appears frightened or withdrawn. The midwife has no power to act, but she is ideally placed to enquire in a general manner after the well-being of other family members. Any suspicions (for that is all that they usually are at this stage) should be passed on to the midwifery supervisor and to the Social Services or NSPCC who will visit and assess the situation (Home Office, Department of Health, Department of Education and Science and the Welsh Office 1991). The Social Services have a duty to investigate. The midwife must always bear in mind the conditions of the United Kingdom's code of conduct on confidentiality (United Kingdom Central Council 1987) which may be breached in the protection of the child's best interests. It is also advisable to document suspicions and the actions taken (Department of Health and Social Security and the Welsh Office 1988).

Types of abuse

Valman (1987) lists four types of abuse:

Physical injury.
Neglect/emotional abuse.
Sexual abuse.
Potential abuse.

Physical injury

Where an injury has been deliberately inflicted, for example, fractures, bruising, poisoning, burns and scalds (Department of Health and Social Security and the Welsh Office 1988).

Neglect

Where food, warmth and clothing are insufficient for normal growth and development (Department of Health and Social Security and the Welsh Office 1988). Such children may be subject to repeated chest, skin or gastrointestinal infections (Skuse 1989a). Where growth is poor, the child is described as 'failing to thrive'

(Skuse 1989a). Admission to hospital for any reason or a period in foster care can result in rapid weight gain, which ceases when the child returns home (Skuse 1989b). Neglect includes inadequate or negligent parenting, which results in accidents (Hobbs 1989a).

Emotional abuse is as damaging to psychological development as love, affection, play and exploration are necessary to it (Scuse 1989a). Emotional rejection can produce a child who has limited social skills and withdraws from human contact. Lack of facilities for play and discovery retard intellectual development (Skuse 1989a). This can be improved if a nursery place can be found (Brooks 1985). Emotional abuse can, like neglect, give rise to failure to thrive; moving the child from the home environment can produce a rapid acceleration in growth (Skuse 1989b).

Sexual abuse

This area has been attracting more attention recently (Wild 1986). Sexual abuse is the involvement of developmentally immature children or adolescents in behaviours they are unable to understand and for which they are therefore in no position to give informed consent (Meadow 1989). Such behaviours break the normal rules of family life and can also be against the criminal law (La Fontaine 1988). Whilst incest is the sexual abuse which most commonly springs to mind, the definition also includes sexual experience and exploitation (Meadow 1989).

The abuser is likely to be male and the abused, female (Wild 1986; Bentovim et al. 1987). Abusers may be older relatives, such as siblings, fathers and step-fathers or family friend's (Wild 1986; Frude 1986; Bentovim et al. 1987). This form of abuse generally affects older children, usually from 8 years upwards and collusion is often used to maintain the child's silence (Frude 1986): for a child to make an allegation of sexual abuse involves much courage, since the outcome is often the break-up of the family unit (sometimes temporarily), and the departure of a person who is not only known and trusted, but also loved.

Potential abuse

Potential abuse (sometimes referred to as grave concern) is the situation where another child in the family has been abused or where, due to the family's lifestyle there are a large number of risk factors (Department of Health and Social Security and the Welsh Office 1988).

When determining risk factors for both the abused and the abusers, it is important to remember that the vast majority of adults and children are neither abusers nor abused (Jones et al. 1987). Children who are abused are more likely to have been born prematurely or to be small for gestational age (Jones et al. 1987). Younger children have more serious injuries than older ones. Except in adolescence, boys are more likely to be abused than girls and the child is more likely than not to be illegitimate (Jones *et al.* 1987). When examining the families where abuse is most likely to occur, the following characteristics may exist: parents younger than average (Meadow 1989); unstable housing; large family size; non-nuclear family structures for example with step-parents; low socio-economic status; marital discord; high unemployment; high rates of criminality (Jones *et al.* 1987). Such characteristics describe many families with problems where abuse does not occur. For this reason they should only be used in the broadest sense to determine at-risk populations, not forgetting that other, more organised families may be able to disguise any problems they have.

The recognition of child abuse causes many difficulties. It may be suspected by neighbours, teachers, social workers, health visitors, midwives, GPs and other family members (Department of Health and Social Security and the Welsh Office 1988). The children themselves may report the abuse to a trusted adult or via an anonymous telephone helpline. Valman (1987) states that child abuse should be suspected where a child (especially if less than 3 years of age) presents in any of the following circumstances:

1. Where there is a delay between an injury happening and the parent seeking help or where no medical help has been sought (Speight 1989).
2. When explanations are given, they are insufficient, implausible, inconsistent or not in keeping with the injuries themselves (Speight 1989). For example, babies not yet able to crawl are unlikely to fall downstairs or fall into a bath of hot water (Hobbs 1989a).
3. Where the child or its sibling has a previous history of child abuse or suspicious injury (Valman 1987).
4. Where, on examination, it is apparent that there have been earlier injuries. This can include faded bruises or on X-ray evidence of healed fractures (Hobbs 1989b).
5. Where the visits to casualty or local GP are for no apparent reason. Such visits may be frequent (Valman 1987).
6. Where the reaction of the parents to the injury and their behaviour to the child appear abnormal (Speight 1989).
7. Where there are obvious signs of neglect or the child fails to thrive (Skuse 1989a).
8. Where the child's interaction with its parents is abnormal (Speight 1989).

When physical abuse is suspected, it is important to act with caution (Speight 1989). The injuries sustained may be similar to those which can occur spontaneously (Hobbs 1989b). In addition, some illnesses can present in a way suspicious of abuse, for example disorders of blood clotting or osteogenesis imperfecta (Wheeler and Hobbs 1988). Care must be taken not to confuse a Mongolian blue spot present in children of non-caucasian or Mediterranean origin with bruising (Wheeler and Hobbs 1988).

One of the most important people involved in the detection and management of child abuse in the United Kingdom is the health visitor (Department of Health and

Social Security and the Welsh Office 1988). She has a duty to visit every new baby after its discharge from the care of the midwife and also to perform developmental assessments (Department of Health and Social Security and the Welsh Office 1988). Whilst much of this work is carried out in clinics, home visits are very important in assessing a child's well-being (Department of Health and Social Security 1988). The health visitor has no rights to enter a house unless invited; indeed some authorities write to parents inviting them to use the services offered by the health visitor. Where admission to a house has been refused, the matter may be referred to the social worker, who is one of the key people in the detection and prevention of child abuse (Department of Health and Social Security and the Welsh Office 1988).

In most cases, the social worker would arrange for the child to have a full medical examination by a paediatrician experienced in these matters (Department of Health and Social Security and the Welsh Office 1988). Where the child is of sufficient age and understanding she may give consent; where the child refuses to be examined this must be accepted (Home Office, Department of Health, Department of Education and Science and the Welsh Office 1991). In the case of a younger child, parental consent to medical examination is required and, if refused, a court order may be sought (Mitchels 1989). This could be an Emergency Protection Order, where the child is deemed to be at direct risk (see later) or a Child Assessment Order which lasts for 7 days and which will contain details of any examinations required (Children's Act 1989).

Teachers and others have a dilemma when faced with suspicions of abuse or when informed about it in confidence (Department of Health and Social Security and the Welsh Office 1988). Health visitors may find it hard to betray a family's trust and teachers can agonise over whether their loyalty is to the child or its parents (Department of Health and Social Security 1988; Department of Health and Social Security and the Welsh Office 1988). The police will be notified of any child abuse, but will only become involved where criminal investigation is required (Home, Office, Department of Health, Department of Education and Science, Welsh Office 1991). The second edition of *Working Together* (Home Office, Department of Health, Department of Education and Science, Welsh Office 1991) recommends that there should be established, locally agreed, procedures which are followed in the event of suspected child abuse. This stresses the importance of sharing information and the problems which can result from not doing so.

Social workers, by their statutory duties and powers have a central role in dealing with child abuse (Department of Health and Social Security and the Welsh Office 1988). Their major responsibility is for the safety and future welfare of the child. They have an obligation/duty to investigate each case and to make decisions as to the course of action. The social worker, however, has concern for the whole family and has to tread lightly to avoid jeopardising future relationships, without putting any child at risk (Jones *et al.* 1987).

Once all the information has been collected, a case conference involving all those in authority and directly involved, is convened (McMurray 1989). Where the situation is more serious, emergency holding action may be required. This can include obtaining an Emergency Protection Order (EPO) under the Children's Act 1989, which can be obtained from a court on application by the police or social services department. This lasts for 8 days although after 48 hours, application can be made for the order to be discharged and it may be renewed on one occasion only, for a further 7 days. The child can then be placed in a protected environment, which may be in hospital, with a relative, a community (children's) home or a foster home. This has the effect of removing the child from imminent danger while investigations are proceeding. Parental responsibilities are shared by the social services department and the parents, the EPO stipulates who can and who cannot have contact with the child while the order is in force. Where a child can be proven to be at significant risk of harm if he or she remains in the family, a police constable is authorised to remove the child to suitable accommodation, but this police protection is for a maximum of 72 hours, after which an EPO must be applied for.

Jones *et al.* (1987) give the reasons for case conferences as follows:

Sharing information
Coordinating intervention
Planning action and defining responsibilities
Searching for legal evidence
Relieving individual stress
Self/agency protection
Formalising assessment processes
Planning future coordination and case review. (Jones *et al.* 1987, p. 167)

It is important that all those in authority with information to give and those who are directly involved with the family attend (McMurray 1989). Good, contemporaneous records are made. Midwives frequently attend such conferences, especially where the mother is pregnant or has a new baby.

Where abuse is proven, decisions will need to be made concerning the welfare of the newest family member when born. Care Orders can be applied on babies immediately after birth preventing their being taken home (Home Office, Department of Health, Department of Education and Science, Welsh Office 1991). Following a ruling by the European Court of Human Rights, arrangements have been made to include parents in the decision-making process where care is being planned for their child (Home Office, Department of Health, Department of Education and Science, Welsh Office 1991).

Actions in the United Kingdom that may be taken following the case conference include:

1. Voluntary Supervision – a system of increased support from the social worker, aimed at restoring the family structure and preventing the need for the child to be taken into care (Department of Health and Social Security and the Welsh Office 1988). The child is placed on the Child Protection Register. Parental agreement is needed for this to be applied. Conditions include that proper development of the child is being prevented or neglected, or her health is being

avoidably impaired or neglected or she is being ill-treated. This may also be applied where the child is not attending school or is out of the control of her parents. A Child Assessment Order may be applied for by the social services department or the NSPCC to permit the child's condition and welfare to be properly assessed. This order remains in force for 7 days (Home Office, Department of Health, Department of Education and Science, Welsh Office 1991).

2. The child may be 'looked after' by the local authority; children cared for in this way are referred to as 'accommodated children'. This may be applied for by the parents or the local authority. Parents have to be involved by the local authority in decision-making and there is an emphasis on rehabilitation and returning the child to the family as soon as possible. Aftercare must be maintained once the child has returned home.

3. Care Proceedings – These can only be instigated if the court is satisfied

   a) 'that the child concerned is suffering or is likely to suffer, significant harm: and
   b) that the harm, or likelihood of harm, is attributable to-
      (i) the care given to the child, or likely to be given to him if the order were not made, not being what it would be reasonable to expect a parent to give to him; or
      (ii) the child being beyond parental control.' (Children's Act 1989, Sec 31)

4. Care Orders – A local authority or NSPCC officer can apply to the court for a Care Order. These give the local authority parental responsibility, which is shared with the parents. The authority can determine the extent to which the parents can exercise their responsibility. Care Orders can continue until the child is 18 years old, although the Order can be discharged by the court on application from the local authority, when the child is freed for adoption or when a residence order is made (Home Office, Department of Health, Department of Education and Science, Welsh Office 1991).

5. Supervision Orders – These Orders have the same criteria as Care Orders (see Part 3 above); they place the child in the care of the local authority putting them under the supervision of that authority or of a probation officer. The child may remain at home while a Supervision Order is in force. A designated supervisor should act as a friend, an advisor and a support for the child. While the Order is in force, either the child or the person with parental authority with whom the child is living must ensure that the child lives in a specified place, attends certain places or sees specified people and undertakes specified activities. Supervision orders remain in force for 1 year, with a possibility of 2 further extensions (Home Office, Department of Health, Department of Education and Science, Welsh Office 1991).

6. Interim Orders – It may be decided that interim measures are more appropriate than the above. Both Interim Care and Interim Supervision Orders can be established to allow more time for the case to be investigated. Interim

Orders last a maximum of 8 weeks, with a possible extension of no more than a further 4 weeks (Home Office, Department of Health, Department of Education and Science, Welsh Office 1991).

7. Contact Orders – These are to ensure reasonable contact between the child and her parents or guardians and to solve issues of access.

8. Residence Orders – These are a method of settling where the child will live. These arrangements can be fairly flexible, allowing the place of residence to be split, for example to permit the child to spend time with each parent.

References

Bentovim A, Boston P and Van Elburg A (1987) 'Child sexual abuse-children and families referred to a treatment project and the effects of intervention' *British Medical Journal* 295: 1453–7

Brooks L (1985) 'A vicious circle' *Nursing Times* 81(10 July): 32–5 Children's Act (1989) HMSO: London

Department of Health and Social Security (1988) *Child Protection: Guidance for Senior Nurses, Health Visitors and Midwives* HMSO: London

Department of Health and Social Security and the Welsh Office (1988) *Working Together: A Guide to Arrangements for Inter-agency Co-operation for the Protection of Children from Abuse* HMSO: London

Frude N (1986) 'Sexual abuse of children' *Midwife, Health Visitor and Community Nurse* 22: 302–4

Gilmour A B (1985) 'The role of the community in the prevention of child abuse' *Maternal and Child Health* 10(12): 358–60

Hobbs C J (1989a) 'Burns and scalds' *British Medical Journal* 298: 1302–5

Hobbs C J (1989b) 'Fractures' *British Medical Journal* 298: 1015–18

Home Office, Department of Health, Department of Education and Science, Welsh Office (1991) *Working Together: Under the Children Act 1989* HMSO: London

Jones D N, Pickett J, Oates M R and Barbor P (1987) *Understanding Child Abuse (2nd edn)* Macmillan: Basingstoke

La Fontaine J S (1988) 'Child sexual abuse and the incest taboo: practical problems and theoretical issues' *Man* 23: 1–18

McMurray J (1989) 'Case conferences' *British Medical Journal* 299: 500–2

Meadow R (1989) 'Epidemiology' *British Medical Journal* 298: 727–30

Mitchels B (1989) 'Protecting the child' *British Medical Journal* 299: 599–662

Royal College of Psychiatrists (1982) 'Emotional abuse' *Bulletin of the Royal College of Psychiatrists, Child Psychiatry Section* 6: 85–7

Skuse D H (1989a) 'Emotional abuse and neglect' *British Medical Journal* 298: 1692–4

Skuse D H (1989b) 'Emotional abuse and delay in growth' *British Medical Journal* 299: 113–5

Speight N (1989) 'Non-accidental injury' *British Medical Journal* 298: 879–81

United Kingdom Central Council (1987) *Advisory Paper on Confidentiality* UKCC: London

Valman H B (1987) 'Child abuse' *British Medical Journal* 294: 633–5

Wheeler D M and Hobbs C J (1988) 'Mistakes in diagnosing non-accidental injury: 10 year's experience' *British Medical Journal* 296: 1233–36

Wild N J (1986) 'Sexual abuse of children in Leeds' *British Medical Journal* 292: 1113–6

Further reading

Department of Health and Social Security (1988) *Diagnosis of Child Sexual Abuse: Guidance for Doctors* HMSO: London

Dingwall R (1987) 'A parental prerogative?' *Nursing Times* 83(17): 51

Edwards K (1987) 'Probing the power struggle' *Nursing Times* 83(17): 47–50

Fraser S (1989) 'Abuse: the experience' *British Medical Journal* 299: 731

Hallet C and Stevenson O (1980) *Child Abuse-Aspects of Interprofessional Cooperation* Allen and Unwin: London

Kempe R S and Kempe C H (1978) *Child Abuse* Fontana: London

Mitchell R (1983) 'Parents anonymous' *Nursing Mirror* 14 Dec: 16–7

Salisbury D M, Wright J D and Bradley S J (1987) *Frozen Awareness – A Guide to the Diagnosis and Management of Child Abuse (4th edn)* Wolverhampton Social Services

Wolfe D A (1987) *Child Abuse* Sage: London

Index

abdominal examination
  attitude 128
  auscultation 126, 135
  denominator 128
  engagement 129, 133
  and fetal growth 125, 126–36
  inspection 126
  lie 127, 130
  palpation 126, 130–1
    fundal 130–1
    lateral 132–3
    pelvic 133–5
  position 128–9
  presentation 128, 129
  techniques 130
  uterine size 131–2
abnormalities 257, 591–606
  of alimentary tract 599–600
  causes of 591
  chromosomal 252, 592–3, 602–3
  congenital 44
    dislocation of hip 390, 516, 600–1
    errors of metabolism 603
    frequency 591

  heart disease 601–2
  and preconception care 52
  prevention 595
  types of 597–606
cystic fibrosis 605
detection 595–7
  amniocentesis 596
  blood 595–6
  chorionic villus sampling 597
  ultrasound 597
effect on parents 606
environmental factors 595
handicapped baby 488, 606
hypothyroidism 605–6
multifactorial inheritance 595
single gene disorders 593–4
  autosomal dominant conditions 593
  autosomal recessive conditions 593–4
  X-linked recessive disorders 594
talipes 601
ABO incompatibility 552
abortion 162, 163–70
  causes 165–6
  classification 164–5

abortion (*continued*)
  counselling 170
  defined 163, 363
  diagnosis 165
  frequency 164
  grief reactions 167–8, 484
  habitual 167
  illegal 48
  management 166
  missed 164
  and mortality 159
  and multiple pregnancy 227, 228
  pill 169
  psychological effects 170
  signs of 166
  therapeutic 151, 152, 168–70
    grounds for 168
    methods 169
    morbidity 170
    numbers of 169
Abortion Act (1967) 151, 168
abruptio placentae 204–8, 409
  causes 205–6
  concealed 206–7
  and fetal well-being 207
  prognosis 207
  revealed haemorrhage 206
  signs and symptoms 206–7
  treatment 207–8
acupuncture 303, 304–5
advice
  acceptance of 444
  baby care 517–18
  and breastfeeding 524–6, 528, 537–8
  contraceptive 156, 465–6
  on diet 90–1, 93, 108–9, 217, 218
  family planning 463, 468
  and multiple pregnancy 228
  in preconception care 55
  and teenage pregnancies 153, 156
age, maternal
  and chromosomal abnormalities 593
  contraceptive advice 465–6
  and mortality 251–2
  and perinatal death 44
  and risk 117, 118
AIDS 244
  related complex 243–4
airway of neonate 315–16
alcohol consumption 52, 54, 113
alimentary tract
  congenital abnormalities 599–600
  pregnancy 85
amenorrhoea 78

amniocentesis 166, 596
amnion/amniotic sac 76, 77, 329
amniotic fluid
  abnormalities of 255–7
  and fetal well-being 309
amniotic fluid embolism 425–7
  causes 426
  diagnosis 426
  and DIC 422
  mortality 418
  treatment 426, 426–7
amniotomy 352
anaemia
  and cephalhaematoma 516
  and heart failure of mother 193, 194
  and multiple pregnancy 228
  and postpartum haemorrhage 409
  in pregnancy 215–21
    causes 216
    folic acid deficiency 218–19
    haemoglobinopathies 219
    iron deficiency 216–18
    sickle cell 219, 220–1
    thalassaemia 219–20
anaesthesia 19, 303, 353
  caesarean section 401, 402
  general
    and breastfeeding 531
    hazards of 427–8
  local/regional 306–8
    and forceps delivery 399
  mortality 418
  and postpartum haemorrhage 410
  see also analgesia; epidural anaesthesia
analgesia 303, 304
  and diet in labour 302
  inhalational 305–6
  and Know Your Midwife Scheme 31
  and slow labour 344
  systemic 306
anencephaly 598
anoxia 44, 390
antenatal care 102–21
  aims of 104–5, 121, 125
  booking examination 114–16
  booking interview 109–13
  by GPs 107–8
  by midwives 12–13, 29, 34–5, 107
  equipment needed 28
  and health visitors 108
  history 102–4
  improving 121
  maternal well-being assessment 118–20,
    121

multiple pregnancy 228
and obstetricians 108
oedema 121
planning 110–13
programme of examinations 119
psychological effects of clinics 95–6
rhesus-negative women 254–5
types available 105–7
weight gain 120–1
antepartum haemorrhage 203–12
    abruptio placentae 204–8
    Apt test 204
    and caesarean section 400
    defined 203
    diagnosis 204
    and induction of labour 349
    and low-birthweight baby 562
    management 207–8
    maternal and fetal blood loss 203–4
    placenta praevia 208–12
    and preterm delivery 364
    see also abruptio placentae; bleeding in
        early pregnancy; placenta praevia
anxiety
    and low-birthweight baby 571
    in puerperium 440, 452
Apgar score 314, 315, 356, 494
apnoea attacks 585
Apt test 204
asphyxia 44
    intrauterine 580
    neonate 314–18
attachment see bonding
attitude 128
auscultation 135
Australia 51, 363

backache in pregnancy 89–90
bacterial infections of vagina 236–8
barrier methods of contraception 467,
    470–2
beds, midwives 13
bereavement see grief
biblical midwifery 2
bilirubin 547, 548
    see also jaundice
birth
    chairs/stools 302, 310, 312
        and forceps delivery 399
    notification and registration 37–8, 336–7
    place of 30–1
    plans 147–8, 289
    position 3, 147, 148
    see also childbirth

birthing kit 20
birthrate 42–3
birthweight see low-birthweight; weight
Bishop score 350, 351
bladder
    during labour 276
    in puerperium 438, 441
bleeding
    control in third stage of labour 281–2
    vulval haematoma 334
bleeding in early pregnancy 159–70
    abortion 162, 163–70
    breakthough bleeding 160
    causes of 160–3
    cervical lesions 161
        carcinoma 161
        erosions 161
        polyps 161
    ectopic 161
    hydatidiform mole 162–3
    implantation bleeding 160
    numbers of women 160
    see also antepartum haemorrhage
blood
    ABO incompatibility 552
    antenatal tests 115, 120
    circulation
        changes at birth 496–7
        fetal 495–6
    composition in pregnancy 215–16
    normal coagulation 421
    sampling of fetal 356, 357
    screening for abnormalities 595–6
    volume in puerperium 439
    see also anaemia; haemolytic disease;
        jaundice; rhesus
blood pressure 174–5
    antenatal care 120
    following delivery 334
    in labour 300
    maintenance of 175
    pregnancy 84, 176
bonding 334, 444–5
    and induction of labour 353
    and multiple pregnancy 231–2
    and SGA babies 570
    and ultrasound scans 96
booking examination 114–16
booking interview 109–13
bowels
    newborn 505–6
    in puerperium 438–9
breastfeeding
    abscess 536–7

breastfeeding (*continued*)
  advantages 520–1
  attachment to breast 532, 535
  breast milk jaundice 553–4
  and cardiac disease 195
  complementary or supplementary feeds
    533–4
  constituents of breast milk 521–3
  contra-indications 196, 198, 537
  contraception 469
  engorgement 534–5
  expressed milk 531
  first feed 532–3
  frequency of feeds 533
  geographical differences 524
  initiation of 334, 436
  insufficient milk 535–6
  keys to success 531–2
  length of feeds 532, 533
  management 530–2
  milk ejection 530
  milk production 528–30
  one or both breasts 534
  and prevention of infection 588
  problems 534–7
  and psychosis 453
  and renal disease 196
  social class differences 523–4
  sore nipples 535, 537
  stopping 537–8
  suck cycle 529, 530
  and uterine contractions 437
  and weight of newborn 508
  winding 517
breasts
  abscess 536–7
  anatomy 526–8
  bras 528
  changes in pregnancy 527–8
  in puerperium 439, 441
  pumps 531
breech presentation 309, 373–4
  care in labour 386–7
  causes 384–5
  conduct of delivery 387–9
  dangers 389–90
  diagnosis 385, 386
  diet in labour 302
  management 385–6
  mechanism 387
  perinatal mortality rate 383–4
  and placenta praevia 210
  types of 384
British Medical Association 5, 103

brow presentation 391–2
Burns-Marshall delivery 388, 389

caesarean section 399–404
  and abruptio placentae 207, 208
  anaesthetic 401, 402
  and diabetes mellitus 191
  and ethnic group 378
  and exercise in pregnancy 146
  and genital warts 241
  and herpes simplex 240–1, 585
  and hypertension 182
  and incoordinate labour 348
  indications for 400
  and malpresentations 392, 393
  and maternal age 252
  mortality 418
  and placenta praevia 210, 211, 212
  post-natal care 442
  post-operative 402
  preparation for 400–1
  and preterm delivery 369
  psychological aspects 402–3
  rise in rate of 403–4
    implications 404
  and unstable lie 253
  and uterine rupture 423, 424
candida albicans 238–9
capillary haemangioma 506
caput succedaneum 515
carcinoma
  of cervix 161, 246
  and hydatidiform mole 162–3
cardiac disease of mother 192–5
  care in pregnancy 193–5
  congenital 192–3
  and labour 275
  rheumatic 192
cardiac massage of neonate 316
cardiac output in pregnancy 83–4
cardiotocography 125, 136–7, 309, 311,
    355
Care Orders 615, 616
care plans, puerperium 435
case conference 614–17
Central Midwives Board (CMB) 5–6, 9
cephalhaematoma 399, 515–16
cephalopelvic disproportion 44, 344, 347,
    374
  and induction of labour 350
cerebral dysfunction 577–80
cervical cerclage 368
cervix 63, 65
  at booking examination 114

carcinoma 161, 246
cervical dystocia 347–8
cervical lesions 161
cervicotomy 348
cytology 235, 245–7
    screening 246–7
dilatation 291, 296, 343, 344
    secondary arrest of 347
    and disordered uterine action 346–7
    during labour 298
        first stage 274, 275
    and prelabour 272–3
    in puerperium 437
    tears 331
child abuse 610–17
    case conference
        possible actions 615–17
        reasons for 615
    emotional 612
    midwives and 611
    needs of child 610
    neglect 611–12
    physical 611
    potential 612–15
    risk factors 612–13
    sexual abuse 612
    and Social Services 611
    and special care unit 445
    suspicions of 613, 614
    types of 611–12
child care system 582
Child Protection Register 615
childbirth
    complications 48
    medicalisation of 357
    natural 94
    philosphies of 9–10
    see also antenatal; birth; labour;
        postnatal
China, family planning 464, 465
chlamydia trachomatis 239, 585, 586
chorion 329–30
chorionic villus sampling 597
chromosomal abnormalities see
    abnormalities
chronic renal disease see renal disease
church 2–3
cleft lip and palate 598–9
clinics, midwives 12–13
clitoris 58
clothing
    during labour 148
    neonate 498
club foot 601

Code of Practice, Midwives' 9, 14
    on home birth 32–3
College of Midwives 5, 8–9
community midwives 25–38
    and antenatal care 116
    place of work 25–6
    referral by 108
    role 34–8
    and vaginal bleeding 159–60
complications of pregnancy and childbirth
    48
    see also antepartum; childbirth; labour;
        postpartum
compound presentation 393
conception, hormones 68–70
condoms 467, 470
condylomata acuminata 241, 246
congenital abnormality see abnormalities
constipation in pregnancy 88
consultant units 30
contraception 463–76
    abstinence 467, 469–70
    barrier methods 467, 470–2
    and breast feeding 469
    and cardiac disease 195
    choice of 466–8
    coitus interruptus 467, 469
    condoms 467, 470, 471
    diaphragms 467, 471
    failure rates 467
    femshield 472
    future 475–6
    history 463–6
    hormonal 467, 473–5
        contra-indications 474
    IUCD 161
    post-coital 475
    and pregnancy 54
    provision of services 468
    and renal disease 196
    sterilisation 476
    and teenage pregnancies 156
    under 16s 151
    vaginal sponge 467, 471–2
contractions, uterine 272, 273–6
    at onset of labour 286, 287
    and posture 301–2
    and progress of labour 291, 295, 296
    in puerperium 437
    see also labour
cord 328–9, 337
    abnormalities 328
    at delivery 313, 315
    clamping 327, 328

cord (*continued*)
  and infant of diabetic mother 576
  and jaundice 554
  and rhesus disease 556
  compression 428
  infection of 586
  and newborn 507
  presentation and prolapse 428–9
  traction 327–8
  and inversion of uterus 425
cot death *see* sudden infant death
  syndrome
counselling
  and abnormality 596, 606
  and abortion 170
  and age risks 252
  bereavement 482, 483, 484
  and cervical screening 247
  genetic 44, 595, 606
  and HIV 244
  and hyperemesis gravidarum 258
  and multiple pregnancy 232
  and postnatal depression 452–3
  sickle cell trait 221
  see also grief
cramp in pregnancy 90
Cranbrook Committee 9
crying of newborn 517
Curve of Carus 271
cystic fibrosis 198–9, 605
cystitis 457
cytomegalovirus 583–4
  and renal disease 196

death rates 41
  targets 42
  see also maternal mortality; perinatal
  mortality; stillbirth
deep transverse arrest 382–3
deep vein thrombosis 442, 459–60
deformities *see* abnormalities
delivery
  checking for cord 313
  conduct of 311–13
  early 43
  of the head 312
    and body 313
  and hypertension 182
  packs 28
  restitution 313
  resuscitation of neonate 314–18
  vulva and perineum 311
  see also labour; preterm

demography *see* maternal mortality;
  perinatal mortality; statistics; stillbirth
Denmark, maternity leave 112
denominator 128
depression
  and abortion 167, 170
  and pregnancy 95
  see also postnatal depression
developing countries
  anaemia 216, 218
  breastfeeding 521, 524
  family size 465
  maternal mortality 48
  syphilis 584
  TBAs 20
  uterine rupture 424
diabetes mellitus 188–91
  and diet 190
  effect on pregnancy 188–90
  and induction of labour 349
  infant of diabetic mother 575–7
    and jaundice 576
  management of 190–1
  types of 188
diet
  advice on 108–9, 217, 218
  after caesarean section 402
  and antenatal care 112–13, 439
  and diabetes 190
  following delivery 334
  in labour 148, 302, 353
  and neural tube defects 597
  onset of labour 289
  in pregnancy 53, 90–3, 217, 218
    calcium 92
    protein 91
    supplementation 91
    vitamins and minerals 92–3
disordered uterine action 345–8
disseminated intravascular coagulation
  421–2
  causes 421–2
  treatment 422
diuretics in pregnancy 194
doctors 26
  antenatal care by GPs 107–8
  control of childbirth 4–5
  GPs expertise 26
  intervention 10, 310
  involvement 8, 13
  and marginalisation of midwives 11–12
  opposition from, US 18
  and role of midwife 11
  see also obstetricians

domiciliary midwifery 9
Domino delivery 30, 31, 36, 105–6, 287
doptone machine 308, 355
Down's syndrome 252, 593, 596, 602, 603
drug-dependent mother, infant of 580–2
   signs of withdrawal 581
drugs and pregnancy 54

early teenage pregnancies *see* teenage
   pregnancies
eclampsia 177, 178, 300, 334
   and DIC 422
   postnatal 183
   prevention and detection 181–2
ectopic gestation 115, 161
   and IUCD 161
Edinburgh Sighthill Scheme 106
education
   and cervical screening 247
   sex 151
   see also advice; parent education
Eisenmenger's syndrome 192, 193, 194
embryonic development 72–8
   cell differentiation 75–8
emergencies 417–18, 423–30
   amniotic fluid embolism 425–7
   cord presentation and prolapse 428–9
   disseminated intravascular coagulation
      421–2
   failed intubation 427–8
   fetal 428–30
   and home birth 32, 36
   hypertonic uterine action 347, 423
   and information giving 427
   inversion of uterus 424–5
   Mendelson's Syndrome 427
   ruptured uterus 423–4
   shock 334, 418–21
   shoulder dystocia 429–30
   thromboembolic disorders 458–60
   see also shock
Emergency Protection Order 614, 615
employment *see* work
encephalocele 598
endotracheal intubation 316–17
enemata 300–1
engagement 129, 133
Entonox machine 305
epidural anaesthesia 306–8
   and breech presentation 387
   by midwives 13
   and cardiac disease 194
   complications 308
   contra-indications 208, 308

and deep transverse arrest 382
following delivery 335
and hypertension 182
and pushing 296
topping-up 307, 308
epilepsy 197–8
episiotomy 58, 329, 331
   anaesthesia 306
   and birth plans 148
   blood loss 413
   breech presentation 387
   direction of 61–2
   and forceps delivery 399
   incidence of 312
   indications for 312, 313
   and Know Your Midwife Scheme 31
   multiple pregnancy 230
   and preterm delivery 369
   repair 332–3
equipment
   of community midwife 27–9
   multiple pregnancy 229
ergometrine 194, 324, 325, 327
   and history of haemorrhage 409
ethnic groups
   at booking examination 111, 115
   caesarean section and forceps deliveries
      378
   and low birthweight 126
   and role of midwife 220, 221
exchange transfusion 576
   and jaundice 555, 556
   management of 557–8
exercise in pregnancy 146–7
exomphalos 600
external cephalic version 385–6
   contra-indications 386

face presentation 390–1
failure to thrive 611–12, 613
fallopian tubes 63, 66–7, 71, 72
Family Planning Association 465
family planning *see* contraception
fathers 96
   and caesarean section 402–3
   and stillbirth 486
feeding, infant 520–42
   artificial 538–41
      advertising of 541
      frequency of feeds 541
      history 538–9
      management of 540–1
      types of milk 539–40
   and diabetic mother 576

feeding, infant (*continued*)
  factors influencing method 523–6
  preterm baby 566–8
  weaning 541–2
  see also breastfeeding
fertilisation 71–2
fertility rate 43, 150
fetus
  activity 119, 125
    assessing 136, 137
  blood circulation 495–6
  blood loss 203–4
  distress 354
    and caesarean section 400
  growth
    and abdominal examination 125
    cardiotocography 136–7
    detecting problems 125–6
    and hypertension 180
  heart 135
  heart rate
    and artificial rupture of membranes 345
    decelerations 356
    during labour 308–9, 311
    monitoring 355–7
  monitoring 354–7
    and birth plans 148
    effectiveness of 356–7
    and pethidine 306
    and rise in caesarean sections 403
  movements 79–80
  position
    determination of 298
    during labour 298
  screening 115
  size 135
  skull 508–14
  well-being
    assessment in labour 291, 308–9, 355–7
    and hypertension 181
    and preterm delivery 369
  see also labour
fibroids 226
  and postpartum haemorrhage 409
fits 197–8
flying squad *see* emergencies
fontanelles 510, 511, 512
footling presentation 384
forceps delivery
  anaesthesia 306
  breech presentation 388
  cephalhaematoma 516

  and deep transverse arrest 382–3
  and ethnic group 378
  first use 3, 4
  and hypertension 182
  and preterm delivery 369
  and pushing 310
  types of forceps 397–8
  see also instrumental delivery
fourth day blues 444
France, maternity leave 112
fungal infections 238–9

galactosaemia 604–5
Gardnerella vaginalis 236
gastroenteritis in newborn 587
gastroschisis 600
general practitioners *see* doctors
genetic counselling 44
genital warts 241, 246
genitalia 57–71
  at booking examination 114
  external 57–9
  internal 62–7
gestational proteinuric hypertension and induction of labour 349
Gillick Ruling 151, 466
gingivitis 85
Glasgow, teenage pregnancies 154
gonococcus 237, 585, 586
GP units 30, 31, 36
Graafian follicle 68, 69
  structure 70–1
grande multipara
  and breech presentation 384
  and risk 252–3
  unstable lie 253
grasp reflex 501
gravidity defined 113
grief 12, 444–5, 480–90
  and abnormality 606
  and abortion 167–8, 170
  adjustment 482
  anticipatory 490
  denial of 481
  experiencing 481–2
  handicapped baby 488
  maternal death 487
  maternity and 482–90
  and miscarriage 483–4
  stages of 481
  stillbirth and 484–7
  and subfertility 483
  sudden infant death syndrome 488–90
  support agencies 482, 483, 484, 487

and termination 484
growth-retarded baby 568–9
  see also intrauterine growth retardation;
    low-birthweight baby
Gynaecologists, International Federation of
  10

haemolytic disease of newborn 551
haemophilia 594
haemorrhage, policy on 422
  see also antepartum haemorrhage;
    bleeding; postpartum haemorrhage
haemorrhoids 89
handicapped baby see abnormalities
health
  defined 41–2
  preventative 41
  and socio-economic class 41
health visitors
  and antenatal care 108
  and child abuse 613–14
  and parent education 145
hearing of newborn 516
heart disease, congenital 601–2
  signs 601
heart failure of mother, risk factors 193
heartburn 88
heat loss of neonate 497–8
heparin 194
hepatitis infections 235, 241–2, 585
  management 242
  and pregnancy 53
  and renal disease 196
herpes simplex 235, 240–1, 246, 585
  and pregnancy 53
  and renal disease 196
high-risk women 106
  cardiotocography 136–7
  diet in labour 302
history of midwifery 1–10
HIV infection 235, 242–5
  and breastfeeding 537
  and pregnancy 53
home birth 30
  advantages and disadvantages 33
  equipment required 34
  guidelines for selection 31
  mortality rate 18
  obtaining 32
  outcomes 30–1
  preparations for 33–4
  role of midwife 34–8
hormonal contraception 467, 473–5
hormone assays 138

hormones
  fetal 271
  and onset of labour 271
  ovarian 68–70, 72
Hospital Activity Analysis 41
hospitals
  births in 31
  length of stay 443
  lying-in 4
  opted-out 15, 16
housing 112, 154
Human Fertilisation and Embryology Act
  (1991) 168
human immuno deficiency virus see HIV
  infection
human papillomavirus 235, 246
hydatidiform mole 162–3
hymen 58
hyperemesis gravidarum 257–8
  management 258
hypertension 174–83
  and caesarean section 400
  diagnosis 176, 179
  and ECV 386
  effects of 179
  and epidural anaesthesia 308
  gestational proteinuric 176, 177–8
    and multiple pregnancy 227
  and heart failure of mother 193
  labour and delivery 182
  and low-birthweight baby 562
  management 179–82
  maternal observations 180–1
  prevention and detection of eclampsia
    181–2
  in pregnancy 176–7
  pregnancy induced 44
  and preterm delivery 364
hypertonic uterine action 347–8
hypnosis 305
hypoglycaemia, neonatal 353, 576
hypothyroidism 605–6
  and jaundice 553
  screening 516
hypotonic baby 580
hypotonic uterine action 343–4, 345–6
hypovolaemia 208, 211, 257, 410
  see also antepartum haemorrhage;
    postpartum haemorrhage
hypoxia 383, 390
  and preterm baby 565
hysterectomy
  and morbidly adherent placenta 413
  and uterine rupture 424

incontinence, urinary 109, 313
    stress 458
incoordinate uterine action 344, 348
independent midwifery 14
induction of labour 11, 348–53
    amniotomy 352
    failure and hazards 352–3
    indications for 349–50
    methods 350–2
    outcomes 352–3
    oxytocin 351–2
    prerequisites for success 350
    prostaglandins 350–1, 352
inefficient uterine action 346–7
Infant Life Preservation Act (1929) 168
infant mortality 42, 45–6, 46
    causes 46
    targets 42
    see also neonatal mortality
infection
    and abortion 166
    and breast-fed babies 521
    and heart failure of mother 193, 194
    in newborn 582–8
    and preterm baby 568
    in puerperium 454–7
    and renal disease 196
    small-for-gestational age baby 569
infectious diseases
    and pregnancy 53, 235–47
    WHO targets 42
information giving, and emergencies 421
    see also advice
injuries, birth 499–500
instrumental delivery 396–9
    complications of 399
    conditions for 398–9
    indications 397
    trauma 413
intermittent positive pressure ventilation
        315, 316–17
intervention 3, 10, 104, 263
    doctors 310
    and midwives 10
    policies 11
    and safety 18
    see also emergencies; induction of labour
intrapartum care
    equipment needed 28
    record keeping 29
    role of midwife 35–6
intrauterine contraceptive device see IUCD
intrauterine death
    and DIC 422

    and induction of labour 349
intrauterine growth retardation 43
    and cardiac disease of mother 192, 194
    detection of 125–6
    and drug abuse 580
    and hypertension 179
    and induction of labour 349
    and multiple pregnancy 228
    and preconception care 52
    and preterm delivery 364
    and ultrasound 135, 139
intrauterine hypoxia 347, 352
intubation, failed 427–8
IPPV 315, 316–17
IUCD 467, 468, 472–3
    failure rate 467
    and renal disease 197

Japan 224, 363
jaundice 352, 383, 430, 547–58
    ABO incompatibility 552
    breast milk 553–4
    causes 549–54
    and cephalhaematoma 516
    exchange transfusion 555, 556
        management of 557–8
    haemolytic disease 551
    hepatic causes 552–3
    and hypothyroidism 553
    and infant of diabetic mother 576
    and infection 552
    management 554–7
    obstruction 553
    phototherapy 555–6, 557, 558
    physiological 554
    physiology 547–8
    red cell abnormalities 552
    rhesus incompatibility 549–51

kernicterus 547, 557
ketoacidosis 191, 302, 348, 353
Kjelland's forceps 382, 391, 398
Kleihauer test 550, 556
Know Your Midwife Scheme 13–14, 26
    future of 16
    results of 31, 106, 287
    risk categories 118

labour
    abnormal 345–8
        deep transverse arrest 382–3
    active management of 342–57
    activity in 301–2, 343, 344
    assessing progress 290–7, 342–3

augmentation of 344–5
  psychological effects 345
and birth plans 148
birth of shoulders 280
breast massage 345
causes of slow 343–4
conditions for normality 276
control of bleeding 281–2
crowning 277–8
defined 261–2
descent 276–7, 278, 343
diet in 148, 302, 353
disordered uterine action 345–8
duration of 262–3
enemata and shaves 300–1
engagement 276
extension of head 278
fetal distress 354
fetal monitoring 354–7
first stage 262, 273–6, 301–9
  phases of 343
flexion 277
fluid intake 353–4
fourth stage 262, 333–5
and hypertension 182
hypertonic uterine action 347–8
hypotonic uterine action 343–4, 345–6
incoordinate, management 348
inefficient uterine action 346–7
internal rotation of head 277, 278
internal rotation of shoulders 279
intervention in 263
length of 290–1, 309–10, 343, 410
maternal care 300–8
maternal distress 353–4
mechanism of 264–71, 276–80
meconium 354–5
multiple pregnancy 229–31
obstructed 423
onset of 271–3, 286–9
pain
  cause of 304
  relief 303–6
partogram 291, 292–5, 296
physiology of 261–82
planning care 289–90
positions in 301–2
precipitate 410
prelabour 262, 272–3
prolonged 410
pushing 296
restitution 279
second stage 262, 296, 309–13
  active phase 309–10

diagnosis and duration 309–10
  fetal skull 514
  latent phase 309
  positions 310
secondary arrest of cervical dilatation
    347
separation of placenta 280–1
stages of 262
third stage 262, 280–2
  active management 327–8
  complications 407–15
  examination of placenta 328
  history of management 324–5
  maternal surface 330
  membranes 329–30
  umbilical cord 328–9
time-scale 343
and trial of labour/trial of scar 404
vaginal examinations 296–9
see also analgesia; delivery; induction of
    labour; postpartum haemorrhage;
    preterm labour
lactation and stillbirth 487
  see also breastfeeding; breasts
lay midwives 18, 19
legislation 5–7
  see also individual Acts
leucorrheoa 236
lie 127, 130
  and grande multipara 253
life chances 41
life expectancy
  and socio-economic class 41
  targets 42
lightening 131–2
lignocaine 306
liquor, abnormalities of 255–7
listeria 584–5
lochia 437, 442, 454
loss see grief
Lovset manoeuvre 388
low-birthweight baby 561–71
  causes 562, 563
  classification of 561–3
  growth-retarded 562
  influence of race 126
  morbidity 570
  numbers of 126
  and perinatal death 43
  and preconception care 52
  and smoking 54
  see also intrauterine growth-retardation;
      preterm baby
lying-in hospitals 4

McRobert's manoeuvre 429
malformed baby *see* abnormalities
malpositions
  care of women with posterior positions
    383
  defined 373
  occipito-posterior 380
    causes 380-1
    diagnosis 381-2
    outcomes 382-3
    pelvic assessment by vaginal examination
      379-80, 381-2
  see also malpresentation
malpractice 16-17
malpresentation 344, 373-93
  brow 391-2
  and caesarean section 400
  compound 393
  defined 373
  face 390-1
  footling presentation 384, 385
  shoulder 392-3
  see also breech presentation;
    malpositions
marital breakdown and teenage pregnancies
  156
massage 303
mastitis 535, 536
maternal distress in labour 353-4
maternal mortality 8, 46-7
  and amniotic fluid embolism 426
  and cardiac disease 193
  causes 47
  Confidential Enquiries into 46-7, 418
  defined 46
  and grief 487
  historically 103, 104
  international 48
  targets 42
Maternal Mortality and Morbidity,
    Committee on (1930) 103
maternal well-being
  assessment in labour 291
  blood pressure 300
  monitoring 299-300
  in puerperium 441, 442
  pulse rate 300
  temperature 299
maternity leave 112
  and breastfeeding 524
Maternity Services Advisory Committee
    287, 288
Maternity Services Advisory Committee
    (1982) 104, 108

Mauriceau-Smellie-Veit manoeuvre 388,
    389
meconium 354-5, 387
medical aid
  postpartum haemorrhage 410-11, 413,
    415
  and shock 420
  see also emergencies
medical disorders of mother 187-99
  see also cardiac disease; cystic fibrosis;
    diabetes mellitus; epilepsy; renal
    disease
medical model 9-10, 11, 262, 310, 357
  see also intervention
membranes 329-30
  artificial rupture 344-5, 352
    and amniotic fluid embolism 426
    and labour 275, 298
  see also labour
Mendelson's Syndrome 427
meningocele 598
menstrual cycle 68-70
midcavity forceps 398
midwives
  autonomy of 11
  beds 13
  biblical 2
  care by
    effectiveness of 18-19
    and mortality rate 18-19
    results of 14
  clinics 12-13
  detecting deviations from normal 12
  early training 4-7
  history 1-10
  men as 4, 9
  and nursing culture 11
  supervision 16-17
  support for 487
  underuse of 107
  see also community midwives; role of
    midwife
Midwives Act (1902) 5-6, 16
Midwives Act (1919) 6, 7
Midwives Act (1926) 7
Midwives Act (1936) 7, 8, 16, 103
Midwives' Institute 5, 7, 8
Midwives, International Confederation of
  10
minor disorders of pregnancy *see*
  pregnancy
Miscarriage Association 168
miscarriage and grief 483-4
  see also abortion

mitral stenosis 192
Mongolian blue spot 613
morbidity statistics 41
morning sickness 87–8, 96
Moro reflex 500
mortality rate
  early teenage pregnancy 150
  home births 18
  hospital births 18
  and maternal age 251–2
  and midwifery care 18–19
  WHO targets 42
  see also infant mortality; maternal
    mortality; neonatal mortality; risk;
    stillbirth
motherhood
  adaptation to 450–1
  coping 450–1
  idealisation of 94
multiple pregnancy 43, 224–32
  antenatal care 228
  and bonding 231–2
  and breech presentation 384
  cardiac output 84
  causes 225–6
  complications 227–8
  diagnosis 226–7
  diet in labour 302
  and heart failure of mother 193
  incidence 224–5
  labour 229–31
    induction 349
  and low-birthweight baby 562
  minor disorders 227
  postpartum care 231
  and postpartum haemorrhage 409
  presentation 229
  and preterm delivery 364
  psychological problems 231–2
  and risk 117
  triplets 226
  twins 225–6
    causes 225–6
    folic acid deficiency 219
    Siamese 225–6
myelomeningocele 598

National Childbirth Trust 304
National Health Service 14
  establishment of 8, 11
  and family planning 465
  future midwifery 14, 15–16
natural childbirth 94
neglect of child 611–12

negligence 16–17
neonatal mortality 45–6
  grief reactions 167
  and resuscitation 354–5
neonate see newborn
Netherlands 17–18, 20
neural tube defects 597–8
  detection 595, 596, 597
  and diet 597
  and folate deficiency 219
  and ultrasound 138
neural tube development 77–8
New Zealand 19–20
newborn
  activity 505
  alertness 494
  birth injuries 499–500
  bowels 505–6
  care of 499, 504–18
    requiring extra 575–88
  clothing 498
  cold injury 499
  cord 507
  crying 517
  daily examination 504–6
  of drug-dependent mother 580–2
  fetal skull 508–14
  hormonal effects 506
  hypotonic 580
  infection in 504, 507, 508, 582–8
    alimentary tract 587
    defences against 582
    and hospital visits 588
    intrapartum 585
    neonatal 585–8
    prevention 588
    skin 587–8
    transplacental 583–5
    urinary tract 587
  initial examination 337–9
  initiation of respiration 493–4
  mouth 506
  neurologically disturbed 577–80
    causes 577–8
    diagnosis 578–9
    midwifery management 579–80
    treatment 579
  reflexes 500–1
  scalp 515–16
  screening tests 516
  skin 505, 506
  sleep 516–17
  sore buttocks 507–8
  temperature 505

newborn (*continued*)
    thermoregulation 497–8
    weight 508
Newcastle Community Midwifery Care
    106–7
Nigeria, twinning 224
nipples, sore 535, 537
    see also breastfeeding
non-specific vaginitis 236
Norway 363
nurse-midwives 19
Nurses, Midwives and Health Visitors Act
    (1979) 9

obesity
    and heart failure of mother 193
    and risk 253
obstetric physiotherapist 109
obstetricians
    and antenatal care 108
    and duplication of care 11–12
    use of forceps 3
Obstetricians and Gynaecologists–Royal
    College of 8
obstetrics
    early 4–5
    technological 9
oedema 121, 178
    pregnancy 82–3
oesophageal atresia 599–600
oestrogens 68–70, 72, 87, 138
oligohydramnios 257
omphalitis 586
omphalocele 600
operative delivery 399–404
    see also caesarean section
operculum 65, 273
ophthalmia neonatorum 586
ovaries 67, 68
ovum 70–1
oxytocic drugs 253, 324, 327, 328, 334,
    347, 348
    indiscriminate use 325
    induction of labour 351–2, 485
    and postpartum haemorrhage 411, 412,
    415

pain relief
    and birth plans 148
    in labour 303–6
    and parent education 143
palpation 130–5
    onset of labour 288–9
parasitic infections 239–40

parent education 142–8
    birth plans 147–8
    classes 142–5
    curriculum 145–6
    exercise in pregnancy 146–7
    multiple pregnancy 228
    parenting skills 450
    and socio-economic class 143–4
parents
    and asphyxiated baby 318
    effect of abnormality 606
    involvement in birth 148
    and low-birthweight baby 570–1
parity
    defined 113
    and perinatal death 44
    and risk 251–2
partogram 291, 292–5, 296, 299, 335, 343
Pawlik's Grip 135
Peel Report 9, 104
pelvic/pelvis
    abnormal 374–8
        causes 374, 377
    android 374–5, 376, 380, 382
    anthropoid 375–7
    assessment 378–80
        and shoe size 378
        vaginal examination 379–80, 381–2
    at booking examination 114–15
    gynaecoid 374, 375
    inclination of 270–1
    palpation 133–5
    pelvic brim 266–8, 271
        diameters of 267–8
    pelvic cavity 268
        pelvic outlet 268–70
    pelvic floor 59–62
        repair of 330–1
    physiology 264–71
    platypelloid 377–8, 390
    in puerperium 438
    and rickets 378
pemphigus 588
perinatal asphyxia 569
perinatal mortality
    breech presentation 383–4
    causes 43–4, 51
    and hypertension 176
    Netherlands 17–18
    rate 43–4
    risk factors 44–5
    Scandinavia 45
    and technology 404
    teenage pregnancies 153

perineal body 61–2
perineum
  and delivery 311, 312–13
  repairs to 331–2
    postnatal care 436
  tears 331
  trauma to 331
pethidine 306
  and breastfeeding 531
phenylketonuria 37, 165, 594, 595, 603–4
  diagnosis 604
  screening 516
phototherapy 555–6, 557, 558, 576
Pinard's stethoscope 135, 308–9, 355
place of birth and outcomes 30–1
placenta
  barrier 74–5
  development of 73–5
  disposal 35
  examination of 328
  functions of 75
  manual removal 412–13
  Mathews Duncan delivery 280, 281
  morbidly adherent 412–13, 425
  Schultz delivery 280, 281
  separation 326
    breech presentation 389, 390
    incomplete 409
  in third stage of labour 280–1
  weight 330
  see also postpartum haemorrhage
placenta praevia 208–12, 409
  and breech presentation 385
  diagnosis 210–11
  and fetal well-being 211
  and grande multipara 252, 253
  management 211–12
  prognosis 211
  risk factors 210
  types of 208–9
placental abruption and DIC 422
placental hypoxia 355
placing reflex 501
plasmaphoresis 255
polyhydramnios 256–7, 352
  and breech presentation 384
  causes 256
  face presentation 390
  and induction of labour 349
  and low-birthweight baby 562
  and multiple pregnancy 226, 228
  and oesophageal atresia 599
  shoulder presentation 392
position 128–9

delivery
  breech presentation 387
  for forceps delivery 398
  in labour 301–2
  see also malpositions
postmaturity 344
  and induction of labour 349
postnatal care 433–46
  6-week examination 445–6
  blues 451
  equipment needed 28–9
  examination 440–4
  multiple pregnancy 231
  psychological disturbances 449–54
  reception on ward 435–6
  record keeping 29
  role of midwife 36–7
  see also puerperium
postnatal depression 451–3
  cause 452
postpartum haemodilution 436
postpartum haemorrhage 383, 407–15
  bleeding from placental site 408–13
    causes 409–10
    diagnosis 410
  clinical trials 325
  coagulation disorders 414
  control of 324–5, 411–12
  man-made causes 325
  manual removal of placenta 412–13
  medical aid 410–11, 413, 415
  physiological management 326
  primary 408–14
  prophylaxis 412
  secondary 414–15
  time periods 408
  trauma 413–14
poverty
  and preterm delivery 364
  and teenage pregnancies 156
  see also socio-economic class
pre-eclampsia 178, 300
preconception care 51–5
  advice giving 55
pregnancy
  adaptation to 82–96
    body water 82–3
    physiological 82–91
    psychological and social 93–6
  alimentary tract 85
  blood 83
  blood pressure 84
  cardiac output 83–4
  cardiovascular system 90

pregnancy (*continued*)
  cerebrovascular system 88–9
  complications 48
  diagnosis of 78–80
    positive 79–80
    presumptive 78–9
  diet in 90–3
  and employment 254
  exercise in 146–7
  gastrointestinal tract 87–8
  guide to healthy 51–5
  influences on 52
  medical model 95
  minor disorders of 82, 86–7, 96, 108–9
    multiple pregnancy 227
  muscoskeletal system 89–90
  oedema 82–3
  progress of 120–1
  renal tract 84–5
  respiration 86
  risk 251–8
    abnormalities of liquor 255–7
    assessment 253–4
  skin 90
  termination *see* abortion
  tests 79
  varicosities 88–9
  weight gain 86, 87
  see also antenatal care; bleeding in early
    pregnancy; hypertension
prelabour 262, 272–3
premature labour 272
prematurity
  and breech presentation 384, 385
  and preconception care 52
presentation 128, 129
  multiple pregnancy 229
  see also breech; malpositions;
    malpresentation
preterm baby 563–8
  care of 563–8
  excretion 568
  hypoglycaemia 569
  hypothermia 569
  nutrition 566–8
  oxygenation 564–6
  protection from harm 568
  temperature control 564
preterm delivery 368–70
  and drug abuse 580
  place of birth 368–9
  and smoking 44
  and transfer to special unit 369–70
  and working women 254

preterm labour 363–8
  bedrest 366
  causes 363–5
  cervical cerclage 368
  corticosteroids 367–8
  diagnosis 365
  drug therapy 366–7
  management 365–70
  and multiple pregnancy 227–8
  psychological care 365–6
  risk factors 364–5
  rupture of membranes 368
preventative health services 41
primary health care team 25, 26–7, 105
primigravida
  defined 113
  and risk 117
primiparous defined 113
private practice of midwives 14
progesterone 68–70, 72, 87
  and varicosities 88–9
prostaglandins 271–2, 275
  and abortion 169
  induction of labour 350–1, 352
  pessaries 194
  and preterm labour 367
  see also hormones
proteinuria 176–7, 179
psychological adjustment to pregnancy
  93–6
psychoprophylaxis 304
psychosis in puerperium 453–4
puerperal fever 5
puerperium 433–46
  6-week examination 445–6
  complication 449–60
  defined 433
  examination 435–6, 440–4
  fourth day blues 444
  infection in 454–7
    signs of 455–6
    treatment 456–7
  physiological changes 436–9
  psychological disturbances 439–40,
    449–54
  psychosis 453–4
  thromboembolic disorders 458–60
  visits in 433–4
pulmonary aspiration syndrome 427
pulmonary embolism 459, 460
pulse rate in labour 300
pushing 311
  prolonged 310
pyodermia 588

Q test 53

record keeping 29–30
  abdominal examination 126
  booking interview 110–13
  examination of neonate 338
  exchange transfusion 558
  in labour 311
    fourth stage 335–6
    third stage 330
  labour ward 336
  onset of labour 288–9
  post-natal care 442, 443
  see also child abuse; partogram
reflexes, neonate 500–1
registration of birth 37–8, 336–7
  stillbirth 37, 38, 486–7
relaxation techniques 146–7, 304
renal disease 195–7
  and induction of labour 350
  and infections 196
  renal transplant 195–6
  risks of 196
renal system and hypertension 177
repairs 331–3
respiration in pregnancy 86
respiratory disease of newborn 576
respiratory distress syndrome of newborn
    and diabetes 190
respiratory failure of newborn 314–18
resuscitation of neonate 314–18, 354–5
retro-placental clot 280
rhesus-negative women 115, 597
  and abortion 166
  antenatal care 254–5
  and ECV 386
  isoimmunisation 550
    haemolytic disease 551
    and induction of labour 349
    prevention of 550–1
  management of disease 556–7
  rhesus incompatibility 549–51
risk/risk factors 116–18
  and grande multipara 252–3
  high 117
  and home births 31
  intermediate 117
  low 118, 119
  and obesity 253
  in pregnancy 251–8
    assessment 253–4
    teenage 150, 152–3
  and socio-economic class 252
role of midwife 10–12

and adaptation to motherhood 450–1
  answering questions 290
  antenatal care 34–5
  and antepartum haemorrhage 208
  assessing progress in labour 290–7
  booking interview 109–13
  care of newborn 517–18
  and child abuse 611
  in community 34–8
  and emotional needs 450–1
  and ethnic groups 220
  and grief 482, 483, 484, 486–7
  and hypertension 180
  intrapartum care 35–6
  and jaundice 558
  and medical disorders of mother 187–8
  multiple pregnancy 228
  and neonate 493–4
  and onset of labour 286–9
    information required 288
  and parent education 144–5
  postnatal care 36–7
  and psychological adjustment to
    pregnancy 96
  and psychological disturbances 449–53
  in puerperium 433–5, 440–4
  supervisor role 16–17
  and teenage pregnancies 156–7
  see also breastfeeding; breasts; epidural
    anaesthesia; feeding, infant
rooting reflex 500–1
rotational forceps 398
Royal College of Midwives 15
rubella 53, 115, 583
Rules, Midwives' 9, 14, 29

Safe Motherhood Initiative 48
scalp of newborn 515–16
Scandinavia 397
  perinatal mortality 45
Scotland 4, 154
seizures of newborn 577–8
septicaemia and DIC 422
Sex Discrimination Act 9
sex education 151
sexual abuse 612
sexually transmitted diseases 115
shaves 300–1
shock 417
  anaphylactic 419
  bacteraemic 419
  cardiogenic 418
  causes 424, 426
  hypovolaemic 418

shock (*continued*)
  low resistence 419
  management 420–1
  physiological effects of 419
  severity classified 420
  signs 334
  and uterine rupture 424
short forceps 397–8
shoulder dystocia 429–30
shouider presentation 392–3
show 296
Siamese twins 225–6
siblings 96, 112
  and SIDS 488
sickle cell disease/trait 111, 219, 220–1,
    594, 595
  at booking examination 115
  screening 516
SIDS *see* sudden infant death
Sighthill Scheme 106
single women 93–4
skin infection in newborn 587–8
skull, fetal 508–14
  diameters 511–12
  fontanelles 510, 511, 512
  internal anatomy 512–13
  moulding 513–14
sleep of newborn 516–17
small-for-gestational age baby 568–70
  infection 569
  perinatal asphyxia 569
  see also low-birthweight baby; preterm
    baby
smoking
  and abortion 165, 170
  and antenatal care 113
  and antepartum haemorrhage 206
  and breastfeeding 524
  and healthy pregnancy 52, 54
  and heart failure of mother 193
  and low birthweight 126, 562
  and perinatal death 44
  and preterm delivery 364
  and risk 117, 118
social security benefits *see* welfare
    provision
social workers 614
socio-economic class
  and breastfeeding 523–4
  and cardiac disease 192
  and cervical cancer 246
  death rate differentials 41
  and infant mortality 46
  and length of stay in hospital 443

  and low birthweight 126
  and parent education 143–4
  and perinatal mortality 44, 51–2
  and preterm delivery 364
  and risk 117, 118, 252
  and stress in puerperium 451
  and teenage pregnancies 152, 153
sonicaid 135, 137
spermicides 467, 470, 471
spina bifida occulta 598
statistics 40
  data collection 40–1
  and maternity care 42–7
stepping reflex 501
stillbirth 46
  choice of labour 485
  defined 363
  diagnosis 485
  grief reactions 167, 484–7
  and hypertension 179
  and lactation 487
  rate 43
    and socio-economic class 41
  registration 37, 38, 486–7
stork's beak mark 506
stress
  and pregnancy 95
  and preterm delivery 364, 366
  in puerperium 450–1
stress incontinence 458
striae gravidarum 90
subfertility and grief 483
sudden infant death syndrome 488–90, 570
  causes 488
  and drug abuse 582
  risk factors 489
supervision, midwifery 16–17
sutures 332–3
syntocinon 324–5, 327, 351–2
  multiple pregnancy 230
syntometrine 327, 388, 399
  and postpartum haemorrhage 411, 413
syphilis 235, 237–8, 584, 595
  screening for 238

talipes 601
Tay Sachs disease 594
TBAs *see* traditional birth attendants
teachers of midwifery *see* training
technology 104
  effectiveness 11
  and perinatal mortality 404
teenage pregnancies 150–7
  finance 153–4

housing 154
major complications 152–3
and marital breakdown 156
numbers 150–1
obstetric aspects 151–3
reasons for 151
risk factors 150, 152–3
and schooling 154–6
social aspects 156–7
telemetry 386
temperature
in labour 299
newborn 497–8, 505
TENS *see* Transcutaneous
termination *see* abortion
thalassaemia 594, 595
screening 516
thermoregulation of neonate 497–8
thromboembolic disorders in puerperium
458–60
thrombophlebitis 458–9
thrush infection in newborn 506, 507, 587
tocolytics 366
toxoplasmosis 584
traction reflex 501
traditional birth attendants 2, 20, 48
training, midwifery 9
early 4–7
future needs 15
history of 2, 8
Transcutaneous Electrical Nerve
Stimulation (TENS) 305
transfusion, intrauterine 255
transient tachypnoea of the newborn 566,
577
trial of labour 404
diet in labour 302
trial of scar 404
trichomonas 239–40
twilight sleep 19
twin pregnancy *see* multiple pregnancy

UKCC 9, 14
role of midwife 10
on supervision 16–17
see also Rules
ultrasound 11, 138–9
and bonding 96, 444
and detection of abnormality 597
Doppler 139
and fetal growth 125
findings 138–9
liquor volume 135
and multiple pregnancy 226

and pregnancy diagnosis 79
umbilical cord *see* cord
United Kingdom Central Council *see*
UKCC
United States 18–19
antenatal care 114
caesarean section 400, 403
doctors in 4
episiotomy 61, 312
family planning 464, 468
HIV infection 245
preterm delivery 368
teenage pregnancies 151, 153
training in 5
urinalysis
antenatal care 120
in labour 300
and proteinuria 179
urinary tract
incontinence 109
and episiotomy 313
infection 84–5
in newborn 552, 587
in puerperium 454, 455, 457, 458
and renal transplant 196
problems in puerperium 457–8
urine retention 331, 438
uterus
and abdominal examination 131–2
abnormality and breech presentation 384
at booking examination 114, 115
atonic 409–10
during pregnancy 65
and embryonic development 74
inversion of 424–5
post-natal care 441–2
in puerperium 436–7
rupture of 423
causes 423–4
mortality 418
signs of 424
traumatic 423
scars 423
structure and function 62–5
subinvolution 437, 456

vagina 65–6
discharges
bacterial 236–8
normal 235–6
examination
pelvic assessment 379–80, 381–2
examination in labour 296–9
indications for 297

vagina (*continued*)
   fungal infections 238–9
   parasitic infections 239–40
   in puerperium 437–8
   tears 331
vaginal bleeding *see* bleeding in early
     pregnancy
varicosities in pregnancy 88–9
vasa praevia 329
ventilation 570
ventouse delivery 397
viral infections in pregnancy 240–5
   see also infections
vitamins and minerals in pregnancy 92–3
vulva 57–9
vulval haematoma 334, 414

weaning 541–2
weight
   of infants and feeding method 521
   of mother 53, 120–1
     gain 86, 87

newborn 508
   see also low birthweight
welfare provision
   historically 102–3
   teenage pregnancies 153–4
Welsh Perinatal Mortality Initiative 45
witchcraft 2
women
   as healers 2
   status of pregnant 94–5
Women's Liberation movement 94
work
   and pregnancy 254
     hazardous 54–5, 112, 254
   and preterm delivery 364
World Health Organization 1, 10, 20
   abortion defined 163
   Health For All 41–2
   on preterm labour 363
   Safe Motherhood Initiative 48

X-rays in pregnancy 380